CRC HANDBOOK SERIES IN CLINICAL LABORATORY SCIENCE

Each section contains one or more volumes.

CRC Handbook Series in Clinical Laboratory Science

David Seligson, Editor-In-Chief

Chairman and Professor
Department of Laboratory Medicine
School of Medicine
Yale University

Section I: Hematology
Volume I

Robert M. Schmidt, Section Editor

Medical Director
International Reference and Research
Center for Blood Diseases
Lihue, Kauai, Hawaii

Formerly: Director, Hematology Division
Center for Disease Control
Atlanta, Georgia

CRC PRESS, INC.
Boca Raton, Florida 33431

Library of Congress Cataloging in Publication Data (Revised)

Main entry under title:

CRC handbook series in clinical laboratory science.
Spine title: Handbook series in clinical laboratory science.
Includes bibliographies and index.
CONTENTS: Section A. Nuclear medicine. v. — Section E. Clinical microbiology. v. — Section I. Hematology.
1. Medical laboratories. 2. Diagnosis, Laboratory. I. Seligson, David. II. Chemical Rubber Company, Cleveland, III. Title: Handbook series in clinical laboratory science.

RB37.C18 616.07'56 76-27688
ISBN 0-8493-7000-0 (set)

This book presents data obtained from authentic and highly regarded sources. Reprinted material is quoted with permission, and sources are indicated. A wide variety of references are listed. Every reasonable effort has been made to give reliable data and information but the editor and the publisher cannot assume responsibility for the validity of all materials or for the consequences of their use.

International Standard Book Number
Complete Set 0-8493-7000-0
Hematology Section, Volume I 0-8493-7091-4

Library of Congress Card No. 76-27688
Printed in the United States

PUBLISHERS PREFACE

In 1913, when the First Edition of the *Handbook of Chemistry and Physics* appeared, scientific progress, particularly in chemistry and physics, had produced an extensive literature but its utility was seriously handicapped because it was fragmented and unorganized. The simple but invaluable contribution of the *Handbook of Chemistry and Physics* was to provide a systematic compilation of the most useful and reliable scientific data within the covers of a single volume. Referred to as the "bible", the Handbook soon became a universal and essential reference source for the scientific community. The latest edition published represents more than 65 years of continuous service to millions of professional scientists and students throughout the world.

In the years following World War II, scientific information expanded at an explosive rate due to the tremendous growth of research facilities and sophisticated analytical instrumentation. The single-volume Handbook concept, although providing a high level of convenience, was not adequate for the reference requirements of many of the newer scientific disciplines. Due to the sheer quantity of useful and reliable data being generated, it was no longer feasible or desirable to select only that information which could be contained in a single volume and arbitrarily to reject the remainder. **Comprehensiveness** had become as essential as **convenience.**

By the late 1960's it was apparent that the solution to the problem was the development of the multi-volume Handbook. This answer arose out of necessity during the editorial processing of the *Handbook of Environmental Control.* A hybrid discipline or, to be more precise, an interdisciplinary field such as Environmental Science could be logically structured into major subject areas. This permitted individual volumes to be developed for each major subject. The individual volumes, published either simultaneously or by some predetermined sequence, collectively became a multi-volume Handbook series.

The logic of this new approach was irrefutable and the concept was promptly accepted by both the scientist and science librarian. It became the format of a growing number of CRC Handbook Series in fields such as Materials Science, Laboratory Animal Science, and Marine Science.

Within a few years, however, it was clear that even the multi-volume Handbook concept was not sufficient. It was necessary to create an information structure more compatible with the dynamic character of scientific information, and flexible enough to accommodate continuous but unpredictable growth, regardless of quantity or direction. This became the objective of a "third generation" Handbook concept.

This latest concept utilizes each major subject within an information field as a "Section" rather than the equivalent of a single volume. Each Section, therefore, may include as many volumes as the quantity and quality of available information will justify. The structure achieves permanent flexibility because it can, in effect, expand "vertically" and "horizontally". Any section can continue to grow (vertically) in number of volumes, and new sections can be added (horizontally) as and when required by the information field itself. A key innovation which makes this massive and complex information base almost as convenient to use as a single-volume Handbook is the utilization of computer technology to produce up-dated, cumulative index volumes.

The *Handbook Series in Clinical Laboratory Science* has the distinction of being the prototype for the "sectionalized, multi-volume Handbook series". Currently underway are additional information programs based on the same organizational design. These include information fields such as Nutrition, Energy, and Agricultural Science which are of critical importance not only to scientific progress but to the advancement of the total quality of life.

We are confident that the "third generation" CRC Handbook comprises a worthy contribution to both information science and the scientific community. We are equally certain that it does not represent the ultimate reference source. We predict that the most dramatic progress in the management of scientific information remains to be achieved.

B. J. Starkoff
President
CRC Press, Inc.

PREFACE
CRC HANDBOOK SERIES IN CLINICAL LABORATORY SCIENCE

According to the *Webster 4 — Merriam Dictionary,* 3rd ed., a handbook is

1a. a book capable of being conveniently carried as a ready reference,
1b. a concise reference book covering a particular field of knowledge,
2a. a bookmaker's book of bets.

In order to accommodate the information in the field of clinical laboratory science we shall need more than 20 volumes. A series of volumes such as these, that will weigh in the order of 24 kg (53 pounds), will not fit the meaning of la: nor will 2a fit, although we are gambling that we can get the appropriate information together in a reasonable time. Definition 1b is more appropriate to our goal which is to accumulate, arrange, and present the qualitative and quantitative clinical laboratory data related to men and women (of all ages), so that anyone who needs to extract some information from the vast amount available will have it at his or her fingertips, provided he or she is within arm's length of these volumes.

To understand the biology of man, to know man, sick and well, requires knowledge of the body constituents and their interrelationships; the dynamic relationships of these constituents; and information about tools, chemicals and techniques used to get these data. Notation of the source of the data is important to scholars. It is our purpose to present this information in tabular and graphic form in a systematic way in order to help readers retrieve it.

If we are successful, we will make it possible for a user to find any information related to constituents of blood, body fluids, body tissues, and so on, whether they be organic or inorganic molecules, viruses, bacteria, or parasites. Users of these volumes should be able to find easily the composition of a buffer, the half-life of an isotope, or the life cycle of a parasite if that information has been used to study man or if the chemicals or particles are found in man.

We shall consider this *Handbook Series in Clinical Laboratory Science* successful if it meets most of our goals and if it provides the nidus for continuing growth. The editor of the series, the executive editor of each volume, the advisory boards, contributors, and publisher will make every effort to improve subsequent editions of this *Handbook.* The user will undoubtedly find errors of omission and commission or will have new information (all of which we hope will be called to our attention). All of us should strive to improve these volumes so that users and contributors the world over will find them useful in knowing more about man.

David Seligson
Editor-in-Chief

DAVID SELIGSON, EDITOR-IN-CHIEF
CRC HANDBOOK SERIES IN CLINICAL LABORATORY SCIENCE

Dr. David Seligson is Professor and Chairman of the Department of Laboratory Medicine (Clinical Pathology) and Professor of Pathology in the School of Medicine at Yale University. He is the Director of the Department of Clinical Laboratories of the Yale-New Haven Hospital. He has an Sc.D. in Biochemistry from Johns Hopkins University (1942) and an M.D. from the University of Utah (1946). He has been a President of the American Association of Clinical Chemists and the Academy of Clinical Laboratory Physicians and Scientists. He is a Fellow of the American Society of Clinical Pathologists, College of American Pathologists, American College of Physicians, and American Board of Clinical Chemistry.

He has been editor of *Standard Methods of the American Association of Clinical Chemists* (Volumes 2,3, and 4) and he is a member of other editorial boards.

Dr. Seligson has an honorary Masters degree from Yale University and has received the following awards:

John G. Reinhold Award, Philadelphia Section of the American Association of Clinical Chemists, 1966

Fellowship of Medici Publici, University of Utah College of Medicine and Medical Alumni Association, 1966

Donald D. Van Slyke Award, American Association of Clinical Chemists 1971 Ames Award, American Association of Clinical Chemists, National Meeting, Seattle, Washington, August 1971

Gerald T. Evans Award, Academy of Clinical Laboratory Physicians and Scientists, June 1974

Honorary Member Association of Clinical Biochemists, London, April 1976

PREFACE
SECTION I: HEMATOLOGY
VOLUME I

The Hematology section of the *CRC Handbook Series in Clinical Laboratory Science* provides a single ready reference for information on hematology which is now found in a wide variety of textbooks, laboratory manuals, monographs and journal articles written to reach specialized audiences. Organization of the section was performed with the assistance of an Editorial Advisory Board whose members represent the subspecialty areas of hematology. The twelve Board members are authorities from the major hematologic disciplines including internal medicine, pathology, pediatrics, laboratory medicine and basic research. Contributors to the Hematology Section are international experts selected by the Advisory Board members. It has been necessary to divide the material into three volumes to ensure in-depth coverage. Volume I includes blood collection, blood volume, hemoglobin and platelets. Board members who edited chapters in the first volume are John A. Koepke, Walter A. Schroeder, Douglas A. Triplett, and Onno W. van Assendelft. The factual contents of each chapter have been chosen by the individual contributors.

Publication of the Hematology Section would not have been possible without the enthusiastic support of the Editorial Advisory Board and the efforts of our contributors. Excellent editorial assistance was provided by Effie M. Brosious and Jessie Knight Schmidt. Wendy L. Clark of CRC Press proved to be a faithful, energetic and patient coordinating editor.

Robert M. Schmidt
Section Editor

ROBERT M. SCHMIDT
SECTION EDITOR
SECTION I: HEMATOLOGY

Robert M. Schmidt, M.D., M.P.H., is Medical Director, International Reference and Research Center for Blood Diseases, Lihue, Kauai, Hawaii, where he is also President of the Board of Trustees of the International Health Resource Center of Hawaii and Medical Director, International Center for Health Education. Prior to accepting these positions in 1979, he was Director, Hematology Division, National Center for Disease Control, U.S. Public Health Service, Department of H.E.W., Atlanta, Georgia. He also holds faculty appointments in Medicine, Preventive Medicine and Community Health, and Pediatrics, at Emory University, Morehouse Medical School, and Tufts University.

Dr. Schmidt received an A.B. degree from Northwestern University, an M.D. degree from Columbia University College of Physicians and Surgeons, where he received several honors including the microbiology, pharmacology, urology, Upjohn Achievement and Borden Undergraduate Medical Research awards, and an M.P.H. degree in health services administration, international health and laboratory medicine from Harvard University. He also trained in internal medicine at the University of California at San Diego and is completing a Ph.D. degree in Law, Medicine and Public Policy at Emory University. He received the United States Public Health Service Commendation Medal while at CDC. He is a diplomate of the National Board of Medical Examiners and the American Board of Preventive Medicine, a Fellow of the American Society of Clinical Pathologists, a Fellow of the American College of Preventive Medicine, and a member of numerous scientific and medical societies including the American Association for the Advancement of Science, the American Society of Hematology, the American Society for Microbiology, the American College of Physicians, the American Public Health Association, the Academy of Clinical Laboratory Physicians and Scientists, and the American Medical Association. He chairs the Area Committee on Hematology of the National Committee for Clinical Laboratory Standards and the Clinical Chemistry and Hematology Committee of the American Public Health Association. He is also a member of the Secretariat and Managing Board of the International Committee for Standardization in Hematology (ICSH) and their representative to the International Committee on Thrombosis and Hemostasis, Secretary of the ICSH Expert Panel on Abnormal Hemoglobins and Thalassemia, Executive Secretary of the ICSH Expert Panel on Oral Anticoagulant Control, and Secretary of the ICSH Committee on Training; he is Secretary of the American Society of Hematology Committee on Clinical Hematology Laboratory Standards and a member of their Education and Training Committee, and numerous other professional, national and international committees, advisory boards and panels. He serves as a consultant to the Biologics, Genetics and Health Laboratory Services units of the World Health Organization. He is a member of the editorial board of the *American Journal of Clinical Pathology* and serves as a referee for other professional journals. His medical interests span a wide area including laboratory medicine, especially hematology, preventive medicine, international health, and the interdisciplinary public health aspects of these fields. He is the author of numerous publications including ten books and manuals.

While continuing these activities, Dr. Schmidt is currently developing the international health centers in Hawaii whose purpose is to promote world health through improved preventive health education, health professional continuing education, and medical laboratory reference services, in an atmosphere of basic and applied research.

ADVISORY BOARD MEMBERS
SECTION I: HEMATOLOGY
VOLUME I

CONTRIBUTORS
SECTION I: HEMATOLOGY
VOLUME I

Ronald C. Barwick
Department of Pediatrics
University of Texas Medical Branch
Galveston, Texas

T. K. Bills
Cardeza Foundation
Thomas Jefferson University
Philadelphia, Pennsylvania

E. J. Walter Bowie
Division of Hematology
Section of Hematology Research
Blood Coagulation Laboratory
Mayo Clinic
Mayo Medical School
Rochester, Minnesota

Barry S. Coller
Division of Hematology
Department of Medicine
Health Sciences Center
State University of New York
Stony Brook, New York

J. L. Daniel
Specialized Center for Thrombosis Research
Temple University
Philadelphia, Pennsylvania

H. James Day
Specialized Center for Thrombosis Research
Temple University
Philadelphia, Pennsylvania

J. Roger Edson
Department of Laboratory Medicine and Pathology
University of Minnesota Medical School
Minneapolis, Minnesota

Georgi D. Efremov
Zemjodelski Fakultet
Odelenie za Biohemija
Autokomanda
Skopje, Yugoslavia

Bruce Lee Evatt
Hematology Division
Center for Disease Control
Atlanta, Georgia

George Grusky
Department of Medicine
New York University Medical Center
New York, New York

Chaim Hershko
Hadassah University Hospital
Jerusalem, Israel

S. Holme
Cardeza Foundation
Thomas Jefferson University
Philadelphia, Pennsylvania

Holm Holmsen
Specialized Center for Thrombosis Research
Temple University
Philadelphia, Pennsylvania

G. Izak
Chief Scientist's Office
Israel Ministry of Health
Hadassah University Hospital
Jerusalem, Israel

Simon Karpatkin
Department of Medicine
New York University School of Medicine
New York, New York

Robert D. Koler
University of Oregon Medical School
Portland, Oregon

Shirley P. Levine
Department of Medicine
Division of Hematology
Audie L. Murphy Memorial Veteran's Hospital and
University of Texas Health Science Center
San Antonio, Texas

S. M. Lewis
Hematology Department
Royal Postgraduate Medical School
London, England

C. Harold Mielke, Jr.
Institute of Health Research
Institutes of Medical Sciences
Pacific Medical Center
San Francisco, California

Stefan Niewiarowski
Specialized Center for Thrombosis Research
Temple University
Philadelphia, Pennsylvania

Kenneth W. Olsen
Department of Biochemistry
University of Mississippi Medical Center
Jackson, Mississippi

Michael B. O'Sullivan
Mayo Medical School
Department of Laboratory Medicine
Mayo Clinic
Rochester, Minnesota

Charles A. Owen, Jr.
Section of Clinical Pathology
Department of Biochemistry
Mayo Clinic
Mayo Graduate School of Medicine
Mayo Medical School
Rochester, Minnesota

Robert Rodvien
Institute of Health Research
Institutes of Medical Sciences
Pacific Medical Center
San Francisco, California

Rose G. Schneider
Department of Pediatrics
University of Texas Medical Branch
Galveston, Texas

Walter A. Schroeder
Division of Chemistry and Chemical Engineering
California Institute of Technology
Pasadena, California

Jean M. Slockbower
Mayo Medical School
Department of Laboratory Medicine
Mayo Clinic
Rochester, Minnesota

J. Bryan Smith
Cardeza Foundation
Thomas Jefferson University
Philadelphia, Pennsylvania

Douglas A. Triplett
Department of Pathology
Ball Memorial Hospital
Muncie, Indiana

Onno W. van Assendelft
Hematology Division
Center for Disease Control
Atlanta, Georgia

Peter N. Walsh
Specialized Center for Thrombosis Research
Temple University
Philadelphia, Pennsylvania

Richard K. Wertz
Department of Laboratory Medicine
Sutter Memorial Hospital
Sacramento, California

William P. Winter
Center for Sickle Cell Disease
Howard University
Washington, D.C.

Ruth N. Wrightstone
Sickle Cell Center
Medical College of Georgia
Augusta, Georgia

Dorothea Zucker-Franklin
Department of Medicine
New York University Medical Center
New York, New York

TABLE OF CONTENTS
SECTION I: HEMATOLOGY
VOLUME I

BLOOD COLLECTION

Introduction 3
Laboratory Hematology Procedures 5
Blood Drawing Techniques 21
Blood Collection Equipment 27

BLOOD VOLUME

Blood Volume 33

HEMOGLOBIN

Hemoglobin 43
Genetics of Hemoglobins 51
The Chromatography of Hemoglobin 67
Electrophoretic Mobilities of Mutant Hemoglobins 87
Starch Gel Electrophoresis 97
The Three-Dimensional Structure of Hemoglobin 105
Hemoglobinopathies 177
Hemoglobinometry 211
Iron Metabolism 221

PLATELETS

Platelet Production 255
Kinetics of Isotopically Labeled Platelets 263
Platelet Biochemistry 273
Platelet Ultrastructure 313
Laboratory Tests in Platelet Function 329
Contributions of Platelets to Intrinsic Coagulation 351
Cell Counting — the Platelet 361
Bleeding Time Procedures 369
Platelet Aggregation by ADP, Collagen, and Ristocetin: a Critical Review of Methodology and Analysis 381
Platelet Retention Procedures 397
Laboratory Evaluation of Platelet Coagulant Activities 403
Platelet Sizing 409
Characterization and Assay of Platelet Secretory Proteins 435
Qualitative Abnormalities of Platelet Function 447
Acquired Qualitative Abnormalities of Platelet Function 463
Von Willebrand's Disease 471
Quantitative Disorders of Platelets 487

Index 505

Blood Collection

BLOOD COLLECTION — INTRODUCTION

Clinical laboratories, including the hematological, are faced with an increasing work load and an ever-broadening range of increasingly complex tests. At the same time, there is an increased demand for a greater validity of test results. This demand can only be met adequately when all factors in the analytical process are adequately controlled. One of the factors to which insufficient attention has been paid — possibly because it is so often outside the jurisdiction of the laboratory performing a specific test — is the proper collection, storage, and transport of blood specimens.

The usual specimen source for hematologic determinations is capillary or venous blood. The specimen must be obtained in a proper manner; must be collected in a proper container, with the correct anticoagulant in a sufficient but not excessive amount; must be properly and correctly labeled; and finally, must be properly transported to the laboratory. Only if these conditions are fulfilled can one expect the laboratory to produce results that are valid and meaningful for the patient.

The first chapter of this section on blood collection provides a listing of tests commonly performed in the hematological laboratory. The author, M. B. O'Sullivan, has grouped these tests in tables relating to erythrocyte measurements, leukocyte measurements, platelet measurements, coagulation factors, and hematopoietic factors. The tables include information on the type of sample, i.e., whole blood, plasma, serum, or red cells; on the usual anticoagulant; and on storage conditions. A discussion of factors to be taken into account in the interpretation of the test results follows each group of tests.

The second section, by J. M. Slockbower, provides guidelines for obtaining venous blood samples, capillary blood samples, and the labeling of specimens.

The final section, by O. W. van Assendelft, deals with certain types of specimen containers and other equipment used in obtaining blood specimens.

LABORATORY HEMATOLOGY PROCEDURES

Michael B. O'Sullivan

Peripheral Blood Erythrocyte Measurements

Table 1
PERIPHERAL BLOOD ERYTHROCYTE MEASUREMENTS

Test title	Principle of methods in current clinical use	Specimen	Additive	Special considerations	Storage and stability
Erythrocyte counts	1. Hemocytometer[1]	Whole blood, venous or capillary[2]	EDTA	Technical errors result from failure to mix blood adequately	Room temp; 24 hr[3]
	2. Automated electronic particle counting[4]	Whole blood, venous or capillary	EDTA	—	Room temp; 24 hr[2,3]
	3. Automated dark-field optical counting[4,5]	Whole blood, venous or capillary	EDTA	—	Room temp; 24 hr
Hemoglobin (Hb)	1. Colorimetric				
	(a) Cyanmethemoglobin[6]	Whole blood, venous or capillary	EDTA	International standard method[6]	Room temp; 24 hr[2,3]
	(b) Oxyhemoglobin[7]	—	—	—	Room temp; 24 hr
Packed cell volume (PCV; hematocrit, Hct)	1. Centrifugation				
	(a) Macromethod of Wintrobe[8]	Whole blood, venous or capillary	EDTA	Trapped plasma, 3—4%	Room temp; 4 hr Refrigerated; 24 hr[3]
	(b) Micromethod[9]	—	—	Trapped plasma, 1—5%	—
	(c) Automated U-tube[4,10]	—	—	—	—
	2. Electrical conductivity[11,12]	Whole blood, venous or capillary	EDTA	Our experience indicates this is an unreliable method	—
	3. Computation from MCV and erythrocyte count[4,13]	Whole blood, venous or capillary	EDTA	—	Room temp; 4 hr Refrigerated; 24 hr[3]
Erythrocyte indices MCV	1. Calculation from PCV and erythrocyte count[14]	Whole blood, venous or capillary	EDTA	—	Room temp; 4 hr Refrigerated; 24 hr[3]
	2. Measured from mean pulse heights of electronic counting[4,13]	Whole blood, venous or capillary	EDTA	—	Room temp; 4 hr Refrigerated; 24 hr[3]
MCH (Mean corpuscular hemoglobin)	Calculated from Hb and erythrocyte count[14]	Whole blood, venous or capillary	EDTA	—	Room temp; 24 hr[3]
MCHC (Mean corpuscular hemoglobin concentration)	Calculated from Hb and Hct[14]	Whole blood, venous or capillary	EDTA	—	Room temp; 4 hr Refrigerated; 24 hr[3]
Reticulocyte count	Microscopic counting of red cells supravitally stained with new methylene blue[15,16]	Well-prepared, well-stained, peripheral blood smear	None	Smear should be made from fresh blood	—
Erythrocyte sedimentation rate	Measures the rate of settling of erythrocytes in vertical column of blood				
	1. Westergren[17]	Whole blood, venous	0.105 molar solution, trisodium citrate, in 1:4 dilution with whole blood	Recommended by NCCLS and ICSH as standard method[18]	Room temp; 4—5 hr Refrigerated; 24 hr[19]
	2. Modified Westergren[19]	Whole blood, venous	EDTA with sodium chloride in 1:4 dilution with whole blood	—	Room temp; 4—5 hr Refrigerated; 24 hr[19]
	3. Wintrobe method[20]	Whole blood, venous	EDTA	—	—
	4. Micro method[2]	Whole blood, capillary	Trisodium citrate in 1:4 dilution with whole blood	—	—

Table 1 (continued)
PERIPHERAL BLOOD ERYTHROCYTE MEASUREMENTS

Test title	Principle of methods in current clinical use	Specimen	Additive	Special considerations	Storage and stability
Zeta sedimentation ratio	Measures degree of packing of erythrocytes during four 45-sec alternating spinning cycles of dispersion and compaction in vertical capillary tubes[21]	Whole blood, venous or capillary	EDTA	Results expressed as vol%. Results not affected by anemia	—
Fragility, osmotic	1. Manual technique: serial dilution in hypotonic saline to the point where all erythrocytes lyse.[22] The percent hemolysis can be plotted for each saline concentration. Further clinically important information can be derived if osmotic fragility is performed both on a fresh specimen and following a 24-hr incubation at 37°C.	Fresh whole blood	Heparin or defibrination	—	Room temp; 1 hr
	2. Automated techniques: Fragiligraph[23]	Fresh whole blood	Heparin	Complete fragility curve can be obtained from single sample in approximately 5 min[24]	Room temp; 1 hr

Biologic and Physiologic Variation

Erythrocyte Count, Hemoglobin, Hematocrit, and Erythrocyte Indices

Effects of age and sex — The erythrocyte count (RBC), hematocrit (Hct), and hemoglobin (Hb), are highest at birth (average hemoglobin value 19.0 g/dℓ), drop to a minimum at about 2 months (average hemoglobin 11.0 g/dℓ, and are relatively constant at this level from ages 2 to 24 months.[25] From 2 to 11 years, the values gradually increase (to about 13 g hemoglobin/dℓ).[26] In the adult, the values for males are higher than for females (mean hemoglobin, male about 15 g/dℓ, mean hemoglobin, female about 13.5 g/dℓ). During the course of adult life, an age effect is seen, with the hemoglobin, hematocrit, and RBC values tending to decrease with age in the male, whereas in the female this trend is reversed (Hb, Hct, and RBC increase).[27-29] The mean cell volume (MCV) is highest at birth (about 120 fℓ),[25] drops to a low of about 72 fℓ at 18 months,[25,26] and reaches adult levels at about 18 years.[26] Thereafter, there are no apparent sex influences. There is a slight gradual increase in the MCV with age (in both sexes) to about 60 years, when the values level off.[29] The mean cell hemoglobin (MCH) follows closely the MCV trend. The mean corpuscular hemoglobin concentration (MCHC) tends to be slightly less in females than in males and is little influenced by age.[29]

Intraindividual variations — The mean physiological hour-to-hour and week-to-week intraindividual variations in terms of percent coefficient of variation were demonstrated in 20 healthy adult volunteers to be for hemoglobin, 2.5 and 2.2% and for hematocrit, 2.6 and 2.7%, respectively. Diurnal variations of the hemoglobin and hematocrit values represent a significant part of the total intraindividual variation, with afternoon values being lower than early morning values by, on the average, 0.3 g Hb/dℓ.[31,32] However, differences as large as 1.5 g/dℓ can occur in individual subjects.[30]

Other factors — Transient strenuous muscular activity raises the red count and hemoglobin,[33] while postural change from the recumbent to the standing position may increase hemoglobin and hematocrit values by as much as 5 to 10%.[34-36] The position of the arm during venipuncture also has been shown to affect erythroid values — the hemacocrit being 2 to 4% lower with the arm held at the atrial level instead of being lowered.[36] Prolonged stasis caused by constriction with a tourniquet for 1 min or longer may result in a falsely high hematocrit of from 2.5 to 5%.[35] Cigarette smokers have higher hemoglobin and hematocrit values, which may in fact lead to frank polycythemia in some subjects as a result of carboxyhemoglobinemia.[37]

Reticulocyte Counts

Effects of age and sex — Newborns have levels of 2 to 6%, but this drops to normal adult levels by the end of the first week of life.[38] The normal range for adults is 0.5 to 1.5% or an absolute count of 25,000 to 75,000 per $\mu\ell$. The normal functioning marrow should predictably respond with increased output of reticulocytes to the degree of anemia or hypoxia. With a peripheral hematocrit value of 35%, red cell production in the unimpaired marrow should be twice normal and at 25%, three times normal.[39]

Erythrocyte Sedimentation Rate (ESR)

Effects of age and sex — The ESR is higher in females and increases with age.[40,41]

Osmotic Fragility

It has been reported[42] that the osmotic resistance of cord blood and adult blood did not differ. The span of hemolysis, however, was greater in cord blood, resistant cells being more numerous than in adult blood. Resistant cells continued in the circulation during childhood. At about puberty, a definite shift to the adult red cell type seemed to occur.

Peripheral Blood Leukocyte Measurements

Table 2
PERIPHERAL BLOOD LEUKOCYTE MEASUREMENTS

Test title	Principle of methods in current clinical use	Specimen	Additive	Special considerations	Storage and stability
Leukocyte counts	1. Hemocytometer, manual, microscopic[43]	Whole blood, venous or capillary	EDTA	—	24 hr at room temp; 48 hr at 4°C
	2. Automated electronic particle counting[4]	Whole blood, venous or capillary	EDTA	—	
	3. Automated dark-field optical[4,5]	Whole blood, venous or capillary	EDTA	—	
Leukocyte differential counts	1. Visual microscopic classification[44,45]	Whole blood; venous, capillary, or finger stick	EDTA None	— —	Slide must be made and stained, preferably immediately from "fingerstick" drop or as soon as possible from EDTA blood to avoid artifacts that develop in 1—3 hr at room temp.[46] Slide can be stored indefinitely
	2. Automated computerized pattern recognition of stained cells[47-49]	Whole blood; venous, capillary, or finger stick	EDTA None	— —	
	3. Automated optical analysis of selective cytochemically stained cells[50-52]	Whole blood, venous or capillary	EDTA	—	30 hr at room temp[53]

Biologic and Physiologic Variation

Effects of age and sex — There is a neutrophilic leukocytosis at birth (white blood cell (WBC) 18,000/$\mu\ell$ with about 65% total neutrophils) that subsides in the first 2 to 3 days of life (WBC approximately 12,000/$\mu\ell$ with about 65% total neutrophils).[54,55] In the early years of childhood, the lymphocyte is the predominant cell until about the 7th year of life.[54-56] In adult population studies, no conclusive patterns related to age and sex have been defined,[29,57,58] although a recent publication suggests a statistically significant decrease in the lymphocyte count in the elderly in comparison to younger adults.[59] A moderate leukocytosis of up to 15,000/$\mu\ell$ is common during pregnancy, peaking about 8 weeks prior to parturition.[60] Onset of labor is accompanied by further neutrophilic leukocytosis, sometimes very pronounced; the count returns to normal levels a week or so after delivery.[60]

Intraindividual variation — Newer automated instruments that produce much more precise counts of the venous leukocyte categories have allowed more reliable definitions of their fluctuating patterns, long suspected but ill-defined by manual techniques. In 20 healthy adults, mean physiologic within-day and week-to-week variations within the same individual, expressed in terms of percent coefficient of variations for white cell counts, were as follows: total WBC 9.4% and 15.7%, neutrophils 12.9% and 26.0%, lymphocytes 10.3% and 13.2%, monocytes 18.6% and 19.3%, eosinophils 19.9% and 26.9%, and basophils 7.4% and 15.0%.[30] Within the same individual, the hour-to-hour variance was overall less pronounced than the variance from day to day. The within-day variance demonstrated diurnal trends that, however, were relatively unique for each individual, but varied considerably from individual to individual. The exceptions were the eosinophils and, to a lesser extent, the basophils, which tended to show a more consistent pattern for the entire group with low afternoon values relative to early morning levels. These latter diurnal fluctuations perhaps parallel diurnal glucocorticoid fluctuations. Of importance was that intraindividual variance was much less than differences between individuals, suggesting that individual human beings maintain their total and specific subclasses of leukocytes within much tighter limits than can be appreciated from "normal value" studies derived from mixed populations of healthy subjects.

Other factors — Marked leukocytosis (both neutrophilia and lymphocytosis) occurs with strenuous exercise.[61] Wintrobe[61] references changes in the leukocyte counts with pain, emotion, and ovulation,[62] while indicating that reported changes in leukocyte levels with digestion, season, and climate are controversial. Granulocytopenia and leukopenia without clinical consequences have been reported in about 25% of blacks.[63]

Platelet Measurements in Peripheral Blood

Table 3
PLATELET MEASUREMENTS IN PERIPHERAL BLOOD

Test title	Principle of methods in current clinical use	Specimen	Additive	Special considerations	Storage and stability
Platelet counts	1. Manual methods				
	(a) Light microscopy[64]	Whole blood, venous or capillary	EDTA	—	5 hr at room temp[65]
	(b) Phase-contrast microscopy[66]	Whole blood, venous or capillary	EDTA	—	—
	2. Automated methods				
	(a) Electronic particle counting[67-69]	Platelet-enriched plasma (venous or capillary)	EDTA	Good drawing technique critical; tissue juice contamination causes platelet aggregation with resultant low platelet count[79]	No data available
	(b) Electro-optical counting[70,71]	Whole blood, venous or capillary	EDTA		
Platelet aggregation	The transmittance of light through stirred platelet-rich plasma in a cuvette is compared to a platelet-poor plasma bank. The increase in transmittance following the addition of an aggregating agent is used as an index of platelet aggregation[72,73]	Whole blood	3.2% Citrate	Technique must be standardized. Many variables including venipuncture technique, anticoagulant effects, centrifugation and cellular	Interval between venipuncture and measurement of platelet aggregation should be fixed and stated with all data documented.[75]

Table 3 (continued)
PLATELET MEASUREMENTS IN PERIPHERAL BLOOD

Test title	Principle of methods in current clinical use	Specimen	Additive	Special considerations	Storage and stability
				contamination, platelet concentration, interval after venipuncture, pH and temperature, vigor of stirring—all can markedly affect platelet aggregation[74]	"Intrinsic variables", e.g., exercise and mental stress, induce plasma instability so that small delays in time of testing radically alter results.[76]
Platelet retention	Decrease in platelet count that occurs when blood contacts a foreign surface for standard period of time — (a) roller flask technique,[76] (b) glass bead columns,[77] (c) adhesion of site of small skin incision	Whole blood, venous	EDTA or heparin	Blood must be handled gently. Platelet retention is decreased if blood is disturbed, but returns to normal if it is allowed to stand for 1 hr before performing test[78]	Allow blood to stand for 1 hr before performing test[78]

Biologic and Physiologic Variation

Effects of age and sex — Platelet counts in normal neonates show little difference from adult values.[80] At birth, there is normal bleeding time and normal platelet retention. However, the time required for maximal platelet aggregation with ADP, collagen, and thrombin has been reported to be prolonged in the newborn.[81] In the adult, there appears to be no age effect,[82] and no sex differences have been reported in the numerous normal value studies published.

Intraindividual variation — The day-to-day variation in platelet counts within the individual is quite small — reported as 3.5% coefficient of variation (C.V.). The week-to-week fluctuations are somewhat larger, 6.6% C.V., but still a good deal less for the individual in comparison to the interindividual variances of the group, 21.9% C.V.[30] Platelet aggregation shows four to five times greater variability between samples drawn several days apart than between those drawn 10 min apart in the same individual. Venous stasis and sampling technique has little or no effect on aggregation results.[74]

Other factors — A thrombocytosis follows exercise with counts returning to normal within 30 min.[83] Platelet adhesion and ADP-induced aggregation are also accentuated by exercise.[84] A change to high altitude or to other forms of hypoxia increases the platelet count.[85] Smoking may produce platelet hyperaggregability[86] and has also been reported to shorten platelet survival. Cyclical changes in platelet concentrations during the menstrual cycle have been reported, with a slightly increased number at ovulation, the levels falling until menstruation, and a rapid increase shortly after the onset of menses.[87]

Coagulation Tests

Introduction

Blood coagulation is a highly involved and delicately balanced process of multiple, interlinked, enzymatic reactions that result in the eventual creation of a gel of fibrin from the soluble protein, fibrinogen. Starting with the venipuncture and ending with the test, coagulation test results can be affected by many variables. These variables affect many of the coagulation tests similarly and are more conveniently discussed as a preamble to the table.

Special Considerations and Storage and Stability Requirements

The venipuncture must be clean, and the flow of blood must be free.[88,89] A two-syringe technique may be employed, or a butterfly can be used. After discarding the first few drops of blood, the sample is allowed to flow directly into the tubes. For some tests the use of evacuated tubes has been discouraged. Hemolysis, aspiration of air, and prolonged application of the tourniquet all affect the clotting tests.[88,90] If blood is obtained from intravenous tubing, it should be established that there is no heparin in the tubing.[89] Sodium oxylate, 0.1*M*, and sodium citrate, 0.11*M*, are the usual anticoagulants. Sodium oxylate allows adsorption of the vitamin K-dependent factors by barium sulfate, but sodium citrate is generally preferred because it allows preservation of factors V and VIII coagulant activities.[90] If the patient has a high hematocrit, there will be proportionately more anticoagulant to plasma volume, and the volume of anticoagulant should be reduced according to the degree of elevation of the hematocrit.[91] In general, the samples should be tested as soon as possible after venipuncture. They should be placed on ice and stoppered to prevent change of pH. The sample can be tested up to 4 hr after the venipuncture if it is treated in this way and taken in citrated anticoagulant. In general, however, it is best to do the tests within 2 hr. Freezing is best avoided; but if the sample must be frozen, it should be quick frozen and stored at −70°C. Factor VII[92] and factor XI[93] may be activated by freezing. It is best to use plastic syringes and test tubes to minimize contact activation of the clotting mechanism (Table 4).

Table 4
COAGULATION TESTS

Test title	Principle of methods in current clinical use	Specimen	Additive
Prothrombin time	Tissue thromboplastin and calcium are added to citrated plasma. The tissue thromboplastin reacts with factors V, VII, and X to form prothrombinase, which converts prothrombin to thrombin. Fibrinogen is converted to fibrin by the thrombin[94]	Plasma	0.11 *M* Sodium citrate
Partial thromboplastin time	The intrinsic coagulant activity of plasma is measured after the addition of calcium and partial thromboplastin as a substitute for platelet factor 3[95]	Plasma	0.11 *M* Sodium citrate
Activated partial thromboplastin time	Contact activation for a standard time is produced by the addition of Celite or kaolin, or other activator, before the clotting time is measured[96]	Plasma	0.11 *M* Sodium citrate (oxalate)
Thrombin time	A standard thrombin solution is added to citrated plasma in order to measure the rate of transformation of plasma fibrinogen to fibrin[97,98]	Plasma	0.11 *M* Sodium citrate
Prothrombin consumption	The residual coagulant activity in serum is measured by doing a prothrombin time on serum. Serum lacks factor V and fibrinogen, so these factors are supplied by adding adsorbed rabbit plasma (factor V is stable in rabbit plasma). If clotting of the plasma has been normal, then the serum will contain little coagulant activity so that the prothrombin consumption time will be long. Conversely, if clotting has been abnormal (as for example, in hemophilia), there will be a lot of residual coagulant activity, and the prothrombin consumption time will be short In thrombocytopenia and certain qualitative platelet diseases, the lack of platelet factor 3 will cause an abnormal prothrombin consumption test. The addition of inosithin or some other substitute for platelet factor 3 to the freshly drawn blood will correct this abnormality[99,100]	Serum	—
Protamine gel	The addition of a solution of protamine sulfate to citrated plasma precipitates the fibrin monomer complexes, and a gel is formed[101,102]	Plasma	0.11 *M* Sodium citrate
Coagulation factor assays			
Fibrinogen (I)	1. Selective precipitation of fibrinogen from plasma with either salt solutions[103] or heat[104]	Plasma	0.11 *M* Sodium citrate
	2. Separation of fibrinogen from other plasma proteins by clotting with excess thrombin. The clot is washed and dissolved in a solution of sodium hydroxide-urea. The amount of protein is then determined spectrophotometrically[105]	—	—
	3. Thrombin-clottable protein technique: when plasma is diluted sufficiently, the fibrinogen concentration becomes the limiting factor in the clotting time after the addition of thrombin[106,107]	—	—
	4. Immunologic procedures[108]	—	—
Factor II (prothrombin)	The anticoagulated plasma is defibrinated by means of the addition of weak thrombin. The prothrombin is converted to thrombin by the addition of thromboplastin and calcium. The amount of thrombin formed is measured at intervals by adding the reaction mixture to the standard solution of fibrinogen[109,110]	Plasma	0.11 *M* Sodium citrate
Factor V, factor VII, factor X	A plasma from a patient known to be deficient in factors V, VII, or X is used as a substrate, and the prothrombin time is performed. The degree to which the unknown plasma corrects the deficiency is compared to the correction of dilutions of a standard plasma[111]	Plasma	0.11 *M* Sodium citrate
Factor VIII, factor IX, factor XI, factor XII	A plasma congenitally lacking factor VIII, IX, XI, or XII is used as a substrate, and the activated partial thromboplastin time is performed. The effectiveness of the patient's plasma is compared with that of normal plasma[111] A two-stage assay for factor VIII can be performed using a modification of the thromboplastin generation test. It is preferred by some workers for measurement of concentrate and is said not to be influenced by the activated coagulation factors present in patients with disseminated intravascular coagulation[112]	Plasma	0.11 *M* Sodium citrate

Table 4 (continued)
COAGULATION TESTS

Test title	Principle of methods in current clinical use	Specimen	Additive
Factor XIII	Factor XIII, or fibrin-stabilizing factor, is a transpeptidase that converts the weak hydrogen bonds between the molecules of fibrin monomer into covalent bonds. If factor XIII is not present, then the clot is soluble in 5 M urea and weak acids. The quantity of factor XIII can be measured by means of a thromboelastogram[113] and also by the dansyl-cadaverine assay[114]	Plasma	0.11 *M* Sodium citrate
Factor VIII-related antigen	The antigen is detected by an antibody made to a purified preparation of factor VIII by the technique of Zimmerman et al.[115] The antibody is almost certainly detecting the von Willebrand moiety of the factor VIII molecule (or molecules). It can also be detected by the Laurell method[115] or by radioimmunoassay	Plasma	0.11 *M* Sodium citrate
Ristocetin cofactor assay (Willebrand factor)	The Willebrand factor can be measured by the degree of platelet aggregation produced by the antibiotic ristocetin[116]	—	0.11 *M* Sodium citrate
Antithrombin III	Antithrombin III is one of the inhibitors of thrombin that can be measured by a functional assay [117] or by immunoelectrophoretic techniques using a precipitating antibody to antithrombin III[118]	Serum or defibrinated plasma	—

Biologic and Physiologic Variability

Effects of age and sex — Results of the prothrombin time vary considerably at birth, and there is a tendency towards prolonged prothrombin times in the first 3 days of life, which usually reverses spontaneously thereafter. While this prolongation can be prevented by administration of vitamin K to the mother or infant, hypoxia seems to compound the problem and contribute to further prolongation.[119] Factors I, II, VII, IX, X, XII, plasminogen, and antithrombin III are decreased in the full-term newborn in comparison with older children or adults, while there are no differences in factors V, VIII, XIII, and fibrin-split products.[119] A number of coagulation factors appear to change with age later on in life. Factors V, VII, VIII, and X all appear to increase with advancing years.[120-124] while factors XI, XII, and antithrombin III appear to increase with age in the male and decrease in the female.[121] No sex differences were demonstrated for factors V and XIII.[122,125] With factor VII, however, though no sex differences were noted at 20, by age 60 females had higher levels.[123]

Other factors — With pregnancy, increases in factors I, II, VII, IX, X, and XII have been noted, with factor V showing no increase and factor XIII declining.[125,126] Factor VIII and plasminogen have been reported to increase with exertion.[127-129]

Peripheral Blood Concentrations of Hematopoietic-Related Factors

Table 5
PERIPHERAL BLOOD CONCENTRATION OF HEMATOPOIETIC-RELATED FACTORS

Test title	Principle of methods in current clinical use	Specimen	Additive	Special considerations	Storage and stability
Ferritin	1. Immunoradiometric[130-133]	Serum or plasma (EDTA or heparin)[133]	—	Nonlinearity of method may lead to erroneous interpretation[133,134]	Stable for 6 months if frozen[133]
	2. Enzyme immunoassay [135]	Serum	—	—	—
	3. Radioimmunoassay [136]	Serum	—	—	—
Folate	1. Microbiologic assay [137,138]	Serum	Ascorbate, 15 mg/m*ℓ*, added to better preserve folate activity[139]	Patient fasting — recent intake may increase serum levels.[140,141] Antimicrobial agents in serum may interfere with bioassay[142]	Serum stable 4—5 days at room temp with 15 mg ascorbic acid added per m*ℓ*. Nonhemolyzed samples show no loss of activity for 7—10 days when stored at 4°C. For storage at −20°C up to 3 months, add 5 mg ascorbic acid per m*ℓ*[139]
	2. Microbiologic assay[143,144]	Red cells	Heparin or EDTA ascorbate	Red cell folate does not fluctuate as readily as serum folate. Provides better assessment of tissue folate isoenzymes[143]	Hemolysates prepared with 1% ascorbic acid solution are stable 3—5 months at −20°C.[139] Must also store serum and have hematocrit determined to estimate RBC folate

Table 5 (continued)
PERIPHERAL BLOOD CONCENTRATION OF HEMATOPOIETIC-RELATED FACTORS

Test title	Principle of methods in current clinical use	Specimen	Additive	Special considerations	Storage and stability
	3. Competitive protein binding[145,146]	Serum	Ascorbate	—	Same as microbiologic assay
	4. Competitive protein binding[147]	Red cells	Ascorbate	—	Same as microbiologic assay
Haptoglobin	1. Hemoglobin-binding techniques				
	Peroxidase activity of haptoglobin-hemoglobin (Hp-Hb) complex[148]	Serum	—	Phenotypes affect binding capacity, which accounts for wide range of values in healthy population.[149] Therefore, a drop in value of two consecutive samples is clinically more significant than a single determination	After separating serum, stable 3 days at 30°C, 7 days at 4°C. If stored longer, freeze[150]
	Electrophoretic separation of Hp-Hb complex[151,152]	Sérum	—	—	—
	Gel-filtration separation of Hp-Hb complex[153]	Serum	—	—	—
	2. Immunologic techniques				
	Radial immunodiffusion[154]	Serum	—	Because of different molecular weight of different phenotypes, this method may give results different from those obtained by hemoglobin binding techniques[150]	—
	Latex agglutination[155]	Serum	—	Used to screen for low levels of haptoglobin	—
	Nephelometric immunoassay[156]	Serum	—	—	—
Iron	1. Spectrophotometric (bathophenanthroline)[157]	Serum	—	Recommended by International Committee for Standardization in Hematology[157]	Separate serum from cells within 2 hr Stable for at least 4 days at room temp and for 1 week at 4°C[158]
	2. Spectrophotometric with other chromogens, e.g., o-phenanthroline, ferrozine, TPTZ terosite[158]	Serum	—	—	—
	3. Atomic absorption[159]	Serum	—	Invalid unless preceded by protein precipitation	—
Iron-binding capacity	1. Spectrophotometric after saturation with excess iron[160]	Serum	—	Separate serum from cells within 2 hr	Stable for at least 4 days at room temp and for 1 week at 4°C. Stable many months if frozen[158]
	2. Radioisotopic after saturation with excess isotopically labeled iron[161,162]	Serum	—	—	—
Transferrin	1. Radial immunodiffusion[163]	Serum	—	—	—
	2. Nephelometric immunoassay[164]	—	—	—	—
Vitamin B12	1. Microbiologic[165]	Serum	—	Antimicrobial agents in serum may interfere with bioassay[166]	Stable at room temp or 4°C for 3 weeks provided no bacterial growth occurs[167]
	2. Competitive protein binding[168,169]	Serum	—	Serum is preferred to plasma because artifacts can be introduced by the use of heparinized or EDTA-treated plasma.[167] Samples should not be collected in ascorbic acid or high concentrations of fluoride, since these agents appear to destroy B12[170] There have been recent reports[171] of patients with megaloblastic bone marrows and low Vitamin B12 levels measured by microbiological methods but with clinically inappropriate	—

Table 5 (continued)
PERIPHERAL BLOOD CONCENTRATION OF HEMATOPOIETIC-RELATED FACTORS

Test title	Principle of methods in current clinical use	Specimen	Additive	Special considerations	Storage and stability
				normal or elevated B12 levels when measured by currently available competitive binding techniques	
Vitamin B12 unsaturated binding capacity	Radioisotope saturation [172]	Serum	—	—	Stable for 4 days at room temp and 7 days at −15°C [167]

Physiologic and Biologic Variability

Ferritin

Immunoradiometric assays are quite recent developments whereby ferritin can be quantitated in human serum; hence, population studies in normal individuals are limited. Studies indicate that serum ferritin levels are three times higher in males than in females,[131,173] and that there is a slight, positive correlation of serum ferritin with age in females but not in males.[173]

Folate

Serum and red cell folate levels, high at birth, fall rapidly in the first 6 weeks of life.[174,175] In the adult, no differences relative to age or sex have been detected.[176] Serum folate falls rapidly after dietary intake declines;[177] however, red cell folate levels are not as sensitively affected by short-term negative folate balances.[178]

Haptoglobin

Haptoglobin (Hp) is a genetically polymorphic serum protein, with three phenotypes generally recognized (Hp 1-1, 2-1, and 2-2). Haptoglobin in human serum has a broad, normal value range. This wide range encompasses the three major phenotypes, there being a different range for each type.[149] Ahaptoglobinemia normal in the first 6 weeks of life[179] persists in the adult in a rare, genetically determined condition. Ahaptoglobinemia is somewhat more common in the black races,[180] occurring in about 3 to 5% of apparently normal adults and in about 12 to 15% of the children of black parents in the U.S.[181] There is a sex difference in haptoglobin serum levels, with females showing a lower level than males.[149]

Iron and Iron-Binding Capacity

Serum iron in umbilical cord blood is high (av 160 μg/dℓ) and rapidly drops to about one-third of that value in the first 24 hr of life. The level recovers during the following 2 weeks. However, from the age of 2 months on, serum iron levels in children tend to be low (20 to 40 μg/dℓ below adult female values). These values seem to be maintained to puberty when adult female levels are attained in both sexes. The further increase in male values apparently occurs between 15 to 20 years.[182,183] In the adult, average serum iron values for males are some 10 μg/dℓ higher than for females, whereas there is little if any sex difference in the total iron-binding capacity.[184] There is a large diurnal variation in serum iron.[185,186] This occurs in children as well as in adults.[183] Maximum values occur in the morning, and the minimum (as much as 30% or more below the morning value) occurs late in the evening. Women show a pronounced fall in serum iron levels during menstruation.[187] The values decrease as much as 30% below the mean value at the onset of menstruation. This decrease may persist for a few days. Serum iron usually decreases, and the iron-binding capacity increases during pregnancy. However, these changes may reflect degrees of iron deficiency.[188]

Vitamin B12

Serum levels of the vitamin may vary within the same individual by as much as 80 pg/mℓ within the same day, 90 pg/mℓ from day to day, and up to 160 pg/mℓ over a period of weeks.[189] There apparently is no sex variation. It has been reported that serum vitamin B_{12} levels decline with age, being below the lower limits of normal in 7% of nonanemic individuals over the age of 65.[190] The significance of low serum B_{12} levels without anemia and with normal B_{12} absorption remains uncertain.[191]

REFERENCES

1. **Davidsohn, I. and Nelson, D. A.,** The blood, in *Todd-Sanford Clinical Diagnosis by Laboratory Methods,* 15th ed., Davidsohn, I. and Henry, J. B., Eds., W. B. Saunders, Philadelphia, 1974, 117.
2. **Stuart, J., Barrett, B. A., and Prangnell, D. R.,** Capillary blood collection in haematology, *J. Clin. Pathol.,* 27, 869, 1974.
3. **Brittin, G. M., Brecher, G., Johnson, C. A., and Elashoff, R. M.,** Stability of blood in commonly used anticoagulants, *Am. J. Clin. Pathol.,* 52, 690, 1969.
4. **Brittin, G. M. and Brecher, G.,** Instrumentation and automation in clinical hematology, *Prog. Hematol.,* 7, 299, 1971.
5. **Mansberg, H. P.,** Optical techniques of particle counting, in *Advances in Automated Analysis,* Vol. 1, Technicon International Congress, New York, Mediad, 1969, 213.
6. **International Committee for Standardization in Hematology,** Recommendations for haemoglobinometry in human blood, *B. J. Haematol.,* 12 (Suppl), 71, 1967.
7. **Davidsohn, I. and Nelson, D. A.,** The Blood, in *Todd-Sanford Clinical Diagnosis by Laboratory Methods,* 15th ed., Davidsohn, I. and Henry, J. B., Eds., W. B. Saunders, Philadelphia, 1974, 106.
8. **Wintrobe, M. M.,** A simple and accurate hematocrit, *J. Lab. Clin. Med.,* 15, 287, 1929.
9. **Strumia, M. M., Sample, A. B., and Hart, E. D.,** An improved microhematocrit method, *Am. J. Clin. Pathol.,* 24, 1016, 1954.
10. **Ohringer, P.,** PCV centrifuge — an automatic microhematocrit, in *Advances in Automated Analysis,* Technicon Instrument Congress, Miami Thurman Associates, 1970, 407.
11. **Davis, R. E., Bresland, R., and Green, R.,** Evaluation of electronically measured hematocrit values, *Lab. Prac.,* 15, 1376, 1966.
12. **Kernen, J. A., Wurzel, H., and Okada, R.,** New electronic method for measuring hematocrit: clinical evaluation, *J. Lab. Clin. Med.,* 57, 641, 1961.
13. **Brittin, G. M., Brecher, G., and Johnson, C. A.,** Evaluation of the Coulter model S, *Am. J. Clin. Pathol.,* 52, 679, 1969.
14. **Wintrobe, M. M.,** Variation in the size and hemoglobin content of erythrocytes in the blood of various vertebrates, *Folia Haematol.,* 51, 32, 1933.
15. **Brecher, G.,** New methylene blue as a reticulocyte stain, *Am. J. Clin. Pathol.,* 19, 895, 1949.
16. **Deiss, A. and Kurth, D.,** Circulating reticulocytes in normal adults as determined by the new methylene blue method, *Am. J. Clin. Pathol.,* 53, 481, 1970.
17. **Westergren, A.,** Studies of the suspension stability of the blood in pulmonary tuberculosis, *Acta Med. Scand.,* 54, 247, 1921.
18. **International Committee for Standardization in Hematology,** Reference method for the erythrocyte sedimentation rate (ESR) test on human blood, *Br. J. Haematol.,* 24, 671, 1973.
19. **Gambino, S. R., Dike, J. J., Monteleone, M., and Budd, D. C.,** The Westergren sedimentation rate using K_3 EDTA, *Am. J. Clin. Pathol.,* 43, 173, 1965.
20. **Wintrobe, M. M. and Landsberg, J. W.,** A standardized technique for the blood sedimentation test, *Am. J. Med. Sci.,* 189, 102, 1935.
21. **Bull, B. S. and Brailsford, J. D.,** The zeta sedimentation ratio, *Blood,* 40, 550, 1972.
22. **Parpart, A. K., Lorenz, P. B., Parpart, E. R., Gregg, J. R., and Chase, A. M.,** The osmotic resistance (fragility) of human red cells, *J. Clin. Invest.,* 26, 636, 1947.
23. **Danon, D.,** A rapid micro method for recording red cell osmotic fragility by continuous decrease of salt concentration, *J. Clin. Pathol.,* 16, 377, 1963.
24. **Danon, D., Fire, Y. F., Rimon, A., and Beu-David, A.,** Simple rapid osmotic fragility test proposed as a routine in blood banks, *Transfusion,* 4, 339, 1964.

25. **Matoth, Y., Zaizon, R., and Varsano, I.,** Postnatal changes in some red cell parameters, *Acta Paediatr. Scand.*, 60, 317, 1971.
26. **Guest, G. M. and Brown, E. W.,** Erythrocytes and hemoglobin of the blood in infancy and childhood, *Am. J. Dis. Child*, 93, 486, 1957.
27. **Wintrobe, M. M., Lee, G. R., Boggs, D. R., Bithell, T., Athens, J. W., and Foerster, J., Eds.,** *Clinical Hematology*, 7th ed., Lea & Febiger, Philadelphia, 1974, 1791.
28. **Natvig, H., Lellar, O. D., and Anderson, J.,** Studies on hemoglobin values in Norway. VII. VIII, *Acta Med. Scand.*, Vol. 182, 183, 1967.
29. **Klee, G. G.,** Decision Rules for Accelerated Hematology Laboratory Investigation, Ph.D. thesis, Graduate School, University of Minnesota, 1974, 54, 67, 126.
30. **Statland, B. E., Winkel, P., Harris, S. C., Burdsall, M. J., and Saunders, A. M.,** Evaluation of biologic sources of variation of leukocyte counts and other hematologic quantities using very precise automated analyzers, *Am. J. Clin. Pathol.*, 69, 48, 1978.
31. **Elwood, P. C.,** Diurnal hemoglobin variation in normal male subjects, *Clin. Sci.*, 23, 379, 1962.
32. **Stengle, J. M. and Schade, A. L.,** Diurnal-nocturnal variations of certain blood constituents in normal human subjects: plasma iron, siderophilin, bilirubin, copper, total serum protein and albumin, hemoglobin and hematocrit, *Br. J. Haematol.*, 3, 117, 1957.
33. **Dacie, S. V. and Lewis, S. M.,** *Practical Haematology*, 5th ed., Churchill Livingstone, Edinburgh, 1975, 15.
34. **Ekelund, L. G., Eklund, B., and Kajserl,** Time course for the change in hemoglobin concentration with change in posture, *Acta Med. Scand*., 190, 335, 1971.
35. **Mollison, P. L.,** *Blood Transfusion in Clinical Medicine*, 4th ed., Blackwell Scientific, Oxford, 1967, 124.
36. **Eisenberg, S.,** The effect of posture and position on the venous sampling site on the hematocrit and serum protein concentration, *J. Lab. Clin. Med.*, 51, 755, 1963.
37. **Smith, J. R. and Landow, S. A.,** Smokers' polycythemia, *N. Engl. J. Med.*, 298, 6, 1978.
38. **Castleman, B., Ed.,** Normal laboratory values, *N. Engl. J. Med.*, 290, 39, 1974.
39. **Hillman, R. S. and Finch, C. A.,** The misused reticulocyte, *Br. J. Haematol.*, 17, 313, 1969.
40. **Klee, G. G.,** Decision Rules for Accelerated Hematology Laboratory Investigation, Ph.D. thesis, Graduate School, University of Minnesota, 1974, 127.
41. **Hilder, R. M. and Gunz, F. W.,** The effect of age on normal values of the Westergren sedimentation rate, *J. Clin. Pathol.*, 17, 292, 1964.
42. **Sjolin, S.,** The resistance of red cells in vitro, *Acta Paediatr.*, Suppl. 98, 43, 390, 1954.
43. **Davidsohn, I. and Nelson, D. A.,** The Blood, in *Todd-Sanford Clinical Diagnosis by Laboratory Methods*, 15th ed., Davidsohn, I. and Henry, J. B., Eds., W. B. Saunders, Philadelphia, 1974, 124.
44. **Wintrobe, M. M., Lee, G. R., Boggs, D. R., Bithell, T., Athens, J. W., and Foerster, J., Eds.,** *Clinical Hematology*, 7th ed., Lea & Febiger, Philadelphia, 1974, 24.
45. **Dacie, J. V. and Lewis, S. M., Eds.,** *Practical Hematology*, 5th ed., Churchill Livingstone, Edinburgh, 1975, 69.
46. **Dacie, J. V. and Lewis, S. M., Eds.,** *Practical Hematology*, 5th ed., Churchill Livingstone, Edinburgh, 1975, 6.
47. **Young, I. T.,** Automated leukocyte recognition, in *Automated Cell Identification*, Weid, G. L. and Bahr, G. F., Eds., Academic Press, New York, 187, 1970.
48. **Ingram, M. and Preston, K., Jr.,** Automatic analysis of blood cells, *Sci. Am.*, 223, 72, 1970.
49. **Bacus, J. W. and Gose, E. E.,** Leukocyte pattern recognition, IEEF, transaction on systems, *Man and Cybernetics*, Vol. SMC-2, 513, 1972.
50. **Mansberg, H. P., Saunders, A. M., and Groner, W.,** The Hemalog D white cell differential system, *J. Histochem. Cytochem.*, 22, 711, 1974.
51. **Pierre, R. V. and O'Sullivan, M. B.,** Evaluation of the Hemalog D automated differential leukocyte counter, *Mayo Clin. Proc.*, 870, 1974.
52. **Simmons, A. and Elbert, G.,** Hemalog D and manual differential leukocyte counts: a laboratory comparison of results obtained with blood of hospitalized patients, *Am. J. Clin. Pathol.*, 64, 512, 1975.
53. **Pierre, R. V.,** personal communications.
54. **Altman, P. L. and Dittmer, D. S., Eds.,** *Biology Data Book*, Vol. 3, 2nd ed., Federation of American Societies of Experimental Biology, Bethesda, Md., 1974, 1856.
55. **Xanthou, M.,** Leukocyte blood picture in healthy full-term and premature babies during neonatal period, *Arch. Dis. Child.*, 45, 1970, 242.
56. **Wintrobe, M. M., Lee, G. R., Boggs, D. R., Bithell, T. C., Athens, J. W., and Foerster, J., Eds.,** *Clinical Hematology*, 7th ed., Lea & Febiger, Philadelphia, 1974, 58.
57. **Zacharski, L. R., Elveback, L. R., and Linman, J. W.,** Leukocyte counts in healthy adults, *Am. J. Clin. Pathol.*, 56, 148, 1971.

58. Simmons, A., Leaverton, P., and Elbert, G., The establishment of normal laboratory values for differential white cell counts by manual and cytochemical methods (Hemalog-D^{TM}), *J. Clin. Pathol.*, 27, 55, 1974.
59. Diaz-Jouanen, E., Strickland, R. G., and Williams, R. C., Studies of human lymphocytes in the newborn and the aged, *Am. J. Med.*, 58, 620, 1975.
60. Cruickshank, J. M. and Alexander, M. K., The effect of parity on the leukocyte count in pregnant and non-pregnant women, *Br. J. Haematol.*, 18, 531, 1970.
61. Wintrobe, M. M., Lee, G. R., Boggs, D. R., Bithell, T. C., Athens, J. W., and Foerster, J., Eds., *Clinical Hematology*, 7th ed., Lea & Febiger, Philadelphia, 1974, 251.
62. Garrey, W. E. and Bryan, W. R., Variation in white blood cell counts, *Physiol. Rev.*, 15, 597, 1935.
63. Brown, G. O., Herbig, F. K., and Hamilton, J. R., Leukopoenia in Negroes, *N. Engl. J. Med.*, 279, 1410, 1966.
64. Rees, H. M. and Ecker, E. E., An improved method for counting blood platelets, *JAMA*, 70, 621, 1923.
65. Davidsohn, I. and Nelson, D. A., The Blood, in *Todd-Sanford Clinical Diagnosis by Laboratory Methods*, 15th ed., Davidsohn, I. and Henry, J. B., Eds., W. B. Saunders, Philadelphia, 1974, 126.
66. Brecher, G. and Cronkite, E. P., Morphology and enumeration of human blood platelets, *J. Appl. Physiol.*, 3, 365, 1958.
67. Bull, B. S., Schneiderman, M. A., and Brecher, G., Platelet counts with the Coulter counter, *Am. J Clin. Pathol.*, 44, 678, 1965.
68. Fry, G. L. and Hoak, J. C., Improved method for electronic counting of platelets, *J. Lab. Clin. Med.*, 74, 536, 1969.
69. Bull, B. S., Aids to electronic platelet counting, *Am. J. Clin. Pathol.*, 54, 707, 1970.
70. Brittin, G. M., Dew, S. A., and Jewell, E. K., Automated optical counting of blood platelets, *Blood*, 38, 422, 1971.
71. Simmons, A., Schwabhauer, M. L., and Earhart, C. A., Automated platelet counting with the autoanalyzers, *J. Lab. Clin. Med.*, 77, 656, 1971.
72. Born, G. V. R. and Cross, M. J., Aggregation of blood platelets, *J. Physiol. (London)*, 168, 178, 1963.
73. Owen, C. A., Jr., Bowie, E. J. W., and Thompson, J. H., Eds., *The Diagnosis of Bleeding Disorders*, 2nd ed., Little, Brown, Boston, 1975, 97.
74. Newhouse, P. and Clark, C., *Platelet Function Laboratory Evaluation and Clinical Application*, Triplett, D. A., Ed., American Society of Clinical Pathologists, Chicago, 1978, 63.
75. Warlow, C., Ogston, D., and Douglas, A. S., The relationship between platelet aggregation and the time interval after venipuncture, *Thromb. Diath. Haemorrh. (Stuttgart)*, 31, 133, 1974.
76. Harrison, M. J. G., Emmons, P. R., and Mitchell, J. R. A., The variability of human platelet aggregation, *J. Atheroscler. Res.*, 7, 197, 1967.
77. Salzman, E. W., Measurement of platelet adhesiveness: a simple in vitro technique demonstrating an abnormality in von Willebrand's disease, *J. Lab. Clin. Med.*, 62, 724, 1963.
78. Bowie, E. J. W. and Owen, C. A., Jr., The value of measuring platelet "adhesiveness" in the diagnosis of bleeding diseases, *Am. J. Clin. Pathol.*, 60, 302, 1973.
79. Coller, B. S. and Zucker, M. B., Reversible decrease in platelet retention by glass bead columns (adhesiveness) induced by disturbing the blood, *Proc. Soc. Exp. Biol.* Med., 136, 769, 1971.
80. Fogel, B. J., et al., Platelet counts in healthy premature infants, *J. Paediatr.*, 73, 108, 1968.
81. Mull, M. M. and Hathaway, W. E., Altered platelet function in newborn, *Pediatr. Res.*, 4, 229, 1970.
82. Shapleigh, J. B., Mayes, S., and Moore, C. V., Hematologic values in the aged, *J. Gerontol.*, 7, 207, 1952.
83. Sarajas, H. S. S., et al., Thrombocytosis evoked by exercise, *Nature (London)*, 192, 721, 1961.
84. Prentice, C. R. M., et al., Studies on blood coagulation, fibrinolysis and platelet function following exercise in normal and splenectomized people, *Br. J. Haematol.*, 23, 541, 1972.
85. Tocantins, L. M., The mammalian blood platelet in health and disease, *Medicine*, 17, 175, 1938.
86. Hawkins, R. I., Smoking, platelets and thrombosis, *Nature (London)*, 236, 450, 1972.
87. McBride, J. A. and Snodgrass, C. A., The effect of the normal menstrual cycle on the total platelet count, adhesive platelet count and platelet adhesiveness, *J. Obstet. Gynnaecol. Br. Commonw.*, 75, 367, 1968.
88. Bowie, E. J. W., Thompson, J. H., Didisheim, P., and Owen, C. A., Jr., *Mayo Clinic Laboratory Manual of Hemostasis*, W. B. Saunders, Philadelphia, 1971, 19.
89. McPhedran, P., Clyne, L. P., Ortoli, N. A., Gagnon, P. G., and Sanders, F. J., Prolongation of the activated partial thromboplastin time associated with poor venipuncture technic, *Am. J. Clin. Pathol.*, 62, 16, 1974.

90. Beller, F. K. and Graeff, H., Equipment and general requirements of the coagulation laboratory, in *Thrombosis and Bleeding Disorders: Theory and Methods,* Bang, N. U., Beller, F. K., Deutsch, E., and Mammen, E. F., Eds., Academic Press, New York, 1971, 57.
91. Hardisty, R. M., Hutton, R. A., Montgomery, D., Richard, S., and Trebilcock, H., Secondary platelet aggregation: a quantitative study, *Br. J. Haematol.,* 19, 307, 1970.
92. Harper, T. A., *Laboratory Guide to Disordered Haemostasis,* New York, Appleton-Century-Crofts, 1970.
93. Hougie, C., Hemophilia and related conditions — congenital deficiencies of prothrombin (factor II), factor V and factors VII to XII, in *Hematology,* 2nd ed., Williams, W. J., Beutler, E., Erslev, A. J., and Rundles, R. W., Eds., McGraw-Hill, New York, 1977, 1416.
94. Quick, A. J., Stanley-Brown, M., and Bancroft, F. W., A study of the coagulation defect in hemophilia and in jaundice, *Am. J. Med. Sci.,* 190, 501, 1935.
95. Langdell, R. D., Wagner, R. H., and Brinkous, K. M., Effect of antihemophilic factor on one-stage clotting tests: a presumptive test for hemophilia and a simple one-stage antihemophilic factor assay procedure, *J. Lab. Clin. Med.,* 41, 637, 1953.
96. Proctor, R. B. and Rapaport, S. I., The partial thromboplastin time with kaolin: a simple screening test for first stage plasma clotting factor deficiencies, *Am. J. Clin. Pathol.,* 36, 212, 1961.
97. Jim, R. T. S., A study of the plasma thrombin time, *J. Lab. Clin. Med.,* 50, 45, 1957.
98. Lewis, J. H. and Didisheim, P., Differential diagnosis and treatment in hemorrhagic disease, *Arch. Intern. Med.,* 100, 157, 1957.
99. Owen, C. A., Jr. and Thompson, J. H., Jr., Soybean phosphatides in prothrombin-consumption and thromboplastin-generation tests: their use in recognizing "thrombasthenic hemophilia," *Am. J. Clin. Pathol.,* 33, 197, 1960.
100. Quick, A. J. and Favre-Gilly, J. E., The prothrombin consumption test: its clinical and theoretic implications, *Blood,* 4, 1281, 1949.
101. Kidder,W. R., Logan, L. J., Rapaport, S. I., and Patch, M. J., The plasma protamine paracoagulation test: clinical and laboratory evaluation, *Am. J. Clin. Pathol.,* 58, 675, 1972.
102. Seaman, A. J., The recognition of intravascular clotting: the plasma protamine paracoagulation test, *Arch. Intern. Med.,* 125, 1016, 1970.
103. Parfentjev, I. A., Johnson, M. L., and Clifton, E. E., The determination of plasma fibrinogen by turbidity with ammonium sulfate, *Arch. Biochem. Biophys.,* 46, 470, 1953.
104. Goodwin, J. F., An evaluation of technics for the separation and estimation of plasma fibrinogen, *Clin. Chem.,* 11, 63, 1965.
105. Ratnoff, O. D. and Menzie, C. A., A new method for the determination of fibrinogen in small samples of plasma, *J. Lab. Clin. Med.,* 37, 316, 1951.
106. Filip, D. J., Eckstein, J. D., and Sibley, C. A., Observations on diagnostic kits for the determination of plasma fibrinogen, *Am. J. Clin. Pathol.,* 62, 32, 1974.
107. Morse, E. E., Panek, S., and Menga, R., Automated fibrinogen determination, *Am. J. Clin. Pathol.,* 55, 671, 1971.
108. Wolf, P. and Walton, K. W., Investigation of a quantitative anomaly encountered in the assay of fibrinogen by immunodiffusion, *Immunology,* 8, 6, 1965.
109. Owen, C. A., Jr., Hurn, M. M., and Mann, F. D., Dextran as a substitute for acacia in assay of plasma prothrombin, *Am. J. Clin. Pathol.,* 25, 1279, 1955.
110. Warner, E. D., Brinkhous, K. M., and Smith, H. P., A quantitative study on blood clotting: prothrombin fluctuations under experimental conditions, *Am. J. Physiol.,* 114, 667, 1936.
111. Bowie, E. J. W., Thompson, J. H., Jr., Didisheim, P., and Owen, C. A., Jr., *Mayo Clinic Laboratory Manual of Hemostasis,* W. B. Saunders, Philadelphia, 1971, 117.
112. Pool, J. G. and Robinson, J., Assay of plasma antihemophilic globulin (AHG), *Br. J. Haematol.,* 5, 17, 1959.
113. Duckert, F., Jung, E., and Shmerling, D. H., A hitherto undescribed congenital haemorrhagic diathesis probably due to fibrin stabilizing factor deficiency, *Thromb. Diath. Haemorrh.,* 5, 179, 1960.
114. Lorand, L., Urayama, T., de Kiewiet, J. W. C., and Nossel, H. L., Diagnostic and genetic studies on fibrin-stabilizing factor with a new assay based on amine incorporation, *J. Clin. Invest.,* 48, 1054, 1969.
115. Zimmerman, T. S., Immunological differentiation of classic hemophilia (factor VIII deficiency) and von Willebrand's disease, *J. Clin. Invest.,* 50, 244, 1971.
116. Olson, J. D., Brockway, W. J., Fass, D. N., Magnuson, M. A., and Bowie, E. J. W., Evaluation of ristocetin-Willebrand factor assay and ristocetin-induced platelet aggregation, *Am . J. Clin. Pathol.,* 63, 21, 1975.
117. Owen, C. A., Jr. and Bollman, J. L., Serum and plasma antithrombin, *Proc. Soc. Exp. Biol. Med.,* 67, 367, 1948.

118. **Mammen, E. F.**, Determination of antithrombin, in *Thrombosis and Bleeding Disorders: Theory and Methods,* Bang, N. U., Beller, F. K., Deutsch, E., and Mammen, E. F., Academic Press, New York, 1971, 268.
119. **Schwartz, E. and Gill, F. M.**, Hematology of the newborn, in *Hematology,* 2nd ed., Williams, W. J., Beutler, E., Erslev, A. J., and Rundles, R. W., Eds., McGraw-Hill, New York, 1977, 44.
120. **Gedde-Dahl, T. W., Jeremic, M., and Weisert, O.**, Factor V (proaccelerin) concentration in 1016 blood donors; the effects of age, sex and ABO blood groups, *Scand. J. Clin. Lab. Invest.,* 35, 25, 1975.
121. **Hamilton, P. J., Allardyce, M., Ogston, D., Dawson, D., and Douglas, A. S.**, The effect of age upon the coagulation system, *J. Clin. Pathol.,* 27, 980, 1974.
122. **Brozovic, M., Chakrabarti, R., Stirling, Y., Fenton, S., North, W. R. S., and Meade, T. W.**, Factor V in an industrial population, *Br. J. Haematol.,* 33, 543, 1976.
123. **Brozovic, M., Stirling, Y., Harricks, C., North, W. R. S., and Meade, T. W.**, Factor VII in an industrial population, *Br. J. Haematol.,* 28, 381, 1974.
124. **Jeremic, M., Weisert, O., and Gedde-Dahl, T. W.**, Factor VIII (AHG) levels in 1016 regular blood donors: effects of age, sex, and ABO blood groups, *Scand. J. Clin. Lab. Invest.,* 36, 461, 1976.
125. **Coapland, A., Alkjaersig, N., and Fletcher, A. P.**, Reduction in plasma factor XIII (fibrin stabilizing factor) concentration during pregnancy, *J. Lab. Clin. Med.,* 73, 144, 1969.
126. **Phillips, L. L., Rosano, L., and Skrodelis, V.**, Changes in factor XI (plasma thromboplastin antecedent) levels during pregnancy, *Am. J. Obstet. Gynecol.,* 116, 1114, 1973.
127. **Rosing, D. R., Brakman, P., Redwood, D. R., Goldstein, R. E., Beiser, G. D., Astrup, T., and Epstein, S. E.**, Blood fibrinolytic activity in man. Diurnal variation and the response to varying intensities of exercise, *Circ. Res.,* 27, 171, 1970.
128. **Britton, B. J., Giddings, J. C., Brooks, L., and Bloom, A. L.**, Fibrinolytic, factor VIII and pulse rate responses to repeated adrenaline infusion followed by haemorrhage, *Thromb. Haemostasis,* 37, 527, 1977.
129. **Stibbe, J.**, Effect of exercise on F-VIII-complex: proportional increase of ristocetin cofactor (von Willebrand factor) and F-VIII-AGN but disproportional increase of F-VIII-AHF, *Thromb. Res.,* 10, 163, 1977.
130. **Addison, G. M., Beamish, M. R., Hales, C. N., Hodgkins, M., Jacobs, A., and Leuwellin, P.**, An immunoradiometric assay for ferritin in the serum of normal subjects and patients with iron deficiency and iron overload, *J. Clin. Pathol.,* 25, 326, 1972.
131. **Jacobs, A., Miller, F., Worwood, M., Beamish, M. R., and Wardrop, C. A.**, Ferritin in the serum of normal subjects and patients with iron deficiency and iron overload, *Br. Med. J.,* 4, 206, 1972.
132. **Lipschitz, D. A., Cook, J. D., and Finch, C. A.**, A clinical evaluation of serum ferritin as an index of iron stores, *N. Engl. J. Med.,* 290, 1213, 1974.
133. **Miles, L. E. M., Lipschitz, D. A., Bieber, C. P., and Cook, J. D.**, Measurement of serum ferritin by a 2-site immunoradiometric assay, *Anal. Biochem.,* 61, 209, 1974.
134. **Green, R., Watson, L. R., Saab, G. A., and Crosby, W.**, "Normal" serum ferritin — a caution, *Blood,* 50, 545, 1977.
135. **Theriault, L. and Page, M.**, A solid phase enzyme immunoassay for serum ferritin, *Clin. Chem.,* 23, 2142, 1977.
136. **Luxton, A. W., Walker, W. H. C., Gauldie, J., Ali, M. A. M., and Pelletier, C.**, A radioimmunoassay for serum ferritin, *Clin. Chem.,* 23, 683, 1977.
137. **Waters, A. H. and Mollin, D. L.**, Studies on the folic acid activity of human serum, *J. Clin. Pathol.,* 14, 355, 1961.
138. **Chanarin, I. and Berry, V.**, Estimation of serum L casei activity, *J. Clin. Pathol.,* 17, 111, 1964.
139. **Demetriou, J. A.**, *Vitamins in Clinical Chemistry: Principles and Techniques,* 2nd ed., Henry, R. J., Cannon, D. C., and Winkelman, J. W., Eds. Harper & Row, Hagerstown, Md., 1974, 1411.
140. **Reizenstein, P.**, Errors and artefacts in serum folic acid assays, *Acta Med. Scand.,* 178, 133, 1965.
141. **Luhby, A. L. and Cooperman, J. M.**, Folic acid deficiency in man and its interrelationships with Vitamin B-12 metabolism, *Adv. Metab. Disorders,* 1, 263, 1964.
142. **Beard, M. E. and Allen, D. M.**, Effect of antimicrobial agents on the Lactobacillus casei folate assay, *Am. J. Clin. Pathol.,* 48, 401, 1967.
143. **Hoffbrand, A. V., Newcombe, B. F. A., and Mollin, D. L.**, Method of assay of red cell folate activity and the value of the assay as a test for folate deficiency, *J. Clin. Pathol.,* 19, 17, 1966.
144. **Spray, G. H.**, Estimation of red cell folate activity, *J. Clin. Pathol.,* 22, 212, 1969.
145. **Dunn, R. T. and Foster, L. B.**, Radioassay of serum folate, *Clin. Chem.,* 19, 1101, 1973.
146. **Waxman, S. and Schreiber, C.**, Measurement of serum folate levels and serum folic acid binding protein by ^{3}H-PGA radioassay, *Blood,* 42, 281, 1976.
147. **Schreiber, C. and Wasman, S.**, Measurement of red cell folate levels by ^{3}H-pteroylglutamic acid (^{3}H-Pte-Glu) radioassay, *Br. J. Haematol.,* 27, 551, 1974.

148. **Jayle, M. F.**, Methode de dosage de l'haptoglobine sérique, *Bull. Soc. Chim. Biol. (Paris),* 33, 876, 1951.
149. **Nyman, M.**, Serum haptoglobin: methodological and clinical studies, *Scand. J. Clin. Lab. Invest.,* Suppl. 39, 11, 1959.
150. **Makarem, A.**, Hemoglobin, Myoglobins and Haptoglobins, in *Clinical Chemistry: Principles and Techniques,* 2nd ed., Henry, R. J., Cannon, D. C., and Winkelman, J. W., Eds., Harper & Row, Hagerstown, Md., 1974, 1205.
151. **Ferris, T. G., Easterling, R. E., Nelson, K. J., and Budd, R.**, Determination of serum-hemoglobin binding capacity and haptoglobin-type by acrylamide gel electrophoresis, *Am. J. Clin. Pathol.,* 46, 385, 1966.
152. **Rowe, D. S.**, A rapid method for the estimation of serum haptoglobin, *J. Clin. Pathol.,* 14, 205, 1961.
153. **Lionetti, F. J., Valerie, C. R., Bond, J. C., and Fortier, N. L.**, Measurement of hemoglobin binding capacity of plasma by means of dextron gels, *J. Lab. Clin. Med.,* 64, 519, 1963.
154. **Braun, H. J. and Aly, F. W.**, Problems in the quantitative estimation of human serum haptoglobin by single radial immunodiffusion, *Clin. Chim. Acta.,* 26, 588, 1969.
155. Kit insert, Cal Biochem-Behring Corporation, La Jolla, California.
156. **Kluthe, R., Faul, J., and Heimpel, H.**, Quantitative estimation of human serum haptoglobins by an immunological method, *Nature (London),* 205, 93, 1965.
157. **International Committee for Standardization in Hematology**, Proposed recommendations for measurement of serum iron in human blood, *Br. J. Haematol.,* 20, 451, 1971.
158. **Weissman, N. and Pileggi, V. J.**, Inorganic ions, in *Clinical Chemistry: Principles and Techniques,* 2nd ed., Henry, R. J., Cannon, D. C., and Winkelman, J. W., Eds., Harper & Row, Hagerstown, Md., 1974, 681.
159. **Rodgerson, D. O. and Helfer, R. E.**, Determination of iron in serum or plasma by atomic absorption spectrophotometry, *Clin. Chem.,* 12, 338, 1966.
160. **Ramsay, W. N. M.**, The measurement of serum transferrin by iron binding capacity, *J. Clin. Pathol.,* 26, 691, 1973.
161. **Tauxe, W. N.**, A rapid radioactive method for the determination of the serum-binding capacity, *Am. J. Clin. Pathol.,* 35, 403, 1961.
162. **Bothwell, T. H., Jacobs, P., and Kamener, R.**, The determination of the unsaturation iron-binding capacity of serum using radioactive iron, *S. Afr. J. Med. Sci.,* 24, 93, 1959.
163. **Burrows, S.**, Comparison of methods designed to measure transferrin and iron-binding capacity of serum, *Am. J. Clin. Pathol.,* 47, 326, 1967.
164. **Eckman, I., Robbins, J. B., Van den Hamer, C. J. A., Lentz, J., and Scheinberg, I. H.**, Automation of a quantitative immunochemical microanalysis of human serum transferrin: a model system, *Clin. Chem.,* 16, 558, 1970.
165. **Matthews, D. M.**, Observations on the estimation of serum Vitamin B-12 using Lactobacillus leichmanii, *Clin. Sci.,* 22, 101, 1962.
166. **Streeter, A. M., Shum, H. Y., and O'Neill, B. J.**, The effects of drugs on the microbiological assay of serum folic acid and Vitamin B-12 levels, *Med. J. Aust.,* i, 900, 1970.
167. **Demetriou, J. A.**, Vitamins, in *Clinical Chemistry: Principles and Techniques,* 2nd ed., Henry, R. J., Cannon, D. C., and Winkelman, J. W., Eds., Harper & Row, Hagerstown, Md., 1974, 1389.
168. **Lan, K.-S., Gottlieb, C., Wasserman, L. R., and Herbert, V.**, Measurement of serum Vitamin B-12 level using radioisotope dilution and coated charcoal, *Blood,* 26, 202, 1963.
169. **Rowen, J. W., Robson, M. B., Morgan, J. O., and Hoffbrand, A. V.**, Comparison of three methods for measuring Vitamin B-12 in serum: radioisotopic Euglena gracilis and Lactobacillus leichmannii, *Br. J. Haematol.,* 22, 21, 1972.
170. **Block, E., Akerkar, A., and Hoholick, M.**, Effect of ascorbic acid in Vitamin B-12 quality control sera, *Clin. Chem.,* 24, 176, 1978.
171. **McIntyre, P. A.**, Newer developments in nuclear medicine applicable to hematology, *Prog. Hematol.,* 10, 361, 1977.
172. **Gottlieb, C., Lan, K.-S., Wasserman, L. R., and Herbert, V.**, Rapid charcoal assays for intrinsic factor (I.F.), gastric juice, unsaturation B-12 binding capacity, antibody to I.F. and serum unsaturated B-12 binding capacity, *Blood,* 25, 6, 1965.
173. **Cook, J. D., Lipschitz, D. A., Miles, L. E., and Finch, C. A.**, Serum ferritin as a measure of iron stores in normal subjects, *Am. J. Clin. Nutr.,* 27, 681, 1974.
174. **Maloth, Y., Pinkas, A., Zamir, R., Mooallem, F., and Grossowicz, N.**, Studies on folic acid in infancy. I. Blood levels of folic and folinic acid in healthy infants, *Paediatrics,* 33, 507, 1964.
175. **Vanier, T. M. and Tyas, J. F.**, Folic acid status in normal infants during the first year of life, *Arch. Dis. Child.,* 41, 658, 1966.
176. **Magnus, E. M.**, Folate activity in serum and red cells of patients with cancer, *Cancer Res.,* 27, 490, 1967.

177. **Herbert, V.**, Experimental nutritional folate deficiency in man, *Trans. Assoc. Am. Phys.*, 65, 307, 1962.
178. **Chanarin, I.**, *The Megaloblastic Anemias*, Blackwell Scientific Publications, Oxford, 1969, 322.
179. **Bergstrand, C. G., Czar, B., and Tarukoski, P. H.**, Serum haptoglobin in infancy, *Scand. J. Clin. Lab. Invest.*, 13, 576, 1961.
180. **Harris, H., Robson, E. B., and Siniscalco, M.**, Atypical segregation of haptoglobin types in man, *Nature (London)*, 182, 1324, 1958.
181. **Giblett, E. R.**, *Genetic Markers in Human Blood*, 1st ed., F. A. Davis, Philadelphia, 169, 86.
182. **Vahlquist, B.**, Das Serumeisen, Eine padiatrisch-Klinische und experimentelle Studie, *Acta Paediatr.*, Suppl. 5, 28, 1, 1941.
183. **Hagberg, B.**, The iron-binding capacity of serum in infants and children, *Acta Paediatr.*, Suppl. 93, 42, 3, 1953.
184. **Fairbanks, V. F., Fahey, J. L., and Beutler, E.**, *Clinical Disorders of Iron Metabolism*, 2nd ed., Grune & Stratton, New York, 1971, 184.
185. **Hoyer, K.**, Physiologic variations in the iron content of human blood serum. I. The variations from week to week, from day to day and through twenty-four hours. II. Further studies of the intradiem variations, *Acta Med. Scand.*, 119, 572 and 557, 1944.
186. **Hamilton, L. D., Gubler, C. J., Cartwright, G. E., and Wintrobe, M. M.**, Diurnal variation in plasma iron level of man, *Proc. Soc. Exp. Biol. Med.*, 75, 65, 1950.
187. **Zilva, J. F. and Patston, V. J.**, Variation in serum iron in healthy women, *Lancet*, i, 459, 1966.
188. **Fairbanks, V. F., Fahey, J. L., and Beutler, E.**, *Clinical Disorders of Iron Metabolism*, 2nd ed., Grune & Stratton, New York, 1971, 186.
189. **Anderson, B. B.**, Investigation into the Euglene method for the assay of the B-12 in serum, *J. Clin. Pathol.*, 17, 14, 1964.
190. **Elwood, P. C., Shinton, N. K., Wilson, C. I. D., Sweetnam, P., and Frazer, A. C.**, Hemoglobin, Vitamin B-12 and folate levels in the elderly, *Br. J. Haematol.*, 21, 557, 1971.
191. **Hughes, D., Elwood, P. C., Shinton, N. K., and Wrighton, R. J.**, Clinical trial of the effect of Vitamin B-12 in elderly subjects with low serum B-12 levels, *Br. Med. J.*, 2, 458, 1970.

BLOOD DRAWING TECHNIQUES

Jean M. Slockbower

Quality Control

The collecting and handling of blood specimens demand the same standards of quality control that have long been applied to the analytical process. Highly sophisticated and controlled laboratory technology is of no avail if the specimens are error-ridden due to faulty identification or poor collection techniques.

To ensure representative, biological specimens for laboratory testing, uniform procedural guidelines and training in the techniques of blood collection should be implemented in every laboratory. Standards for blood collection procedures and equipment are being developed by the National Committee for Clinical Laboratory Standards (NCCLS) and the International Committee for Standardization in Hematology (ICSH).

Specimen Labeling

Organization is essential in areas where blood specimens are collected so that records of patients seen and specimens drawn may be maintained in an accurate manner. Studies indicate that 8% of errors in patient name, age, sex, and identification number go undetected even with extensive, manual checking procedures.[1]

Record, in order of acquisition, each request for a blood specimen. This accessioning provides a means of identifying all paperwork and supplies associated with each patient. Use the assigned accession number on all specimens taken from the patient at one time. On labels, record the information given on the blood request form. Include the following:

1. Patient's *full name*
2. Patient's identification number
3. Accessioning number
4. Date
5. Time

Other information may be added, i.e., the physician, room number, test name, and initials of the person drawing the specimen. Print labels in ink, indelible pencil, or by imprinted computer.

Patient Identification

Before drawing any specimens, positively identify the patient to ensure that the blood specimen is being taken from the same individual designated on the blood request form. Ask the patient to state his or her full name (including middle name). Do not merely have the patient confirm the name. If the patient request form contains a home address, ask for this information; compare it with the information given on the blood request form and labels. Check the bracelet identification usually issued by hospitals. If the patient is unable to speak, ask a member of the family, a doctor, or a nurse for assistance in identification. If there is even a minor discrepancy, such as the slight misspelling of the name or the reversal of the identifying numbers, have the nurse in charge identify the patient by name and number. Label all specimen tubes *immediately* before or after drawing the blood.

Venous Blood Sampling

After identifying the patient, fulfill other basic requirements prior to venipuncture:

verify diet restrictions, position the patient comfortably, verify tubes, assemble necessary supplies, and select the appropriate system for drawing the blood specimen. There are two systems used in drawing venous blood samples: the syringe and the evacuated system.

In general, a syringe is used when difficulty is anticipated in drawing a specimen, e.g., from patients with fragile vein walls, thready, or "roley" veins.

The evacuated system is the most commonly used means of collecting specimens today. It is generally preferable to the syringe method, since it allows blood to pass directly from the vein into the evacuated tube. The evacuated system is composed of three basic elements: (1) a sterile blood collection needle, (2) a holder securing both the needle and the evacuated tube, and (3) an evacuated tube containing a premeasured vacuum and, if applicable, a premeasured additive.

Venipuncture Procedure

The act of venipuncture itself consists of a number of steps that occur simultaneously. These are (1) applying the tourniquet, (2) closing the patient's hand, (3) selecting the vein site, (4) cleaning the site, (5) inspecting the needle and container, (6) grasping the patient's arm, (7) performing the venipuncture, (8) releasing the tourniquet, (9) opening the patient's hand, (10) placing the gauze, (11) removing the needle, (12) applying pressure, and (13) bandaging the arm.

1. Applying the tourniquet: use a tourniquet to increase venous pressure to facilitate vein identification and entry. Apply the tourniquet 3 to 4 in. above the venipuncture site. Never apply the tourniquet for longer than 1 min. To do so may invalidate test results as a consequence of fluid shifts and altered metabolism due to prolonged stagnation. Gerbrandy et al. found that in venous blood specimens taken before, during, and after the upper arm was compressed for over 7 min, the plasma protein concentration was increased by an average of 20%.[2] The differences found in measurements of blood constituents from prolonged tourniquet application may partly be due to hemoconcentration.
2. Closing the patient's hand: the patient can accentuate the arm veins by making a fist. Avoid vigorous hand exercise or "pumping."
3. Selecting the vein site: the veins of a patient may provide an avenue of entry for various therapeutic agents as well as blood transfusions. Select the vein site carefully in order to preserve vein patency. Use the superficial veins of the anterior surface of the arm for drawing specimens. The antecubital veins — especially the median cubital and the cephalic — are used most frequently, since they are larger, fuller, and fixed. Palpate the selected vein to identify its course and depth. Judiciously avoid nearby arteries that have thicker and firmer walls as well as other vital structures in the arm. Complete the palpation before the sterile preparation of the site.
4. Cleansing the site: cleanse the vein site to prevent any chemical or microbiological contamination. A satisfactory antiseptic agent in which to soak the gauze pad is a 70% alcohol solution. In a circular motion, clean the vein site from the center to the periphery. Allow the area to dry to prevent hemolysis and/or a burning sensation when the venipuncture is performed. Contamination may result if an ungloved finger is used to palpate the vein after the site has been cleansed. If the venipuncture proves difficult and the vein must be touched again in order to draw blood, cleanse the finger with alcohol before touching the site.
5. Inspect the needle and container.
6. Grasping the patient's arm: hold the patient's arm. If right handed, firmly grasp the patient's arm with the left hand. Using the left thumb to draw the skin taut

anchors the vein. The thumb should be 1 or 2 in. below and to the side of the venipuncture site.

7. Performing the venipuncture: syringe system — apply the appropriate needle to the syringe. The patient's arm should be in a downward position. Align the needle and syringe with the vein from which the blood will be drawn. With the bevel side in an upward position, push the needle into the vein. A sensation of resistance will be felt, followed by ease of penetration as the vein is entered. Withdraw the desired amount of blood. Replace the first syringe with another if additional blood is needed. The needle should remain in the vein as long as this is being done. When transferring blood from a syringe to a vacuum tube, *do not* remove the rubber stopper of the tube beforehand. The blood must be removed from the syringe by the action of the vacuum. It must not be "injected" into the vacuum tube. This technique is extremely important if the tube contains an anticoagulant or additive. The vacuum ensures the correct proportion of blood to the anticoagulant additive. Evacuated system — thread the appropriate needle into the holder until it is secure. Insert the appropriate tube into the holder up to the recessed guideline on the needle holder. The patient's arm should be in a downward position to prevent the possibility of backflow. Align the needle with the vein from which the blood will be drawn. With the bevel in an upward position, push the needle into the vein. Depress the tube to the end of the holder, thereby puncturing the diaphragm of the stopper. Remove the tube from the holder as soon as the blood flow ceases. If multiple samples are needed, other tubes are placed in the holder.
8. Release the tourniquet.
9. Opening the patient's hand: release the tourniquet before removing the needle from the vein. Then ask the patient to open his or her hand. This allows the blood circulation to return to normal and reduces the amounts of pressure and bleeding at the venipuncture site.
10. Place gauze.
11. Remove the needle.
12. Apply pressure.
13. Bandaging the arm: place a gauze pad above the venipuncture site and remove the needle slowly, while keeping the bevel in an upward position. Slip the gauze pad down over the site and apply slight pressure. Wrap a gauze bandage tightly around the arm over the pad.

Hematoma Prevention

Fully penetrating, yet only puncturing the uppermost wall of the vein will prevent a hematoma while performing a venipuncture. Partial penetration may allow blood to leak into the soft tissues surrounding the vein by way of the needle bevel. Use only major veins. Release the tourniquet before removing the needle.

Hemolysis Prevention

Avoid drawing blood from a hematoma. Avoid using a needle with too small a bore size. To avoid frothing, make sure the needle is fitted securely on a syringe. Ascertain the venipuncture site before puncturing. Avoid drawing the plunger back too forcefully when using a needle and syringe. Mix anticoagulated samples gently but thoroughly.

Capillary Blood Sampling

For small quantities of blood required for hematologic procedures or some chemical tests, adequate samples can be collected by doing a skin puncture. Collection of skin puncture blood is particularly important in pediatrics, because adequate blood samples can be obtained without drawing large quantities of venous blood. Drawing large quantities of venous blood may result in anemia, especially in premature infants, and it can be hazardous to patients, especially when deep veins are punctured.

Skin puncture blood specimens from adults may be desirable from (1) severely burned patients, (2) extremely obese patients, (3) patients with thrombotic tendencies, (4) patients with malignancies with venipuncture reserved for or limited to therapeutic purposes, and (5) geriatric patients.

Studies have shown that there is no significant difference between individual capillary and venous blood values for PCV, RCC, MCV, WCC, and platelet count.[3]

However, specimens from skin punctures of newborns may have a higher incidence of hemolysis than specimens from venipuncture, due to the increased red blood cell fragility of infants and high hematocrit.[4]

Sites for Puncture

1. The lateral or posterolateral portion of the heel
2. The big toe
3. The palmar (palm side) surface of the last digit of the finger
4. The dorsal surface of the last digit of the finger just proximal of the nail bed
5. The ear lobe

The heel is most often used prior to age 1 year. Take care to prevent the point of the lancet from penetrating the bone of the newborn. The puncture of the calcaneous can increase the risk of osteomyelitis with all its serious consequences.[5] After 1 year of age, the finger is most often used. The ear lobe has been found to contain a higher concentration of hemoglobin than finger tip or venous blood so its use is not advisable. The site must be nonedematous, since the tissue fluid can cause abnormal results. The skin puncture must bleed freely.

Containers

There are a variety of containers that are used for collection of capillary blood.

1. Capillary pipettes are most often used for collection of routine blood test specimens. An advantage of this type of collection is that the specimen is collected in several tubes and can be distributed easily. However, the pipettes are hard to label and must be broken after centrifugation to obtain sera or plasma.
2. A microcontainer composed of a small polypropylene tube with a capillary tube in the lid has been developed. The specimen is collected by capillary action and then flows into the tube. Little hemolysis results with the use of this microcontainer.[6]
3. "Unopettes" — disposable diluting pipettes consisting of a capillary tube and a reservoir containing a premeasured volume of diluent — are convenient to use for many hematological procedures.[7]
4. Small conical glass or plastic tubes can be used for collection. In order to move the blood toward the bottom of the tube, the technologist must flick her or his wrist after each drop is collected. This drop-by-drop collection increases the chance of hemolysis of the specimen.

Puncture Procedure

Skin puncture consists of a number of related steps. These are puncture location site, site warming, cleansing site, skin puncture, removal of first drop of blood, collection of the specimen, and pressure application.

1. The skin puncture site should be warm. This can be done by gently massaging the area or applying a warm, wet washcloth to the site for approximately 3 min.
2. Cleanse the site to be punctured very well with 70% alcohol, and dry it with a clean gauze pad. Alcohol left on the skin can cause elevation in glucose results and can also cause hemolysis of the blood. Skin normally contains sodium and potassium. If the skin is not properly cleansed, the sample may be contaminated and the test results may be false.
3. Grasp the finger or heel firmly.
4. Make a quick puncture with a sterile lancet. Remove the first drop of blood with a gauze pad because it is most likely contaminated with tissue fluid. Then collect the specimen.
5. After a drop of blood forms over the puncture site, place the tip of a capillary tube against the side of the drop. The blood will flow readily into the tube by capillary action. Blood should not be collected by "scooping" it from the skin. Rapid pipetting is necessary to collect the sample before coagulation begins. One half to 1 mℓ of blood may be collected if an adequate puncture has been performed.
6. Hold the puncture site downward and gently apply pressure to the surrounding tissue. Excessive squeezing will cause contamination of the blood with tissue fluid.
7. After collection, prevent further bleeding by applying slight pressure with a gauze pad. The puncture site may be bandaged for protection.
8. If necessary, seal the capillary tubes with commercially available sealing material. If Unipets with diluent are used for collection, wash the specimen completely into the diluent immediately after collection and before coagulation occurs.

Blood Films

The reliability of the information obtained depends to a considerable extent on the quality of the smears. Properly spread films are essential for accurate work. Slides and cover glasses must be scrupulously clean and free of grease and dust, so that they will wet and allow uniform spreading of the blood.

1. Two slide method: place a small drop of blood about 2 mm in diameter on slide A 2 cm from the end. Place the edge of another slide B, on the surface of the first at a 30 to 40° angle. Draw slide B back against the drop of blood until the drop runs across the end of slide B. Push slide B forward at a moderate speed and spread the blood evenly on the slide A into a moderately thin film. Air dry rapidly by waving the slide or by using a fan.
2. Cover slip method: using No. 1 cover slips of 2 cm square, place a small drop of capillary or venous blood on one cover slip. Place the second cover slip diagonally over the first to allow the blood to spread out evenly. Then smoothly slide the slips apart (parallel to their surfaces) and air dry.

Expert morphologic evaluation of the peripheral blood cells is one of the most vital procedures in laboratory hematological diagnosis. Thus it is essential that the blood film be of ideal thickness. For routine hematological purposes, moderately thin smears are desirable. The viewing area must be carefully selected. The head, tail, and edges of a slide are not satisfactory for counting, due to overlap or paucity of cells. Uniformity of the blood film is especially critical in computerized pattern recognition systems. Automatic devices are now available that use the traditional wedge principle or centrifugation of the slide to spread the drop of blood.

REFERENCES

1. **Taswell, H. F., Smith, A. M., Sweatt, M. A., and Pfaff, K. J.,** Quality control in the blood bank: a new approach, *Am. J. Clin. Pathol.*, 62, 491, 1974.
2. **Gerbrandy, J., vanLeeuwen, A. M., Hellendoorn, H. B. A., deVries, L. A., and technical assistance from van Daatselaar, J. J.,** The binding between electrolytes and serum proteins calculated from an in vivo filtration method, *Clin. Sci.*, 19, 181, 1960.
3. **Stuart, J., Barrett, B. A., and Prangnell, D. R.,** Capillary blood collection in haematology, *J. Clin. Pathol.*, 27, 869, 1974.
4. **Blumenfeld, T. A., Hertelendy, W. G., and Ford, S.,** A study of simultaneously obtained skin puncture serum, skin puncture plasma and venous serum and the effects of warming the skin prior to puncture, *Clin. Chem.*, submitted, 1977.
5. **Lilien, L. D., Harris, V. J., Ramausthy, R. S., and Pildes, R. S.,** Neonatal osteomyelitis of the calcaneus: complication of heel procedure, *J. Pediatr.*, 88, 478, 1976.
6. **Hicks, J. R., Rowland, G. L., and Buffone, G. J.,** Evaluation of a new blood-collection device (Microtainer) that is suited for pediatric use, *Clin. Chem.*, 22, 2034, 1976.
7. **Gerarde, H. W. and Anderson, E.,** *Hematology Manual — Unopette — Disposable Diluting Pipette*, 6th ed. (revised), Becton, Dickinson, 1973.

BLOOD COLLECTION EQUIPMENT

O. W. van Assendelft

Because much of the equipment used for obtaining blood specimens has already been covered in the chapter "Blood Drawing Techniques", only a short summary of some containers and skin puncture materials will be given in this section.

The Container

Containers into which blood samples are collected must meet certain basic requirements. As a minimum, they must not leak the specimen, either on closing or on opening, and the material from which the containers are manufactured must not alter or damage the contents. Most specimens drawn in the U.S. involve the use of evacuated tubes for which a standard[1] has been published by the National Committee for Clinical Laboratory Standards (NCCLS).* This standard describes the tube size (compare Table 1), color coding, and additives (compare Table 2). Because adverse reactions after blood drawing — caused by microbial contamination — have been described, it has been proposed that all evacuated tubes used should be sterile. Specific information about evacuated tubes may be obtained from the manufacturers.** Especially in pediatric hematology, blood specimens are preferably obtained by skin puncture.[2] The blood is collected, drop by drop, into a small tube or, by capillary action, into a capillary tube. Test tubes may be straight walled or conical, glass or plastic, heparinized or nonheparinized; capillaries may be small bore, small volume, or large bore, large volume. Collection of blood in capillary tubes is usually preferred, because with this method, there is less danger of hemolysis. A standard for micro-blood-collection devices is not yet available. Specific information on capillary tubes may be obtained from the manufacturers.*** Many types of lancets are used in the skin puncture procedure. No study is known to have been performed to determine optimal blade design or optimal depth of puncture. Care must always be taken to prevent the point of the instrument from penetrating the bone.

Table 1
SPECIFICATIONS FOR EVACUATED TUBES USED IN DRAWING BLOOD SPECIMENS[1]

Nominal size (mm)	Outside tube diameter (mm)	Maximum draw (m*l*)
10 × 65	10—11	3
13 × 75	11.5—13	5
13 × 100	11.5—13	7
16 × 100	15—16	10
16 × 127	15—16	15

* 771 E. Lancaster Avenue, Villanova, Pa., 19085. Tel. (215) 515-2435.

** e.g., Becton-Dickinson Company, Stanley Rd., Rutherford, N.J., 07070; Corning Glass Works, Medfield Industrial Park, Medfield, Mass., 02052; Jelco Laboratories, Johnson Drive, Raritan, N.J., 08869; Kimble-Terumo, Inc., Box 605, Elkton, Md., 21921; Sherwood Medical Industries, Inc., 1831 Olive St., St. Louis, Mo., 63103.

***e.g., Clay-Adams, 299 Webro Rd., Parsippany, N.J., 07054; Dade, Division American Hospital Supply Company, P.O. Box 520672, Miami, Fla., 33152.

Table 2
COLOR CODING AND ANTICOAGULANTS (ADDITIVES) USED WITH EVACUATED BLOOD COLLECTION TUBES[1]

Color	Tube use	Anticoagulant	Amount	Code
Gray	Plasma or whole blood (glycolysis inhibition)	Potassium oxalate, sodium fluoride	2.0 mg/mℓ, 2.5 mg/mℓ	NFX
Yellow	Sterile tube interior	—	—	—
Green	Plasma or whole blood	Lithium heparin	10—30 IU/mℓ	LIH
Red	Serum	—	—	—
Blue	Plasma or whole blood	Trisodium citrate $2H_2O$[a]	1:9, 1:4	NC9, NC4
Lavender	Plasma or whole blood	EDTA(K_3)	1.5 mg/mℓ, (±10%)	K3E

[a] Trisodium citrate · $2H_2O$, 0.109 mol/ℓ; 32 g/ℓ solution. Used in ratio 1 volume plus 9 volumes in coagulation studies, 1 volume plus 4 volumes for the erythrocyte sedimentation rate.

Table 3
PLASMA FLOW RATE, NEEDLE DIAMETER, AND NEEDLE LENGTH

Gauge	Internal diameter (mm)	Length (mm)	Plasma flow[a] rate (mℓ/s)
19 } Thin wall	0.79	25	1.17
19 } Thin wall	0.79	40	0.96
19	0.65	40	0.75
19	0.65	50	0.66
20	0.56	25	0.56
20	0.56	40	0.32
21	0.5	40	0.29
21	0.5	50	0.27

[a] Flow rates obtained with reconstituted plasma under a constant head of pressure of 100 mm of mercury.

With permission from Sacker, L. S., *Quality Control in Haematology,* Lewis, S. M. and Coster, J. F., Eds., Academic Press, London, 1975, 211.

Needles

Needles of many gauges and lengths are manufactured. Care should be taken in selecting the appropriate needle for drawing blood. The most commonly used sizes for drawing blood by venipuncture are gauge 19 through 22.[3] No attempt at uniformity of color coding has been made. No systematic study of blood-flow rates with different sizes and lengths of needles is available. Some indication of blood flow rates to be expected, however, may be obtained from Table 3.

REFERENCES

1. National Committee for Clinical Laboratory Standards, NCCLS Approved Standard: ASH-1, Standard for Evacuated Tubes for Blood Specimen Collection, Villanova, Pa., 1977.
2. National Committee for Clinical Laboratory Standards, NCCLS Proposed Standard: PSH-4, Standard Procedures for the Collection of Diagnostic Blood Specimens by Skin Puncture, Villanova, Pa., 1977.
3. National Committee for Clinical Laboratory Standards, NCCLS Proposed Standard: PSH-3, Standard Procedures for the Collection of Diagnostic Blood Specimens by Venipuncture, Villanova, Pa., 1977.
4. **Sacker, L. S.,** Specimen collection, in *Quality Control in Haematology,* Lewis, S. M. and Coster, J. F., Eds., Academic Press, London, 1975, 211.

Blood Volume

BLOOD VOLUME

S. M. Lewis

Blood volume measurement is based on the principle of dilution analysis performed with a suitable marker. In practice, isotopes have superseded other markers such as Evans blue dye (Tables 1 and 2), and standard techniques in which isotopes are used have been recommended by the International Committee for Standardization in Haematology (ICSH).[1] Total blood volume comprises the summation of red cell mass and plasma volume. These can be measured individually, or one may be calculated from the other if the body hematocrit is known. However, body hematocrit cannot be measured directly. It differs from venous hematocrit (PCV) by a factor which is usually said to be 0.9, but which actually varies by ±10% or even more in certain diseases and in pregnancy. Thus it is preferable to measure both red cell mass and plasma volume by direct methods. Combinations of isotopes suitable for simultaneous red cell mass and plasma volume estimation are listed in Table 3.

Peripheral blood hemoglobin content, red cell count, and PCV do not always closely reflect the red cell mass, especially outside the normal range.[2] Discrepancy is even more marked if the plasma volume is reduced or increased disproportionately (Table 4). Pathological (and physiological) states which cause variation in blood volume are listed in Tables 5 and 6.

Blood volume can be expressed in several ways (Table 7). Expression as milliliters per kilogram body weight may be misleading in obese subjects, as fat is relatively avascular; nonetheless, for clinical purposes, it is the most practical method, as none of the various prediction formulae give 95% confidence limits better than ±10%. Normal ranges based on weight alone are given in Table 8, and Tables 9 and 10 present data which appear to be relatively reliable for predicting normal values.

Table 1
RADIOACTIVE ISOTOPES SUITABLE FOR ESTIMATING RED CELL MASS

Isotope	Available form	Half-life	Principle radiations (keV)	Usual dose (μCi/kg)	Ref.
^{51}Cr	Sodium citrate	27.8 days	EC → X; γ (320)	0.2	1
^{11}CO	Cyclotron	0.34 hr	β^+ (980) → γ (511)	5—10	3
^{32}P	Sodium phosphate	14.3 days	β^-(1710)	0.05	1
$^{99}Tc^m$ [a]	^{99}Mo generator	6 hr	γ (140)	1—2	4,5,17

[a] Not suitable if mixing time is delayed, e.g., in splenomegaly.[4,6]

Table 2
RADIOACTIVE ISOTOPES SUITABLE FOR ESTIMATING PLASMA VOLUME

Isotope	Half-life	Principle radiations (keV)	Usual dose (μCi/kg)
^{123}I	13.3 hr	EC → X; γ (159)	0.05
^{131}I	8.05 days	β^- (606); γ (364)	0.05
^{125}I	60 days	EC → X; γ (35)	0.05
^{99}Tc^m	6 hr	γ (140)	1—2
^{113}In^m	1.67 hr	γ (390)	1—2

Human serum albumin[1]
IgM globulin[7]
(Transferrin)[8,a]

[a] May be unreliable, as plasma clearance rate depends on erythropoietic activity.

Table 3
COMBINATIONS OF THE MORE COMMON ISOTOPES USED FOR SIMULTANEOUS PLASMA AND RED CELL VOLUME ESTIMATIONS

Tracers: Plasma	Tracers: Red cells	Comment
^{125}I-albumin	^{32}P	^{125}I measured in plasma by well-type scintillation counter; ^{32}P measured in whole blood G-M counter; small correction needed for contribution of ^{125}I to counting rate of whole blood sample
	^{51}Cr	^{125}I measured in plasma by well-type scintillation counter; ^{51}Cr measured in whole blood by same counter
	^{99}Tc^m	^{125}I measured in plasma by well-type scintillation counter; ^{99}Tc^m measured in whole blood by same counter
^{131}I-albumin	^{32}P	^{131}I measured in plasma by well-type scintillation counter; ^{32}P measured in whole blood by end-window G-M counter with absorber or thick-walled G-M counter; small correction needed for contribution of ^{131}I to counting rate of whole blood sample
	^{51}Cr	^{131}I measured in plasma by well-type scintillation counter; ^{51}Cr measured in whole blood by same counter; large correction needed for contribution of ^{131}I to counting rate of whole blood sample; this may be based on venous hematocrit (PCV) or measurement of 0.64 MeV gamma rays
	^{99}Tc^m	^{131}I measured in plasma by well-type scintillation counter; ^{99}Tc^m measured in whole blood by same counter; correction needed for contribution of ^{131}I to counting rate of whole blood sample

From International Committee for Standardization in Haematology, *Br. J. Haematol.*, 25, 801, 1973. With permission.

Table 4
CLINICAL EFFECT OF VARIABLE BLOOD VOLUME

Plasma volume	Red cell volume	Blood count
Normal	Low	Accurately reflects degree of anemia
	High	Accurately reflects state of polycythemia
High	Normal	Pseudoanemia
	Low	Exaggerates extent of anemia
	High (PCV > 0.5)	Polycythemia more severe than apparent
Low	Normal	Pseudopolycythemia
	Low (in acute hemorrhage or chronic anemia when PCV < 0.2)	Anemia more severe than apparent
	High	Exaggerates degree of polycythemia

Table 5
VARIATIONS IN RED CELL MASS

Increased

- Polycythemia vera
- Secondary polycythemia (''erythrocytosis'')
  - Physiological
    - High altitude (after 3 weeks)
    - Chronic obstructive pulmonary disease
    - Cardiovascular shunt
    - Massive obesity (''Pickwickian'' syndrome)
    - Hypoventilation
    - High oxygen-affinity hemoglobinopathy
    - Congential decrease in red cell 2, 3- diphosphoglycerate (DPG)
    - Smoking
  - Excessive erythropoietin production
    - Renal carcinoma
    - Renal cysts
    - Hydronephrosis
    - Renal transplantation
    - Cerebellar hemangioblastoma
    - Hepatoma
    - Uterine fibroid
    - Ovarian carcinoma
    - Adrenal cortical hyperplasia
  - Familial polycythemia

Reduced

- Anemias
- Acute hemorrhage
- Post partum

Table 6
VARIATIONS IN PLASMA VOLUME

Increased	Reduced
Congestive cardiac failure	Stress polycythemia ("spurious polycythemia")
Nephritis	Peripheral circulatory failure
Myeloma	Essential hypertension
Macroglobulinemia	Dehydration
Cirrhosis	Edema
Primary hypersplenism	Prolonged bed rest
Tropical splenomegaly	High altitude (in first 2 weeks)
Nontropical idiopathic splenomegaly	Severe anemia[a]
Secondary splenomegalies	Acute hemorrhage[a]
Pregnancy (2nd and 3rd trimesters)	
Polycythemia[a]	

[a] See Table 4.

Table 7
EXPRESSION OF BLOOD VOLUME

In mℓ/kg body weight
In mℓ/kg ideal body weight
  From standard tables (e.g., Documenta Geigy)[9]
  From calculation: weight (kg) = height (cm) − 100
  From fat-free lean body weight[10,11]
As fraction of normal volume based on prediction formulas[a]

[a] See Tables 9 and 10.

Table 8
NORMAL BLOOD VOLUME

Parameter	(95% confidence limits)[a]
Red cell mass	
Men, 30 mℓ/kg	± 5 mℓ/kg
Women, 25 mℓ/kg	± 5 mℓ/kg
Plasma volume	b
ca. 40 mℓ/kg	
Total blood volume	
Men and women, 70 mℓ/kg	± 10 mℓ/kg

[a] Measurement has precision of ± 2%.
[b] As plasma volume is labile, level of precision has not been established, and there are no well-based confidence limits for normal plasma volume measurement.

Table 9
FORMULAE FOR PREDICTING NORMAL BLOOD VOLUME

From height (H) and weight (W)[12]
  Red cell mass
    Men, 8.2H + 173W − 693
    Women, 16.4H + 5.7W − 1649
Plasma volume
    Men, 23.7H + 9.0W − 1709
    Women, 40.5H + 8.4W − 4811
From surface area (SA)[12]
  Red cell mass
    Men, 1100 SA
    Women, 840 SA
Plasma volume
    Men, 1630 SA
    Female, 1410 SA
From cube of height (H^3) and weight (W)[13]
  Blood volume
    Men, $0.3669H^3 + 0.03219W + 0.6041$
    Women, $0.3561H^3 + 0.03308W + 0.1833$
From log height (H) (in children) [14]
  Log blood volume
    0.247 + 2.14 log H
From surface area (SA) and weeks of gestation (P)[15]
  Plasma volume
    673 + 32.9P + 1857.2SA
From surface area (direct observation)[16]
  See Table 10

Table 10
MEAN VALUES FOR RED CELL MASS (RCM) AND PLASMA VOLUME (PV) RELATED TO BODY SURFACE AREA (SA) FOR MEN AND WOMEN[a]

	Men		Women			Men		Women	
SA	RCM	PV	RCM	PV	SA	RCM	PV	RCM	PV
1.39	—	—	1136	1964	1.77	1907	2922	1588	2666
1.40	—	—	1148	1982	1.78	1917	2940	1599	2682
1.41	—	—	1162	2000	1.79	1927	2958	1610	2702
1.42	—	—	1172	1018	1.80	1938	2976	1622	2720
1.43	—	—	1184	2039	1.81	1951	2994	1634	2740
1.44	—	—	1196	2058	1.82	1964	3013	1645	2760
1.45	—	—	1208	2076	1.83	1977	3031	1657	2778
1.46	—	—	1220	2094	1.84	1990	3050	1670	2796
1.47	—	—	1232	2112	1.85	2003	3069	1681	2815
1.48	—	—	1242	2132	1.86	2016	3087	1692	2838
1.49	—	—	1254	2148	1.87	2029	3106	1704	2854
1.50	1684	2498	1268	2168	1.88	2042	3125	—	—
1.51	1692	2513	1280	2184	1.89	2055	3144	—	—
1.52	1699	2529	1291	2204	1.90	2070	3164	—	—
1.53	1707	2544	1302	2222	1.91	2087	3183	—	—
1.54	1715	2560	1315	2252	1.92	2104	3202	—	—
1.55	1722	2575	1326	2258	1.93	2212	3222	—	—
1.56	1730	2591	1338	2278	1.94	2138	3242	—	—
1.57	1737	2606	1349	2296	1.95	2156	3261	—	—
1.58	1745	2621	1362	2314	1.96	2173	3280	—	—

Table 10 (continued)
MEAN VALUES FOR RED CELL MASS (RCM) AND PLASMA VOLUME (PV) RELATED TO BODY SURFACE AREA (SA) FOR MEN AND WOMEN[a]

	Men		Women			Men		Women	
SA	RCM	PV	RCM	PV	SA	RCM	PV	RCM	PV
1.59	1752	2637	1376	2336	1.97	2191	3299	—	—
1.60	1760	2652	1386	2354	1.98	2208	3318	—	—
1.61	1768	2667	1398	2374	1.99	2226	3337	—	—
1.62	1776	2682	1408	2392	2.00	2244	3358	—	—
1.63	1784	2697	1421	2410	2.01	2266	3390	—	—
1.64	1792	2712	1434	2428	2.02	2288	3402	—	—
1.65	1800	2727	1445	2444	2.03	2310	3424	—	—
1.66	1809	2742	1458	2462	2.04	2332	3446	—	—
1.67	1817	2757	1468	2480	2.05	2354	3468	—	—
1.68	1826	2772	1480	2500	2.06	2375	3490	—	—
1.69	1834	2787	1492	2520	2.07	2397	3513	—	—
1.70	1842	2802	1504	2538	2.08	2419	3536	—	—
1.71	1851	2819	1516	2558	2.09	2441	3558	—	—
1.72	1861	2837	1527	2576	2.10	2463	3580	—	—
1.73	1870	2854	1540	2592	2.11	2486	3604	—	—
1.74	1880	2971	1552	2612	2.12	2510	3628	—	—
1.75	1889	2888	1563	2630	2.13	2535	3653	—	—
1.76	1898	2905	1576	2648	2.14	2560	3679	—	—
					2.15	2586	3704	—	—

Note: Range of normal values: RCM — men, ± 24% of mean value; women, ± 25% of mean value; PV — men, ± 22% of mean value; women, ± 22% of mean value.

[a] RCM and PV in milliliters, SA in square meters.

From Hurley, P. J., *J. Nucl. Med.*, 16, 46, 1975. With permission.

REFERENCES

1. **International Committee for Standardization in Haematology,** Standard techniques for the measurement of red-cell and plasma volume, *Br. J. Haematol.*, 25, 801, 1973.
2. **Bentley, S. A. and Lewis, S. M.,** The relationship between total red cell volume, plasma volume and venous haematocrit, *Br. J. Haematol.*, 33, 301, 1976.
3. **Glass, H. I., De Garreta, A. C., Lewis, S. M., Grammaticos, P., and Szur, L.,** Measurement of splenic red-blood-cell mass with radioactive carbon monoxide, *Lancet*, 1, 669, 1968.
4. **Farrant, A., Lewis, S. M., and Szur, L.,** The elution of $^{99}Tc^{m}$ from red cells and its effect on red cell volume measurement, *J. Clin. Pathol.*, 27, 983, 1974.
5. **Eckelman, W. C., Reba, R. C., and Albert, S. N.,** A rapid simple improved method for the preparation of Tc^{99m} red blood cells for the determination of red cell volume, *Am. J. Roentgenol.*, 118, 861, 1973.
6. **Schmidt, R. M., Lehmann, H., and Heimpel, H.,** Sodium pertechnate as a red cell label: in vitro and in vivo studies, *Br. J. Haematol.*, 32, 411, 1976.

7. **Valeri, C. R., Cooper, A. G., and Pivacek, L. E.,** Limitations of measuring blood volume with iodinated I^{125} serum albumin, *Arch. Intern. Med.*, 132, 534, 1973.
8. **Wochner, R. D., Adatepe, M., Van Amburg, A., and Potchen, E. J.,** New method for estimation of plasma volume with the use of the distribution space of transferrin-113m Indium, *J. Lab. Clin. Med.*, 75, 711, 1970.
9. **Diem, K. and Lentner, C., Eds.,** Body measurements, in Documenta Geigy, *Scientific Tables*, 7th ed., J. R. Geigy, Basel, 1970, 712.
10. **Huff, R. L. and Feller, D. D.,** Relation of circulating red cell volume to body density and obesity, *J. Clin. Invest.*, 35, 1, 1956.
11. **Muldowney, F. P.,** The relationship of total red cell mass to lean body mass in man, *Clin. Sci.*, 16, 163, 1957.
12. **Retzlaff, J. A., Tauxe, W. N., Kieley, J. M., and Stroebel, C. F.,** Erythrocyte volume, plasma volume and lean body mass in adult men and women, *Blood,* 33, 649, 1969.
13. **Nadler, S. B., Hidalgo, J. U., and Bloch, T.,** Prediction of blood volume in normal human adults, *Surgery,* 51, 224, 1962.
14. **Gross, S. and Godel, J. C.,** Comparative studies of height and weight as a blood volume reference standard in normal children and children with sickle cell anaemia, *Am. J. Clin. Pathol.*, 55, 662, 1971.
15. **Smith, R. W. and Yarbrough, C. J.,** Plasma volume prediction in normal pregnancy, *Am. J. Obstet. Gynecol.*, 99, 18, 1967.
16. **Hurley, P. J.,** Red cell and plasma volumes in normal adults, *J. Nucl. Med.*, 16, 46, 1975.
17. **Jones, J. and Mollison, P. L.,** A simple and efficient method of labelling red cells with 99m TC for determination of red cell volume, *Br. J. Haematol.*, 38, 141, 1978.

Hemoglobin

HEMOGLOBIN

W. A. Schroeder

Hemoglobin has probably been subjected to more experiments and more probably is known about it than about any other protein. These few pages give a broad background for the detailed information of many kinds that will be provided in the following sections. The emphasis is on human hemoglobins.

The information about hemoglobin is far more extensive than could possibly be included in this chapter. Of the many books and reviews on the topic of hemoglobin, the following are cited as sources of additional information: Antonini and Brunori,[1] Huisman,[7] Weatherall and Clegg,[17] Kitchen and Boyer,[9] Lehmann and Huntsman,[11] Ranney,[12] Weatherall,[18,19] and Bunn et al.[3]

General Properties of Hemoglobin

Nomenclature

The function of hemoglobin is to combine with oxygen in the lungs and to release that oxygen in the tissues. In this process, oxygen combines with (but does not oxidize in the chemical sense) the ferrous iron of the heme group. In this form it is commonly called "oxyhemoglobin." Many other ligands, such as carbon monoxide, will also combine. When the ligand is carbon monoxide, the proper name is carbonmonoxyhemoglobin, although it is commonly incorrectly called carboxyhemoglobin in the literature. When oxygen is released, deoxyhemoglobin results; the incorrect designation "reduced" hemoglobin appears in the older literature. When oxidation to the ferric form occurs either spontaneously or by chemical means, the product is methemoglobin. Oxygen no longer combines, but many ions such as cyanide, fluoride, etc, will combine.

Molecular Weight and Subunit Status

Human and other mammalian hemoglobins have molecular weights of the order of 64,500 daltons. The actual molecular weight does not vary more than a few hundred units from hemoglobin to hemoglobin and depends on the actual amino acid composition and the state of liganding.

Normally, hemoglobins are composed of two pairs of different subunits. These subunits are designated α and non-α chains. This distinction is made because in any one species the α chains are combined with various non-α (β,γ, δ, etc.) chains. Thus, for normal adult human hemoglobin A (HbA), the subunit structural formula is $\alpha_2\beta^A{}_2$, where the subscripts have the usual chemical significance and the superscript identifies the hemoglobin. Variant hemoglobins such as HbS are designated as $\alpha_2\beta^S{}_2$ because the aberration is in the β chain, or as $\alpha^X{}_2\beta_2$ if it is in the α chain. Human fetal hemoglobin (HbF) is $\alpha_2\gamma_2$, and a minor component called hemoglobin A_2 (HbA_2) is $\alpha_2\delta_2$. Alpha chains are usually five residues shorter than non-α chains and have a molecular weight that is 700 to 800 daltons less than that of non-α chains.

Functional Properties

Because of the pickup and release of oxygen by hemoglobin, its functional properties can be described in terms of certain parameters of the "oxygen dissociation" or "oxygen equilibrium" curve. It has long been known that this curve has the sigmoid shape shown in Figure 1 whether the determination is done with blood or hemoglobin solution. The curve is usually plotted with percent saturation or fractional saturation on the ordinate and partial pressure or log of the partial pressure of oxygen on the abscissa.

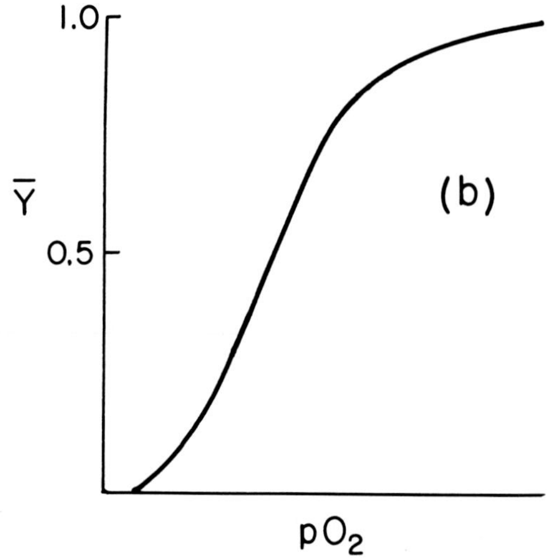

FIGURE 1. Schematic representation of the oxygen association-dissociation curve of hemoglobin. Y is the fractional saturation of the protein with oxygen, and pO_2 is the partial pressure of oxygen.

One parameter of function is termed "p_{50}," "$p_{1/2}$," "log p_{50}," or "log $p_{1/2}$." All of these are merely different forms of defining the pressure at 50% or half-saturation. Thus, in studying a hemoglobin variant, a comparison of its p_{50} with that of HbA under identical conditions would determine whether the oxygen affinity is normal, increased, or decreased. The smaller the p_{50} is, the greater is the affinity of oxygen and vice versa.

Another parameter of function is the so-called "n of the Hill equation." Hill considered the reaction of oxygen with hemoglobin in terms of the equation

$$Hb_n + nO_2 \rightleftharpoons (HbO_2)_n$$

and converted this by the mass law to

$$\bar{Y}/(1 - \bar{Y}) = Kp^n$$

where Y is the fractional saturation, p the partial pressure of oxygen, and K the equilibrium constant. Although n does not yield the information about mechanism or order of reaction that Hill had hoped to obtain, it is a convenient means of representing the shape of the curve or, more precisely, its slope at p_{50}. Normally, n is 2.7 ± 0.2. It does not rise above this value, but decrease below it is a measure of abnormality.

The abscissa in Figure 1 has been given no values because p_{50} and, therefore, the position of the curve along this axis is dependent on pH, temperature, ion concentration, and cofactors. However, n (the shape of the curve) is independent of these variables.

The effect of pH, or the Bohr effect, is another parameter of function and is reported as $\Delta p_{50}/\Delta pH$. The maximum value of p_{50} (minimum affinity) occurs at approximately pH 6.2 and decreases at pH above or below. Below the maximum, this is termed the "acid" Bohr effect and above the maximum the "alkaline" Bohr effect. Only the latter is of any physiological significance.

Because the p_{50} is dependent on several factors, it is important that the exact conditions of pH, temperature, and ion concentration be stated. Since 1967, another factor, the concentration of 2,3-diphosphoglyceric acid (2, 3-DPG), has had to be considered. Chanutin and Curnish[4] and Benesch and Benesch[2] discovered that the presence of 2,3-DPG decreases the oxygen affinity (increases p_{50}) of hemoglobin and that the n does not change. 2,3-DPG is a glycolytic intermediate that normally approximately equals hemoglobin in millimolar concentration in the red cell. In any determination of p_{50}, the concentration of 2,3-DPG cannot be ignored. Either it must be removed ("stripped") or its concentration must be known. Consequently, data on oxygen equilibrium curves published before the effect of 2,3-DPG was discovered in 1967 must be examined with caution because its concentration in such studies is unknown. (See Huisman and Schroeder[6] for a review of this topic.)

Time Course of Hemoglobins in the Individual

Hemoglobins appear and disappear in sequence from the first production of hemoglobin in the developing fetus until the infant is 6 months to 1 year old, at which time it has attained the hematological status of an adult. Toward the middle of the first trimester of gestation, when sufficient blood for study can be obtained, four chains make up most of the hemoglobin; they are the α, γ, ε, and ζ chains in the combinations $\alpha_2\gamma_2$ (HbF), $\alpha_2\varepsilon_2$ (Hb-Gower-2), $\zeta_2\varepsilon_2$ (Hb-Gower-1), and $\zeta_2\gamma_2$ (Hb-Portland-1). Although Hb-Gower-1 was first thought to be ε_4, it is probably $\zeta_2\varepsilon_2$, and the ζ chain is a type of α chain. The ε and ζ chains are not detectable after the end of the first trimester.

The β chains (hence, $\alpha_2\beta_2$ or HbA) may be detected early in pregnancy, and during the second trimester HbA makes up 5 to 10% and HbF the remainder of the hemoglobin. During the last trimester, HbA production increases and that of HbF decreases so that at birth HbA approximates 25% (with considerable variation) and HbF the remainder of the hemoglobin, except for 0.2 to 0.5% of HbA_2.

Postnatally, the reciprocal rise of HbA and HbA_2 and the fall of HbF continue. By the time an infant is approximately 6 months old, the HbF has decreased to a few percent, HbA is the preponderant hemoglobin, and HbA_2 makes up 2 to 3% of the total hemoglobin.

Amino Acid Sequences in the Human Hemoglobin Chains

The amino acid sequences of the α, β, γ, and δ chains follow below. Very little is known about the ε chain. A partial sequence of the ζ chain has been reported.[8]

Human α Chain

				5					10					15
Val-	Leu-	Ser-	Pro-	Ala-	Asp-	Lys-	Thr-	Asn-	Val-	Lys-	Ala-	Ala-	Trp-	Gly-
				20					25					30
Lys-	Val-	Gly-	Ala-	His-	Ala-	Gly-	Glu-	Tyr-	Gly-	Ala-	Glu-	Ala-	Leu-	Glu-
				35					40					45
Arg-	Met-	Phe-	Leu-	Ser-	Phe-	Pro-	Thr-	Thr-	Lys-	Thr-	Tyr-	Phe-	Pro-	His-
				50					55					60
Phe-	Asp-	Leu-	Ser-	His-	Gly-	Ser-	Ala-	Gln-	Val-	Lys-	Gly-	His-	Gly-	Lys-
				65					70					75
Lys-	Val-	Ala-	Asp-	Ala-	Leu-	Thr-	Asn-	Ala-	Val-	Ala-	His-	Val-	Asp-	Asp-

80 85 90

Met- Pro- Asn- Ala- Leu- Ser- Ala- Leu- Ser- Asp- Leu- His- Ala- His- Lys-

95 100 105

Leu- Arg- Val- Asp- Pro- Val- Asn- Phe- Lys- Leu- Leu- Ser- His- Cys- Leu-

110 115 120

Leu- Val- Thr- Leu- Ala- Ala- His- Leu- Pro- Ala- Glu- Phe- Thr- Pro- Ala-

125 130 135

Val- His- Ala- Ser- Leu- Asp- Lys- Phe- Leu- Ala- Ser- Val- Ser- Thr- Val-

140

Leu- Thr- Ser- Lys- Tyr- Arg

Human β Chain

5 10 15

Val- His- Leu- Thr- Pro- Glu- Glu- Lys- Ser- Ala- Val- Thr- Ala- Leu- Trp-

20 25 30

Gly- Lys- Val- Asn- Val- Asp- Glu- Val- Gly- Gly- Glu- Ala- Leu- Gly- Arg-

35 40 45

Leu- Leu- Val- Val- Tyr- Pro- Trp- Thr- Gln- Arg- Phe- Phe- Glu- Ser- Phe-

50 55 60

Gly- Asp- Leu- Ser- Thr- Pro- Asp- Ala- Val- Met- Gly- Asn- Pro- Lys- Val-

65 70 75

Lys- Ala- His- Gly- Lys- Lys- Val- Leu- Gly- Ala- Phe- Ser- Asp- Gly- Leu-

80 85 90

Ala- His- Leu- Asp- Asn- Leu- Lys- Gly- Thr- Phe- Ala- Thr- Leu- Ser- Glu-

95 100 105

Leu- His- Cys- Asp- Lys- Leu- His- Val- Asp- Pro- Glu- Asn- Phe- Arg- Leu-

110 115 120

Leu- Gly- Asn- Val- Leu- Val- Cys- Val- Leu- Ala- His- His- Phe- Gly- Lys-

125 130 135

Glu- Phe- Thr- Pro- Pro- Val- Gln- Ala- Ala- Tyr- Gln- Lys- Val- Val- Ala-

140 145

Gly- Val- Ala- Asn- Ala- Leu- Ala- His- Lys- Tyr- His

Human γ Chain

				5					10					15
Gly-	His-	Phe-	Thr-	Glu-	Glu-	Asp-	Lys-	Ala-	Thr-	Ile-	Thr-	Ser-	Leu-	Trp-
				20					25					30
Gly-	Lys-	Val-	Asn-	Val-	Glu-	Asp-	Ala-	Gly-	Gly-	Glu-	Thr-	Leu-	Gly-	Arg-
				35					40					45
Leu-	Leu-	Val-	Val-	Tyr-	Pro-	Trp-	Thr-	Gln-	Arg-	Phe-	Phe-	Asp-	Ser-	Phe-
				50					55					60
Gly-	Asn-	Leu-	Ser-	Ser-	Ala-	Ser-	Ala-	Ile-	Met-	Gly-	Asn-	Pro-	Lys-	Val-
				65					70					75
Lys-	Ala-	His-	Gly-	Lys-	Lys-	Val-	Leu-	Thr-	Ser-	Leu-	Gly-	Asp-	Ala-	Ile-
				80					85					90
Lys-	His-	Leu-	Asp-	Asp-	Leu-	Lys-	Gly-	Thr-	Phe-	Ala-	Gln-	Leu-	Ser-	Glu-
				95					100					105
Leu-	His-	Cys-	Asp-	Lys-	Leu-	His-	Val-	Asp-	Pro-	Glu-	Asn-	Phe-	Lys-	Leu-
				110					115					120
Leu-	Gly-	Asn-	Val-	Leu-	Val-	Thr-	Val-	Leu-	Ala-	Ile-	His-	Phe-	Gly-	Lys-
				125					130					135
Glu-	Phe-	Thr-	Pro-	Glu-	Val-	Gln-	Ala-	Ser-	Trp-	Gln-	Lys-	Met-	Val-	Thr-
				140					145					
Gly-	Val-	Ala-	Ser-	Ala-	Leu-	Ser-	Ser-	Arg-	Tyr-	His				

Normally, HbF has a mixture of γ chains which are the products of nonallelic genes. Thus, position 136 may have either glycine or alanine.[15] In some instances, isoleucine at position 75 may be replaced by threonine.[13] If threonine is in position 75, it is not yet determined whether glycine or alanine is in position 136.

Human δ Chain

				5					10					15
Val-	His-	Leu-	Thr-	Pro-	Glu-	Glu-	Lys-	Thr-	Ala-	Val-	Asn-	Ala-	Leu-	Trp-
				20					25					30
Gly-	Lys-	Val-	Asn-	Val-	Asp-	Ala-	Val-	Gly-	Gly-	Glu-	Ala-	Leu-	Gly-	Arg-
				35					40					45
Leu-	Leu-	Val-	Val-	Tyr-	Pro-	Trp-	Thr-	Gln-	Arg-	Phe-	Phe-	Glu-	Ser-	Phe-

50 55 60

Gly- Asp- Leu- Ser- Ser- Pro- Asp- Ala- Val- Met- Gly- Asn- Pro- Lys- Val-

65 70 75

Lys- Ala- His- Gly- Lys- Lys- Val- Leu- Gly- Ala- Phe- Ser- Asp- Gly- Leu-

80 85 90

Ala- His- Leu- Asp- Asn- Leu- Lys- Gly- Thr- Phe- Ser- Gln- Leu- Ser- Glu-

95 100 105

Leu- His- Cys- Asp- Lys- Leu- His- Val- Asp- Pro- Glu- Asn- Phe- Arg- Leu-

110 115 120

Leu- Gly- Asn- Val- Leu- Val- Cys- Val- Leu- Ala- Arg- Asn- Phe- Gly- Lys-

125 130 135

Glu- Phe- Thr- Pro- Gln- Met- Gln- Ala- Ala- Tyr- Gln- Lys- Val- Val- Ala-

140 145

Gly- Val- Ala- Asn- Ala- Leu- Ala- His- Lys- Tyr- His

Postsynthetic Changes

A portion of the β and γ chains is modified after the biosynthesis is complete. In the hemoglobin designated as HbA$_{Ic}$, which accounts for 5 to 6% of the total hemoglobin in the normal adult, the β chains have a carbohydrate in Schiff's base linkage to the N-terminal valyl residue.[5,10]

The hemoglobin known as HbF$_1$ or HbF$_I$ has γ chains that are acetylated on the N-terminal glycyl residue.[14,16] The ratio of HbF$_1$ to HbF is approximately 1:4.

REFERENCES

1. **Antonini, E.and Brunori, M.,** *Hemoglobin and Myoglobin in Their Reactions with Ligands,* Elsevier, New York 1971.
2. **Benesch, R. and Benesch, R. E.,** The effect of organic phosphates from the human erythrocyte on the allosteric properties of hemoglobin, *Biochem. Biophys. Res. Commun.,* 26, 162, 1967.
3. **Bunn, H. F., Forget, B. G., and Ranney, H. M.,** *Human Hemoglobins,* W. B. Saunders, Philadelphia, 1977.
4. **Chanutin, A. and Curnish, R. R.,** Effect of organic and inorganic phosphates on the oxygen equilibrium of human erythrocytes, *Arch. Biochem. Biophys.,* 121, 96, 1967.
5. **Holmquist, W. R. and Schroeder, W. A.,** A new N-terminal blocking group involving a Schiff base in hemoglobin A$_{Ic}$, *Biochemistry,* 5, 2489, 1966.
6. **Huisman, T.H.J. and Schroeder, W. A.,** New aspects of the structure, function, and synthesis of hemoglobins, *CRC Crit. Rev. Clin. Lab. Sci.,* 1, 490, 1970.
7. **Huisman, T. H. J.,** Normal and abnormal human hemoglobins, *Adv. Clin. Chem.,* 15, 149, 1972.
8. **Kamuzora, H., Jones, R. T., and Lehmann , H.,** The ζ-chain, an α-like chain of human embryonic haemoglobin, *FEBS Lett.,* 46, 195, 1974.
9. **Kitchen, H. and Boyer, S., Eds.,** Hemoglobin: comparative molecular biology models for the study of disease, *Ann. N. Y. Acad. Sci.,* 241, 1, 1974.

10. **Koenig, R. J. , Blobstein, S. H., and Cerami, A.**, Structure of carbohydrate of hemoglobin A_{Ic}, *J. Biol. Chem.*, 252, 2992, 1977.
11. **Lehmann, H. and Huntsman, R. G.**, *Man's Hemoglobins*, 2nd ed., North-Holland, Amsterdam, 1974.
12. **Ranney, H. M., Ed.**, Hemoglobinopathies, *Semin. Hematol.*, 11, 383, 1974.
13. **Ricco, G., Mazza, V., Turi, R. M., Pich, P. G., Camaschella, C., Saglio, G., and Bernini, L. F.**, Significance of a new type of human fetal hemoglobin carrying a replacement isoleucine → threonine at position 75 (E19) of the γ chain, *Hum. Genet.*, 32, 305, 1976.
14. **Schroeder, W. A., Cua, J. T., Matsuda, G., and Fenninger, W. D.**, Hemoglobin F_I, an acetyl-containing hemoglobin, *Biochim. Biophys. Acta*, 63, 532, 1962.
15. **Schroeder, W. A., Huisman, T. H. J., Shelton, J. R., Shelton, J. B., Kleihauer, E. F., Dozy, A. M., and Robberson, B.**, Evidence for multiple structural genes for the γ chain of human fetal hemoglobin, *Proc. Natl. Acad. Sci. U.S.A.*, 60, 537, 1968.
16. **Stegink, L. D., Meyer, P. D., and Brummel, M. C.**, Human fetal hemoglobin F_1 — acetylation status, *J. Biol. Chem.*, 246, 3001, 1971.
17. **Weatherall, D. J. and Clegg, J. B.**, *The Thalassemia Syndromes*, Blackwell Scientific, Oxford, 1972.
18. **Weatherall, D. J., Ed.**, Abnormal hemoglobins, *Clin. Haematol.*, 3, 215, 1974.
19. **Weatherall, D. J., Ed.**, Hemoglobin: structure, function, and synthesis, *Br. Med. Bull.*, 32, 193, 1976.

GENETICS OF HEMOGLOBINS

Robert D. Koler

Phylogeny

One or more globin gene products are found in all vertebrates as well as in mollusks, annelids, and some plants. All globins share the same homologous structure; they all provide a pocket for the binding of heme and have the common property of reversible combination with oxygen. The most recent of the reviews on the comparative biochemistry of globins are those by Fitch,[1] Dayhoff et al.,[2] Goodman, Moore, and Matsuda,[3] and Coates.[4]

Comparison of the amino acid sequences of globins has led to the construction of an evolutionary tree such as that found in Figure 1. It is based on the maximum parsimony method, which ascribes the descent of related protein amino acid sequences to the fewest number of mutational changes. The result is in general agreement with paleontologic dating of the divergence from common ancestors. The primitive gene that gave rise to all existing globin genes may be as ancient as the time plant life diverged from animal lineages about 1 billion years ago.

A schematic model of the formation of the earth and its atmosphere is shown in Figure 2. A predominately reducing environment was present until about 3 billion years ago when the earliest living forms appeared. Organic evolution resulted in organisms that were able to trap energy from sunlight by photosynthesis. One product of photosynthesis — oxygen — then accumulated and reached its present atmospheric concentration by about 1 billion years ago. This chronology is consistent with the known function of all hemoglobins, i. e., to transport oxygen in those metazoans in which it occurs. The absence of a globin counterpart in more primitive protozoans is also in keeping with an age of less than 3 billion but more than 1 billion years. This chapter will review what has happened to that common ancestral globin gene.

Change in Amino Acid Composition

Dickerson[6] has plotted the number of amino acid changes per 100 sites against the time elapsed since the divergence of two lines as determined by the geologic record. As shown in Figure 3, the rate of change is constant over long time periods for a given protein but differs between proteins. Thus the time required for a 1% change for hemoglobin is 5.8 million years. As compared with histone IV or cytochrome C, hemoglobin has changed at a much more rapid rate.

Change in Function

There are species differences among vertebrates in the hemoglobin-oxygen equilibrium and the kinetics that describe the basic reaction:

$$Hb + n0_2 \rightleftharpoons Hb\,(0_2)_n$$

Coates[4] has proposed a model (Figure 4) suggesting that a sequence of minor modifications of globin structure will account for the evolutionary differences among species. His model begins with a primitive monomer that successively becomes:

1. A dimer in the deoxy form, thus acquiring a Bohr effect and cooperative rather than hyperbolic binding of oxygen (hagfish → lamprey)
2. A tetramer with a greater Bohr effect, greater cooperativity, and further reduction in oxygen affinity (cyclostoma → elasmobranchii)

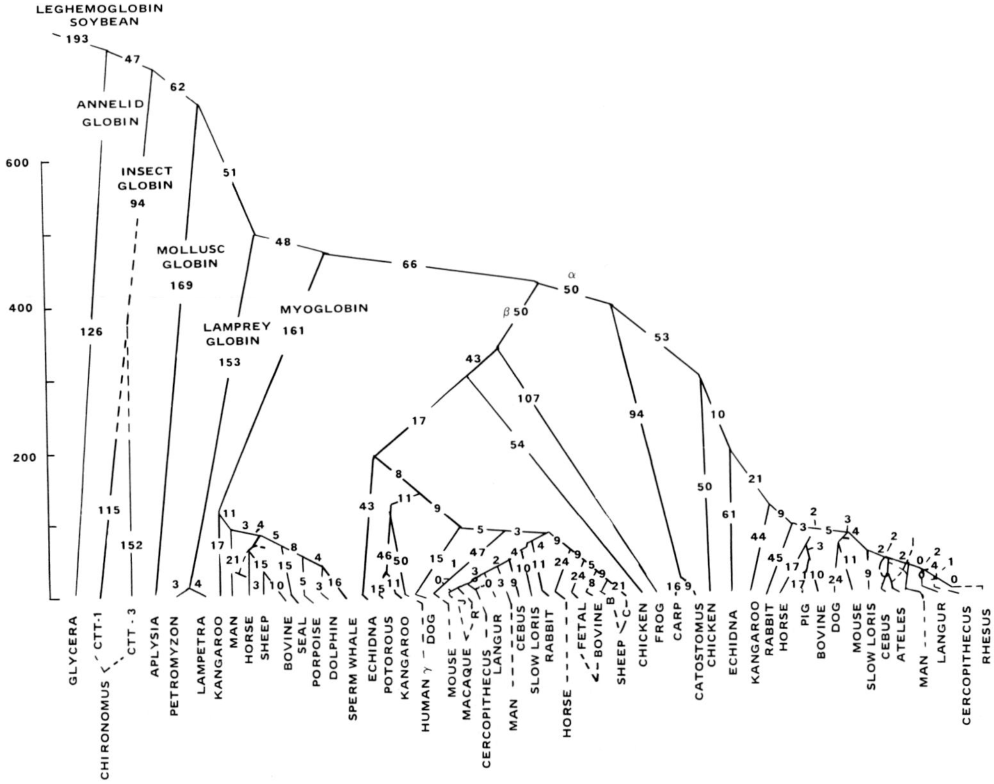

FIGURE 1. Maximum parsimony tree of 55 more adequately sequenced globins. (From Goodman, M., Moore, G. W., and Matsuda, G., *Isozymes. IV. Genetics and Evolution,* Markert, C. L., Ed., Academic Press, New York, 1975, 181. With permission.)

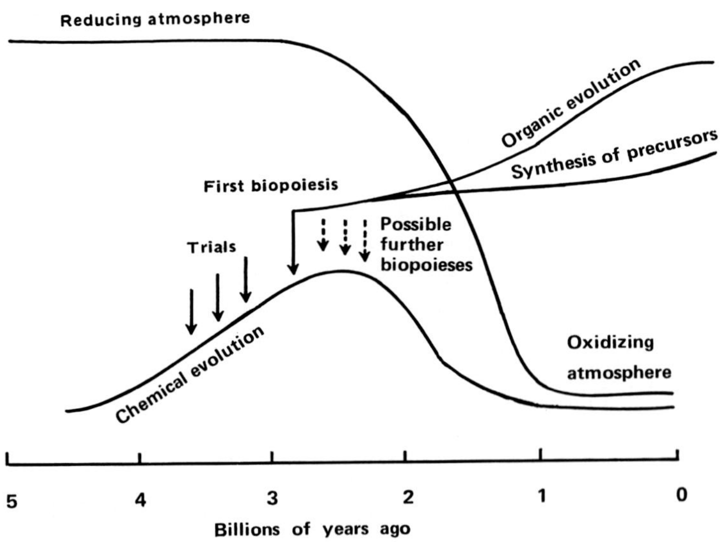

FIGURE 2. Probable origin of life and course of evolutionary events. (From *HEREDITY, EVOLUTION, AND SOCIETY,* Second Edition, by I. Michael Lerner and William J. Libby. W. M. Freeman and Company. Copyright © 1976.

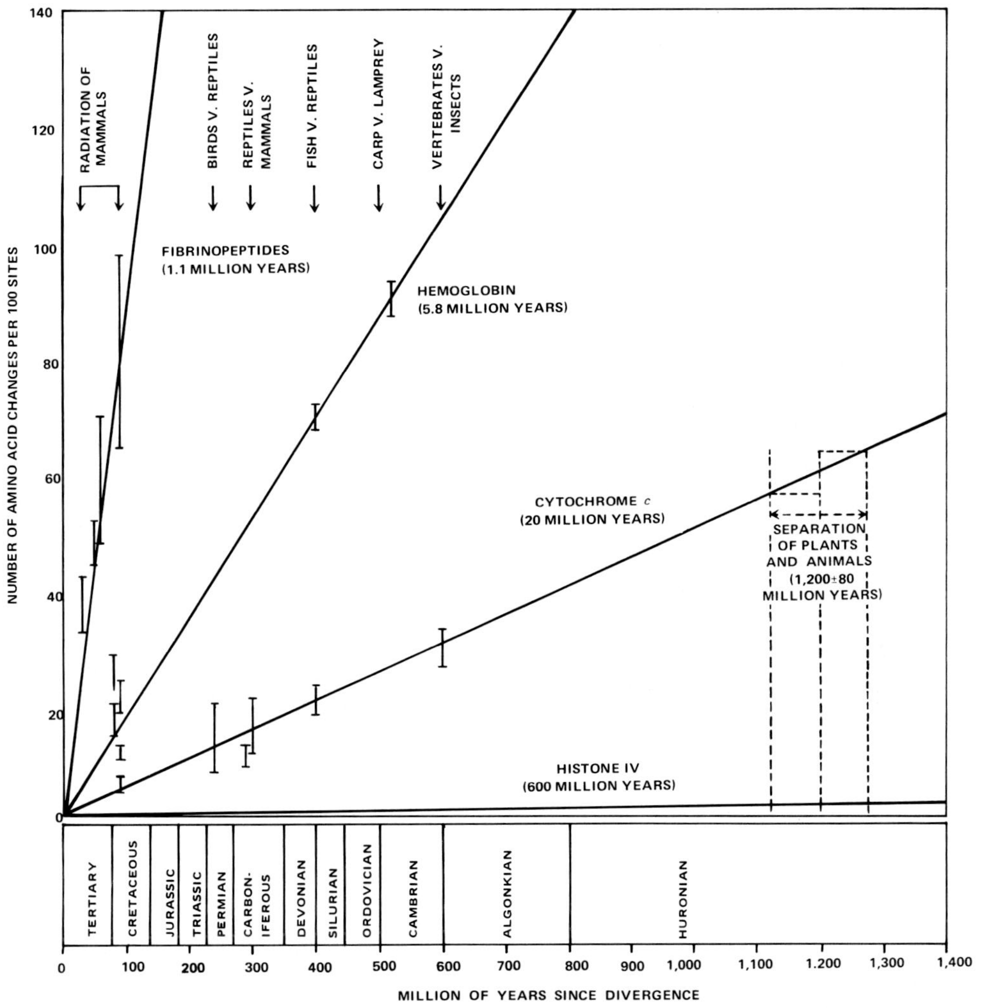

FIGURE 3. Rates of evolution of proteins. (From Dickerson, R. E., *Sci. Am.*, 226, 58, 1972. With permission.)

3. A tetramer that acquires a phosphate-binding site leading to a further increase in Bohr effect and a decrease in oxygen affinity (elasmobranchii → bony fishes and all higher forms)

There has also been a progression in the type of organic phosphate bound. More primitive forms use only ATP. Amphibia, birds, and mammals use 2,3-DPG; after hatching, birds use myoinositol pentaphosphate.[7]

Gene Duplication

Duplication of the ancestral globin gene has resulted in two classes and six different types of globin genes found in the human haploid complement. Ohno[8] has reviewed both the teleologic reasons for gene duplication and the evidence that it has happened. Comparative studies of both phylogenetic and ontogenic development are in keeping with a progressive adaptation of hemoglobins[4,8] by both gene duplication and amino acid substitutions. Human globin genes and their active period during development are listed in Table 1.

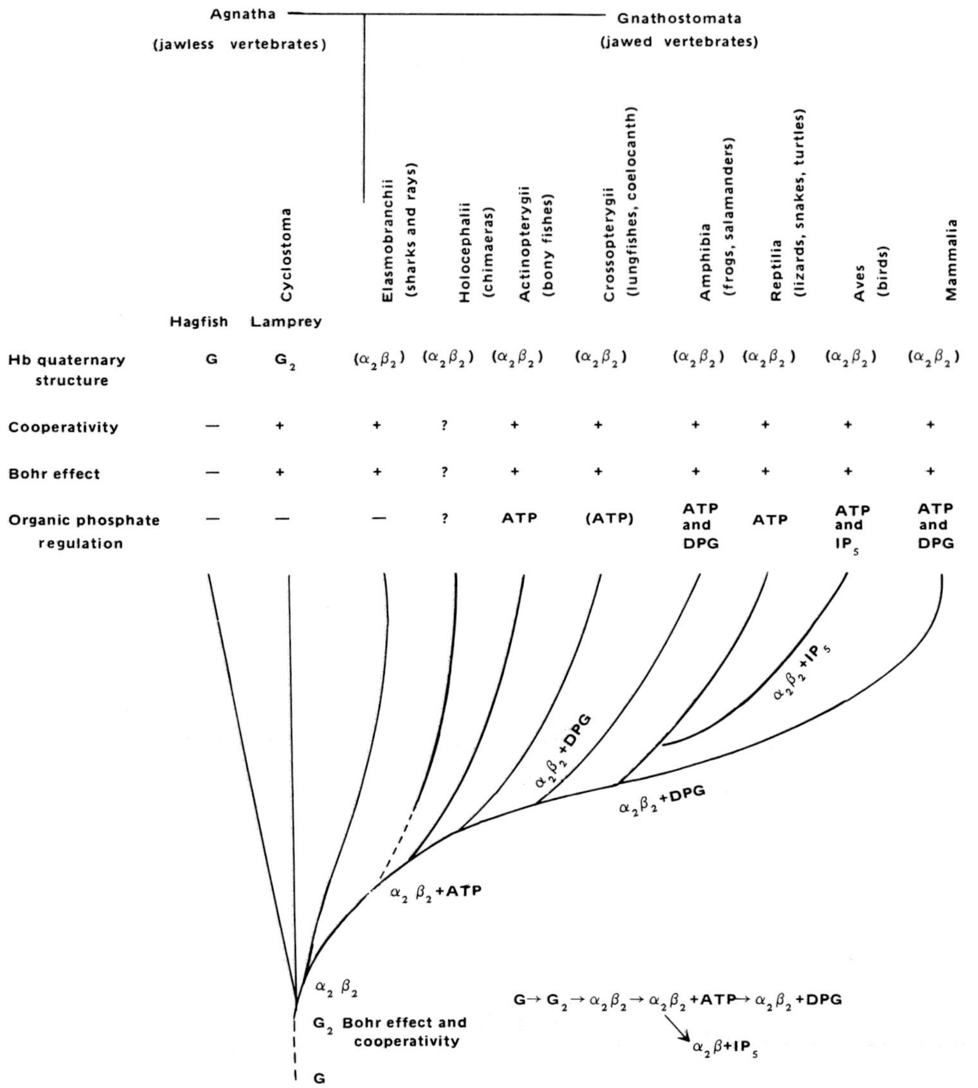

FIGURE 4. Evolution of hemoglobin function in vertebrates. (From Coates, M., *J. Mol. Evol.*, 6, 285, 1975. With permission.)

Alpha and nonalpha classes of globin genes are found in all vertebrates beyond the agnatha or jawless forms. They probably resulted from polyploidization or doubling of the entire chromosome complement early in the evolution of vertebrates.[8] Tandem duplication then resulted in two subtypes at the nonalpha cistron.

More than one alpha subtype has been found in many mammals,[9] including all primates;[10] this suggests that this duplication is relatively ancient or that it has occurred more than once. Boyer et al.[9] have proposed that a number of duplications and subsequent deletions of the alpha globin locus have occurred and that this has assured preservation of the optimum alpha chain structure required to form a tetramer with nonalpha globins.

At the nonalpha cistron, a minimum of three tandem duplications would account for the human subtypes $^{A}\gamma$, $^{G}\gamma$, β, and δ. Duplication of the nonalpha locus is also found in other species. A δ-globin is present in a number of primate species[11] but not in other mammals. A fetal gamma globin analogous to that in humans has been struc-

Table 1
HUMAN GLOBIN GENES[a]

Class	Type	Subtype	Ontogeny	Tetramer	Name
Alpha	ζ	ζ	Embryo	$\zeta_2\varepsilon_2$	Gower I
	α	$^{Buda}\alpha$		$\alpha_2\varepsilon_2$	Gower II
		$^{Pest}\alpha$		$\zeta_2\gamma_2$	Portland
Nonalpha	ε	ε	Fetus	$\alpha_2{}^A\gamma_2$	Fetal
	γ	$^A\gamma$		$\alpha_2{}^G\gamma_2$	Fetal
		$^G\gamma$	Adult	$\alpha_2\beta_2$	Hb A
	β	β		$\alpha_2\delta_2$	Hb A_2
	δ	δ			

[a] Two classes of globin genes with the presently known types and subtypes within each class, the names assigned to tetramers and the time during development that they appear. There is still uncertainty as to whether two subtypes of α chain occur in all human populations.[63-66]

turally characterized in cattle, sheep, goats,[12] and mice [13] and may occur in elephants and rats;[14] none has been found in dogs[14] and pigs.[15]

Human fetal hemoglobin consists of tetramers with two gamma globins that differ only at the 136th amino acid position. One contains glycine and is termed $^G\gamma$; the other contains alanine and is termed $^A\gamma$.[16-21] In addition, Ricco et al.[60] have recently reported further heterogeneity due to the presence of threonine or isoleucine at the 75th amino acid position. The substitution of threonine for isoleucine was found in about one third of cord blood samples from a variety of ethnic groups. It is uncertain, however, whether this will be the marker for a third gamma globin locus or whether it represents a polymorphism with two different alleles at the $^G\gamma$ locus. More than two γ-globin loci have been postulated by Huisman et al.[23] to account for the varying proportions of $^A\gamma$ and $^G\gamma$ chains at different stages of development. A recent direct measurement using hybridization of highly radioactive complementary DNA to total human DNA, however, indicates two or, at most three, γ-globin genes.[24]

Embryonic globins from rabbit and mouse embryos[25] contain a ζ-like chain based on partial amino acid sequences. The time of divergence and classification of embryonic hemoglobins is still tentative, however, because these gene products have not been sought systematically in other species.

Organization of Globin Genes

The arrangement of globin genes on human chromosomes is known in part, but there are still areas of both uncertainty and controversy. This information has been reviewed by Kabat and Koler,[26] and, more recently, in a comprehensive treatment of human hemoglobins by Bunn, Forget, and Ranney.[27]

Absence of Linkage Between Alpha and Nonalpha Cistrons

Independent segregation of allelic genes at the alpha and beta loci has been found in all families in which structural variants of both globins occur.

The annealing of radioactive globin mRNA to metaphase human chromosomes[29] indicated placement of the two cistrons on the proximal long arm of chromosomes 2 and 4 or 5. This result has been criticized[30] because of skepticism about the specificity of such labeling with the small number of globin DNA sequences likely to be present at each cistron. Similar annealing of radioactive mRNA to DNA extracted from human X mouse cell hybrids[28,61,62] suggests that the α cistron is on chromosome 16 and the nonalpha cistron is on chromosome 11. Although the latter results are in conflict with

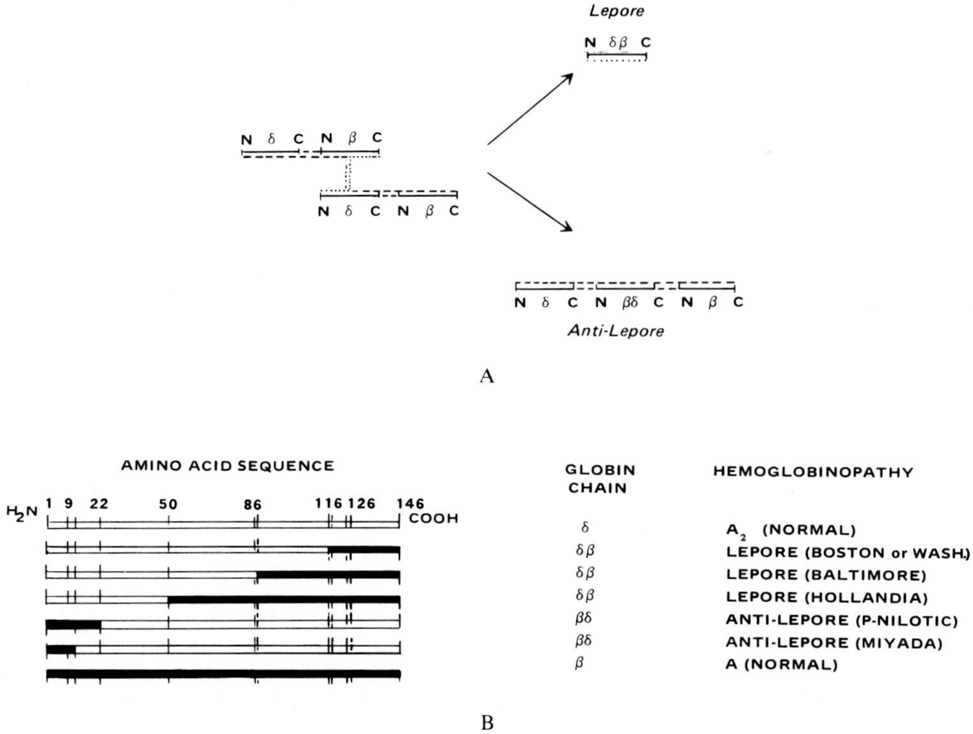

FIGURE 5. (A) Origin of the Lepore and anti-Lepore globin chains by crossing over between misaligned δ- and β-globin genes. N and C refer to the extremities of the gene coding for the amino-terminal and carboxy-terminal ends of the globin chains, (B) Different types of Lepore and anti-Lepore globin chains. (From Benz, E. J. and Forget, B. G., *Progress in Hematology,* Vol. 9, Brown, E. B., Ed., Grune & Stratton, New York, 1975, 107. By permission.)

the in situ labeling of metaphase preparations, and with specific activity measurements of alpha and globin chains synthesized by subjects trisomic for the long arm of chromosome 4,[31] the methodology is more direct and probably more sensitive.

Polarity of Linked Globin Genes in the Nonalpha Cistron

The alignment of nonalpha globin genes is based on the study of rare fusion gene products. The first was found in members of a family who had a thalassemia-like phenotype, and it was designated Hb Lepore.[32] This abnormal hemoglobin was chemically characterized by Baglioni,[33] who found the N-terminal amino acid sequence to be identical with that of the normal δ chain and the C-terminal sequence identical to that of the normal β chain. The mechanism he proposed to explain this finding proved to be consistent with all of the fusion globin genes since discovered. It involves mispairing during meiosis and crossing-over* at a region in the DNA sequence that codes for amino acid sequence, as illustrated in Figure 5. Three different Lepore hemoglobins with differing points of crossover have been reported, as have two different anti-Lepore variants. The recombinant chromosomes differ in that the normal δ and β globin loci are absent from the chromosome carrying the Lepore fusion gene and are retained on the chromosome with the anti-Lepore βδ fusion gene.

* Use of the adjective "nonhomologous" to describe the crossover is ambiguous. The parental chromosomes involved are homologues. The tandemly duplicated globin loci are homologous because of common evolutionary ancestry. The retention of homology, in fact, probably accounts for the similarity in DNA sequence that permits the mispairing. To the extent that they represent separate replicates of the common ancestral globin gene, the pairing is out of register and abnormal, but it is between homologous DNA sequences. Thus it is incestuous, perhaps, but not nonhomologous.

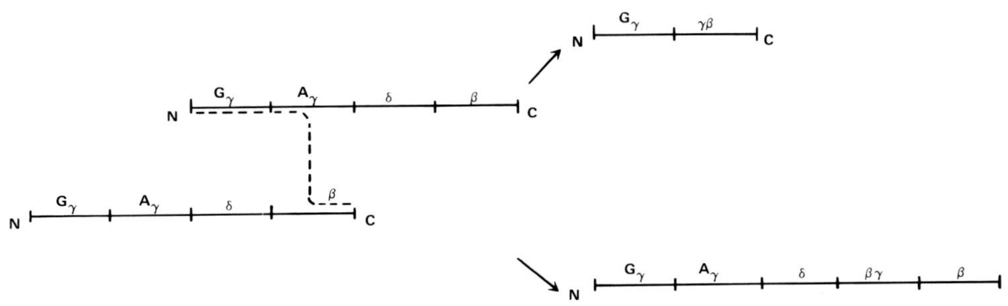

FIGURE 6. Origin of the Kenya globin chain by crossing over between misaligned $^{A}\gamma$ and β globin genes.

Another abnormal hemoglobin, Hb Kenya, has an N-terminal amino acid sequence identical to the $^{A}\gamma$ globin and a C-terminal sequence identical to the normal β chain.[35,36] This fusion gene product, like that for Hb Lepore, is thought to result from a crossover product of mispaired $^{A}\gamma$ and β loci. Figure 6 illustrates the two theoretical products, of which the Hb Kenya chromosome lacks the genetic loci for $^{A}\gamma$, δ, and β globins. This interpretation is in keeping with the phenotypes of subjects heterozygous for Hb Kenya and one individual doubly heterozygous for Hb Kenya and Hb S.

In addition to structural characterization of the fusion gene products, the key information supporting the polarity as diagrammed is that the individual homozygous for Hb Lepore produces no Hb A or Hb A_2,[37] and the individual doubly heterozygous for Hb Kenya and Hb S produces no Hb A and half normal amounts of Hb A_2.[36] These observations indicate that the polarity of globin structure genes within the nonalpha cistron is probably as diagrammed in Figure 6, although the $^{G}\gamma$ locus could alternatively be situated at the C-terminal side of the β globin gene. Close linkage between the δ and β loci is supported by the absence of any recombination in 41 opportunities in families carrying both a δ-chain and a β-chain hemoglobin variant.[38]

Polarity of Linked Globin Genes in the Alpha Cistron

As noted above, there is still uncertainty about how general the tandem duplication of the alpha globin locus may be. The first family reported to have two different α-chain variants, Hb J-Buda and Hb G-Pest, and approximately 50% Hb A,[39-40] led to the designation in Table 1. Since then Hb Rampa and Hb Koya Dora in individuals from a tribe in India[41] and Hb G-Philadelphia and Hb Seal Rock[42] in one individual have been described in which Hb A is also present. These reports do not permit any conclusion about polarity at this cistron, and no fusion gene products are known. In fact, they would not be detectable if they existed, because there has been no structural divergence of duplicated loci like that at the nonalpha cistron.

Genetic Mechanisms Accounting for Abnormal Globin Synthesis

Abnormalities in globin synthesis may be in amount, resulting in an imbalance of chain production, or in structure.

Imbalance of Chain Production

Shortly after the subunits of hemoglobin were identified, it became apparent that the biosynthesis of globin chains and their assembly into tetramers is normally balanced. The progression of hemoglobin types from embryonic to adult life (Table 1) presupposes equal rates of production of subunits of the alpha and nonalpha class. This balance could theoretically be upset if an increase or decrease in production differentially affected either class of globin genes.

Decreased or absent production of alpha chains results in a spectrum of phenotypes designated alpha thalassemia. These range in severity from a "silent carrier" to a lethal form, the hydrops fetalis phenotype in which no alpha chain is produced. At the non-alpha cistron, defects in biosynthesis of beta and/or delta chains have been recognized and the corresponding phenotypes designated beta or delta thalassemia, or hereditary persistance of fetal hemoglobin. The molecular basis of thalassemias has proven to be a productive model for questioning the control of human genes. This information has been collected in several recent reviews, including those by Bunn, Forget, and Ranney,[27] Kabat and Koler,[26] and Weatherall and Clegg.[37]

Documented mechanisms accounting for decreased synthesis of a particular globin chain are deletion of the gene, instability of the globin mRNA, and lack of one or more factors necessary for translation of the globin message. Of interest is the recent report by Boyer et al.[43] demonstrating allelic exclusion of the gene product from one chromosome in subjects heterozygous for hereditary persistance of fetal hemoglobin. If this mechanism, previously known to operate only for genes on the X chromosome and for immunoglobulins, also applies to genes at the hemoglobin loci, many conclusions based on the amount of globin gene product found in mature erythrocytes will need to be reexamined.

Altered Globin Structure

The structure of human globin chains, both normal and abnormal, is well known. It encompasses a large literature beginning with the classic papers by Pauling et al.[44] and Ingram.[45] Since 1976, the International Hemoglobin Information Center has provided periodically updated lists of hemoglobin variants.[46] At this writing, the total includes 80 different alleles at the α-globin loci and 163 different alleles at the β-globin locus that differ from the wild type by a single amino acid substitution. These variants and the normal β-chain codons, as determined by Marotta and co-workers[47-49] are presented in Table 2, together with the functional role of the amino acid side chains as worked out by Perutz and co-workers.[50-53] Given the expected publication of amino acid codons for the alpha globin genes that should soon be available from the M.I.T.-Yale group, the two classes of globin cistrons and the gene products they encode are the best known for any eukaryotic locus. Questions dealing with the relationship of structure to function are treated elsewhere in this handbook. Questions dealing with population genetics, selective advantage, and mutation rates require continued collection of more data describing gene frequencies and incidence of sporadic cases.[54]

The agreement of the codon changes that account for hemoglobin variants with the genetic code has been reviewed by Perutz and Lehmann,[55] Bunn, Forget and Ranney,[27] and Wilson et al.[49] With rare exceptions, all amino acid substitutions can be accounted for as a single base change, and the autosomal dominant inheritance of these variants indicates a change in the DNA of the structure gene. As might be expected, a number of mutations that result in marked instability of the globin chain and severe hemolytic anemia have occurred as sporadic cases.[27,56]

In addition to the single-base change and the fusion gene products discussed above, two other types of variant have been found. Deletions of one or more adjacent amino acid residues have thus far been detected only for the β-chain (Table 3). These are believed to result from meiotic errors in synapsis of the homologous β-globin genes with crossing-over similar to that described for fusion gene products. One variant, Hb McKees Rock,[57] lacks the two C-terminal amino acids, Tyr-His. This could have resulted from a frame shift during synapsis, or it could represent a "nonsense" mutation or termination (UAU → UAA/G) mutation at the 145th codon.

Additions of amino acids to the normal globin sequence have also been discovered. Most of these represent elongations beyond the normal C-terminal residue due either

Table 2
HUMAN GLOBIN VARIANTS[a]

Variant residues	Codon	Amino acid	Homologous sequence alignment α-chain			β-chain	Amino acid	Codon	Variant residues
—	—	V	1	NA	1	1	V[b]	GUG	—
—	—	—	—		2	2	H[b]	CAC	R
—	—	L	2		3	3	L	CUG	—
—	—	S	3	A	1	4	T	ACU	—
—	—	P	4		2	5	P	CCU	—
D	—	A	5		3	6	E	GAA/G	A, K, V
A	—	D	6		4	7	E	GAG	G, K
—	—	K	7		5	8	K	AAG	—
—	—	T	8		6	9	S	UCY	C
—	—	N	9		7	10	A	GCN	D
—	—	V	10		8	11	V	GUU	—
E	—	K	11		9	12	T	ACU	—
D	—	A	12		10	13	A	GCN	—
—	—	A	13		11	14	L	YUN	R, P
—	—	W	14		12	15	W	UGG	R
R, D	—	G	15		13	16	G	GGC	R, D
E	—	K	16		14	17	K	AAG	E
—	—	V	17		15	18	V	GUG	—
—	—	G	18		16	—	—	—	—
D	—	A	19	AB	1	—	—	—	—
—	—	H	20	B	1	19	N	AAC	K
D	—	A	21		2	20	V	GUG	M, D
D	—	G	22		3	21	D	GAU	—
V, K, Q	—	E	23	B	4	22	E	GAA	A, G, K, Q
—	—	Y	24		5	23	V	GUU	—
—	—	G	25		6	24	G	GGU	R, V, D
—	—	A	26		7	25	G	GGU	R
V, G	—	E	27		8	26	E	GAG	K, V
—	—	A	28		9	27	A	GCC	D
—	—	L	29		10	28	L	CUG	P, Q
K, Q	—	E	30		11	29	G	GGC	—
—	—	R	31		12	30	R	AGG	S
—	—	M[c]	32		13	31	L[c]	CUG	—
—	—	F	33		14	32	L	CUG	P, R
—	—	L	34		15	33	V	GUG	—
—	—	S	35		16	34	V	GUC	—
—	—	F	36	C	1	35	Y	UAC	F
—	—	P	37		2	36	P[d]	CCU	—
—	—	T[d]	38		3	37	W[d]	UGG	S
—	—	T[c]	39		4	38	T[c]	ACC	—
—	—	K[d]	40		5	39	Q[d]	CAG	K, E
—	—	T[d]	41		6	40	R[d]	AGG	K, S
—	—	Y[d]	42		7	41	F[c]	UUC	Y
L, V	—	F[c]	43	CD	1	42	F[c]	UUU	S,L
—	—	P	44		2	43	E	GAG	A
—	—	H[c]	45		3	44	S[c]	UCC	—
—	—	F[c]	46	CD	4	45	F[c]	UUU	—
—	—	—	—		5	46	G	GGG	E
N, H	—	D	47		6	47	D	GAU	N
R	—	L	48		7	48	L	CUG	R
—	—	S	49		8	49	S	UCC	—
D	—	H	50	D	1	50	T	ACU	K
—	—	—	—		2	51	P	CCU	R
—	—	—	—		3	52	D	GAU	N, A
—	—	—	—		4	53	A	GCA	—
—	—	—	—		5	54	V	GUU	—

Table 2 (continued)
HUMAN GLOBIN VARIANTS[a]

Variant residues	Codon	Amino acid	Homologous sequence alignment α-chain	Helix position	Homologous sequence alignment β-chain	Amino acid	Codon	Variant residues
—	—	—	—	6	55	M	AUG	—
D, R	—	G	51	7	56	G	GGC	D, R
—	—	S	52	E 1	57	N	AAC	K
D	—	A	53	2	58	P	CCU	R
E, R	—	Q	54	3	59	K	AAG	E, T
—	—	V	55	4	60	V	GUG	—
—	—	K	56	5	61	K	AAG	N, E
D, R	—	G	57	6	62	A	GCU	P
Y	—	H[c]	58	7	63	H[c]	CAU	R, Y, P
—	—	G	59	8	64	G	GGC	D
N	—	K	60	9	65	K	AAG	N, Q
N	—	K	61	10	66	K[c]	AAA	E
—	—	V[c]	62	11	67	V[c]	GUG	A, D, E
—	—	A	63	12	68	L	CUC	—
Y, H, N	—	D	64	13	69	G	GGU	D
—	—	A	65	14	70	A[c]	GCC	D
—	—	L	66	15	71	F[c]	UUU	S
—	—	T	67	16	72	S	AGU	—
K, D	—	N	68	17	73	D	GAU	N, V
—	—	A	69	18	74	G	GGC	D, V
—	—	V	70	19	75	L	CUG	P
E	—	A	71	20	76	A	GCU	D
R	—	H	72	EF 1	77	H	CAC	D
—	—	V	73	2	78	L	CUG	—
G, N, H	—	D	74	3	79	D	GAC	G
N, Y, H	—	D	75	4	80	N	AAC	K
—	—	M	76	5	81	L	CUC	R
—	—	P	77	6	82	K[b]	AAG	D, T, M
K	—	N	78	7	83	G	GGC	C, D
—	—	A	79	8	84	T	ACC	—
R	—	L	80	F 1	85	F	UUU	S
—	—	S	81	2	86	A	GCC	—
—	—	A	82	3	87	T	ACA	K
—	—	L[c]	83	4	88	L[c]	CUG	R, P
R	—	S	84	5	89	S	AGU	N, R
V, Y, N	—	D	85	6	90	E	GAG	K
—	—	L[c]	86	7	91	L[c]	CUG	P, R
Y	—	H[c]	87	F 8	92	H[c]	CAC	Y, Q, D, P
—	—	A	88	9	93	C	UGU	—
—	—	H	89	FG 1	94	D	GAC	—
T, N	—	K	90	2	95	K	AAG	E
—	—	L[c,d]	91	3	96	L[c]	CUG	—
L, Q	—	R[d]	92	4	97	H[d]	CAC	Q, L
—	—	V[c,d]	93	5	98	V[c,d]	GUG	M, G, A
N, Y	—	D[d]	94	G 1	99	D[d]	GAU	N, H, Y
R, A, S, L	—	P[d]	95	2	100	P	CCU	L
—	—	V[d]	96	3	101	E[d]	GAG	K, Q, G
—	—	N[c]	97	4	102	N[c,d]	AAC	K, T, S
—	—	F[c]	98	5	103	F[c]	UUC	L
—	—	K	99	6	104	R	AGG	S
—	—	L	100	7	105	L	CUC	—
—	—	L[c]	101	8	106	L[c]	CUG	P, Q
R	—	S	102	9	107	G	GGC	R
—	—	H	103	10	108	N	AAC	D
—	—	C	104	11	109	V	GUG	M
—	—	L	105	12	110	L	CUG	—
—	—	L	106	13	111	V	GUC	F

Table 2 (continued)
HUMAN GLOBIN VARIANTS[a]

Variant residues	Codon	Amino acid	Homologous sequence alignment: α-chain	Helix	Helix position	Homologous sequence alignment: β-chain	Amino acid	Codon	Variant residues
—	—	V	107		14	112	C	UGU	—
—	—	T	108		15	113	V	GUG	E
—	—	L	109		16	114	L	CUG	—
—	—	A	110		17	115	A	GCC	P
—	—	A	111	G	18	116	H	CAU	—
R, D	—	H	112		19	117	H	CAC	R
—	—	L	113	GH	1	118	F	UUU	—
R	—	P	114		2	119	G	GGC	D
D	—	A	115		3	120	K	AAA	E, N
K	—	E	116		4	121	E	GAA	Q, K, V
—	—	F	117		5	122	F	UUC	—
G	—	T	118	H	1	123	T	ACC	—
—	—	P	119		2	124	P	CCA	R
E	—	A	120		3	125	P	CCA	—
—	—	V	121		4	126	V	GUG	E
—	—	H	122		5	127	Q	CAG	E
—	—	A	123		6	128	A	GCU	—
—	—	S	124		7	129	A	GCC	D, E
—	—	L	125		8	130	Y	UAU	D
N	—	D	126		9	131	Q	CAG	E
N, T	—	K	127		10	132	K	AAA	Q
—	—	F	128		11	133	V	GUG	—
—	—	L[c]	129		12	134	V	GUG	—
—	—	A	130		13	135	A	GCU	P
—	—	S	131		14	136	G	GGU	D
—	—	V[c]	132		15	137	V[c]	GUG	—
—	—	S	133		16	138	A	GCU	—
—	—	T	134		17	139	N	AAU	—
—		V	135	H	18	140	A	GCC	—
P		L[c]	136		19	141	L[c]	CUG	R
—		T	137		20	142	A	GCC	—
—		S	138		21	143	H[b]	CAC	R, Q, P
—		K	139	HC	1	144	K	AAG	N
—		Y	140		2	145	Y	UAU	H, C, D,—
H, P		R	141		3	146	H	CAC	D, P, R
—		—	142	Term		147	—	UAA	—

Note: One and three letter abbreviations for amino acids:

Alanine	Ala	A	Leucine	Leu	L
Arginine	Arg	R	Lysine	Lys	K
Aspartic Acid	Asp	D	Methionine	Met	M
Asparagine	Asn	N	Phenylalanine	Phe	F
Cysteine	Cys	C	Proline	Pro	P
Glycine	Gly	G	Serine	Ser	S
Glutamic Acid	Glu	E	Threonine	Thr	T
Glutamine	Gln	Q	Tryptophan	Trp	W
Histidine	His	H	Tyrosine	Tyr	Y
Isoleucine	Ile	I	Valine	Val	V

[a] The normal structure of human alpha and beta globins, with homologous alignment of helical and nonhelical regions,[50–52] the RNA codons for the β chain[47] and the single amino acid substitutions[46] using the single letter amino acid code.

[b] = 2,3-DPG contact.

[c] = heme contact.

[d] = $\alpha_1\beta_2$ contact.

Table 3
DELETED AMINO ACID RESIDUES

Name	Missing residue(s)	Synaptic error in meiotic pairing[a]		
Hb Leiden	β6 or β7	4 GAA/G -ACU-CCU -GAG-AAG- -ACU-CCU-GAA/G AAG- 4 GAG		
Hb Lyon	β17—18	15 AAG-GUG -UGG-GGC AAC-GUG-GAU- -UGG-GGC-AAG-GUG GAU- 15 AAC-GUG		
Hb Freiburg	β23	21 GUU -GAU-GAA GGU-GGU -GAU-GAA-GUU GGU- 21 GGU	or	21 GUU -GAU-GAA GGU-GGU- -GAU GUU-GGU-GGU- 21 GAA
Hb Niteroi	β43—45 or β42—44	41 GAG-UCC-UUU -UUC-UUU GGG-GAU-CUG- -UUC-UUU-GAG GAU-CUG- 41 UCC-UUU-GGG		
Hb Tochigi	β56—59	54 GGC-AAC-CCU-AAG -GUU-AUG GUG-AAG-GCU- -GUU-AUG-GGC AAG-GCU- 54 AAC-CCU-AAG-GUG		
Hb St. Antoine	β74—75	72 GGC-CUG -AGU-GAU GCU-CAC- -AGU-GAU-GGC CAC- 72 CUG-GCU		
Hb Tours	β87	84 ACA -ACC-UUU-GCC CUG- -ACC-UUU ACA-CUG- 84 GCC		
Hb Gun Hill	β91—95 or β92—96	89 CUG-CAC-UGU-GAC-AAG AGU-GAG CUG-CAC-GUG -AGU-GAG-CUG CAC-GUG- 89 CAC-UGU-GAC-AAG-CUG		
Hb Leslie	β131	129 CAG GCC-UAU AAA-GUG- GCC-UAU-CAG GUG- 129 AAA	or	129 CAG -GCC-UAU AAA-GUG- -GCC CAG-AAA-GUG- 129 UAU
Hb Coventry	β141	139 CUG -AAU-GCC GCC-CAC- -AAU-GCC-CUG CAC- 139 GCC	or	139 CUG -AAU-GCC GCC-CAC- -AAU-CUG GCC-CAC- 139 GCC
Hb McKees Rock	β145—146	143 UAU-CAC -CAC-AAG UAA-GCU-CGC- -CAC-AAG-UAU GCU-CGC- 143 CAC-UAA		

[a] The RNA codons as determined by Marotta et al.[47-49] are aligned to show the most likely synaptic error that would allow crossing over between the corresponding DNA codons to account for the deleted residue(s).

Table 4
HUMAN HEMOGLOBIN VARIANTS

Extended Chains

	Residue	Name
α141	140 (31 Additional residues) Try-Arg-Gln-Ala-Gly-Ala-Ser- 150 Val-Ala-Val-Pro-Pro-Ala-Arg-Trp-Ala-Ser-Glen-Arg-Ala- 160 170 Leu-Leu-Pro(His,Ser,Leu)-Arg-Pro-Phe-Leu-Val-Phe-Glu	Hb Constant Spring
α141	31 Additional residues — identical to Hb Constant Spring except for residue 142, which is lysine instead of glutamine	Hb Icaria
α141	Probably 31 additional residues — identical to Hb Constant Spring except for residue 142, which is serine instead of glutamine	Hb Koya Dora
α139—141	140 Thr-Ser-Asn-Thr-Val-Lys-Leu-Glu-Pro-Arg (Frame shift)	Hb Wayne
β145	144 Lys-Ser-Ile-Thr-Lys-Leu-Ala-Phe-Leu-Leu-Ser-Asn-Phe- 157 Tyr-COOH (Frame shift)	Hb Cranston
β147	144 Lys-Tyr-His-Thr-Lys-Leu-Ala-Phe-Leu-Leu-Ser-Asn-Phe- 157 Tyr-COOH (Frame shift)	Hb Tak
α115—118	117 118 119 Ala-Glu-Phe-Thr-*Glu-Phe-Thr*-Pro (Insertion)	Hb Grady

to a frame-shift mutation or a base change in the normal termination codon to a triplet that permits translation. Hb Constant Spring[58] was the first such example; others are listed in Table 4. The final mechanism, illustrated by Hb Grady,[59] represents an insertion of three repeating residues, Glu-Phe-Thr, between the 118th and 119th positions in the normal α-globin sequence.

Addendum

Following preparation of this review, there have been a number of reports concerning the DNA structure of globin genes. These are based on restriction endonuclease cleavage and recombinant DNA cloning methods, and have demonstrated a much larger map than was anticipated. The β-globin gene of rabbit,[67] mouse,[68] and man,[69] as well as the human γ-globin gene[70] share DNA segments that are transcribed but not translated. One of these comprised of 500 to 900 nucleotides is located between the DNA codons for the 104th and 105th amino acid residues.

The occurrence of such "intervening" or "inserted" DNA segments within DNA sequences that code for the ultimate gene product may be a common property of eukaryotic genes. Darnell[71] has reviewed this evidence. He proposes that RNA·RNA splicing of nuclear RNA transcripts to smaller mRNA's is an enzymatic process[72] which distinguishes eukaryotes from prokaryotes. The similarity in size and position of a large, silent segment of DNA in the non-alpha globin sequences for rabbit, mouse, and human genes suggests that a mechanism to recognize and delete it from the functional mRNA is relatively ancient.

Flavell et al.[73] have examined the DNA sequence of the Lepore globin gene. It is in fact the product of recombination between misaligned δ-globin and β-globin genes as Baglioni suggested from globin amino acid sequences in 1962.

REFERENCES

1. **Fitch, W. M.,** Evolutionary variability in hemoglobins, *Haematol. Bluttransfus.*, 10, 199, 1972.
2. **Dayhoff, M. O., Hunt, L. T., McLaughlin, P. J., and Jones, D. D.,**Gene duplications in evolution: the globins, in *Atlas of Protein Sequence and Structure 1972*, Dayhoff, M. O. Ed., National Biomedical Research Foundation, Washington, D. C., 1972, 17.
3. **Goodman, M., Moore, G. W., and Matsuda, G.,** Evolution of vertebrate hemoglobin amino acid sequences, in *Isozymes. IV. Genetics and Evolution*, Markert, C. L., Ed., Academic Press, New York, 1975, 181.
4. **Coates, M.,** Hemoglobin function in the vertebrates: an evolutionary model, *Aust. J. Biol. Sci*., 28, 367, 1975.
5. **Lerner, I. M.,** *Heredity, Evolution and Society*, W. H. Freeman, San Francisco, 1968, 22.
6. **Dickerson, R. E.,** The structure and history of an ancient protein, *Sci. Am.*, 226, 58, 1972.
7. **Isaacks, R. E., Harkness, D. R., Goldman, P. H., Adler, J. L., and Kim, C.-Y.,** Studies on avian erythrocyte metabolism. VII. Effect of inositol pentaphosphate and other organic phosphates on oxygen affinity of the embryonic and adult-type hemoglobins of the turkey embryo, *Hemoglobin*, 1, 577, 1977.
8. **Ohno, S.,** *Evolution by Gene Duplication*, Springer-Verlag, New York, 1970, 59.
9. **Boyer, S. H., Smith, K. D., and Noyes, A. N.,** Immunologic purification and characterization of hemoglobin chain-synthesizing polysomes: a derivative hypothesis for regulatory and evolutionary interrelationships in hemoglobin biosynthesis, *Ann. N. Y. Acad. Sci.*, 241, 204, 1974.
10. **Nute, P. E ,** Multiple hemoglobin α-chain loci in monkeys, apes, and man, *Ann. N. Y. Acad. Sci.*, 241, 39, 1974.
11. **Boyer, S. H., Crosby, E. F., Noyes, A. N., Fuller, G. F., Leslie, S. E., Donaldson, L. J., Vrablik, G. R., Schaefer, E. W., Jr., and Thurman, L. F.,** Evolution of primate hemoglobin β and δ chains, *Biochem. Genet.*, 5, 405, 1971.
12. **Huisman, T. H. J.,** Structural aspects of fetal and adult hemoglobins from nonanemic ruminants, *Ann. N. Y. Acad. Sci.*, 241, 392, 1974.
13. **Gilman, J. G.,** Rodent hemoglobin structure: a comparison of several species of mice, *Ann. N. Y. Acad. Sci.*, 241, 416, 1974.
14. **Dhindsa, D. S., Hoversland, A. S., and Templeton, J. W.,** Postnatal changes in oxygen affinity and concentrations of 2,3-diphosphoglycerate in dog blood, *Biol. Neonat.*, 20, 226, 1972.
15. **Novy, M. J., Hoversland, A. S., Koler, R. D., and Metcalfe, J.,** A comparison of oxygen affinity and hemoglobin type in the adult and fetal minitiature pig, *Fed. Proc.*, 26, 485, 1967.
16. **Schroeder , W. A., Huisman, T. H. J., Shelton, J. R., Shelton, J. B., Kleihauer, E. F., Dozy, A. M., and Robberson, B.,** Evidence for multiple structural genes for the γ chain of human fetal hemoglobin, *Proc. Natl. Acad. Sci. U.S.A.*, 60, 537, 1968.
17. **Huisman, T. H. J., Schroeder, W. A., Dozy, A. M., Shelton, J. R. , Shelton, J. B., Boyd, E. M., and Apell, G.,** Evidence for multiple structural genes for the gamma chain of human fetal hemoglobin in hereditary persistance of fetal hemoglobin, *Ann. N. Y. Acad. Sci.*, 165, 320, 1969.
18. **Schroeder, W. A., Huisman, T. H. J., Shelton, J. R., Shelton, J. B., Apell, G., and Bouver, N.,** Heterogeneity of fetal hemoglobin in β-thalassemia of the Negro, *Am. J. Hum. Genet.*, 22, 505, 1970.
19. **Huisman, T. H. J., Schroeder, W. A., Stamatoyannopoulos, G. , Bouver, N., Shelton, J. R., Shelton, J B., and Apell, G.,** Nature of fetal homoglobin in the Greek type of hereditary persistence of fetal hemoglobin with and without concurrent β-thalassemia, *J. Clin. Invest.*, 49, 1035, 1970.
20. **Stamatoyannopoulos, G., Schroeder, W. A., Huisman, T. H. J., Shelton, J. R., Shelton, J. B., Apell, G., and Bouver, N.,** Nature of foetal haemoglobin in F-thalassemia, *Br. J. Haematol.*, 21, 633, 1971.
21. **Schroeder, W. A., Shelton, J. R., Shelton, J. B., Apell, G., Huisman, T. H. J., and Bouver, N. G.,** World-wide occurrence of nonallelic genes for the γ chain of human foetal haemoglobin in newborns, *Nature (London) New Biol*., 240, 273, 1972.
22. **Schroeder, W. A.,** The human γ-chain variants. A review, *Hemoglobin*, 1, 513, 1977.
23. **Huisman, T. H. J., Schroeder, W. A., Bannister, W. H., and Grech, J. L.,** Evidence for four nonallelic structural genes for the γ chain of human fetal hemoglobin, *Biochem. Genet.*, 7, 131, 1972.
24. **Old, J., Clegg, J. B., Weaherall, D. J., Ottolenghi, S., Comi, P., Giglioni, B., Mitchell, J., Tolstoshev, P., and Williamson, R.,** A direct estimate of the number of human γ-globin genes, *Cell*, 8, 13, 1976.
25. **Melderis, H., Steinheider, G., and Ostertag, W.,** Evidence for a unique kind of α-type globin chain in early mammalian embryos, *Nature (London)*, 250, 774, 1974.
26. **Kabat, D. and Koler, R. D.,** The thalassemias: models for analysis of quantitative gene control, *Adv. Hum. Genet.*, 5, 157, 1975.
27. **Bunn, H. F., Forget, B. G., and Ranney, H. M.,** *Human Hemoglobins*, W. B. Saunders, Philadelphia, 1977, 101.

28. Deisseroth, A., Velez, R., and Nienhuis, A. W., Hemoglobin synthesis in somatic cell hybrids: independent segregation of the human alpha- and beta-globin genes, *Science,* 191, 1262, 1976.
29. Price, P. M., Conover, J. H., and Hirschhorn, K., Chromosomal localization of human haemoglobin structural genes, *Nature (London),* 237, 340, 1972.
30. Bishop, J. D. and Jones, K. W., Chromosomal localization of human haemoglobin structural genes, *Nature (London),* 240, 149, 1972.
31. Gandini, E., Dallapiccola, B., Laurent, C., Suerinc, E. F., Forabosco, A., Conconi, F., and Del Senno, L., Evidence for localization of genes for human α-globin on the long arm of chromosome 4, *Nature (London),* 265, 65, 1977.
32. Gerald, P. S. and Diamond, L. K., The diagnosis of thalassemia trait by starch block electrophoresis of the hemoglobin, *Blood,* 13, 61, 1958.
33. Baglioni, C., The fusion of two peptide chains in hemoglobin Lepore and its interpretation as a genetic deletion, *Proc. Natl. Acad. Sci. U.S.A.,* 48, 1880, 1962.
34. Benz, E. J. and Forget, B. G., The molecular genetics of the thalassemia syndromes, in *Progress in Hematology,* Vol. 9, Brown, E. B., Ed., Grune & Stratton, New York, 1975, 107.
35. Huisman, T. H. J., Wrightstone, R. N., Wilson, J. B., and Schroeder, W. A., Hemoglobin Kenya, the product of fusion of γ and β polypeptide chains, *Arch. Biochem. Biophys.,* 153, 850, 1972.
36. Kendall, A. G., Ojwang, P. J., Schroeder, W. A., and Huisman, T. H. J., Hemoglobin Kenya, the product of a γ-β fusion gene: studies of the family, *Am. J. Hum. Genet.,* 25, 548, 1973.
37. Weatherall, D. J. and Clegg, J. B.,*The Thalassemia Syndromes,* 2nd ed., Blackwell Scientific Productions , Oxford, 1972, 176.
38. Boyer, S. H., Rucknagel, D. L., Weatherall, D. J., and Watson-Williams, E. F., Further evidence for linkage between the β and δ loci governing human hemoglobin and the population dynamics of linked genes, *Am. J. Hum. Genet.,* 15, 438, 1963.
39. Hollan, S. R., Szelenyi, J. G., Brimhall, B., Duerst, M., Jones, R. T., Koler, R. D., and Stocklen, Z., Multiple alpha chain loci for human haemoglobins: Hb J-Buda and Hb G-Pest, *Nature (London),* 235, 47, 1972.
40. Brimhall, B., Duerst, M., Hollan, S. R., Stenzel, P., Szelenyi, J., and Jones, R. T., Structural characterizations of hemoglobins J-Buda [α61 (E10) Lys → Asn] and G-Pest [α74 (EF3) Asp → Asn], *Biochim. Biophys. Acta,* 336, 344, 1974.
41. DeJong, W. W. W., Khan, P. M., and Bernini, L. F., Hemoglobin Koya Dora: high frequency of a chain termination mutant, *Am. J. Hum. Genet.,* 27, 81, 1975.
42. Bradley, T. B., Wohl, R. C., and Smith, G. J., Elongation of the α-globin chain in a black family: interaction with Hb G-Philadelphia, *Clin. Res.,* 23 (Abstr.), 131, 1975.
43. Boyer, S. H., Margolet, L., Boyer, M. L., Huisman, T. H. J. , Schroeder, W. A., Wood, W. G., Weatherall, D. J., Clegg, J. B., and Cartner, R., Inheritance of F cell frequency in heterocellular hereditary persistance of fetal hemoglobin: an example of allelic exclusion, *Am. J. Hum. Genet.,* 29, 256, 1977.
44. Pauling, L., Itano, H. A., Singer, S. J., and Wells, I. C., Sickle-cell anemia, a molecular disease, *Science,* 110, 543, 1949.
45. Ingram, V. M., Abnormal human haemoglobins. II. The chemical difference between normal and sickle cell haemoglobins, *Biochim. Biophys. Acta,* 36, 402, 1959.
46. Wrightstone, R. N., International hemoglobin information center, *Hemoglobin,* 1, p. 219, 301, 401' and 601, 1977.
47. Marotta, C. A., Wilson, J. T., Forget, B. G., and Weissman, S. M., Human β-globin messenger RNA. III. Nucleotide sequences derived from complementary DNA, *J. Biol. Chem.,* 252, 5040, 1977.
48. Wilson, J. T., de Riel, J. K., Forget, B. G., Marotta, C. A., and Weissman, S. M., Nucleotide sequence of 3′ untranslated portion of human alpha globin mRNA, *Nucleic Acid Res.,* 4, 2353, 1977.
49. Wilson, J. T., Marotta, C. A., Forget, B. G., and Weissman, S. M., Structure of human hemoglobin messenger RNA and its relation to hemoglobinopathies, *Trans. Am. Assoc. Phys.,* 1977, in press.
50. Perutz, M. F., Stereochemistry of cooperative effects in haemoglobin, *Nature (London),* 228, 726, 1970.
51. Perutz, M. F , The Bohr effect and combination with organic phosphates, *Nature (London),* 228, 734, 1970.
52. Perutz, M. F., Nature of haem-haem interaction, *Nature (London) New Biol.,* 237, 495, 1972.
53. Arnone, A., X-Ray diffraction study of binding of 2,3-diphosphoglycerate to human deoxyhaemoglobin, *Nature (London),* 237, 146, 1972.
54. Koler, R. D., Human hemoglobin mutations, *Ann. N. Y. Acad. Sci.,* 241, 736, 1974.
55. Perutz, M. F. and Lehmann, H., Molecular pathology of human haemoglobin, *Nature (London),* 219, 902, 1968.
56. Jones, R. T., Koler, R. D., Duerst, M., and Stocklen, Z., Hemoglobin Casper, G8 β106 Leu → Pro: further evidence that hemoglobin mutations are not random, in *Hemoglobin and Red Cell Structure and Function,* Brewer, G., Ed., Plenum Publishing, New York, 1972, 79.

57. Winslow, R. M., Swenberg, M. L., Gross, E., Hemoglobin McKees Rock ($\alpha_2\beta_2$ $^{145\ Tyr \rightarrow Term}$). A human "nonsense" mutation leading to a shortened β-chain, *J. Clin. Invest.*, 57, 772, 1976.
58. Clegg, J. B., Weatherall, D. J., and Milner, P. F., Haemoglobin Constant Spring. A chain termination mutant? *Nature (London)*, 234, 337, 1971.
59. Huisman, T. H. J., Wilson, J. B., Gravely, M., and Hubbard M., Hemoglobin Grady: the first example of a variant with elongated chains due to an insertion of residues, *Proc. Natl. Acad. Sci. U.S.A.*, 71, 3270, 1974.
60. Ricco, G., Mazza, U., Turi, R. M., Pich, P. G., Camaschella, C., Saglio, G., and Bernini, L. F., Significance of a new type of human fetal hemoglobin carrying a replacement isoleucine → threonine at position 75 (E19) of the γ chain, *Hum. Genet.*, 32, 305, 1976.
61. Deisseroth, A., Nienhuis, A., Turner, P., Velez, R., and Anderson, W. F., Localization of the human α-globin structural gene to chromosome 16 in somatic cell hybrids by molecular hybridization assay, *Cell*, 12, 205, 1977.
62. Diesseroth, A., Nienhuis, A., Ruddle, F., Lawrence, J., and Turner, P., Chromosomal localization of the human β globin gene to human chromosome 11, *Blood*, 50 (Suppl. 1), 105, 1977.
63. Milner, P. F. and Huisman, T. H. J., Studies on the proportion and synthesis of haemoglobin G Philadelphia in red cells of heterozygotes, a homozygote, and a heterozygote for both haemoglobin G and α thalassemia, *Br. J. Haematol.*, 34, 207, 1976.
64. Baine, R. M , Rucknagel, D. L., Dublin, P. A., Jr., and Adams, J. G., Trimodality in the proportion of hemoglobin G Philadelphia in heterozygotes: evidence for heterogeneity in the number of human α chain loci , *Proc. Natl. Acad. Sci. U.S.A.*, 73, 3633, 1976.
65. Abramson, R. K., Rucknagel, D. L., Schreffler, D. C , and Saave, J. J., Homozygous Hb J Tongariki: evidence for only one α chain structural locus in Melanesians, *Science*, 169, 194, 1970.
66. Huisman, T. H. J., Trimodality in the percentages of β chain variants in heterozygotes: the effect of the number of active Hb α structural loci, *Hemoglobin*, 1, 349, 1972.
67. Jeffreys, A. J. and Flavell, R. A., The rabbit β-globin gene contains a large insert in the coding sequence, *Cell*, 12, 1097, 1977.
68. Tilghman, S. M., Tiemeier, D. C., Seidman, J. G., Peterlin, B. M., Sullivan, M., Maizel, J. V., and Leder, P., Intervening sequence of DNA identified in the structural portion of a mouse β-globin gene, *Proc. Natl. Acad. Sci. U.S.A.*, 75, 725, 1978.
69. Mears, J. G., Ramirez, F., Liebowitz, D., and Bank, A., Organization of human δ-dash and β-dash globin genes in cellular DNA and the presence of intragenic inserts, *Cell*, 15, 15, 1978.
70. Smithies, O., Blechl, A. E., Thompson, K. D., Newell, N., Richards, J. E., Slightom, J. L., Tucker, P. W., and Blattner, F. R., Cloning human fetal γ-globin and mouse α-type globin DNA: characterization and partial sequencing, *Science*, 202, 1279, 1978.
71. Darnell, J. E., Jr., Implications of RNA·RNA splicing in evolution of eukaryotic cells, *Science*, 202, 1257, 1978.
72. Blanchard, J-M., Weber, J., Jelenik, W., and Darnell, J. E., Jr., *In vitro* RNA·RNA splicing in adenovirus 2 formation, *Proc. Natl. Acad. Sci. U.S.A.*, 75, 5344, 1978.
73. Flavell, R. A., Kooter, J. M., DeBoer, E., Little, P. F. R., and Williamson, R., Analysis of the β-δ-globin gene loci in normal and Hb Lepore DNA: direct determination of gene linkage and intergene distance, *Cell*, 15, 25, 1978.

THE CHROMATOGRAPHY OF HEMOGLOBIN

William P. Winter

Introduction

Of the methods available to the investigator for separating hemoglobin either from nonhemoglobin proteins or from other hemoglobin types, some form of ion exchange chromatography is most often the method of choice. Preparative electrophoresis is capable of yielding high purity hemoglobin preparations, but the amount of material which can be accommodated per run is small and the dilution factor is large, necessitating a concentration step after the run. Isoelectric focusing affords very high purity and can be adapted to preparative runs, as can polyacrylamide gel electrophoresis. However, in most cases chromatography remains the quickest, simplest, and most economical method to obtain large quantities of specific hemoglobins.

Ion exchange chromatography refers to any liquid chromatography system in which the molecules being separated are partitioned between a soluble and an insoluble ion of the opposite charge to that of the molecule whose purification is desired. Generally, all molecular species in the sample — hemoglobins in this discussion — start out bound to the column, i.e., to the insoluble ion. When the conditions are adjusted, usually either pH or ionic strength, the equilibrium is shifted so that the hemoglobin dissociates from the stationary ion and associates with the soluble or mobile ion. The value of the equilibrium constant for this reaction for any hemoglobin type is a function of the hemoglobin net surface charge or pK_a and hence, a separation occurs. The actual value of the equilibrium constant or the pK_a is of little practical consequence in the purification.

Three other types of chromatography are in widespread use although their applications in hemoglobin purification are somewhat limited. These are gel filtration, affinity chromatography, and paper chromatography. Paper chromatography has no current applications in hemoglobin purification. It is used in fingerprinting tryptic peptides of hemoglobin in the course of structural studies, but that goes beyond the scope of this chapter. For a discussion, see Winter and Rucknagel.[66]

Since gel filtration entails a separation based on molecular size,[1] this technique has relatively little application in hemoglobin work. The variant Hb Porto Alegro, (β 9 Ser → Cys) forms dimers of tetramers (octomers) which separate well from Hb A on gel filtration with Sephadex G-100.[2] Sephadex G-75 has also been used to separate free hemoglobin subunits, primarily α subunits, from hemoglobin tetramers.[3] Occasionally, a sample may be encountered in which extensive hemolysis has taken place before the plasma was removed. Gel filtration on Sephadex G-200 can be used in such cases to separate hemoglobin from the plasma proteins.[4]

Affinity chromatography[5] similarly has relatively few applications in hemoglobin chromatography. Affinity chromatography of heme-proteins has been reported,[6] but the technique was designed for separating heme-proteins from nonheme proteins and requires the conversion of heme proteins to their apo-form. A novel method based on affinity chromatography has been devised for the purification of high oxygen affinity variants.[7] With this method, the exposure of SH groups in high affinity hemoglobin variants, which results from their being stabilized in the R conformational state, is used as the basis of their separation from Hb A.

Choice of Ion Exchanger

There are two primary considerations in choosing an ion exchange medium: the exchange properties (anionic vs. cationic) and the properties of the polymer or resin. The term "resin" in this context is technically inappropriate since it is borrowed from the synthetic polymer field and does not apply to natural carbohydrate polymers whose use is quite widespread. However, the term is in wide use in this context and will be used in this discussion to denote polymeric material, natural or synthetic, which forms the insoluble matrix for ion exchange chromatography.

There are few firm rules to guide the user in choosing between anionic and cationic exchangers. Some investigators prefer to have the hemoglobin of interest elute first from the column. This would dictate an anion exchanger such as DEAE for hemoglobins, S, C, E, D, G, O, and other slow* types but a cation exchanger such as CM for hemoglobins J, I, H, and other fast variants. However, the quality of the separation is of paramount importance and should be the first consideration in selecting an ion exchange media. In general, DEAE probably is the best, and it is the most widely used. However, for the separation of hemoglobin A_2 from slow-moving variants such as hemoglobin C, C-Harlem, O-Arab, O-Indonesia, and Agenogi, CM is the medium of choice.

There are three basic types of resin to choose from: cellulose, dextran, and polystyrene. As a rule, polystyrene-based resins (Dowex®, Amberlite®, Aminex®, and Duolite®) do not work well for chromatography of proteins. An important exception to this is Amberlite® IRC-50 (BioRex®-70) which gives superb separation of some hemoglobins. In most polystyrene resins, however, the cross-linked beads have pores which are extremely small and are not well penetrated by macromolecules. Thus most of the exchange groups are inaccessible to the proteins. Moreover, there is some evidence that proteins on the surface are denatured, and the resin is extremely slow in coming to equilibrium with the starting buffer. For this reason, the Amberlite® is most often used in conjunction with equilibrium elution where there is no change in the buffer pH or ionic strength during the course of elution.

The cyclic dextrans (Sephadex®) are natural carbohydrate polymers produced by bacteria of the genus *Leuconostoc* which are available as ion exchange resins, both anion (A) and cation (C) exchangers, in two porosity grades, 50 and 25. For protein chromatography, the A-50 or C-50 (anion and cation exchangers, respectively) are the desired grades. DEAE and CM Sephadex yield very good, high resolution separations. The principal drawbacks to Sephadex in comparison to cellulose are the initial swelling time, the annoying tendency of the swollen Sephadex to stick to glassware, sinks, pH electrodes, etc., and the striking volume changes it undergoes as the result of pH or ionic strength changes (Figures 1 and 2). Both DEAE Sephadex and CM Sephadex shrink to about half their original volume in going from 0.01 to 0.5 ionic strength. DEAE Sephadex shrinks with increasing pH, while CM Sephadex expands under the same conditions. Volume changes in turn lower the flow rate by increasing the resistance to flow; if the column is being pumped, this often results in the build-up of excessive back pressure, compression of the resin bed, and ultimately the complete cessation of flow with concommitant "blow-out" of the supply lines on the high pressure side.

Cellulose ion exchangers are available in several grades according to the uniformity of the particle dimensions. The best grade — microgranular — has high uniformity and an expanded fibril structure which maximizes the exposure of the charged groups to the solvent. Cellulose requires no significant swelling time to rehydrate and does not exhibit any swelling or shrinking during the run. The Whatman Company produces a grade called CM 52 or DE 52 which has never been dried and hence, needs no rehydrating at all. It is considered by many to be the grade of choice for high resolution separations although it is somewhat more costly than the dry grades CM 32 or DE 32 (Figures 3 and 4).

An ion exchanger with properties similar to both cellulose and Sephadex is the newly

* "Slow" and "fast" in this context refer to the rate of migration relative to Hb A on electrophoresis at alkaline pH.

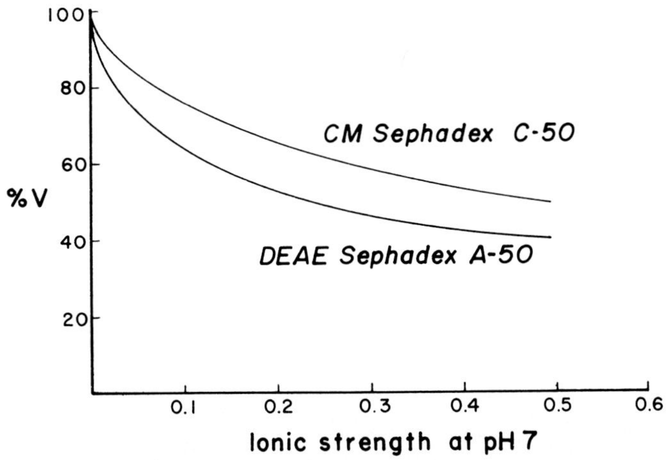

FIGURE 1. Effect of ionic strength on the column volume of ion exchange Sephadexes at pH 7. The volume at ionic strength 0.01 has arbitrarily been taken as 100%. (Redrawn from manufacturer's data.)

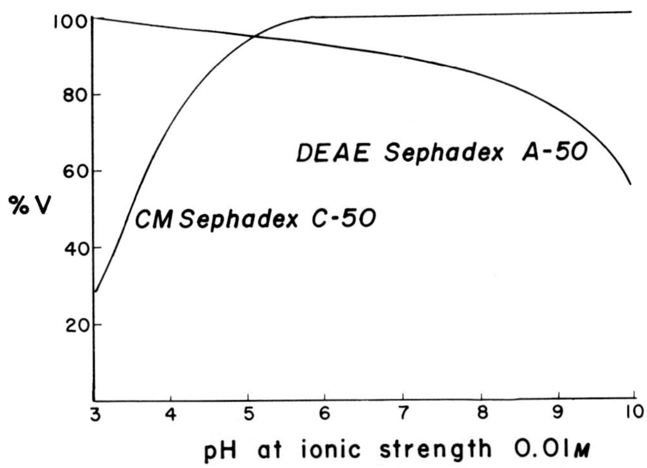

FIGURE 2. Effect of pH on the column volume of ion exchange Sephadexes at ionic strength 0.01. The volume of DEAE Sephadex was taken to be 100% at pH 3 while that of CM Sephadex was taken as 100% at pH 10. (Redrawn from manufacturer's data.)

introduced DEAE-Sephacel (Pharmacia). This material is a beaded cellulose gel matrix which, according to the manufacturer, possesses flow properties superior to either Sephadex or cellulose. Because of its very recent introduction onto the market, no reported applications of this ion exchanger for hemoglobin purification have appeared in the literature. However, the material appears to hold considerable promise.

Choice of Buffer

In theory any buffer system capable of maintaining the pH should be usable in ion exchange chromatography. However, the rule of thumb is that best results can be obtained by using cationic buffers (Tris-HCl, etc.) with anion exchangers and anionic buffers (phosphate, acetate, etc.) with cation exchangers. As previously explained, the reason for this is that elution from an ion exchange column is the result of the competition between the stationary ion and a mobile ion of the same charge for association with the protein. Thus, in a DEAE column, Tris is a better cation to compete with

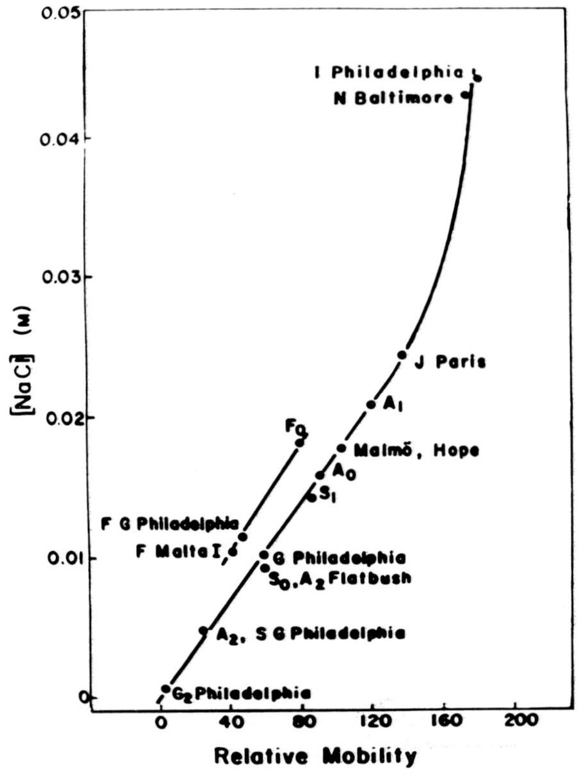

FIGURE 3. Chromatographic properties of selected hemoglobin variants of DE-52 in glycine-NaCl buffers. The abcissa is relative electrophoretic mobility on cellulose acetate at alkaline pH. The mobility of Hb A is taken arbitrarily as 100. Ordinant gives NaCl concentration in milliosmolarity. (Redrawn from Abraham, E. C., Reese, A., Stallings, M., and Huisman, T. H. J., *Hemoglobin,* 1, 27, 1976.)

DEAE than is, for example, sodium which would be the cation if sodium phosphate or acetate were used. However, this is not a ''hard'' rule and there are some examples in the literature in which phosphate buffers have been used with great success in DEAE columns.

In a recent article, a novel buffer system was reported to have widespread applicability with DEAE cellulose in the purification of hemoglobins.[8] A high resolution and compact symmetrical zones have been described. The buffer is 0.2 M glycine, 0.01% KCN, pH 7.7—7.9. Varying amounts of NaCl [0.005 M (0.293 g/ℓ) to 0.2 M (11.7 g/ℓ)] are added to eluting buffers. From the standpoint of convenience, the buffers are attractive since the zwitterionic glycine is a natural buffer and requires no pH adjustment. However, as was pointed out in the discussion of Sephacel, no reported applications outside of an original report have appeared. Hence, it is too early to determine whether this buffer will prove superior to others.

An important — in fact essential — consideration in choosing a buffer is that its pH lies below the pK of the resin for anion exchangers or above it for cation exchangers. If DEAE cellulose is used at pH 10, for example, the ion exchange groups will be almost totally uncharged and binding capacity of the resin will be greatly reduced. Titration curves of typical anion and cation exchangers are shown in Figures 5, 6, and 7.

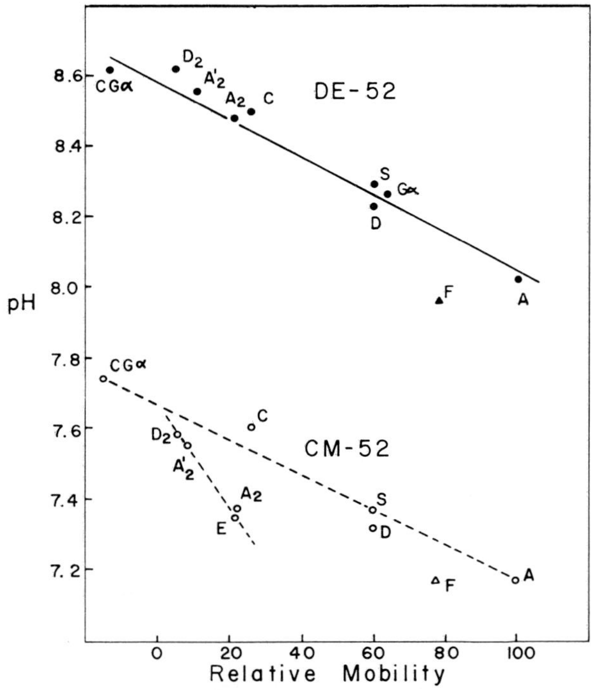

FIGURE 4. Relationship between chromatographic behavior and electrophoretic mobility of selected hemoglobin variants. Electrophoresis is indicated on the abcissa as relative mobility on cellulose acetate at alkaline pH. Hb A = 100. Chromatography was carried out on preswollen microgranular celluloses DE-52 and CM-52 in tris and phosphate buffers, respectively. (Redrawn from Huisman, T. H. J., *Standardization of Laboratory Reagents and Methods for Detection of Hemoglobinopathies,* Schmidt, R. M., Huisman, T. H. J., and Lehmann, M., Eds., CRC Press, Cleveland, 1974, 73.)

Gradients

In theory, the number of column volumes of starting buffer required to elute a protein is equal to the equilibrium constant for the association of the proteins to the immobile phase. If this value is on the order of 1,000 or greater, as is often the case, the volume of starting buffer required to effect an elution would be prohibitively large. Therefore, it is convenient to bring about the elution of the protein by gradually changing the properties of the buffer to lower the equilibrium constants to a value of approaching 1. Under these conditions, the elution of the protein becomes rapid and quantitative.

Numerous types of gradients have been used successfully in hemoglobin chromatography. One of the simplest gradients to construct and use is a 2-chamber gradient (Figure 8). If the vessels are of equal size and identical shape, the gradient will be linear in concentration from the buffer in chamber 1 (the mixing chamber) to that in chamber 2 (the reservoir). If the volumes or shapes are not identical, the instantaneous concentration can be calculated from Equation 1.

$$C_{(t)} = C_2 - (C_2 - C_1)(1 - V)\, A_2/A_1$$

where $C_{(t)}$ = concentration at time t, C_2 = reservoir concentration, C_1 = initial concentration in mixing vessel, V = volume fraction used at time t, and A_2/A_1 = ratio of cross-sectional areas of reservoir (A_2) and mixer (A_1).

The most commonly employed gradients are pH gradients. While in most cases a linear pH change is desired, a simple 2-chamber gradient between two pH values is

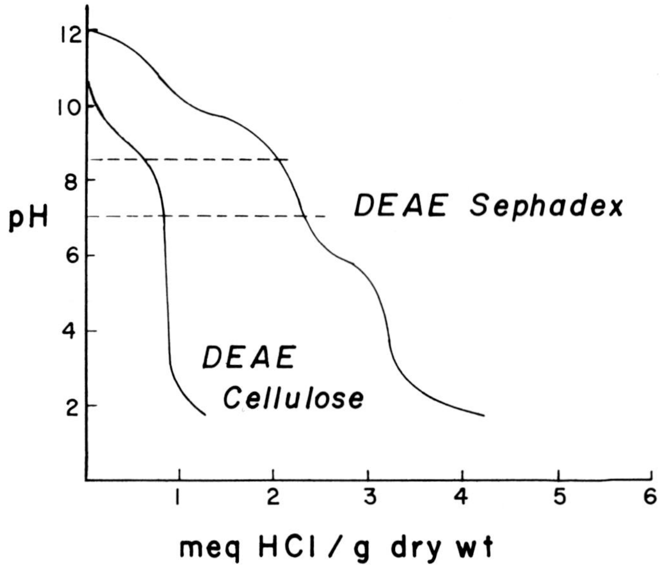

FIGURE 5. Titration curves of diethylaminoethyl ion exchangers. The broken lines indicate the pH range over which the exchangers are normally used. The apparently greater binding capacity of the Sephadex is offset by the much greater water regain of that resin. (Redrawn from manufacturer's data.)

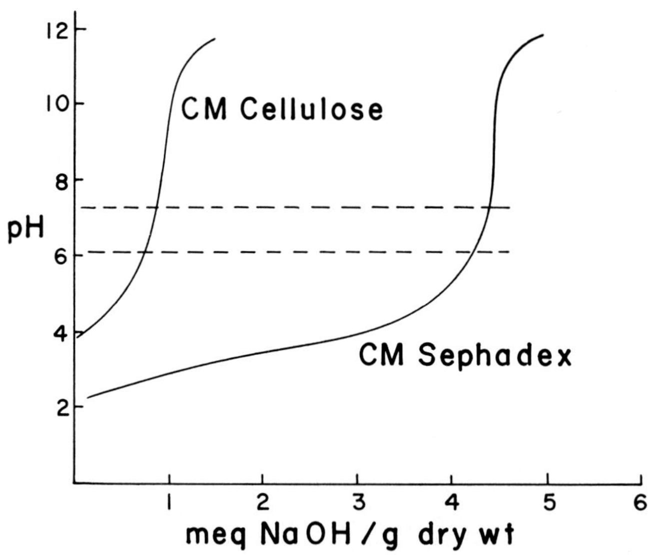

FIGURE 6. Titration curves of carboxymethyl ion exchangers. The broken lines indicate the pH range over which the exchangers are normally used. The apparently greater binding capacity of the Sephadex is offset by the much greater water regain of that resin. (Redrawn from manufacturer's data.)

often unsatisfactory because the capacities of the two buffers may differ. The result is a gradient which tends to maintain the pH of the buffer at higher capacity. Therefore, an approach linearity is employed either by a multichamber gradient or by a series of convex gradients using different limit buffers which are changed at specified times. In the use of the multichamber gradient a Varigrad or its equivalent is employed.[9] The

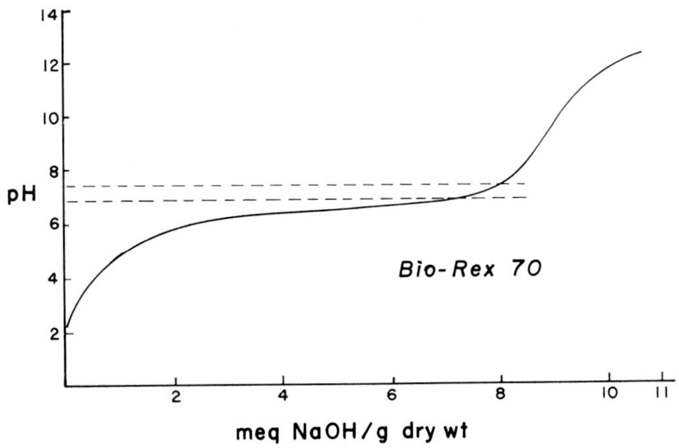

FIGURE 7. Titration curve of carboxymethylated polystyrene resin. A similar curve would be obtained from other resins of this group such as Amberlite IRC-50 and CG-50. (Redrawn from manufacturer's data.)

chambers are filled with buffers approximately 0.2 pH units apart. A typical multi-chamber gradient for DEAE column involves buffers at pH 8.3, 8.1, 7.9, 7.7, 7.5, 7.3, 7.1, 6.9, and 6.7. Equal volumes of each are generally used.

In the multiple convex gradient, a closed mixing chamber is constructed as shown in Figure 9. The chamber is filled with starting buffer, and the reservoir vessel is filled with a second buffer. The column is started, and after a specified volume has passed through the column (most readily measured as a time interval at constant flow rate), the buffer in the reservoir is replaced by a third buffer. A typical schedule of reservoir buffers and changeover times is shown in Table 1. For use with anion exchangers (DEAE), decreasing pH gradients are used; for use with cation exchangers (CM), rising pH gradients are used. Salt gradients are always rising gradients whether they are used with anion or cation exchangers.

Sample Preparation

The sample should be in solution in a buffer whose pH and ionic strength are close to or identical with that of the column. In order to promote good binding to the top of the bed, the sample pH may be slightly higher (for anion exchangers) or lower (for cation exchangers) than that of the column. For example DEAE columns are often equilibrated at pH 8.3 with the sample prepared at pH 8.5

The best general method for sample preparation is dialysis. This ensures that, within differences due to Donnan equilibrium, the pH and ionic strength will be that which is desired. However, if time does not permit lengthy dialysis, the sample may be diluted in the starting buffer to approximate the correct values. There is no advantage to highly concentrated samples in ion exchange chromatography; in fact, a more dilute sample may have better flow properties and may be easier to apply.

Column Size

In ion exchange chromatography, the column dimensions are much less critical than in gel filtration, where a pure equilibrium process is taking place. Length-to-diameter ratios of 10:1 to 20:1 are generally satisfactory, and highly satisfactory results can often be obtained with even shorter columns. However, to achieve desired resolution, still higher length-to-diameter ratios such as 50:1 or 60:1 are frequently specified. Table 2 gives some frequently specified column dimensions together with typical applications

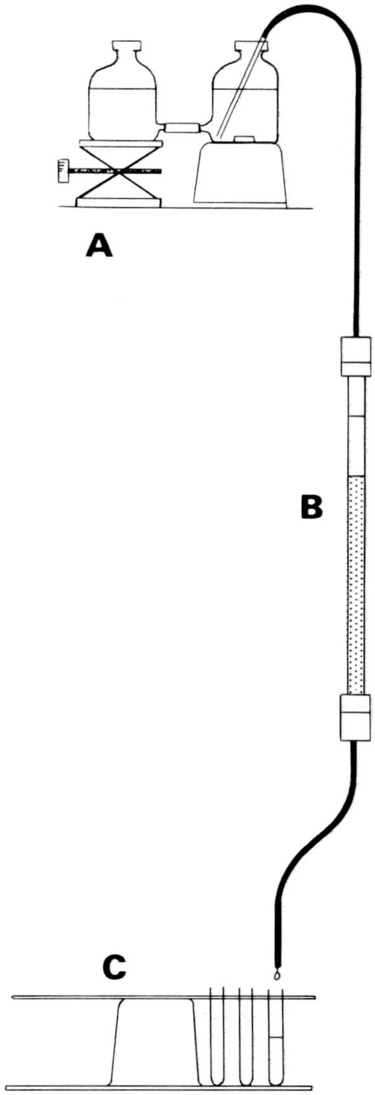

FIGURE 8. Typical equipment assembly for gravity flow chromatography: (A) linear gradient mixer, (B) column, and (C) fraction collector.

of columns of that size and the approximate sample size of hemoglobin accommodated on such columns.

In general, in modifying an existing column to achieve desired results, or in designing a column system for a particular application, the following rules apply to choice of dimensions:[10]

1. The sample capacity is proportional to the *square* of the column diameter. It is largely unaffected by length.
2. The flow rate is proportional to the *square* of the column diameter for any constant bed height.
3. The resolution (relative separation between peaks) is proportional to the *square root* of the bed height.
4. The pressure is proportional to the bed height.

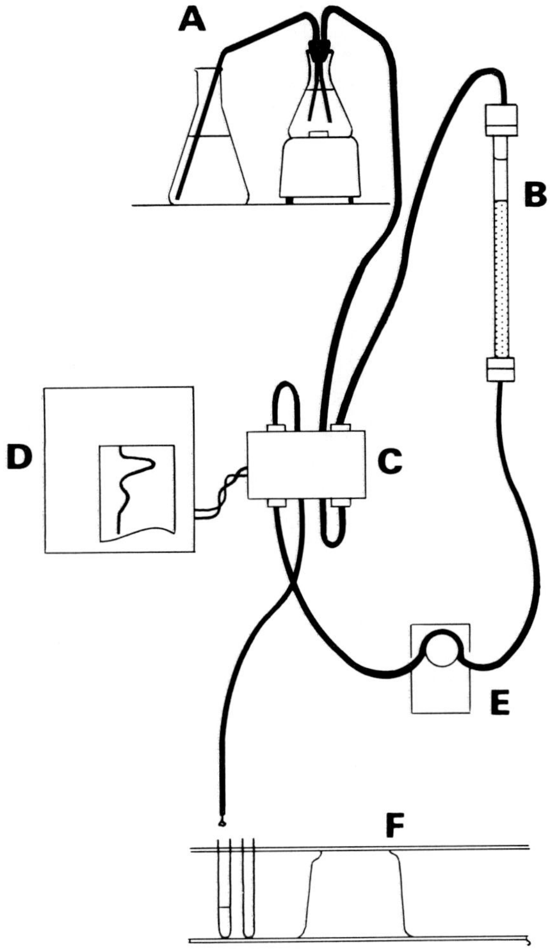

FIGURE 9. Typical equipment assembly for pumped chromatography: (A) constant volume gradient mixer, (B) column, (C) monitor, (D) recorder, (E) pump, and (F) fraction collector. Note that in this assembly, the pump is *below* the column generating a *negative* pressure on the bottom of the column.

Thus if one wished to double the sample load with little or no loss of resolution, he should increase the column diameter by the $\sqrt{2}$, keep the bed height constant, and allow for a doubling of the flow rate at the same back pressure. The total volume of buffer would also be approximately doubled.

Column Preparation

In order to produce satisfactory and reproducible columns, careful attention must be given to the preparation of the columns. Generally, manufacturer's directions for the preparation and the equilibration of the resin of choice should be followed. It is important to realize that equilibration has been achieved only when the pH and ionic strength of the buffer flowing into a column are exactly equal to the pH and ionic strength of the buffer leaving the column. The use of high concentrations of acid or base to adjust the pH in equilibrating ion exchange resins must be avoided. If an exchanger is being equilibrated at pH 8.5 in 0.05 M tris HCl buffer, for example, and it becomes necessary to raise the pH, this may be done by adding 0.05 M tris HCl buffer or simply 0.05 M tris. Adjustment with 1 M tris or, worse yet, with NaOH will change

Table 1
SCHEDULE OF BUFFER CHANGES FOR CONSTANT VOLUME MIXING CHAMBER GRADIENT

	Column diameter and flow rate		
V_i	0.9 cm @ 15 mℓ/hr	15 cm @ 25 mℓ/hr	Change buffer reservoir to:
After	55[a] mℓ (3.6 hr)[a]	110[a] mℓ (4.6 hr)	pH 7.7
After	130 mℓ (8.6 hr)	260 mℓ (10.6 hr)	pH 7.4
After	425 mℓ (28.3 hr)	850 mℓ (34 hr)	pH 7.0
After	550 mℓ (36.6 hr)	1100 mℓ (44 hr)	pH 6.5[b]

Note: In constant volume mixing chamber (For details of gradient assembly, see Figure 9.) V_i pH 8.3 buffer. (All buffers are 0.05 M Tris HCl containing 10^{-4} M EDTA and 0.01% KCN) In reservoir: pH 8.0 buffer.

[a] Times and volumes are cumulative rather than interval.
[b] Continue with the final buffer until the column is fully developed.

Table 2
SOME FREQUENTLY SPECIFIED COLUMN DIMENSIONS, THEIR TYPICAL APPLICATIONS, APPROXIMATE SAMPLE SIZE OF HEMOGLOBIN ACCOMODATED ON SUCH COLUMNS, AND APPROXIMATE FLOW RATE

Column size				
Diameter (cm)	Length (cm)	Application	Sample size (mg)	Approximate flow rate (cc/hr)
0.5	6—8	Microanalytical	2—5	25
0.9—1.0	30—50	Analytical or small scale prep	50—100	15—25
1.8—2.0	35	Prep	100—200	75—90
5.0	35	Large scale prep	300—500	500—600

the ionic strength of the buffer and may adversely affect the performance of the column.

In packing a column, best results will be achieved when the bed is uniform, both from top to bottom and side to side. Channeling, hard spots, cracks, air bubbles, and other irregularities are to be assiduously avoided. The problem of irregularities is relatively minor in small columns (1.5 cm diameter or smaller) but is greatly magnified in large columns. The best slurry from which to pour the column is a 1:1 or 50% slurry in which after a reasonable time (30 min) the settled resin volume (depth) approximately equals the supernatant volume (depth).

In order to avoid air entrapment, it is advisable to place a few centimeters of buffer in the column and open the bottom briefly so as to fill the dead space with liquid. The slurry is then poured. If an extension tube can be arranged, the whole bed may be poured at once. Otherwise, at intervals before the bed has settled, clear supernatant is aspirated and more slurry is added. When the bed is partially settled, the drain is opened and packing is begun. When the packing is complete, the column is run at flow rate or pressure head to be used until the bed is stabilized. The effluent pH should be checked and compared with that of the initial buffer.

REFERENCES FOR TABLES 4 TO 10

a. Huisman, T. H. J. and Dozy, A. M. M., *Chromatography,* 19, 160, 1965.
b. Dozy, A. M. J., Kleihauer, T., and Huisman, T. H. J., *J. Chromatogr.,* 32, 723, 1968.
c. Huisman, T. H. J. and Meyring, C. A., *Clin. Chem. Acta,* 5, 103, 1960.
d. Allen, D. W., Schroeder, W. A., and Balog, J., *J. Am. Chem. Soc.,* 80, 1628, 1958.
e. Jones, R. T. and Schroeder, W. A. J., *Chromatography,* 10, 421, 1963.
f. Huisman, T. H. J. and Prins, H. K., *J. Lab. Clin. Med.,* 46, 255, 1955.
g. Ranney, H. M., Nagel, R., Heller, P., and Udem, L., *Biochim. Biophys. Acta,* 160, 112, 1968.
h. Efremov, G. D., Huisman, T. H. J., Bowman, K., and Wrightstone, R. N., *J. Lab. Clin. Med.,* 83, 657, 1974.
i. Chernoff, A. I., Pettit, N., and Northrop, O., *J. Blood,* 25, 646, 1965.
j. Charache, S., Weatherall, D. J., and Clegg, J. B., *J. Clin. Invest.,* 45, 813, 1966.
k. Hayashi, A., Suzuki, T., Schimizu, T., and Yamamura, Y., *Biochim. Biophys. Acta,* 160, 262, 1968.
l. Vettore, L., DeSandre, G., Dilorio, E. E., Winterhalter, K. H., Lan, A., and Lehman, K., *Blood,* 44, 869, 1974.
m. Van Ros, G., Beale, D., and Lehmann, H., *Br. Med. J.,* 4, 92, 1968.
n. Bromberg, P. A., Alben, J. O., Bare, G. H., Balcerzak, S. P., Jones, R. T., Brimhall, B., and Padilla, F., *Nature London New Biol.,* 243, 177, 1973.
o. Jensen, M., Oski, F. A., Nathan, D. G., and Bunn, H. F., *J. Clin. Invest.,* 55, 469, 1975.
p. Huisman, T. H. J., Martis, E. A., and Dozy, A. M., *J. Lab. Clin. Med.* 52, 312, 1958.
q. Clegg, M. D. and Schroeder, W. A., *J. Am. Chem. Soc.,* 81, 6065, 1959.
r. Dozy, A. M. and Huisman, T. H. J., *J. Chromatogr.,* 40, 62, 1969.
s. Bernini, L. F., *Biochem. Genet.,* 2, 305, 1969.
t. Bonaventura, J. and Riggs, A., *J. Biol. Chem.,* 243, 980, 1968.
u. Huisman, T. H. J., *Standardization of Laboratory Reagents and Methods for Detection of Hemoglobinopathies,* Schmidt, R. M., Huisman, T. H. J., and Lehmann, H., Eds., CRC Press, Cleveland, 1974, 73.
v. Abraham, E. C., Reese, A., Stallings, M., and Huisman, T. H. J., *Hemoglobin,* 1, 27, 1976.
w. Ahern, E., Holder, W., Ahern, V., Serjeant, G. R., Serjeant, B. E., Forbes, M., Brimhall, B., and Jones, R. T., *Biochim. Biophys. Acta,* 393, 188, 1975.

Table 5
CHROMATOGRAPHY OF HEMOGLOBIN S-LIKE VARIANTS

Variant	Substitution	Ref.	Chromatography system	Ref.
Ottawa	α 15 gly → arg	19	DEAE Sephadex A-50	a
Arya	α 47 asp → asn	20	DEAE Sephadex A-50	a
Hasharon	α 47 asp → his	21	DEAE Sephadex A-50	a
			IRC-50	f
Shimonoseki	α 54 glu → arg	22	CG-50	d
L Persian Gulf	α 57 gly → lys	23	IRC-50	f
Daneshgan Tehran	α 72 his → arg	24	DEAE Cellulose	a
G Taichung	α 74 asp → his	25	DEAE Sephadex A-50	a
Q Iran	α 75 asp → his	25	DEAE Sephadex A-50	a
Stanleyville II	α 78 asn → lys	26	IRC-50	m
G Norfolk	α 85 asp → asn	27	DEAE Sephadex A-50	a
G Georgia	α 95 pro → leu	69	DEAE Cellulose	v
Chiapas	α 114 pro → arg	28	IRC-50	e
Bibba	α 136 leu → pro	29	DEAE Sephadex A-50	a, b
S	β 6 glu → val	—	DEAE Cellulose	v
D Iran	β 22 glu → gln	30	DEAE Cellulose	a
Alabama	β 39 gln → lys	31	DEAE Sephadex A-50	a
D Ibadan	β 87 thr → lys	32	IRC-50	f
Tours	β 87 thr → O	33	Biorex-70	k
D Punjab	β 121 glu → gln	34	DEAE Cellulose	a
Richmond	β 102 asn → lys	35	DEAE Sephadex A-50	a, b

Table 6
CHROMATOGRAPHY OF HEMOGLOBIN A-LIKE VARIANTS

Variant	Substitution	Ref.	Chromatography system	Ref.
Aida	α 64 asp → asn	36	DEAE Sephadex A-50	—
Rampa	α 95 pro → ser	37	DEAE Cellulose	s
Denmark Hill	α 95 pro → ala	38	CM Sephadex C-50	r
St. Lukes	α 95 pro → arg	39	DEAE Sephadex A-50	a
Athens-Georgia	β 40 arg → lys	71	DEAE Cellulose	v
M Saskatoon	β 63 his → tyr	40, 41	Biorex-70, CG-50	g
M Milwaukee	β 67 his → tyr	41, 42	CG-50, Biorex-70	g
M Hyde Park	β 92 his → tyr	43	CG-50	—
Malmö	β 97 his → gln	70	DEAE Cellulose	v
Kansas	β 102 asn → thr	44	CM Cellulose	t
San Diego	β 109 val → met	45	CM Sephadex C-50	a
Hope	β 136 gly → asp	46	IRC-50, DEAE Cellulose	f, v
Little Rock	β 143 his → gln	47	CM Cellulose	n
Syracuse	β 143 his → pro	48	CM Cellulose	o

Table 7
CHROMATOGRAPHY OF HEMOGLOBIN J-LIKE VARIANTS

Variant	Substitution	Ref.	Chromatographic system	Ref.
J Paris	α 12 ala → asp	72	DEAE Cellulose	v
J Kurosh	α 19 ala → asp	49	DEAE Sephadex A-50	a
J Nyanza	α 21 ala → asp	50	DEAE Sephadex A-50	a
Norfolk	α 57 gly → asp	51	CM Cellulose	c
Lyon	β 17, 18 lys,val → O	52	Biorex-70	q
J Sicilia	β 65 lys → asn	53	DEAE Sephadex A-50	a
J Cairo	β 65 lys → gln	54	DEAE Sephadex A-50	—
J Chicago	β 76 ala → asp	55	DEAE Sephadex A-50	b
J Habana	β 71 ala → glu	56	DEAE Sephadex A-50	a
J Meerut	β 120 ala → glu	57	DEAE Sephadex A-50	a

Table 8
CHROMATOGRAPHY OF HEMOGLOBIN I-LIKE VARIANTS

Variant	Substitution	Ref.	Chromatography system	Ref.
I	α 16 lys → glu	58	CM Cellulose, DEAE Cellulose	p, v
Nagasaki	β 17 lys → glu	59	CM Cellulose	p, q
Hikari	β 61 lys → asn	60	IRC-50	f
N Baltimore	β 95 lys → glu	11	DEAE Cellulose	v

an example of one possible way — not as the only way or even the best way — in which the equipment could be arranged. The investigator should use these drawings as guides and adapt whatever equipment he has at hand to the job.

Table 9
CHROMATOGRAPHY OF MINOR HEMOGLOBIN TYPES

Hemoglobin	Chain notation	Ref.	Chromatography system	Ref.
Portland	$\xi_2\gamma_2$	61, 62	DEAE Sephadex A-50	a
A_2	$\alpha_2\delta_2$	—	DEAE Cellulose	a, v
F	$\alpha_2\gamma_2$	—	CM Sephadex, DEAE Cellulose	b, r, u, v
Kenya	$\alpha_2\gamma\beta_2$	63	DEAE Sephadex A-50	b
Lepore	$\alpha_2\delta\beta_2$	—	DEAE Cellulose, DEAE Sephadex A-50	a
Constant Spring	α Extension	64	IRC-50	d
Icaria	α Extension	65	IRC-50	d
F Port Royal	g_γ 125 glu → ala		CM Sephadex C-50	r

Table 10
COMPOSITION AND PROPERTIES OF THE SCHROEDER DEVELOPERS (d,q)

Number	pH @ 25°C	Na^+ (M)	KCN (M)	$NaH_2PO_4\,H_2O$* g/4 L	Na_2HPO_4* g/4 L	KCN g/4 L
1	7.22 ± 0.02	0.075	0.01	13.80	14.20	2.6
2	7.18 ± 0.02	0.0625	0.01	13.80	10.65	2.6
3	7.02 ± 0.02	0.050	0.01	13.80	7.10	2.6
4	6.91 ± 0.02	0.050	0.01	16.56	5.68	2.6
5	6.85 ± 0.05	0.055	0.01	16.56	7.10	2.6
6	6.70 ± 0.02	0.055	0.01	18.37	4.74	2.6

* It is recommended by Dr. Schroeder that for best results the hydrates specified be used.

REFERENCES

1. **Porath, J. and Flodin, P.**, Gel filtration, in *Protides of the Biological Fluids,* Vol. 10, Elsevier, Amsterdam, 1963, 290.
2. **Seid-Akhaven, M., Ayres, M., Salzano, F. M., Winter, W. P., and Rucknagel, D. L.**, Two more examples of Hb Porto Alegre, $\alpha_2\beta_2$ 9 ser → cys, in Belem, Brazil, *Hum. Hered.,* 23, 175, 1973.
3. **Gill, F. M. and Schwartz, E.**, Free α-globin pool in human bone marrow, *J. Clin. Invest.,* 52, 3057, 1973.
4. **Killander, J.**, Separation of human heme- and hemoglobin-binding plasma proteins, ceruloplasmin and albumin by gel filtration, *Biochim. Biophys. Acta,* 93, 1, 1964.
5. **Cuatrecasas, P. and Anfinsen, C. B.**, Affinity chromatography, *Ann. Rev. Biochem.,* 40, 259, 1971.
6. **Olsen, K. W.**, Affinity chromatography of heme binding proteins, *Fed. Proc. Abstr.,* 36, 2550, 1977.
7. **Brennen, S. O., Winterbourn, C. C., and Carrell, R. W.**, Isolation of high oxygen affinity hemoglobins, *Hemoglobin,* 1, 479, 1977.
8. **Abraham, E. C., Reese, A., Stallings, M., and Huisman, T. H. J.**, Separation of human hemoglobin by DEAE cellulose chromatography using glycine-KCN-NaCl developers, *Hemoglobin,* 1, 27, 1976.
9. **Peterson, E. A. and Sober, H. A.**, A variable gradient device for chromatography, *Anal. Chem.,* 31, 857, 1959.
10. **Kirkland, J. J.**, *Modern Practice of Liquid Chromatography,* Wiley-Interscience, New York, 1971.
11. **Clegg, J. B., Naughton, M. A., and Weatherall, D. J.**, An improved method for the characterization of human hemoglobin mutants: identification $\alpha_2\beta_2^{95glu}$, Hb N Baltimore, *Nature (London),* 207, 945, 1965.
12. **Vettore, L., DeSandre, G., Dilorio, E. E., Boyer, S. H., Crosby, E. F., Fuller, G. F., Ulenurm, L., and Buck, A. A.**, A survey of hemoglobin in the republic of Chad and characterization of Hb Chad: $\alpha_2^{23\ glu \rightarrow lys}\beta_2$, *Am. J. Hum. Genet.,* 20, 570, 1969.

13. **Vettore, L., DeSandre, G., Dilorio, E. E., Winterhalter, K. H., Lang, A., and Lehmann, H.,** A new abnormal hemoblobin O Padova α30 (B11) glu → lys and a dyserythropoietic anemia with erythroblastic multinuclearity coexisting in the same patient, *Blood*, 44, 869, 1974.
14. **Bunn, H. F., Meriwether, W. D., Balcerzak, S. P., and Rucknagel, D. L.,** Oxygen equilibria of hemoglobin E, *J. Clin. Invest.*, 51, 2984, 1972.
15. **Gossens, M., Garel, M. C., Aurinet, J., Basset, P., Gomes, P., and Rosa, J.,** Hemoglobin C Ziguinchor $\alpha 2^A\beta 2$ 6(A3) $^{glu \rightarrow val}$K 58(E2) pro → arg. The second sickling variant with amino acid substitutions in 2 residues of the polypeptide chain, *FEBS Lett.*, 58, 149, 1975.
16. **Beuzard, Y., Courvalin, J. C., Cohen-Solal, M., Garel, M. C., Rosa, J., Brizand, C. P., and Giband, A.,** Structural studies of hemoglobin St. Etienne β92(F8) his → gln: a new abnormal hemoglobin with loss of proximal histidine and absence of heme in the chains, *FEBS Lett.*, 27, 76, 1972.
17. **Aksoy, M., Erdem, S., Efremov, G. D., Wilson, J. B., Huisman, T. H. J., Schroeder, W. A., Shelton, J. R., Shelton, J. B., Ulitin, O. N., and Muftuoglu, A., Hemoglobin Istanbul:** substitution of glutamine for histidine in a proximal histidine (F8(92)β), *J. Clin. Invest.*, 51, 2380, 1977.
18. **Bradley, T. B., Jr., Wohl, R. C., and Reider, R. F.,** Hemoglobin Gunn Hill: deletion of five amino acid residues and impaired heme-globin binding, *Science*, 157, 1581, 1967.
19. **Vella, F., Casey, R., Lehmann, H., Labossiere, A., and Jones, T. G.,** Hb Ottawa, α_2 15 (A13)gly → arg β_2, *Biochim. Biophys. Acta*, 336, 25, 1974.
20. **Rahbar, S., Mahdavi, N., Nowzari, R., and Mustafaus, I.,** Hemoglobin Arya: α_2 47(CD 5) asp→asn, *Biochim. Biophys. Acta*, 386, 525, 1975.
21. **Halbrecht, I., Issacs, W. A., Lehmann, H., and Ben-Porat, F.,** Hemoglobin Hasharon (α 47 asp → his), *Isr. J. Med. Sci.*, 3, 827, 1967; **Schneider, R. G., Veda, S., Alperin, J. B., Brimhall, B., and Jones, R. T.,** Hemoglobin Sealey ($\alpha_2{}^{47\ his}\ \beta_2$): a new variant in a Jewish family, *Am. J. Hum. Gen.*, 20, 151, 1968.
22. **Hanada, M. and Rucknagel, D. L.,** The abnormality in the primary structure of Hb Shimonoseki, *Biochem. Biophys. Res. Comm.*, 11, 229, 1963.
23. **Rahbar, S., Kinderlehrer, J. L., and Lehmann H.,** Hemoglobin L Persian Gulf, α 57 (E6) gly → arg, *Acta Haematol.*, 42, 169, 1969.
24. **Rahbar, S., Nowzari, G., and Daneshmand, P.,** Hb Daneshgah-Tehran α_2 72 (EFI) his → arg $\beta_2{}^A$, *Nature New Biol.*, 245, 268, 1973.
25. **Lorkin, P. A., Charlesworth, D., Lehmann, H., Rahbar, S., Tuchinda, S., and Lie Injo Luan Eng.,** Two haemoglobins Q, α 74 (EF3) and α 75 (EF4) asp → his, *Br. J. Haematol.*, 19, 117, 1970.
26. **Van Ros, G., Beale, D., and Lehmann, H.,** Haemoglobin Stanleyville II (α 78 asn → lys), *Br. Med. J.*, 4, 92, 1968.
27. **Lorkin, P. A., Huntsman, R. G., Ager, J. A. M., Lehmann, H., Vella, F., and Darbre, P. D.,** Haemoglobin G Norfolk α 85 (F6) asp → asn, *Biochim. Biophys. Acta*, 379, 22, 1975.
28. **Jones, R. T., Brimhall, B., and Lisker, R.,** Chemical characterization of Hb Mexico and Hb Chiapas, *Biochim. Biophys. Acta*, 154, 488, 1968.
29. **Smith, L. L., Barton, B. P., and Huisman, T. H. J.,** Subunit dissociation of the unstable hemoglobin Bibba (α_2 136 pro (H19) β_2), *J. Biol. Chem.*, 245, 2185, 1970.
30. **Rahbar, S.,** Haemoglobin D Iran: β2 22 glutamic acid → glutamine (β4), *Br. J. Haematol.*, 24, 31, 1973.
31. **Brimhall, B., Jones, R. T., Schneider, R. G., Hosty, J. S., Tomlin, G., and Atkins, R.,** Hemoglobin Alabama (β39(C5) glyn → lys) and Hb Montgomery (α48 (CD6) leu → arg), *Biochim. Biophys. Acta*, 379, 28, 1975.
32. **Watson-Williams, E. J., Beale, D., Irvine, D., and Lehmann, H.,** A new hemoglobin D Ibadan, (β87 thr → lys) producing no sickle cell — Hb D disease with Hb S, *Nature (London)*, 205, 1273, 1965.
33. **Wajcman, H., Labie, D., and Schapira, G.,** Hemoglobin Tours: Thr β87 (F3) deleted and hemoglobin St. Antoine, Gly → leu β74—75 (E18—19) deleted. Consequences for oxygen affinity and protein stability, *Biochim. Biophys. Acta*, 295, 495, 1973.
34. **Schneider, R. G., Veda, S., Alperin, J. B., Levin, W. C., Jones, R. T., and Brimhall, B.,** Hemoglobin D Los Angeles in two Caucasian families. Hemoglobin SD disease and Hemoglobin D Thalassemia, *Blood*, 32, 250, 1968.
35. **Efremov, G. D., Huisman, T. H. J., Smith, L. L., Wilson, J. B., Kitchens, J. L., Wrightstone, R. N., and Adams, H. R., Hemoglobin Richmond,** a human hemoglobin which forms assymetric hybrids with other hemoglobins, *J. Biol. Chem.*, 244, 6105, 1969.
36. **Blackwell, R. Q., Jim, R. T. S., Tan, I. G. H., Weng, M.-I., Liu, C.-S., and Wang, C.-L.,** Hemoglobin G Waimanalo α 64 asp → asn, *Biochim. Biophys. Acta*, 322, 27, 1973.
37. **DeJong, W. W. W., Bernini, L. F., and Khan, P. M.,** Hemoglobin Rampa: α 95 pro → ser, *Biochim. Biophys. Acta*, 236, 197, 1971.
38. **Wiltshire, B. G., Clark, K. G. A., Lorkin, P. A., and Lehmann, H.,** Haemoglobin Denmark Hill α 95 (G2) pro → ala; a variant with unusual electrophoretic and oxygen binding properties, *Biochim. Biophys. Acta*, 278, 459, 1972.

39. **Bannister, W. H., Grech, J. L., Plese, C. F., Smith, L. L., Barton, B. P., Wilson, J. B., Reynolds, C. A., and Huisman, T. H. J.**, Hemoglobin St. Luke's or $\alpha_2^{95\ Arg\ (G2)}\ \beta_2$, *Eur. J. Biochem.*, 29, 301, 1972.
40. **Byckova, V., Wajcman, H., Labie, D., and Travers, F.**, Hemoglobin M Saskatoon: further data on biophysics and oxygen equilibrium, *Biochim. Biophys. Acta*, 243, 117, 1971.
41. **Gerald, P. S. and Efron, M. L.**, Chemical studies of several varieties of Hb M, *Proc. Natl. Acad. Sci. U.S.A.*, 47, 1758, 1961.
42. **Udem, L., Ranney, H. M., Bunn, H. F., and Pisciotta, A.**, Some observations on the properties of hemoglobin M Milwaukee I, *J. Mol. Biol.*, 48, 489, 1970.
43. **Heller, P., Coleman, R. D., and Yakulis, V.**, Hemoglobin M Hyde Park: a new variant of abnormal methemoglobin, *J. Clin. Invest.*, 45, 1021, 1966.
44. **Bonaventura, J. and Riggs, A.**, Hemoglobin Kansas, a human hemoglobin with a neutral amino acid substitution and an abnormal oxygen equilibrium, *J. Biol. Chem.*, 243, 980, 1968.
45. **Nute, P. E., Stamatoyannopoules, G., Hermodson, M. A., Roth, D., and Hornung, S.**, Hemoglobinopathic erythrocytosis due to a new electrophoretically silent variant hemoglobin San Diego (β 109 (G11) val → met), *J. Clin. Invest.*, 53, 320, 1974.
46. **Minnich, V., Hill, R. J., Khuri, P. D., and Anderson, M. E.**, Hemoglobin Hope: a beta chain variant, *Blood*, 25, 830, 1965.
47. Bromberg, P. A., Alben, J. O., Bare, G. H., Balcerzak, S. P., Jones, R. T., Brimhall, B., and Padilla, F., High oxygen affinity variant of haemoglobin Little Rock with unique properties, *Nature London New Biol.*, 243, 177, 1973.
48. **Jensen, M., Oski, F. A., Nathan, D. G., and Bunn, H. F.**, Hemoglobin Syracuse ($\alpha_2\ \beta_2$ 143 (H21) his → pro) a new high affinity variant detected by special electrophoretic methods, *J. Clin. Invest.*, 55, 469, 1975.
49. **Rahbar, S., Ala, F., Akhavan, E., Nowzari, G., Shoai, I., and Zamanianpoor, M. H.**, Two new haemoglobins: haemoglobin Perspolis (α 64 (E13) asp → tyr) and haemoglobin J Kurosh (α 19 (AB1) ala → asp), *Biochim. Biophys. Acta*, 119, 1976.
50. **Kendall, A. G., Barr, R. D., Lang, A., and Lehmann, H.**, Haemoblobin J Nyanza: α 21 (B2) ala → asp, *Biochim. Biophys. Acta*, 310, 357, 1973.
51. **Baglioni, C. A.**, Chemical study of Hemoglobin Norfolk, *J. Biol. Chem.*, 237, 69, 1962.
52. Cohen **Solal, M., Bloquit, Y., Garel, M. C., Thillet, J., Gaillard, L., Creyssel, R., Gibaud, A., and Rosa, J.**, Haemoglobin Lyon (β 17—18 (A14—15) lys val → O). Determination by sequenator analysis, *Biochim. Biophys. Acta*, 351, 306, 1974.
53. **Ricco, G., Pich, P. G., Mazza, U., Rossi, G., Ajmar, F., Arese, P., and Gallo, E.**, Hb J Sicilia: β 65 (E9) lys → asn, a beta chain homologue of Hb Zambia, *FEBS Lett.*, 39, 200, 1974.
54. **Garel, M. C., Hassan, W., Coquelet, M. T., Gossens, M., Rosa, J., and Arous, N.**, Hemoglobin J Cairo: β 65 (E9) lys → gln, a new hemoglobin variant discovered in an Egyptian family, *Biochim. Biophys. Acta*, 420, 97, 1976.
55. **Romain, P. L., Schwartz, A. D., Shamsuddin, M., Adams, J. G., Mason, R. G., Vidda, L. N., and Honig, G. R.**, Hemoglobin J Chicago (β 76 (E20) ala → asp): a new variant resulting from substitution of an external residue, *Blood*, 45, 387, 1975.
56. **Colombo, B., Vidal, H., Kamuzora, H., and Lehmann, H.**, A new Haemoglobin J Habana α 71 (E20) alanine → glutamic acid, *Biochim. Biophys. Acta*, 351, 1, 1974.
57. **Blackwell, R. Q., Wong, H. B., Wang, C.-L., Weng, M.-I., and Liu, C.-S.**, Hemoglobin J Meerut: α 120 ala → glu, *Biochim. Biophys. Acta*, 351, 7, 1974.
58. **Schneider, R. G., Alperin, J. B., Beale, D., and Lehmann, H.**, Hemoglobin I in an American Negro family: structural and hematological studies, *J. Lab. Clin. Med.*, 68, 940, 1966.
59. **Maekawa, M., Maekawa, T., Fujiwara, N., Tabara, K., and Matsuda, G.**, Hemoglobin Nagasaki: ($\alpha_2^A\beta_2^{17\ glu}$). A new abnormal hemoglobin found in one family in Nagasaki, *Int. J. Prot. Res.*, 2, 147, 1970.
60. **Shibata, S., Miyaji, T., Iuchi, I., Veda, S., and Takeda, I.**, Hemoglobin Hikari: ($\alpha_2^A\beta_2{}^{61asn}$) a fast moving hemoglobin found in two unrelated Japanese families, *Clin. Chem. Acta*, 10, 101, 1964.
61. **Capp, G. L., Rigas, D. A., and Jones, R. T.**, Hemoglobin Portland I: a new human haemoglobin in structure, *Nature (London)*, 228, 278, 1970.
62. **Kamuzora, H. and Lehmann, H.**, Human embryonic haemoglobins including a comparison by homology of the human ζ and α chains, *Nature (London)*, 256, 511, 1975.
63. **Smith, D. H., Clegg, J. B., Weatherall, D. J., and Giles, H. M.**, Hereditary persistance of foetal haemoglogin associated with a $\gamma\beta$ fusion variant Haemoglobin Kenya, *Nature London New Biol.*, 246, 184, 1973.
64. **Clegg, J. B., Weatherall, D. J., and Milner, P. F.**, Haemoglobin Constant Spring, a chain termination mutant? *Nature (London)*, 234, 337, 1971.

65. **Clegg, J. B., Weatherall, D. J., Contopolou, I., Caroutsos, K., Poungouras, P., and Tsevrenis, H.,** Haemoglobin Icaria, a new chain termination mutant which causes α thalassemia, *Nature (London),* 251, 245, 1974.
66. **Winter, W. P. and Rucknagel, D. L.,** Peptide mapping, in *Standardization of Laboratory Reagents and Methods for the Detection of Hemoglobinopathies,* Schmidt, R. M., Huisman, T. H. J., and Lehmann, H., Eds., CRC Press, Cleveland, 1974, 81.
67. **Baglioni, C. and Lehmann, H.,** Chemical heterogeneity of Haemoglobin O, *Nature (London),* 196, 229, 1962.
68. **Miyaji, T., Suzuki, H., Ohba, Y., and Shibata, S.,** Hemoglobin Agenogi ($\alpha_2\beta_2^{90lys}$), a slow moving hemoglobin of a Japanese family resembling Hb E, *Clin. Chem. Acta,* 14, 624, 1966.
69. **Huisman, T. H. J., Adams, H. R., Wilson, J. B., Efremov, G. D., Reynolds, C. A., and Wrightstone, R. N.,** Hemoglobin G Georgia or $\alpha_2{}^{95leu\ (G2)}\beta_2$, *Biochim. Biophys. Acta,* 200, 578, 1970.
70. **Lorkin, P. A., Lehmann, H., Fairbanks, V. F., Berglund, G., and Leonhardt, T.,** Two new pathological haemoglobins: Olmsted, β 141 (H19) leu → arg and Malmö, β 97 (FG4) his → gln, *Biochem. J.,* 119 68P, 1970.
71. **Brown, W. J., Niazi, G. A., Jayakalshmi, M., Abraham, E. C., and Huisman, T. H. J.,** Hemoglobin Athens-Georgia or $\alpha_2\beta_2$ 40 (C6) arg → lys. A hemoglobin variant with an increased oxygen affinity. To be published; cited in **Lehmann, H. and Kynoch, P. A. M.,** *Human Hemoglobin Variants and their Characteristics* North-Holland, Amsterdam, 1976.
72. **Rosa, J., Maleknia, N., Vergoz, D., and Dumet, R.,** Une nouvelle hemoglobine abnormale: l'hemoglobine Jα_{Paris} 12 ala → asp, *Nouv. Rev. Fr. Hematol.,* 6, 423, 1966.

ELECTROPHORETIC MOBILITIES OF MUTANT HEMOGLOBINS

Rose G. Schneider and Ronald Barwick

Electrophoresis in alkaline buffers (most conveniently on cellulose acetate) and on citrate agar are two especially useful, complementary procedures for the identification of abnormal hemoglobins. The rationale of these methods differs substantially; in the former, mobility is largely a function of the net charge of the hemoglobin, whereas on citrate agar, mobilities are related to many additional factors, particularly the molecular location of the substituted residue.[1] Because these analyses reveal different aspects of molecular structure, the combined data often provide presumptive or, in some cases, highly specific identifications of mutant hemoglobins. (When the data are supplemented by those of globin chain electrophoresis at acidic and alkaline pH, the scope of the identifications is greatly enlarged.)

Previous evaluations of mobilities have usually depended on direct visual comparisons of the hemoglobin being tested with reference samples analyzed simultaneously and recorded by lines representing comparative distances. In an attempt to make the comparisons more uniform and objective, we now present a system of calculating relative mobilities:

1. The mobility of Hb A is designated as zero (0).
2. The distance between the mutant and Hb A is measured from the middle of each electrophoretically separated fraction (or the corresponding densitometric peak), divided by the distance between Hb A and C, and then arbitrarily multiplied by 10. This procedure is expressed in the equation:

$$N = \frac{D\ (A\ to\ X) \times 10}{D\ (A\ to\ C)}$$

   where N = ratio, X = mutant being analyzed, and D = distance between electrophoretically separated fractions.
3. Mobilities of hemoglobins anodic to Hb A are marked plus (+); those cathodic to Hb A are marked minus (−).

Hb C was chosen because it moves farther from Hb A than any other readily available mutant, both in cellulose acetate and citrate agar electrophoresis. In the latter method, cathodic and anodic mobilities may vary independently, according to electrophoretic conditions; we measured each in relation to its own control, the anodic control being Hb C (the equation applied is the same as above) and the cathodic control, Hb F. The distance between Hb A and the mutant was divided by the distance between Hb A and Hb F, and the quotient was multiplied by 4.4, which was generally the relationship of the Hb F control to the 10 value of the Hb C control. The equation for cathodic mobilities on citrate agar electrophoresis is:

$$N = \frac{D\ (A\ to\ X) \times 4.4}{D\ (A\ to\ F)}$$

In areas where Hb C is not available, Hb E or A_2 may be substituted in electrophoresis on cellulose acetate, and Hb S may be substituted on citrate agar. The latter is apt to be a less useful method in areas where Hb S and C are not found.

The ratios provide a more objective measure of comparative mobilities than visual comparisons. They also make it possible to compare hemoglobins analyzed at different times and to computerize the data.

Qualifications

Relative electrophoretic mobilities on citrate agar vary considerably according to technique. Mobilities on cellulose acetate may also vary, especially according to: (1) type of buffer and its ionic strength, (2) electrical conditions, (3) duration of electrophoresis, (4) temperature, (5) method of preparation of hemolysate, and (6) kind and amount of accompanying hemoglobin. These conditions should be kept as constant as possible.

The mobilities of the hemoglobins examined in this laboratory are marked with an asterisk. At least ten measurements were made for each of the more frequent ones, but some rare mutants were only examined once or twice. The mobilities of those hemoglobins not examined here were obtained either from the data compiled by Lehmann and Kynoch[2] or from the original description of the mutant. These figures are approximations and are so marked; however, when the mobility was described as being like that of Hb S (or C), it was given the numerical designation of HB S (or C). A dash (—) indicates that the data were not available. Citrate agar mobilities were generally rounded to the nearest quarter unit.

Data derived from the literature were obtained with a variety of methods (including filter paper or, in a few cases, starch gel). Descriptions, however, are often scanty, with some hemoglobins characterized merely as "slow" or "fast". Data from different laboratories are therefore not strictly comparable.

Methods

Cellulose acetate electrophoresis[1]

Apparatus — Details of technique may vary slightly with the type of apparatus, which generally consists of: Mylar®-backed cellulose acetate plates, a zone electrophoresis chamber, applicators, and a power supply with variable voltage control.

Reagents — All procedures use deionized water.

1. Tris, EDTA borate buffer (TEB) — 10.2 g tris, 0.6 g EDTA, and 3.2 g boric acid per liter
2. Ponceau S — 0.3 g Ponceau S in 100 mℓ of 3% trichloracetic acid
3. Three grams glacial acetic acid per 100 mℓ H_2O
4. Tolidine reagent — 1.0 g O-Tolidine dihydrochloride in 25 mℓ glacial acetic acid made up to 100 mℓ with H_2O
5. Tolidine stain — 20 mℓ tolidine reagent, 10 mℓ 3 to 5% acetic acid, and 2 mℓ 30% H_2O_2

Procedures — Hemolysates (containing 5 to 10 g Hb per 100 mℓ) may be prepared by any of the standard methods.

1. Pour TEB buffer into chambers; soak and position wicks.
2. Soak cellulose acetate plates in TEB buffer for at least 20 min before use.
3. Blot plate between two pieces of absorbent paper quickly and evenly to absorb excess buffer.
4. Apply samples with an applicator to the cellulose acetate at about 2.5 cm from the cathodic end.
5. Put plates on wicks in chamber with glass plate on top to assure even contact. Three plates may be analyzed simultaneously.
6. Apply 450 V for 20 min at room temperature.
7. Remove plates from chamber and stain immediately 1 to 3 min in Ponceau S stain.
8. Remove plate from stain and place in three consecutive 3-min washes in 3% acetic acid or until background is clear.

9. Optional; counterstain in freshly made tolidine stain about 1 to 2 min. Rinse in distilled water for at least 20 min.
10. If desired, clear plate by soaking in absolute methanol 2 min then in 25% glacial acetic acid in absolute methanol for 10 min. Allow plate to dry.

Citrate Agar Electrophoresis[3]

Many methods are available. The following is the method used in this study:

Apparatus — The apparatus used is the same as was implemented for cellulose acetate.

Reagents — The reagents used include:

1. Sodium citrate buffer — 0.5 M, stock solution: 147 g sodium citrate ($Na_3C_6H_5O_7$-$2H_2O$) per liter; adjust to pH 6 with citric acid, 300 g/ℓ.
2. Working buffer — 0.05 M, dilute stock buffer tenfold with water and adjust to pH 6 with the citric acid solution (300 g/ℓ). All solutions should be stored at 4°C.
3. Dilute hemolysate to 1 g/100 mℓ for adult samples and 3 g/100 mℓ for umbilical cord blood samples.
4. Tolidine stain — same as for cellulose acetate; make fresh just before use.

Procedures — Preparation of citrate agar plates is as follows:

1. Soak Mylar-backed cellulose acetate plates (Helena or Gelman) in working buffer for at least 30 min. A rack to hold the plates is convenient.
2. Add 1.0 g Bacto Agar® (Difco® certified) to 100 mℓ working buffer; add 2 drops 5% KCN as preservative. Heat in boiling water bath until agar is completely dissolved.
3. Cool agar to 60 to 70°C.
4. Remove rack of cellulose acetate plates from buffer and drain for about 30 sec. Place rack into melted agar for 30 min; maintain the temperature between 60 and 70°C
5. Remove plates. Place individually (or two, back to back) in plastic bag with 1 to 2 mℓ of working buffer added.
6. Store in tightly closed box in refrigerator. They may be stored for several weeks.

Electrophoresis procedures are as follows:

1. Add working buffer to each side of electrophoresis chamber. Volume depends on type of chamber. Position wicks.
2. Remove citrate agar plate from package and blot to remove excess buffer and agar.
3. Apply sample lightly with applicator approximately 3 cm from anodic end of plate.
4. Immediately invert plate on wicks in electrophoresis chamber and apply 80 V for 30 min. The cellulose acetate plate is covered with a glass plate to assure proper contact with the wicks. Several plates may be analyzed simultaneously.
5. Stain in freshly made tolidine stain until bands become distinct, about 1 to 2 min.
6. Rinse in distilled water for at least 20 min.
7. Remove from water. Clear in clearing solution (80% methanol, 20% acetic acid) for 7 min. Place on hot plate until clear (4 to 5 min).

Table 1
RELATIVE ELECTROPHORETIC MOBILITIES OF MUTANT HEMOGLOBINS

Residue	Substitution	Name	Cellulose acetate pH 8.5 (I, + 8.5; N Baltimore, + 6.6; J Balt., + 4.3; A, 0; F, − 2.6; S, − 5.2; C, −10.0)	Citrate agar pH 6.0 (F, −4.4; A, 0; S, + 5.8; C, + 10.0)
		α Chains		
5	Ala → Asp	J. Toronto*	+4.5	0
6	Asp → Ala	Sawara*	−3.8	+ 1.25
11	Lys → Glu	Anantharaj*	+5.8	0
12	Ala → Asp	J Paris*	+4.7	0
15	Gly → Asp	J Oxford*	+4.8	0
15	Gly → Arg	Ottawa	∼+4	0
16	Lys → Glu	I*	+8.5	0
19	Ala → Asp	Kurosh	∼+4	—
21	Ala → Asp	J Nyanza	∼+4	—
22	Gly → Asp	J Medellin	∼+4	0
23	Glu → Gln	Memphis	−5.2	∼+6.25
23	Glu → Lys	Chad	−10.0	—
23	Glu → Val	Audhali	∼−5	—
27	Glu → Gly	Fort Worth*	−2.7	0
27	Glu → Val	Spanish Town	∼−2.8	0
30	Glu → Lys	O Padova	−10.0	—
30	Glu → Gln	G Chinese	−5.0	0
43	Phe → Val	Torino	0	—
43	Phe → Leu	Hirosaki	0	0
47	Asp → Gly	Kokura, Umi*	−5.8	+2.0
47	Asp → His	Hasharon*	−5.5	+6.25
47	Asp → Asn	Arya*	−5.2	0
48	Leu → Arg	Montgomery*	−4.6	+2.5
50	His → Asp	J Sardegna	∼+4	0
51	Gly → Asp	J Abidjan	∼+2	—
51	Gly → Arg	Russ*	−5.2	0
53	Ala → Asp	J Rovigo*	+4.5	0
54	Gln → Arg	Shimonoseki*	−5.6	+0.5
54	Gln → Glu	J Mexico*	+4.6	0
57	Gly → Arg	L Persian Gulf	∼−5	0
57	Gly → Asp	Norfolk	∼+4	—
58	His → Tyr	M Boston	0	—
60	Lys → Asn.	Zambia	∼+4	—
61	Lys → Asn	J Buda	∼+4	—
64	Asp → Asn	G Waimanalo (Aida)	∼−1	—
64	Asp → His	Q India*	−4.8	+0.75
64	Asp → Tyr	Perspolis	∼−5	—
68	Asn → Asp	Ube-2*	+4.4	0
68	Asn → Lys	G Philadelphia*	−5.2	0
71	Ala → Glu	J Habana	∼+4	—
72	His → Arg	Daneskgah-Tehran*	−4.9	0
74	Asp → His	Mahidol*	−4.3	+2.25
74	Asp → Asn	G Pest	∼−5	—
74	Asp → Gly	Chapel Hill	—	—
75	Asp → His	Q Iran*	−4.8	+1.0
75	Asp → Tyr	Winnipeg*	−4.9	0
75	Asp → Asn	Matsue-Oki*	−5.1	+1.5
78	Asn → Lys	Stanleyville-II*	−5.1	0
80	Leu → Arg	Ann Arbor	∼−6	—
82	Ala → Asp	Garden State	—	—
84	Ser → Arg	Etobicoke	0	0
85	Asp → Asn	G Norfolk*	−5.3	0
85	Asp → Tyr	Atago*	+4.2	0
85	Asp → Val	Inkster*	−5.0	0
87	His → Tyr	M Iwate*	−1.9	0
90	Lys → Asn	J Broussais*	+3.4	0
90	Lys → Thr	J Rajappen	∼+4	—
92	Arg → Gln	J Cape Town*	+3.3	0
92	Arg → Leu	Chesapeake*	+3.1	+0.75
94	Asp → Tyr	Setif*	−5.6	+6.5
94	Asp → Asn	Titusville*	−5.4	+6.0
95	Pro → Leu	G Georgia*	−4.7	−1.5
95	Pro → Ser	Rampa*	−4.8	−1.5

Table 1 (continued)
RELATIVE ELECTROPHORETIC MOBILITIES OF MUTANT HEMOGLOBINS

Residue	Substitution	Name	Cellulose acetate pH 8.5 (I, + 8.5; N Baltimore, + 6.6; J Balt., + 4.3; A, 0; F, − 2.6; S, − 5.2; C, − 10.0)	Citrate agar pH 6.0 (F, -4.4; A, 0; S, + 5.8; C, + 10.0)
95	Pro → Ala	Denmark Hill	∼−1	—
95	Pro → Arg	St. Lukes	∼−1	—
102	Ser → Arg	Manitoba	0	—
112	His → Asp	Hopkins-II*	+4.1	0
112	His → Arg	Strumica (Serbia)	∼−3	—
114	Pro → Arg	Chiapas	∼−5	—
115	Ala → Asp	J Tongariki	∼+4	—
116	Glu → Lys	O Indonesia*	−7.1	2.5
120	Ala → Glu	J Meerut, J Birmingham	∼+4	—
126	Asp → Asn	Tarrant*	−2.3	+5.4
127	Lys → Thr	St. Claude	∼+4	—
127	Lys → Asn	Jackson*	+3.3	0
136	Leu → Pro	Bibba	∼−5	—
141	Arg → Pro	Singapore	∼−2	—
141	Arg → His	Suresnes	—	—
		β Chains		
1	Val → Ala	Raleigh*	0	−4.2
2	His → Arg	Deer Lodge*	−2.6	0
6	Glu → Val	S*	−5.2	+5.8
6	Glu → Lys	C*	−10.0	+10.0
6	Glu → Ala	G Makassar	∼−5	—
7	Glu → Gly	G San Jose*	−3.6	+7.5
7	Glu → Lys	C Siriraj	∼−4	+10.0
9	Ser → Cys	Porto Alegre	∼0.4	+10.0
10	Ala → Asp	Ankara	∼+4	—
14	Leu → Arg	Sögn	−5.2	—
14	Leu → Pro	Saki*	−5.2	0
15	Trp → Arg	Belfast*	−5.5	0
16	Gly → Asp	J Baltimore*	+4.3	0
16	Gly → Arg	D Bushman	−5.2	—
17	Lys → Glu	Nagasaki	∼+5	—
19	Asn → Lys	D Ouled Rabah	−5.2	—
20	Val → Met	Olympia	0	0
20	Val → Asp	Strasbourg*	+0.5	0
22	Glu → Lys	E Saskatoon	−10.0	0
22	Glu → Gly	G Taipei	∼−5	—
22	Glu → Ala	G Coushatta*	−4.8	0
22	Glu → Gln	D Iran*	−5.2	0
24	Gly → Arg	Riverdale-Bronx	∼−5	0
24	Gly → Val	Savannah	∼−3	—
24	Gly → Asp	Moscva	∼+2	0
25	Gly → Arg	G Taiwan Ami	∼−5	—
26	Glu → Lys	E*	−10.0	0
26	Glu → Val	Henri Mondor*	−5.2	0
27	Ala → Asp	Volga	0	0
28	Leu → Gln	St. Louis*	−3.1	0
28	Leu → Pro	Genova	0	—
29	Gly → Asp	Lufkin*	+2.8	0
30	Arg → Ser	Tacoma*	+0.9	0
32	Leu → Pro	Perth	0	0
32	Leu → Arg	Castilla*	−5.0	0
35	Tyr → Phe	Philly	0	—
37	Trp → Ser	Hirose	∼−5	0
39	Gln → Lys	Alabama*	−4.9	0
39	Gln → Glu	Vaasa	—	—
40	Arg → Lys	Athens-Ga (Waco)*	−0.4	−2.0
40	Arg → Ser	Austin*	+2.5	−3.1
41	Phe → Tyr	Mequon	—	—
42	Phe → Ser	Hammersmith*	0	0
42	Phe → Leu	Bucuresti	0	—
43	Glu → Ala	G Galveston*	−4.8	0
46	Gly → Glu	K Ibadan	∼+0.5	—
47	Asp → Asn	G Copenhagen	∼−5	—

Table 1 (continued)
RELATIVE ELECTROPHORETIC MOBILITIES OF MUTANT HEMOGLOBINS

Residue	Substitution	Name	Cellulose acetate pH 8.5 (I, + 8.5; N Baltimore, + 6.6; J Balt., + 4.3; A, 0; F, − 2.6; S, − 5.2; C, − 10.0)	Citrate agar pH 6.0 (F, -4.4; A, 0; S, + 5.8; C, + 10.0)
48	Leu → Arg	Okaloosa*	−4.7	0
50	Thr → Lys	Edmonton	−5.2	0
51	Pro → Arg	Willamette*	−5.1	0
52	Asp → Asn	Osu Christiansborg*	−5.2	0
52	Asp → Ala	Ocho Rios	−5.2	0
56	Gly → Asp	J Bangkok*	+3.3	0
56	Gly → Arg	Hamadan*	−5.1	+0.25
57	Asn → Lys	G Ferrara*	−5.2	0
58	Pro → Arg	Dhofar	~−5	—
59	Lys → Glu	I High Wycombe	~+7	—
59	Lys → Thr	J Kaohsiung	~+4	—
61	Lys → Glu	N Seattle*	+7.4	0
61	Lys → Asn	Hikari	~+6	0
62	Ala → Pro	Duarte	0	—
63	His → Arg	Zurich	~−5	—
63	His → Tyr	M Saskatoon*	0	0
63	His → Pro	Bicetre	—	—
64	Gly → Asp	J Calabria*	+3.6	0
65	Lys → Asn	Sicilia	~+4	—
65	Lys → Gln	J Cairo*	+4.7	0
66	Lys → Glu	J Toulouse	~+5	—
67	Val → Asp	Bristol	0	—
67	Val → Glu	M Milwaukee	0	—
67	Val → Ala	Sydney	−5.2	—
69	Gly → Asp	J Cambridge	~+4	—
70	Ala → Asp	Seattle	~+4	—
71	Phe → Ser	Christchurch	0	—
73	Asp → Tyr	Vancouver*	−4.9	+0.55
73	Asp → Asn	Korle Bu*	−4.9	+0.5
73	Asp → Val	Mobile*	−4.9	+0.5
74	Gly → Val	Bushwick	~−8	—
74	Gly → Asp	Shepherds Bush	~+0.5	0
75	Leu → Pro	Atlanta	0	—
76	Ala → Asp	J Chicago	~+4	0
77	His → Asp	J Iran	~+4	—
79	Asp → Gly	G Hsi-Tsou	~−5	—
80	Asn → Lys	G Szuhu*	−3.0	+6.25
81	Leu → Arg	Baylor*	−4.4	+2.75
82	Lys → Asn → Asp	Providence*	+1.6, +2.2	−3.0, −4.2
82	Lys → Thr	Rahere	0	~−4.4
82	Lys → Met	Helsinki	0	—
83	Gly → Cys	Ta-Li	0	—
83	Gly → Asp	Pyrgos*	+3.2	−2.75
85	Phe → Ser	Bryn Mawr, Buenos Aires	~−0.4	—
87	Thr → Lys	D Ibadan*	−4.9	+1.0
88	Leu → Arg	Boras	~−2.5	—
88	Leu → Pro	Santa Ana	~−2.5	—
89	Ser → Asn	Creteil*	+0.2	0
89	Ser → Arg	Vanderbilt	—	—
90	Glu → Lys	Agenogi*	−8.2	+6.8
91	Leu → Pro	Sabine*	−5.9, −8.6	0
91	Leu → Arg	Carribean	−5.2	0
92	His → Tyr	M Hyde Park	~+0.3	—
92	His → Gln	St. Etienne (Istanbul)*	−8.9	0
92	His → Asp	J Altgeld Gardens	~+5	—
92	His → Pro	Newcastle	~−2.6	0
95	Lys → Glu	N Baltimore*	+6.6	0
97	His → Gln	Malmo*	+0.5	−1.1
97	His → Leu	Wood*	0	−2.25
98	Val → Met	Koln*	−7.53	−2.2
98	Val → Gly	Nottingham*	−8.4, −9.1	0
98	Val → Ala	Djelfa*	0	0
99	Asp → Asn	Kempsey*	−3.1	+4.3

Table 1 (continued)
RELATIVE ELECTROPHORETIC MOBILITIES OF MUTANT HEMOGLOBINS

Residue	Substitution	Name	Cellulose acetate pH 8.5 (I, + 8.5; N Baltimore, + 6.6; J Balt., + 4.3; A, 0; F, − 2.6; S, − 5.2; C, − 10.0)	Citrate agar pH 6.0 (F, -4.4; A, 0; S, + 5.8; C, + 10.0)
99	Asp → His	Yakima*	−2.3, −1.0	+6.5
99	Asp → Tyr	Ypsilanti	∼−3.4, ∼−2.2	—
100	Pro → Leu	Brigham	0	—
101	Glu → Lys	British Columbia*	−2.7	+10.75
101	Glu → Gln	Rush	∼−0.4, ∼−4.9	∼+0.5
101	Glu → Gly	Alberta	—	—
102	Asn → Lys	Richmond*	−0.5, −2.7	0, +5.75
102	Asn → Thr	Kansas	—	—
102	Asn → Ser	Beth Israel	∼+0.3	—
103	Phe → Leu	Heathrow	0	0
104	Arg → Ser	Camperdown	0	—
106	Leu → Pro	Casper, Southhampton	0	—
106	Leu → Gln	Tübingen	∼−3.1	—
107	Gly → Arg	Burke*	−2.2	+5.75
108	Asn → Asp	Yoshizuka	—	—
109	Val → Met	San Diego	0	—
111	Val → Phe	Peterborough	0	−5
113	Val → Glu	New York*	+1.5	0
115	Ala → Pro	Madrid	0	0
117	His → Arg	P Galveston*	−5.2	0
119	Gly → Asp	Fannin-Lubbock*	+¼.¾	0
120	Lys → Glu	Hijiyama*	+6.6	0
120	Lys → Asn	Riyadh*	+3.1	0
121	Glu → Gln	D Punjab, D Los Angeles*	−5.2	0
121	Glu → Lys	O Arab*	−9.7	+1.75
121	Glu → Val	Beograd	—	—
124	Pro → Arg	Khartoum	—	—
126	Val → Glu	Hofu*	+4.5	0
127	Gln → Glu	Hacettepe	∼+4	—
129	Ala → Asp	J Taichung	∼+4	—
129	Ala → Glu or Asp	K Cameroon	—	—
130	Tyr → Asp	Wien	0	—
131	Gln → Glu	Camden*	+1.6	−2.5
132	Lys → Gln	K Woolwich*	+2.7	−3.5
135	Ala → Pro	Altdorf	0	—
136	Gly → Asp	Hope*	+0.8	−4.0
141	Leu → Arg	Olmsted	0	—
143	His → Arg	Abruzzo	∼−5	—
143	His → Gln	Little Rock	∼+0.1	∼−4.25
143	His → Pro	Syracuse	0	—
144	Lys → Asn	Andrew-Minneapolis	"Anodic"	—
145	Tyr → His	Bethesda*	0	+2.75
145	Tyr → Cys	Rainier	0	∼+3
145	Tyr → Asp	Ft. Gordon, Nancy, Osler*	+2.1	−2.0
145	Tyr → Term	Mckees Rocks	—	—
146	His → Asp	Hiroshima*	+2.4	−4.4
146	His → Pro	York	0	∼−2
146	His → Arg	Cochin-Port Royal*	−2.7	+0.5
	β_4	H*	+10.0	0
		Fusion Hemoglobins		
	δβ	Lepore-Hollandia	∼−5	0
	δβ	Lepore-Baltimore	∼−5	0
	δβ	Lepore-Washington-Boston*	−5.2	0
	βδ	Miyada	—	—
	βδ	P Congo	∼−5	0
	β	P Nilotic*	−4.9	0
	γβ	Kenya*	−6.9	0
		Deleted residues		
β6 or 7	Glu → 0	Leiden	—	—
β17—18	(Lys-Val) → 0	Lyon	∼+3.3	—
β23	Val → 0	Freiburg	—	—
β42—44 or	Phe-Glu-Ser	Niteroi	∼−0.5	—

Table 1 (continued)
RELATIVE ELECTROPHORETIC MOBILITIES OF MUTANT HEMOGLOBINS

Residue	Substitution	Name	Cellulose acetate pH 8.5 (I, + 8.5; N Baltimore, + 6.6; J Balt., + 4.3; A, 0; F, − 2.6; S, − 5.2; C, − 10.0)	Citrate agar pH 6.0 (F, -4.4; A, 0; S, + 5.8; C, + 10.0)
43—45	→ 0 or Glu-Ser-Phe → 0			
β56—59	Gly-Asn-Pro-Lys → 0	Tochigi	—	—
β74—75	Gly-Leu → 0	St. Antoine	—	—
β87	Thr → 0	Tours	—	—
β91—95	Leu-His-Cys-Asp-Lys → 0	Gun Hill*	−6.0, −9.4	+ 3.0
β131	Gln → 0	Deaconess*	−2.8	+ 6.75
β141	Leu → 0	Coventry	0	—
		Extended chains		
α141	31 Added	Constant Spring	—	—
α141	31 Added	Icaria	—	—
α141	16 or 17 Added	Koya Dora	—	—
β146	10 Added	Tak	∼−3	∼ + 5
α139—141	Frame shift	Wayne	—	—
β145	Frame shift	Cranston	−5.2	—
α115—118	Insertion	Grady*	+ 3.0	0
		More than one mutation in one chain		
β6 β73	Glu → Val Asp → Asn	C Harlem*	−10.0	+ 5.8
α78 α79	Asn → Asp Ala → Gly	J Singapore	—	—
β6 β58	Glu → Val Pro → Arg	C Ziguinchor*	−10.3	+ 5.8
β6 β142	Glu → Val Ala → Val	Travis*	−5.1	+ 4.0
β6 β95	Glu → Lys Lys → Glu	Arlington Park	0	0
		δ Chains		
2	His → Arg	A_2 Sphakia	—	—
12	Asn → Lys	A_2 NYU	∼−10.8	—
16	Gly → Arg	A_2' (B_2)*	−11.1	0
20	Val → Glu	A_2 Roosevelt	—	—
22	Ala → Glu	A_2 Flatbush*	−4.5	0
43	Glu → Lys	A_2 Melbourne	∼−11.7	—
69	Gly → Arg	A_2 Indonesia	—	—
116	Arg → His	A_2 Coburg	∼−3.4	—
136	Gly → Asp	A_2 Babinga*	−9.2	−4.0
		γ Chains		
1	Gly → Cys	F Malaysia	—	—
5	Glu → Lys	F Texas-I*	−10.6	−3.5
6	Glu → Lys	F Texas-II*	∼−10.5	—
7	Asp → Asn	F Auckland	—	—
12	Thr → Lys	F Alexandra	∼−9.2	—
22	Asp → Gly	F Kuala Lumpur	∼−10.9	0
61	Lys → Glu	F Jamaica	—	—
75	Ile → Thr	F Sardinia	−2.6	—
80	Asp → Tyr	F Victoria Jubilee	∼−5.4	—
97	His → Arg	F Dickinson*	−5.45	−4.4
117	His → Arg	F Malta-I	∼−7.5	—
121	Glu → Lys	F Hull	∼−10.1	—
125	Glu → Ala	F Port Royal	—	−4.4
130	Trp → Gly	F Poole	—	—
	γ_4	Bart's*	+ 7.6	−4.0

REFERENCES

1. **Schneider, R. G. and Hightower, B. J.,** Structure in relation to behavior of mutant hemoglobins in citrate agar electrophoresis, *Hemoglobin,* 1, 427, 1977.
2. **Lehmann, H. and Kynoch, P. A. M.,** *Human Haemoglobin Variants and Their Characteristics,* Elsevier/North-Holland, Amsterdam, 1976.
3. **Schneider, R. G., Hosty, T. S., Tomlin, G., and Atkins, R.,** Identification of hemoglobins and hemoglobinopathies by electrophoresis on cellulose acetate plates impregnated with citrate agar, *Clin. Chem.,* 20, 74, 1974.

STARCH GEL ELECTROPHORESIS

Georgi D. Efremov

The electrophoretic method that uses starch gel as a supporting medium[1] is considered to be the most accurate and reliable procedure, even for routine screening for hemoglobinopathies. This method provides higher resolution and greater reproducibility than any other electrophoretic technique.

Equipment

A vertical electrophoretic apparatus[2] is most commonly used. It consists of (1) electrode tanks with a baffle and either platinum or silver-silver chloride electrode, (2) plastic trays with an inside depth of 6 to 7 mm and plastic lids, (3) a plastic cutting tray with either a blade or wire-cutting device, (4) glass or plastic staining tanks, and (5) a power supply capable of providing 500 to 600 V.

Several commercial models, some of which are more elaborate than is necessary, are available for detection of abnormal hemoglobins. A simple, inexpensive, horizontal system can be constructed in every laboratory.[3] Two pairs of plastic food-storage boxes, each connected with filter paper wicks, can be used as electrode tanks. Platinum wire, which is used for the electrodes, is placed in the outer boxes and connected by cables to a power supply. The tray for containing the starch gel is a plastic plate measuring 24 × 14 × 0.5 cm to which plastic edges (22 × 1 × 0.5 cm and 14 × 1 × 0.5 cm) are fixed on the sides of the plate with plastic or metal clamps. For cutting the gel, the two long edges are replaced with edges of the dimensions 20 × 1 × 0.2 cm; a tightly stretched nylon fishing thread will cut the gel when it is drawn over these lower edges. For routine screening purposes, it is advisable to use a longer tray (45 × 14 × 0.5 cm) so that 30 to 40 samples (in three rows) can be analyzed simultaneously.

Source of Starch

Partially hydrolyzed starch can be obtained from the following sources: BDH Chemicals, Poole, England; Connaught Medical Research Laboratories, Toronto, Canada; or Otto Hiller, Madison, Wisconsin, who manufactures the starch under the trade name Electro-Starch®. Electro-Starch® has certain physical properties that allow superior separation of hemoglobin variants.

Hydrolyzed potato starch can also be prepared in any laboratory. Hydrolysis is best performed in batches of 1 kg as follows. In a 5-ℓ Erlenmeyer® flask, 1 kg of potato starch is thoroughly mixed with 1 ℓ of 2% HCl in acetone which has been warmed to 38°C. The Erlenmeyer flask is closed with a stopper and left in a water bath at 38°C for 45 min (or 60 min). After this time the supernatant is decanted, and 400 mℓ 1-N sodium acetate is added to the starch. The mixture is well shaken, poured on a large Buchner® funnel, and washed with 10 ℓ of tap water and 10 ℓ of distilled water. Finally, the starch is washed with 200 mℓ of acetone and dried in an oven at 40 to 45°C.

Buffer Systems

Any of several different buffer systems may be used to separate hemoglobin variants. The buffers that have been used most successfully are listed in Table 1. Routine screening can best be carried out with either tris-EDTA-borate system. Other systems are valuable for specific separations. Thus the discontinuous tris-citrate-borate system gives a slightly improved resolution of slowly migrating, minor hemoglobin components. The phosphate buffer system (pH 6.5 to 7.0) is useful for detecting small quan-

Table 1
BUFFER SYSTEMS FOR STARCH GEL ELECTROPHORESIS OF HEMOGLOBINS

Stock buffer	Buffer for preparation of gel	Buffer for electrode vessels	Time (hr)	V/cm
	Tris-EDTA-borate system, pH 8.6[4]			
Tris 110 g EDTA (acid) 5.85 g Boric acid 30.9 g Final volume 1000 mℓ	Dilute stock 1:20	Dilute stock 1:7	3—4	15—18
	Tris-EDTA-borate system, pH 9.0[5]			
Tris 20.2 g EDTA 2.0 g Boric acid 1.5 g Final volume 1000 mℓ	Dilute stock 1:4	Use stock buffer	4—5	20—25
	Discontinuous tris-citrate-borate system, pH 9.0[6]			
Tris 9.2 g Citric acid 1.05 g Final volume 1000 mℓ		Boric acid 18.55 g NaOH 2.4 g Final volume 1000 mℓ	2—3	15—18
	Phosphate system, pH 6.5—7.0[7]			
$Na_2HPO_4 \cdot 2H_2O$ 7.2 g Titrate with H_3PO_4 to pH 6.5—7.0 Final volume 1000 mℓ	Dilute stock 1:7.5	Use stock buffer	3—4	15—18
	Phosphate system, pH 7.0[8]			
$Na_2HPO_4 \cdot 2H_2O$ 3.3 g KH_2PO_4 1.075 g Final volume 1000 mℓ	Dilute stock 1:5	Use stock buffer	3—4	15—18

tities of hemoglobins (Hb) H and Bart's. Under these conditions, both variants will move toward the anode, while Hb A remains at the origin. The phosphate buffer system at pH 7.0 gives a satisfactory separation of abnormal methemoglobins, because at this pH the imidazole ring of the histidyl residue carries a charge. Hemoglobin solutions, both treated and untreated with ferricyanide, must, however, be applied. Figure 1 provides some examples of separations that can be obtained with the starch gel electrophoretic method using the tris-EDTA-borate system at pH 9.0.[5]

Gel Preparation

The procedure for preparing the gel is described in detail by Smithies.[2] The concen-

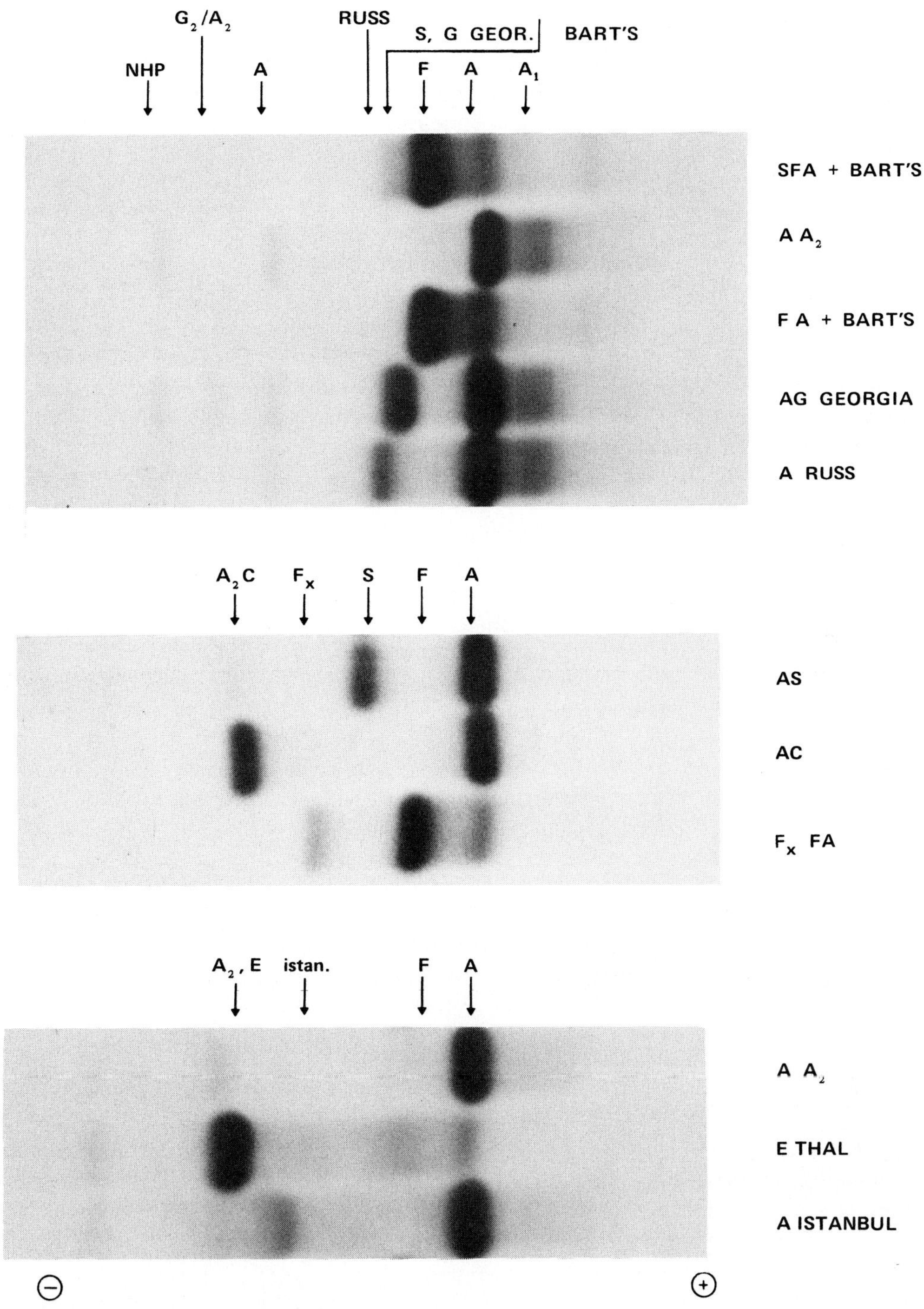

FIGURE 1. Starch gel electrophoresis of hemolysates with various types of hemoglobin. Tris-EDTA-boric acid buffer, pH 9.0.

tration of starch in the gel may need to be varied somewhat with the individual lots, although for separation of hemoglobins, the concentration is not critical. Usually 11 to 13 g of hydrolyzed starch per 100 mℓ of buffer provides a gel of suitable strength. The starch, suspended in the appropriate buffer, is thoroughly shaken in a 1000-mℓ vacuum flask and heated to boiling with continuous shaking until a translucent gel appears. In a more simple and less physically demanding alternative procedure, three fourths of the total volume of buffer is brought to boiling and then added, with vigorous shaking, to a vacuum flask containing a suspension of the starch in the remaining one fourth of the buffer. Regardless of the method of preparation, the content of the flask is degassed under vacuum, and the gel is poured into the tray. A preheated glass plate or special cover is placed over the gel, and a weight is added so that the cover is held tightly in place during cooling. The volume of gel to be prepared will depend upon the volume of the tray.

Sample Insertion

The simplest method of inserting the sample employs small pieces of filter paper. With a surgical knife or razor blade, a cut is first made across the gel about 5 cm from one end. A piece of filter paper (Whatman® no. 3 mm) about 8 × 12 mm is then dipped into hemolysate (about 10% solution). This saturated paper is blotted slightly and placed between the cut edges of the starch. When older samples are used, one drop of 2% KCN should be added to four drops of hemolysate before the hemoglobin is applied to the filter paper. Eight to twelve pieces of paper can be applied on a tray 12 to 14 cm wide. Electrophoresis is begun with the samples nearer the cathode. As soon as the hemoglobin has migrated into the gel, the electrophoresis is stopped, the papers are removed, the cut edges of the gel are brought into contact, and the gel is covered with cellophane or Saran Wrap®.

Vertical electrophoretic methods usually employ a slot-forming mold, so that the hemolysates (about 25 $\mu\ell$ of a 10% solution) are placed into the slots of the gel with the use of disposable Pasteur® pipettes. Each slot is completely filled with the buffer that is used to prepare the gel and to which 0.2 mℓ of 2% KCN in 10 mℓ buffer is added. The latter step is necessary to prevent the occurrence of more slowly moving ferrihemoglobin zones. The slots are finally covered with petroleum jelly, and the remainder of the gel surface is covered with Saran Wrap®.

Electrophoretic Conditions

Electrophoresis can be carried out vertically or horizontally. The duration of electrophoresis varies and depends upon the buffer and the voltage. For screening purposes, it is advisable to use high voltage (500 to 600 V) and a short period (4 to 5 hr) for electrophoresis. When horizontal electrophoresis is used, rapid loss of heat is foiled by placing a plastic frame on top of the gel. Both gel and frame are then covered with Saran Wrap®, and about 200 mℓ of cold water is added.

Gel Slicing

At the end of the electrophoresis, the gel is placed in a plastic tray that has sides 2 to 3 mm high. Alternatively, the 0.5-cm plastic edges that were used for preparing the gel are removed and replaced with 0.2—0.3 cm edges. When either a microtome knife or a nylon fishing line is drawn over these edges, the gel is neatly sliced.

Staining

Half of the gel is stained with a 1% solution of amido black 10 B dissolved in a mixture of methanol, water, and glacial acetic acid (5:5:1 by volume) for 5 to 10 min. Excess dye is removed by repeated washings with the methanol, water, and glacial acetic acid mixture. The second half may be stained with a benzidine reagent. A suitable stain is prepared by adding 0.1 to 0.2 mℓ of 30% hydrogen peroxide to a solution of 100 mg of o-dianisidine in 70 mℓ of ethanol and 30 mℓ of 0.5 M sodium acetate buffer, pH 4.7.[4,9,10] After the gel is stained for approximately 1 hr, the stain is decanted and the gel is washed thoroughly with water. Gels can also be made transparent by

Table 2
RELATIVE ELECTROPHORETIC POSITIONS OF α-CHAIN VARIANTS ON STARCH GEL ELECTROPHORESIS AT pH 8.6—9.0

Relative position	Variants
Slower than Hb A_2	Constant Spring,[a,b] Icaria,[a,b] Koya Dora[b]
Like Hb A_2	Chad, O-Padova, O-Indonesia
Between Hb A_2 and Hb S	Ann Arbor[c]
Like Hb S	Hasharon,[c] Arya, Montgomery, Memphis, Russ, Shimonoseki, Q-India, G-Philadelphia, Daneshgan Tehran, Mahidol, Chapel Hill, Stanleyville II, Etobicoke,[c] Inkster, Setif,[c] Titusville, St. Luke's, Bibba[c]
Between Hb S and Hb F	Sawara, Ottawa, G-Honolulu, L-Persian Gulf, Perspolis, G-Pest, Q-Iran, Winnipeg, Atago, G-Norfolk, G-Georgia, Rampa, Strumica, Chiapas
Like Hb F	Pore Phillip, Denmark Hill, Manitoba
Like Hb A	Torino,[c] Hirosaki,[c] M-Boston, M-Iwate
Between Hb A and Hb J	K, Hopkins 2, Grady, St. Claude, Singapore, Wayne[a,b]
Like Hb J	J-Toronto, Anantharaj, J-Paris, J-Oxford, J-Kurosh, J-Nianza, J-Medellin, J-Sardegna, Mexico, Zambia, J-Buda, Ube-2, Broussais, J-Rajappen, Chesapeake, J-Cape Town, J-Tongariki, Camaguey, J-Cubujuqui, Suresnes, J-Birmingham, Koelliker

[a] Appears as two bands.
[b] Variant with extended chain.
[c] Unstable.

immersion in undiluted glycerol overnight at 4 to 8°C.[11] Quantitation of hemoglobin fractions by either elution of the dye or with a scanning device does not seem very satisfactory.

A simple method for obtaining hemoglobin bands from starch gel is to cut out the required unstained band and to place it into a suitable slot of previously prepared small starch block. A piece of cellophane or dialysis membrane is inserted vertically into the block at a distancc of about 1 cm anodally of thc inscrted starch gel band. Migration of the hemoglobin from the starch gel to the block takes about 1 hr, whereupon the hemoglobin is eluted from the block.

Preservation of the Gels

Gels stained with amido black can be kept indefinitely in cellophane wrappers or in a covered box which contains the destaining solution (methanol, water, glacial acetic acid, 5:5:1 by volume).

Electrophoretic Mobilities of Hemoglobin Variants

The relative electrophoretic mobilities on starch gel electrophoresis at pH 8.5 to 9.0 of many α, β, δ, and γ chain variants are listed in Tables 2, 3, and 4. Their positions are estimated relative to hemoglobins, A_2, S, F, A, J, and I (in order of increasing mobility).

Chain Separation

Starch gel electrophoresis can be used for identifying an abnormal globin chain.[12]

Table 3

RELATIVE ELECTROPHORETIC POSITIONS OF β CHAIN VARIANTS ON STARCH GEL ELECTROPHORESIS AT pH 8.6 to 9.0

Relative position	Variants
Like Hb A_2	C,[a] E, E Saskatoon, C Harlem, Agenogi, Gun Hill,[b] O Arab, Miyada[c]
Between Hb A_2 and Hb S	Siriraj,[b] Porto Alegro, Bushwick,[b] Tours, Santa Ana, Sabine,[b] Istanbul,[b] Newcastle,[b] M Hyde Park, Köln,[b] Kenya,[d] Steinheim[d]
Like Hb S	Sogn,[b] D Bushman, D Ouled Rabah, G Coushatta, D Iran, Riverdale-Bronx,[b] Okaloosa,[b] Ocho Rios, Hamadan, Sidney,[b] Ta-Li,[b] Tours,[b] Boras,[b] Nottingham,[b] P, D Punjab, Beograd, Khartum, Olmsted,[b,e] Lepore[f]
Between Hb S and Hb F	G Makassar, Leiden,[b] G San Jose, G Taiwan-Ami, G Galveston, G Copenhagen, Zurich,[b] H Hsi-Tsou, G Szuhu, Radcliffe, Kempsey, Alberta, Tübingen,[b] Cochin-Port-Royal
Like Hb F	Freiburg,[b] Savannah,[b] Hirose, Yakima, Ypsi,[g] Richmond, Beth Israel,[b] Leslie, Tak[b]
Between Hb F and Hb A	St. Louis,[b] Athens-Georgia, Kansas, Abruzzo
Like Hb A	Saki,[b] Olympia, Volga,[b] Genova,[b] Perth,[b] Philly,[b] Hammersmith,[b] Louisville,[b] Duarte,[b], Bicetre,[b] M Saskatoon,[b] Bristol,[b] Christchurch,[b] St. Antoine,[b] Atlanta,[b] Creteil, Arlington Park, Brigham, Heathrow, Casper,[b] San Diego, Peterborough,[b] Madrid,[b] Altdorf, Hope, Coventry,[b] Little Rock, Syracuse, Rainier, Bethesda, York
Between Hb A and Hb J	Alamo, Moscva,[b] Tacoma,[b] Seattle, Helsinki, Rahere, Malmo, Wood, Camperdown, Yoshizuka, New York, Wien,[b] Camden, Andrew-Minneapolis, North Shore
Like Hb J	Ankara, J Baltimore, J Bangkok, J Kaoshiung, Seattle,[b] Rambam, Shepherds Bush, J Chicago, J Iran, Pyrgos, Hacettepe, Hofu, J Taichung, J Guantanamo, Fort Gordon, Hiroshima, Lyon
Between Hb J and Hb I	Nagasaki, Hikari, N Seattle, N Baltimore, Hijiyama
Like Hb I	I Toulouse[b]

[a] At pH 8.1, migrates slightly more slowly than Hb A_2.
[b] Unstable.
[c] Fusion (βδ) Hb.
[d] Fusion (γβ) Hb.
[e] Small fraction in the position of Hb F.
[f] Fusion (δβ) Hb.
[g] Multiple "hybrid" and polymer bands.

Table 4
RELATIVE ELECTROPHORETIC POSITIONS OF γ AND δ CHAIN VARIANTS ON STARCH GEL ELECTROPHORESIS AT pH 8.6—9.0

Relative position	γ-Chain variants	δ-Chain variants
Slower than Hb A_2	F Texas I, F Texas II, F Hull, F Carlton	A_2 Sphakia, Nyu, B_2, A_2 Melbourne, A_2 Indonesia
Between Hb A_2 and Hb S	F Kuala Lumpur, F Victoria Jubilee, F Port Royal, F Alexandra, F Melbourne, F Malta-I	A_2 Babinga
Like Hb S	F Auckland	A_2 Roosevelt
Between Hb S and Hb F	—	A_2 Flatbush, A_2 Coburg
Like Hb A	F Poole	—
Between Hb A and Hb J	F Malaysia	—
Like Hb J	F Jamaica	—

The buffer used is either a barbital or a tris-EDTA-borate buffer (pH 8.0 to 8.6), and contains 6 M urea and β-mercaptoethanol. A barbital buffer is prepared by dissolving 18.4 g of diethylbartituric acid in 600 mℓ of boiling distilled water, whereupon 15 mℓ of 4 N NaOH is added with mixing. The volume is adjusted to 1000 mℓ with distilled water, and the pH is brought to 8.0 with 1 N NaOH.

To prepare a gel, 90 g of starch (18% instead of 12% suspension of hydrolyzed starch) is mixed thoroughly with 180 g of urea, and the mixture is added to 300 mℓ of barbital or tris-EDTA borate buffer. This material is held at 70 to 80°C in a water bath for 5 to 10 min with constant stirring until it is smooth and clear and then poured into a starch gel tray. The same 6 M urea-barbital or 6 M urea-tris-EDTA-borate buffer with 2 mℓ of β-mercaptoethanol per one liter is used as a bridge buffer. The samples to be applied to the gel should contain approximately 2 mg globin in 0.1 mℓ of the same buffer used for preparing the gel, to which 0.1 mℓ β-mercaptoethanol per 10 mℓ of buffer is added. The samples are applied to the gel in the usual manner, and electrophoresis is carried out at 4°C for about 20 hr at 300 to 350 V. The gels are sliced and stained with amido black in the usual manner. The α chains migrate cathodally, whereas the β and γ chains migrate toward the positive pole. The δ chain remains near the area of application.

REFERENCES

1. **Smithies, O.**, Zone electrophoresis in starch gels: group variations in the serum proteins of normal adults, *Biochem. J.*, 61, 629, 1955.
2. **Smithies, O.**, An improved procedure for starch gel electrophoresis: further variation in the serum proteins of normal adults, *Biochem. J.*, 71, 585, 1959.
3. **Giblett, E. R.**, *Genetic Markers in Human Blood,* Davis, Philadelphia, 1969, 101.
4. **Weatherall, D. J.**, *The Thalassaemia Syndromes,* Blackwell Scientific, Oxford, 1965, 211.
5. **Efremov, G. D., Huisman, T. H. J., Smith, L. L., Wilson, J. B., Kitchens, J. L., Wrightstone, R. N., and Adams, H. R.**, Hemoglobin Richmond, a human hemoglobin which forms asymmetric hybrids with other hemoglobins, *J. Biol. Chem.*, 244, 6105, 1969.
6. **Poulik, M. D.**, Starch gel electrophoresis in a discontinuous system of buffers, *Nature (London),* 180, 1477, 1957.
7. **Gammack, D. B., Huehns, E. R., and Shooter, E. M.**, Identification of the abnormal polypeptide chain of hemoglobin G_{Ib}, *J. Mol. Biol.*, 2, 372, 1960.

8. **Gerald, P. S.**, The electrophoretic and spectroscopic characterization of hemoglobin M, *Blood*, 13, 936, 1958.
9. **Huisman, T. H. J.**, Normal and abnormal human hemoglobins, in *Advances in Clinical Chemistry*, Vol. 6, Sobotka, H. and Stewart, C. P., Eds., Academic Press, New York, 1963, 649.
10. **Lehmann, H. and Huntsman, R. G.**, *Man's Haemoglobins*, North-Holland, Amsterdam, 1966, 275.
11. **Gratzer, W. B. and Beaven, G. H.**, Transparent starch gels: preparation, optical properties, and application to hemoglobin characterization, *Clin. Chim. Acta*, 5, 577, 1960.
12. **Chernoff, A. I. and Pettit, N. M.**, The amino acid composition of hemoglobin. III. A qualitative method for identifying abnormalities of the polypeptide chains of hemoglobins, *Blood*, 24, 750, 1964.

THE THREE-DIMENSIONAL STRUCTURE OF HEMOGLOBIN

K. W. Olsen

The determination of the three-dimensional structure of hemoglobin by Perutz and co-workers is a major milestone in the progress of biochemistry. This work makes possible the study of the stereochemical role of each amino acid residue in the function of hemoglobin. As a result, many physiologically and chemically important aspects of hematology, such as the Bohr effect, the allosteric mechanism of oxygen binding, and the nature of abnormal hemoglobins, can be explained by the three-dimensional structure of this protein. The subject has been reviewed numerous times[1-5] and is discussed in every modern biochemistry text.[6-10] In this chapter, the structure of hemoglobin will be briefly described and related to its function. The three-dimensional data will be tabulated, so that it can be applied to future problems involving hemoglobin.

The globin fold is the characteristic tertiary structure of the oxygen-binding hemoproteins. It has been demonstrated by X-ray crystallography (Tables 1 and 2), not only in hemoglobins and myoglobins[11-36] of several different species, but also in the globins of the sea lamprey,[23] the midge larva,[19,20] and the bloodworm.[21,22] Although the sequences of these proteins differ by as much as 87%,[37] the tertiary structure is maintained, as can be seen in the stereo-pair drawings of Figure 1.* There are over 50 known globin sequences that have internal gaps when compared with each other. Thus it is necessary to have a residue numbering system based on the three-dimensional structure. The globin fold (Figure 2) consists of eight helical segments, labeled A through H, which are connected by nonhelical regions and are named for the helices that they connect. For example, the region between helices A and B is the AB section. The region from amino terminus to the start of the first helical is named NA, while that from the end of the H helix to the carboxyl terminus is called HC. The first residue of the A helix is designated as A1, the second as A2, and so forth. The sequences of the human myoglobin[38] and hemoglobin[39-42] chains are given in Table 3 with these designations. The advantage of this numbering system is that homologous residues will always have the same designation. Thus the proximal histidine that binds the iron of the heme is at position F8, although it is residue 87 in the α chain and 92 in the β chain. Since the horse methemoglobin is the most accurately determined of these crystal structures, it will be described first, and the other proteins will be related to it.

The globin fold (Figure 2) is a compact structure with dimensions of 45 × 35 × 25 Å.[11] The eight helical segments of the globin fold account for about 75% of the residues. The differences between myoglobin and the α and β chains of hemoglobin are summarized in Table 4. Helix D is not present in the α chain, and the AB connecting segment is absent in the β chain. Most of the segments are α helices, but segment C is a 3_{10} helix in both hemoglobin chains, and segment F is followed by one turn of π helix,[4,29] as shown in Figures 6 and 7. The conformational parameters for the three types of helices are given in Table 5, and they are illustrated in Figures 3 to 5. Some of the globin helices have irregular hydrogen bonds. This is particularly true of the heme-linked helices E and F and of the FG corner (Figures 6 to 10). These helices contain few linear hydrogen bonds, and several bifurcated hydrogen bonds are formed. Helix E is more regular in the α subunit than in the β subunit (Figures 8 and 9). The π

* All figures and tables for this chapter follow text.

** Stereoviewers are available from Edmond Scientific Company, Barrington, New Jersey 08007; Taylor-Merchant Corporation, 25 West 45th Street, New York, New York 10036; and Lansing Instrument Corporation, Lansing, Michigan. A pair of enlarging lenses with 85 mm focal lengths, mounted 70 mm apart in cardboard, is also adequate.

helix involving residues F7 to FG3 is stabilized by a hydrogen bond, from the side chain of Arg FG4(92)α to the main chain carbonyl of Lys FG2(90)α (Figure 6) in the α subunit, and by a hydrogen bond from the imidazole of His FG4(97)β to the carbonyl of Cys F9(93)β in the β chain. The entire hydrogen bonding network for the horse methemoglobin molecule is given in Figures 11 and 12.* The secondary and tertiary structures of the α and β chains of methemoglobin are shown in Figures 13 and 14.

The major forces that determine the tertiary structures of proteins are thought to be hydrophobic interactions.[47,48] The strength of these interactions depends on the increase in the entropy of the solution, when the nonpolar side chains are packed together on the interior of the protein. Thus the hydrophobic residues are found on the interior of the globin fold, and the hydrophilic ones are on the exterior (Figure 15). Serine and threonine residues that are occasionally found on the interior form hydrogen bonds with other residues, but nonpolar residues are not generally found at internal positions, as shown in Table 6.[49] In contrast, only a few of the surface or surface-crevice residues are consistently nonpolar (Table 7). The variation in the hydrophobicity of partially buried residues may be a source of species variation in the stability of the tertiary structure.[50] The residue variability due to species differences in myoglobins and hemoglobins is summarized in Table 8. These data emphasize the importance of having nonpolar residues at internal positions for the maintenance of the globin fold. Thus a mutation that introduces a charged residue into one of these positions will produce an unstable, abnormal hemoglobin.[51]

The structure and environment of the heme groups is critically important to the function of hemoglobin. The porphyrin rings in methemoglobin appear to be planar, although small deformations may be present, since they would not be detectable in a 2.0 Å resolution electron density map. The distance that the iron atom is displaced from the plane of the porphyrin ring depends on both the ligands and the spin state of the iron. A detailed discussion of spin states can be found in Reference 3. The spin states of various hemoglobin derivatives are listed in Table 9. The high-spin iron atom in both deoxy- and methemoglobin should have a radius that is too large to fit into the plane of the porphyrin. This effect is seen only in deoxy- and metmyoglobin, deoxyhemoglobin, and the model compound 2-methylimidazole iron (11) tetraphenylporphin, and is not seen in methemoglobin (Table 10). The small displacement seen in the α subunits of methemoglobin[29] could be most easily explained if the pyrrole rings were ruffled, so that the nitrogens would be on either side of the iron. When the crystallographic studies of hemoglobin were begun, the significance of spin states was not apparent, and the methemoglobin was assumed to be very similar to oxyhemoglobin. In most respects this assumption still seems to be true. Thus the comparison of the deoxy- and methemoglobin structure should show us the changes that occur during oxygenation.

The environment of the hemes is shown in Figures 16 and 17 for horse methemoglobin and in Figures 18 and 19 for human deoxyhemoglobin. The hemes are bound to the globin by a covalent bond between the nitrogen atom of the proximal His F8 and the iron atom, and by a large number of nonpolar interactions between the porphyrin and the hydrophobic residues that form its binding pocket. A list of these interactions is given in Table 11. The propionic acid side chains of the α heme form salt links with

* The amino acid residues discussed in this chapter are abbreviated with the normal three letter code, the segment name and number, the sequence position number in parentheses, and the chain designation. Figures 11 and 12 use the one-letter code for the amino acids. The codes are as follows: alanine, Ala, A; arginine, Arg, R; asparagine, Asn, N; aspartic acid, Asp, D; cysteine, Cys, C; glutamine, Gln, Q; glutamic acid, Glu, E; glycine, Gly, G; histidine, His, H; isoleucine, Ile, I; leucine, Leu, L; lysine, Lys, K; methionine, Met, M; phenylalanine, Phe, F; proline, Pro, P; serine, Ser, S; threonine, Thr, T; tryptophan, Trp, W; tryosine, Try, Y; and valine, Val, V. Asx refers to either aspartic acid or asparagine (not established).

His CD3(45)α and Lys E10(61)α, but those of the β heme do not. If methemoglobin is used as a model for oxyhemoglobin, the heme environments change upon deoxygenation. Table 12 compares the distances between various points on the hemes to the surrounding residues in horse methemoglobin and human deoxyhemoglobin. The relative movements of the hemes and the various helices are quite similar in the α and β subunits. Figure 20 shows the changes in the distance from the heme center to the surrounding residues between methemoglobin and deoxyhemoglobin for both subunits. Helix E is closer to the hemes in the deoxy state; however, this change is greater in the β subunits than in the α subunits. On the other hand, helix B and the CD segment have moved further away from the heme axis in all subunits of deoxyhemoglobin. One of the most significant movements that occurs during deoxygenation involves helix F, which contains the proximal histidine at position F8. This helix rotates clockwise, as seen from the FG corner. The imidazole group of F8 moves approximately 0.4 Å away from the porphyrin in the deoxy structure. As a result of this rotation, Leu F7 moves away from the heme, but Leu F4 moves toward the heme. The FG segment also moves toward the heme, particularly Leu FG3. The movements of the tertiary structure are summarized in Figure 21. Obviously, the largest movements are those involving the FG corner and the HC segment. The carboxyl terminal residues appear to be free in solution in methemoglobin, but they make several interchain salt linkages in deoxyhemoglobin.[55,56] The changes in these salt bridges are an important aspect of the heme-heme interactions. Helix A, which is remote from the heme group, also moves; however, the importance of this movement is difficult to assess, since the position of this helix differs in human and horse deoxyhemoglobins.[25] Data showing the extent of this species difference in the three-dimensional structure of deoxyhemoglobin are presented in Table 13.

During deoxygenation both heme groups rotate slightly clockwise, as viewed from their propionic acid side chains. The β heme moves toward the solvent, but the α heme is held somewhat more rigidly, because of the interactions of His CD3(45)α and Lys E10(61)α with its propionate groups.

An important difference between the α and β subunits is the position of valine E11 relative to the heme-linked water. The distance between the water molecule and gamma carbon of Val E11 is 3.8 Å in the α subunit, but only 3.3 Å in the β subunit.[29] The resulting steric interference between the β chains and the ligands explains why the β hemes are more easily reduced than the α hemes in the oxy quaternary structure. In the deoxy quaternary structure, the β hemes are less readily autoxidized than the α hemes for the same reason.[25]

Many of the physiologically important properties of hemoglobin depend on the changes in its quaternary structure. The basic quaternary structure is shown in Figure 22. To form the quaternary structure, the subunits bury approximately one fifth of their surface area in the interfaces between them.[54] The $\alpha_1\beta_1$ contact accounts for 60% of that area, and the $\alpha_1\beta_2$ contact accounts for 33%. The other 7% is in $\alpha_1\alpha_2$ and $\beta_1\beta_2$ contacts. The stability of the tetramer comes largely from hydrophobic interactions in the subunit interfaces.[54] However, these interfaces are far more polar than earlier studies[57,58] indicated. In methemoglobin there are 15 bound water molecules in the $\alpha_1\beta_1$ contact and 4 bound water molecules in the $\alpha_1\beta_2$ contact.[29] There are 17 to 19 hydrogen bonds present in the $\alpha_1\beta_1$ interface, and 6 to 7 hydrogen bonds in the $\alpha_1\beta_2$ interface.[29] The amount of surface area buried in the subunit contacts, and the percentage of polar interactions in the contract regions, which was estimated from the number of nitrogen and oxygen atoms found there, is given in Table 14.

The $\alpha_1\beta_1$ dimer of methemoglobin is seen in Figure 23. More detailed views of this contact are given in Figures 24 and 25. The residues involved in this interface and their interactions are summarized in Table 15A for methemoglobin, and in Table 16A for deoxyhemoglobin. The α carbon coordinates for this dimer in the deoxy- and methemoglobins can be superimposed on each other as a rigid body,[54] demonstrating that there are no major changes in the $\alpha_1\beta_1$ contact during the allosteric transition. The relative rotation of the α_1 and β_1 subunits by 3.7°, found in earlier reports,[59] appears to result from the changes in tertiary structure.

The $\alpha_1\beta_2$ dimer is shown in Figure 26. Two points are immediately obvious from this stereodiagram. First, the FG corner, which is subject to a large movement during the deoxygenation, is intimately involved in this subunit contact, which can be seen in detail in Figure 27. Second, the heme groups are closer and more directly connected through the protein structure in this dimer than in the $\alpha_1\beta_1$ dimer. The residues and interactions involved in this contact are summarized in Table 15B. The differences in the $\alpha_1\beta_2$ interfaces in deoxy- and methemoglobin can be seen by comparing Table 16B and Figures 28 to 30 with Table 15B and Figures 26 and 27. The contact region of deoxyhemoglobins is shown diagrammatically in Figure 31. The changes in this dimer are much more dramatic than in the $\alpha_1\beta_1$ dimer. The two subunits have turned 13° relative to each other. The contact is dovetailed, so that the C helix of one subunit fits into the FG segment of the other. Thus there are two C-FG interactions per $\alpha_1\beta_2$ interface, related to each other by the pseudo-dyad. In both met- and deoxyhemoglobin, Trp C3(37)β fits into a V-shaped groove formed by the alpha carbon of Val FG5(93)α, but the two residues move slightly relative to one another. The other C-FG interaction, however, changes greatly during the transition of the quaternary structure. In methemoglobin, the side chain of Thr C3(38)α fits into the groove of Val FG5(98)β, but in deoxyhemoglobin this threonine is replaced by Thr C6(41)α. This change is shown diagrammatically in Figure 32. These two threonines are on successive turns of the C helix. Thus there is no intermediate residue that could fit into the groove at Val FG5(98)β. In addition, Asp G1(94)α forms a hydrogen bond with Asn G4(102)β in methemoglobin, while Tyr C7(42)α forms one with Asp G1(99)β in deoxyhemoglobin. No intermediate hydrogen bonding patterns are possible. Thus the hemoglobin molecule is constrained to be in one of only two possible quaternary structures, by the dovetailing and the intersubunit hydrogen bonding.

The resulting two-state model provides a structural explanation for many of the physiological properties, including diphosphoglycerate binding, the Bohr effect, and heme-heme interaction.

The binding of diphosphoglycerate (DPG) to deoxyhemoglobin has been studied by X-ray crystallography.[60] One molecule of DPG per tetramer binds in the central cavity between the β subunits, which can be seen in Figure 22A. The phosphate groups form salt bridges to the cationic groups of Val NA1(1)β, His NA2(2)β, Lys EF6(82)β, and His H21(143)β, as shown in Figure 33. In methemoglobin the amino termini move further apart, while the EF segments move closer together. The complementarity of the binding site and DPG is lost, and the affinity for DPG drops 150-fold. Since DPG can bind only to the deoxy conformation of hemoglobin, it stabilizes this form, resulting in a lower oxygen affinity in the presence of DPG. This phenomenon explains the difference in the oxygen affinity of fetal and adult blood. In fetal hemoglobin, the γ chain has serine rather than histidine at position H21, decreasing the affinity for DPG. In the presence of DPG, adult hemoglobin has a lower oxygen affinity than fetal hemoglobin, even though they have similar affinities when stripped of DPG. Inositol hexaphosphate can also occupy the DPG-binding site in deoxyhemoglobin[61] and in fluoromethemoglobin,[62] which has the same conformation as deoxyhemoglobin.

The Bohr effect is the lowering of the oxygen affinity of hemoglobin with decreasing pH. At the present time, approximately 60% of the alkaline Bohr effect, which operates above pH 7, can be accounted for by structural explanations. Carbamylation of the α amino groups of Val NA1(1)α with cyanate demonstrated that this group accounted for about 20% of the Bohr effect.[63] The X-ray structure of this carbamylated deoxyhemoglobin shows that the anion normally bound between the α-amino group and the positively charged guanidinium of Arg HC3(141)α of the second α chain (Figure 34) is missing.[64] In the oxy conformation, this salt bridge is not formed and the anion is released, causing the pK of the α-amino group to decrease by 0.8 units.[65] His HC3(146)β is also involved in the Bohr effect. The imidazole of this residue forms a salt linkage to the carboxyl group of Asp FG1(94)β in the deoxy structure only. When the pK of His HC3(146)β was measured by proton nuclear magnetic resonance, it was found to be 8.0 in deoxyhemoglobin and 7.1 in carboxyhemoglobin. This change in pK would account for 40% of the total Bohr effect. It had been suggested that His H5(122)α was responsible for the remaining 40% of the Bohr effect, since it appeared to have different interactions in deoxy and methemoglobin.[55] However, more recent results at higher resolution show that this histidine has identical interactions in both structures.[25,29] Measurements of the Bohr effects of mutant and animal hemoglobins that lacked particular histidines could not attribute the remainder of the Bohr effect to any of these residues.[66] Thus the groups responsible for the last 40% are still unknown.

Carbon dioxide can react reversibly with the α-amino groups of hemoglobin to form carbamino compounds.[67] Since the deoxy structure reacts more readily than does the oxy structure, CO_2 binding lowers oxygen affinity. The β-chain carbamate group probably forms a salt linkage with Lys EF6(82)β, but it does not appear that this interaction would differ between the oxy and deoxy conformation.[68] The α-chain carbamate group probably displaces the inorganic anion and interacts directly with Arg HC3(141) on the other α subunit. Thus the deoxy structure is stabilized, but the oxy structure is not.

The heme-heme interaction of hemoglobin is the positive cooperativity of oxygen binding to the tetramer. This type of allosteric binding behavior is often explained by the Monod-Wyman-Changeux[69] or by the Koshland-Nemethy-Filmer[70] models. Both of these models were developed by applying certain assumptions to the equilibrium equations for binding oxygen. The Monod-Wyman-Changeux model assumes that there are only two possible quaternary structures, which differ in oxygen affinity. Oxygen binding would affect the equilibrium between the two quaternary structures, but the binding to one subunit is not affected by the oxygenation state of the other subunits in the same molecule. The Koshland-Nemethy-Filmer model differs, by assuming that binding of oxygen to one subunit increases the affinity of a neighboring subunit. Perutz,[55,56,71] on the other hand, has developed a stereochemical theory that explains heme-heme interactions on the basis of the known conformational differences between oxy- and deoxyhemoglobin. Figure 35 illustrates this theory. In this diagram, oxygen binds to the α subunit first. While it is not necessary to assume this binding order, there is some evidence supporting a sequential order with the α subunits reacting before the β subunits.[72] The α heme pocket is open enough to allow oxygen to enter and bind to the iron, whereas in the β chain, the entrance is closed and must be opened by thermal energy. When the oxygen binds to the α_1 subunit, the iron changes from high spin to low spin with a simultaneous decrease in its radius, so that it can move into the plane of the porphyrin. This movement triggers a sequence of conformational changes, since the iron atom pulls the proximal histidine (F8) with it. As a result, helix F moves toward helix H, and Tyr HC2(140)α_1 is expelled from its position between these helices. This is illustrated diagrammatically in Figure 36. The movement of this tyrosine causes the displacement of the carboxyterminal Arg HC3(141)α_1. This, in turn, breaks the salt linkages to the α_2 chain shown in Figures 34 and 35. The dissolution of the salt bridges allows the release of a Bohr proton from the α-amino group of Val NA1(1)α_2. The α_1 chain now has an oxy tertiary structure, but the quaternary structure is still in the deoxy conformation. The process is essentially identical for the β subunits, except for the changes in the intersubunit salt linkages, shown in Figure 34. The successive transitions of the subunits from the deoxy to the oxy tertiary structure, and the associated rupturing of the ionic bonds between subunits, increases the strain until a transition to the oxy quaternary structure occurs. In Figure 35 this transition happens between steps 3 and 4. The central idea of the stereochemical theory is that the positive cooperativity is directly linked to this change in the quaternary structure. Once the molecule is in the oxy quaternary conformation, the remaining deoxy subunits can more easily adopt the oxy tertiary structure, which means that oxygen can be bound more readily.

The three-dimensional structure of hemoglobin also provides us with an understanding of the changes in the functional properties of abnormal hemoglobins.[73] Perutz, Lehmann, and co-workers have investigated the molecular pathology of human hemoglobin[51,74] and have concluded that there are four basic types of mutant proteins. First, there are mutations of the residues that are in contact with the heme group. These substitutions often have a direct effect on oxygen affinity and sometimes result in an unstable hemoglobin. In some cases, replacement of a nonpolar contact between the heme group and the globin will eliminate the heme-binding affinity of the protein. Other changes, characteristic of the hemoglobins M, stabilize the ferric form of the iron. The effects of some mutations of this type are summarized in Table 17.

The second type of mutation that causes major functional changes involves replacements in the subunit contacts. Some of these substitutions trap the molecule into either the oxy or deoxy quaternary structure, resulting in the loss of allosteric properties. Alterations in the subunit interfaces also promote dissociation of the tetramer into dimers and monomers. Examples of this type of abnormal hemoglobin are given in Table 18.

The other two types of mutation involve changes in the positions that are not directly involved in the heme pockets or the subunit interactions. In one class, an altered tertiary is the result of a substitution that prevents the polypeptide chain from folding into the normal tertiary structure. If a hydrophobic, internal residue is replaced by an ionic amino acid, the resulting hemoglobin is generally unstable, as illustrated by hemoglobin Wien in Table 19. The positions of mutations that lead to instability are shown in Figure 37. The second type of mutation in a general position is one that causes an alteration to the exterior of the tetramer. Nearly all of these substitutions are harmless, but hemoglobin S is an obvious exception. The conclusions obtained by examining the effect of several changes in general positions on the three-dimensional structure of hemoglobin, are listed in Table 19.

The explanations of Perutz and Lehmann[51,74] for the altered functional properties of abnormal hemoglobins have proven to be generally correct. Investigations of these mutant proteins by X-ray crystallography, however, have provided additional details. In several cases, such as oxy hemoglobin Chesapeake[115] and deoxy hemoglobin Kansas,[119,120] the structural effects are not limited to the area surrounding the replacement, but are spread throughout the tetramer. Thus these diffraction studies not only provide a greater understanding of the abnormal physiological properties of the mutant hemoglobins, but also allow an investigation of the relationship between the amino acid sequence and the three-dimensional structure of a protein. The results of the X-ray determinations of abnormal hemoglobin structures are summarized in Table 20.

Acknowledgment

The author wishes to thank Miss Martha E. Hutchinson for her assistance in checking the references and the Mississippi Heart Association for their grant support.

Table 1
X-RAY STRUCTURE DETERMINATIONS OF MONOMERIC GLOBINS

Species	Derivative	Resolution ($Å^{-1}$)	Ref.
Sperm-whale myoglobin	Aquomet	2.0	11,12
	Deoxy	2.0	13
	Azidomet	2.8	14
	Cyanmet	2.8	15
	CO	1.8	16
Seal myoglobin	Aquomet	5.0	17
Tuna myoglobin	Aquomet	6.0	18
Chironomus	Aquomet	2.5	19
erythrocruorin	CO	2.5	20
	Deoxy	2.5	20
Glycera hemoglobin	Cyanmet	5.5	21,22
Lamprey hemoglobin	Cyanmet	2.5	23
Leghemoglobin	Aquomet	5.0	24

From Perutz, M. F., *Br. Med. Bull.*, 32, 195, 1976. Reproduced by permission of the Medical Department, the British Council.

Table 2
X-RAY STRUCTURE DETERMINATIONS OF TETRAMERIC HEMOGLOBINS

Species	Derivative	Resolution ($Å^{-1}$)	Ref.
Human Hb A	Deoxy	2.5	25,26
	CO	2.8	27
Human Hb F	Deoxy	3.5	28
Horse	Aquomet	2.0	29
	Deoxy	2.8	30
	CO	2.8	31
	Azidomet	5.5	32
	Cyanmet	2.8	33
	Fluoromet	2.8	34
	Deuteromet	2.8	35
	Metmangano	2.8	36

From Perutz, M. F., *Br. Med. Bull.*, 32, 195, 1976. Reproduced by permission of the Medical Department, The British Council.

Table 3
AMINO ACID SEQUENCES AND POSITIONS OF HUMAN HEMOGLOBINS AND MYOGLOBIN

Structural Position		α-Chain		β, γ and δ Chains				Myoglobin	
		Number	Sequence	Number	β Sequence	γ Sequence	δ Sequence	Number	Sequence
NA	1			1	Val	Gly	Val		
	2	1	Val	2	His	His	His	1	Gly
	3	2	Leu	3	Leu	Phe	Leu	2	Leu
A	1	3	Ser	4	Thr	Thr	Thr	3	Ser
	2	4	Pro	5	Pro	Glu	Pro	4	Asp
	3	5	Ala	6	Glu	Glu	Glu	5	Gly
	4	6	Asp	7	Glu	Asp	Glu	6	Glu
	5	7	Lys	8	Lys	Lys	Lys	7	Trp
	6	8	Thr	9	Ser	Ala	Thr	8	Gln
	7	9	Asn	10	Ala	Thr	Ala	9	Leu
	8	10	Val	11	Val	Ile	Val	10	Val
	9	11	Lys	12	Thr	Thr	Asn	11	Leu
	10	12	Ala	13	Ala	Ser	Ala	12	Asn
	11	13	Ala	14	Leu	Leu	Leu	13	Val
	12	14	Trp	15	Trp	Trp	Trp	14	Trp
	13	15	Gly	16	Gly	Gly	Gly	15	Gly
	14	16	Lys	17	Lys	Lys	Lys	16	Lys
	15	17	Val	18	Val	Val	Val	17	Val
	16	18	Gly	—	—	—	—	18	Glu
AB	1	19	Ala	—	—	—	—	19	Ala
B	1	20	His	19	Asn	Asn	Asn	20	Asp
	2	21	Ala	20	Val	Val	Val	21	Ile
	3	22	Gly	21	Asp	Glu	Asp	22	Pro
	4	23	Glu	22	Glu	Asp	Ala	23	Gly
	5	24	Try	23	Val	Ala	Val	24	His
	6	25	Gly	24	Gly	Gly	Gly	25	Gly
	7	26	Ala	25	Gly	Gly	Gly	26	Gln
	8	27	Glu	26	Glu	Glu	Glu	27	Glu

Table 3 (continued)
AMINO ACID SEQUENCES AND POSITIONS OF HUMAN HEMOGLOBINS AND MYOGLOBIN

Structural Position		α-Chain		β, γ and δ Chains				Myoglobin	
		Number	Sequence	Number	β Sequence	γ Sequence	δ Sequence	Number	Sequence
	9	28	Ala	27	Ala	Thr	Ala	28	Val
	10	29	Leu	28	Leu	Leu	Leu	29	Leu
	11	30	Glu	29	Gly	Gly	Gly	30	Ile
	12	31	Arg	30	Arg	Arg	Arg	31	Arg
	13	32	Met	31	Leu	Leu	Leu	32	Leu
	14	33	Phe	32	Leu	Leu	Leu	33	Phe
	15	34	Leu	33	Val	Val	Val	34	Lys
	16	35	Ser	34	Val	Val	Val	35	Gly
C	1	36	Phe	35	Tyr	Tyr	Tyr	36	His
	2	37	Pro	36	Pro	Pro	Pro	37	Pro
	3	38	Thr	37	Trp	Trp	Trp	38	Glu
	4	39	Thr	38	Thr	Thr	Thr	39	Thr
	5	40	Lys	39	Gln	Gln	Gln	40	Leu
	6	41	Thr	40	Arg	Arg	Arg	41	Glu
	7	42	Tyr	41	Phe	Phe	Phe	42	Lys
CD	1	43	Phe	42	Phe	Phe	Phe	43	Phe
	2	44	Pro	43	Glu	Asp	Glu	44	Asp
	3	45	His	44	Ser	Ser	Ser	45	Lys
	4	46	Phe	45	Phe	Phe	Phe	46	Phe
	5	—	—	46	Gly	Gly	Gly	47	Lys
	6	47	Asp	47	Asp	Asn	Asp	48	His
	7	48	Leu	48	Leu	Leu	Leu	49	Leu
	8	49	Ser	49	Ser	Ser	Ser	50	Lys
D	1	—	—	50	Thr	Ser	Ser	51	Ser
	2	—	—	51	Pro	Ala	Pro	52	Glu
	3	—	—	52	Asp	Ser	Asp	53	Asp
	4	—	—	53	Ala	Ala	Ala	54	Glu
	5	—	—	54	Val	Ile	Val	55	Met

Table 3 (continued)
AMINO ACID SEQUENCES AND POSITIONS OF HUMAN HEMOGLOBINS AND MYOGLOBIN

Structural Position		α-Chain		β, γ and δ Chains				Myoglobin	
		Number	Sequence	Number	β Sequence	γ Sequence	δ Sequence	Number	Sequence
	6	50	His	55	Met	Met	Met	56	Lys
	7	51	Gly	56	Gly	Gly	Gly	57	Ala
E	1	52	Ser	57	Asn	Asn	Asn	58	Ser
	2	53	Ala	58	Pro	Pro	Pro	59	Glu
	3	54	Gln	59	Lys	Lys	Lys	60	Asp
	4	55	Val	60	Val	Val	Val	61	Leu
	5	56	Lys	61	Lys	Lys	Lys	62	Lys
	6	57	Gly	62	Ala	Ala	Ala	63	Lys
	7	58	His	63	His	His	His	64	His
	8	59	Gly	64	Gly	Gly	Gly	65	Gly
	9	60	Lys	65	Lys	Lys	Lys	66	Ala
	10	61	Lys	66	Lys	Lys	Lys	67	Thr
	11	62	Val	67	Val	Val	Val	68	Val
	12	63	Ala	68	Leu	Leu	Leu	69	Leu
	13	64	Asp	69	Gly	Thr	Gly	70	Thr
	14	65	Ala	70	Ala	Ser	Ala	71	Ala
	15	66	Leu	71	Phe	Leu	Phe	72	Leu
	16	67	Thr	72	Ser	Gly	Ser	73	Gly
	17	68	Asn	73	Asp	Asp	Asp	74	Gly
	18	69	Ala	74	Gly	Ala	Gly	75	Ile
	19	70	Val	75	Leu	Ile	Leu	76	Leu
	20	71	Ala	76	Ala	Lys	Ala	77	Lys
EF	1	72	His	77	His	His	His	78	Lys
	2	73	Val	78	Leu	Leu	Leu	79	Lys
	3	74	Asp	79	Asp	Asp	Asp	80	Gly
	4	75	Asp	80	Asn	Asp	Asn	81	His
	5	76	Met	81	Leu	Leu	Leu	82	His
	6	77	Pro	82	Lys	Lys	Lys	83	Glu

Table 3 (continued)
AMINO ACID SEQUENCES AND POSITIONS OF HUMAN HEMOGLOBINS AND MYOGLOBIN

Structural Position	α-Chain		β, γ and δ Chains				Myoglobin	
	Number	Sequence	Number	β Sequence	γ Sequence	δ Sequence	Number	Sequence
7	78	Asn	83	Gly	Gly	Gly	84	Ala
8	79	Ala	84	Thr	Thr	Thr	85	Glu
F 1	80	Leu	85	Phe	Phe	Phe	86	Ile
2	81	Ser	86	Ala	Ala	Ser	87	Lys
3	82	Ala	87	Thr	Gln	Gln	88	Pro
4	83	Leu	88	Leu	Leu	Leu	89	Leu
5	84	Ser	89	Ser	Ser	Ser	90	Ala
6	85	Asp	90	Glu	Glu	Glu	91	Gln
7	86	Leu	91	Leu	Leu	Leu	92	Ser
8	87	His	92	His	His	His	93	His
9	88	Ala	93	Cys	Cys	Cys	94	Ala
FG 1	89	His	94	Asp	Asp	Asp	95	Thr
2	90	Lys	95	Lys	Lys	Lys	96	Lys
3	91	Leu	96	Leu	Leu	Leu	97	His
4	92	Arg	97	His	His	His	98	Lys
5	93	Val	98	Val	Val	Val	99	Ile
G 1	94	Asp	99	Asp	Asp	Asp	100	Pro
2	95	Pro	100	Pro	Pro	Pro	101	Val
3	96	Val	101	Glu	Glu	Glu	102	Lys
4	97	Asn	102	Asn	Asn	Asn	103	Tyr
5	98	Phe	103	Phe	Phe	Phe	104	Leu
6	99	Lys	104	Arg	Lys	Arg	105	Glu
7	100	Leu	105	Leu	Leu	Leu	106	Phe
8	101	Leu	106	Leu	Leu	Leu	107	Ile
9	102	Ser	107	Gly	Gly	Gly	108	Ser
10	103	His	108	Asn	Asn	Asn	109	Glu
11	104	Cys	109	Val	Val	Val	110	Cys
12	105	Leu	110	Leu	Leu	Leu	111	Ile

Table 3 (continued)
AMINO ACID SEQUENCES AND POSITIONS OF HUMAN HEMOGLOBINS AND MYOGLOBIN

Structural Position		α-Chain		β, γ and δ Chains				Myoglobin	
		Number	Sequence	Number	β Sequence	γ Sequence	δ Sequence	Number	Sequence
	13	106	Leu	111	Val	Val	Val	112	Ile
	14	107	Val	112	Cys	Thr	Cys	113	Gln
	15	108	Thr	113	Val	Val	Val	114	Val
	16	109	Leu	114	Leu	Leu	Leu	115	Leu
	17	110	Ala	115	Ala	Ala	Ala	116	Gln
	18	111	Ala	116	His	Ile	Arg	117	Ser
	19	112	His	117	His	His	Asn	118	Lys
GH	1	113	Leu	118	Phe	Phe	Phe	119	His
	2	114	Pro	119	Gly	Gly	Gly	120	Pro
	3	115	Ala	120	Lys	Lys	Lys	121	Gly
	4	116	Glu	121	Glu	Glu	Glu	122	Asp
	5	117	Phe	122	Phe	Phe	Phe	123	Phe
H	1	118	Thr	123	Thr	Thr	Thr	124	Gly
	2	119	Pro	124	Pro	Pro	Pro	125	Ala
	3	120	Ala	125	Pro	Glu	Gln	126	Asp
	4	121	Val	126	Val	Val	Met	127	Ala
	5	122	His	127	Gln	Gln	Gln	128	Gln
	6	123	Ala	128	Ala	Ala	Ala	129	Gly
	7	124	Ser	129	Ala	Ser	Ala	130	Ala
	8	125	Leu	130	Tyr	Trp	Tyr	131	Met
	9	126	Asp	131	Gln	Gln	Gln	132	Asn
	10	127	Lys	132	Lys	Lys	Lys	133	Lys
	11	128	Phe	133	Val	Met	Val	134	Ala
	12	129	Leu	134	Val	Val	Val	135	Leu
	13	130	Ala	135	Ala	Thr	Ala	136	Glu
	14	131	Ser	136	Gly	Gly	Gly	137	Leu
	15	132	Val	137	Val	Val	Val	138	Phe

Table 3 (continued)
AMINO ACID SEQUENCES AND POSITIONS OF HUMAN HEMOGLOBINS AND MYOGLOBIN

Structural Position	α-Chain		β, γ and δ Chains				Myoglobin	
	Number	Sequence	Number	β Sequence	γ Sequence	δ Sequence	Number	Sequence
16	133	Ser	138	Ala	Ala	Ala	139	Arg
17	134	Thr	139	Asn	Ser	Asn	140	Lys
18	135	Val	140	Ala	Ala	Ala	141	Asp
19	136	Leu	141	Leu	Leu	Leu	142	Met
20	137	Thr	142	Ala	Ser	Ala	143	Ala
21	138	Ser	143	His	Ser	His	144	Ser
HC 1	139	Lys	144	Lys	Arg	Lys	145	Asn
2	140	Tyr	145	Tyr	Tyr	Tyr	146	Tyr
3	141	Arg	146	His	His	His	147	Lys

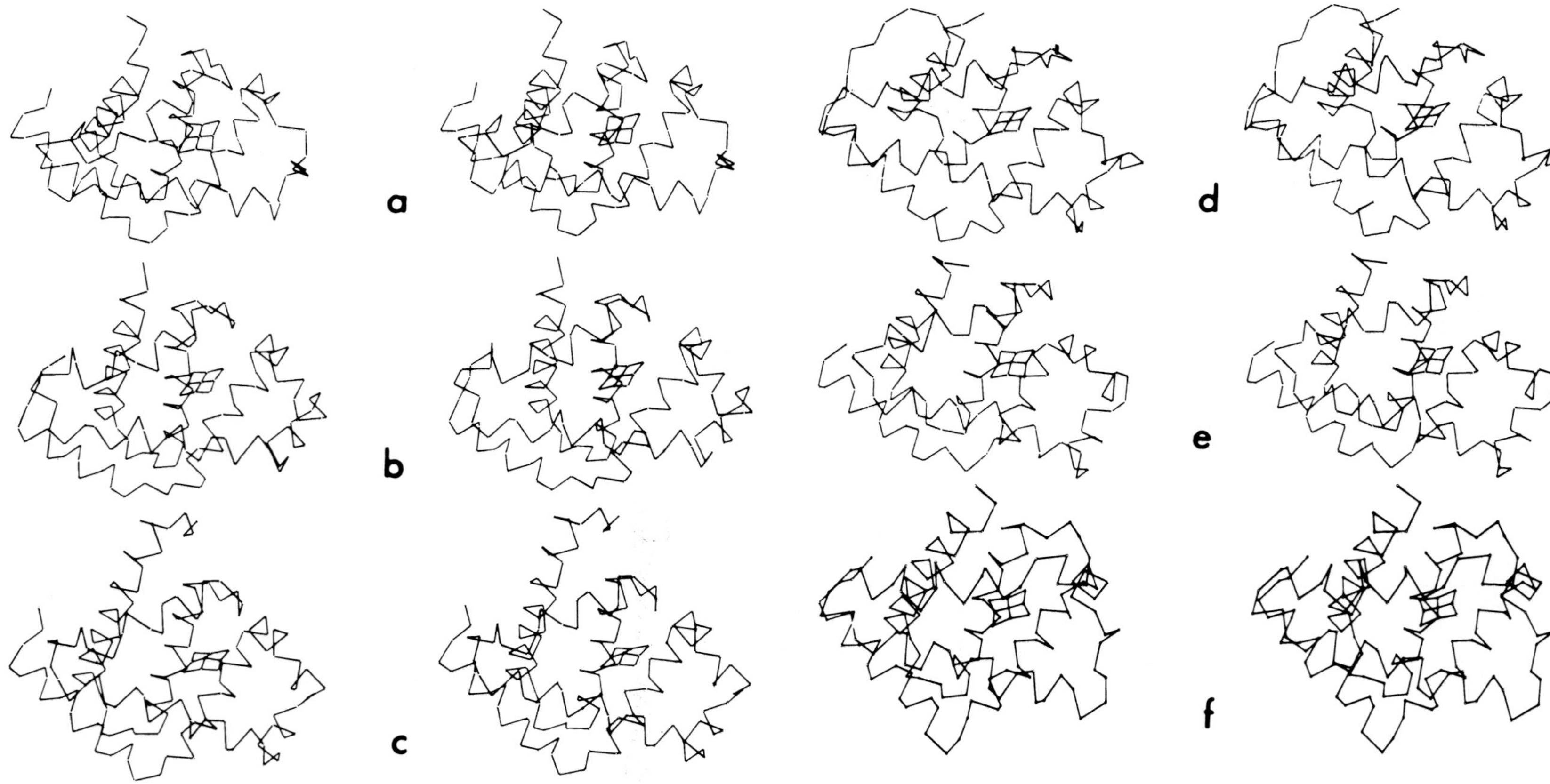

FIGURE 1. Stereo-pair drawings of the α-carbon backbones of six globins. All have the same orientation to demonstrate the conservation of the three-dimensional structure. (1) horse hemoglobin α-chain, (2) horse hemoglobin β-chain, (3) sperm whale myoglobin, (4) sea lamprey glovin V, (5) midge larva glovin CTT-III (erythrocruorin), and (6) bloodworm major monomeric globin. (From Padlan, E. A. and Love, W.E., *J. Biol. Chem.*, 249, 4067, 1974. With permission.)

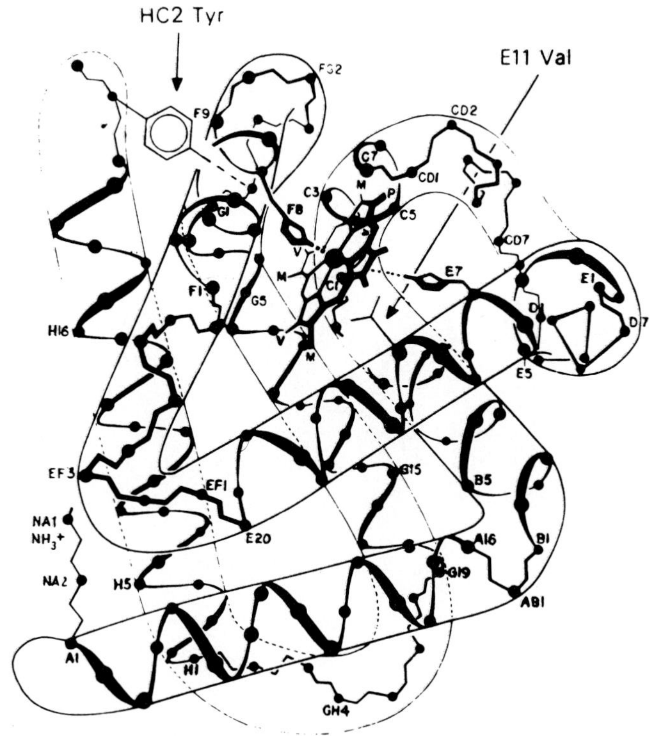

FIGURE 2. The globin fold. This diagram shows the secondary and tertiary structure that is common to all of the globins. Proximal His F8, distal His E7, Val E11, and Tyr HC2 are important residues in the mechanism of mammalian hemoglobins. The letters M, V, and P refer to the methyl, vinyl, and propionate side chains of the heme. (From Perutz, M. F., *Br. Med. Bull.*, 32, 195, 1976. Reproduced by permission of the Medical Department, The British Council.)

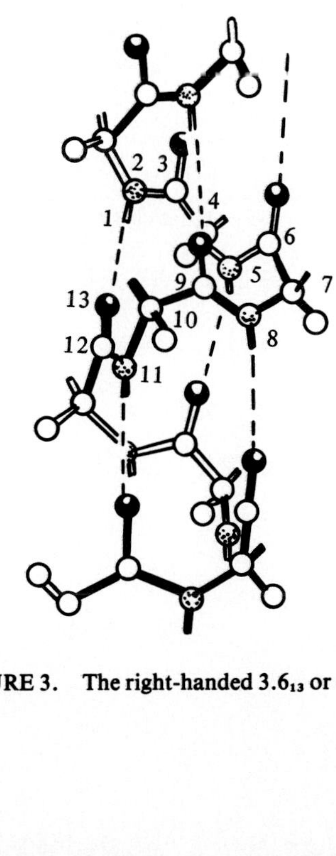

FIGURE 3. The right-handed 3.6_{13} or α helix.

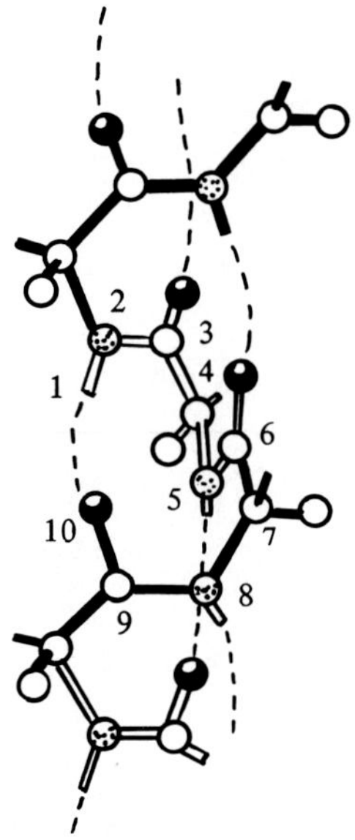

FIGURE 4. The right-handed 3_{10} helix.

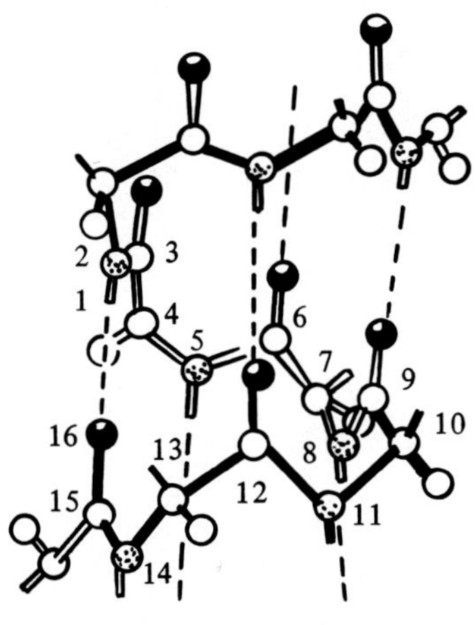

FIGURE 5. The right-handed 4.4_{16} or π helix.

Table 4
DIFFERENCES BETWEEN THE α- AND β-CHAINS AND MYOGLOBIN (M)

Number of residues	α 141	β 146	M 153
Segment			
NA	= M	Contains 3 residues	Contains 2 residues
A	= M	= M	—
AB	2 amides A16-B1 differ	−2 Residues	—
B	= M	= M	—
BC	= M	= M	—
C	$3 \cdot 0_{10}$ Helix	$3 \cdot 0_{10}$ Helix	α-Helix
CD	All different	2 Amides CD5—7 differ	—
D	Absent	= M	—
E	Irregular	E18—20 irregular	1 Kink
EF	3 Amides EF2—5 differ, but α = β	—	—
F	= M	= M	—
FG	= M	= M	—
G	—	G1—3 in $3 \cdot 0_{10}$ Helix differ	—
GH	= M	Amide GH1—2	—
H	Contains 21 residues	Contains 21 residues	Contains 26 residues
HC	Contains 3 residues	Contains 3 residues	Contains 4 residues

From Perutz, M. F., *Proc. Roy. Soc. Ser. B.*, 173, 113, 1969. With permission.

Table 5
CONFORMATIONAL PARAMETERS OF HELICES

Type	Residues/turn	Atoms/turn	ϕ^a	ψ^b	h (Å)^c	Ref.
3_{10}	3	10	130.7	154.3	2.00	44,46
α	3.615	13	133.0	122.8	1.495	43,46
π	4.4	16	122.9	110.3	1.15	45,46

[a] Dihedral angle between the plane of the peptide bond containing the amino group of a residue, and the plane containing amino nitrogen atom, the alpha carbon atom, and the carbonyl carbon atom of the same residue. See Reference 46 for a detailed explanation.

[b] Dihedral angle between the plane of the peptide bond containing the carbonyl group of a residue, and the plane containing amino nitrogen atom, the alpha carbon atom, and the carbonyl carbon atom of the same residue. See Reference 46 for a detailed explanation.

[c] Height of one residue along the axis of the helix.

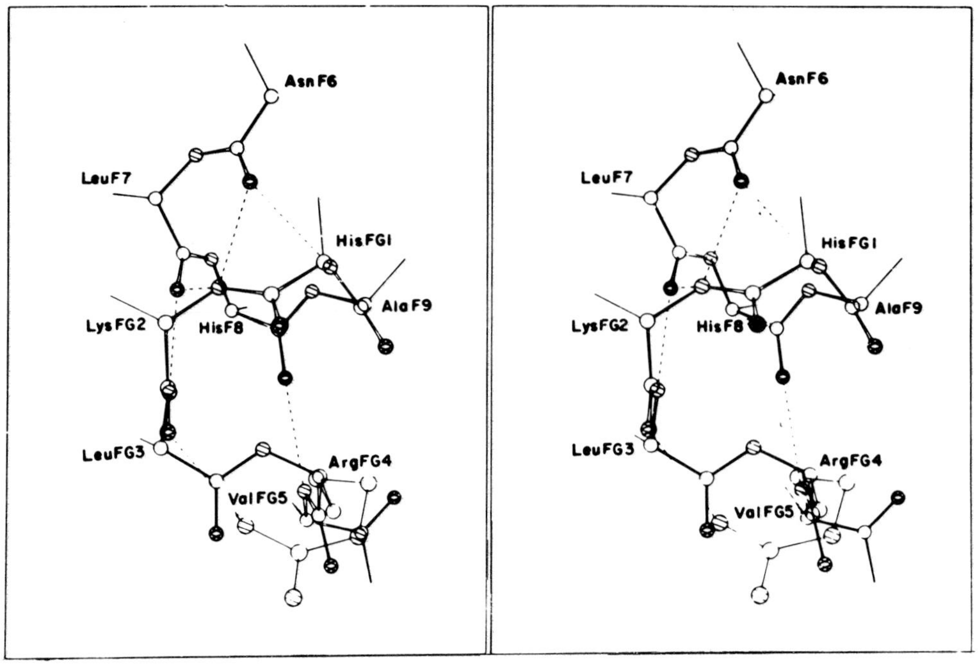

FIGURE 6. Stereo-pair drawing of the transition from α helix to π helix at the end of segment F in the α subunit of horse methemoglobin. (With permission from Ladner, R. C., Heidner, E. J., and Perutz, M. F., *J. Mol. Biol.*, 114, 385, 1977. Copyright by Academic Press Inc. (London) Ltd.)

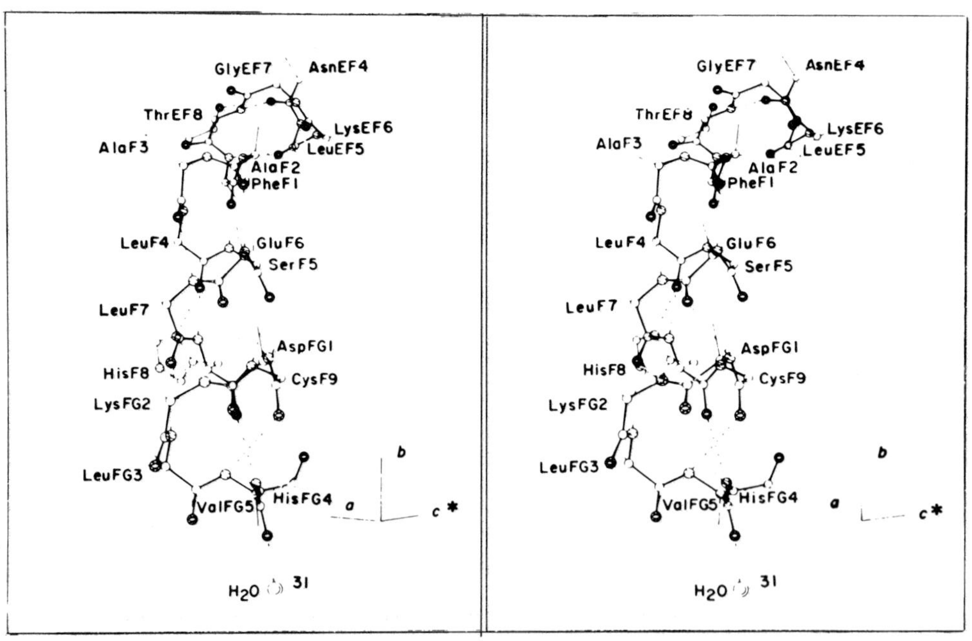

FIGURE 7. Stereo-pair drawing of helix F and segment FG in the β subunit of horse methemoglobin. (With permission from Ladner, R. C., Heidner, E. J., and Perutz, M. F., *J. Mol. Biol.*, 114, 385, 1977. Copyright by Academic Press Inc. (London) Ltd.)

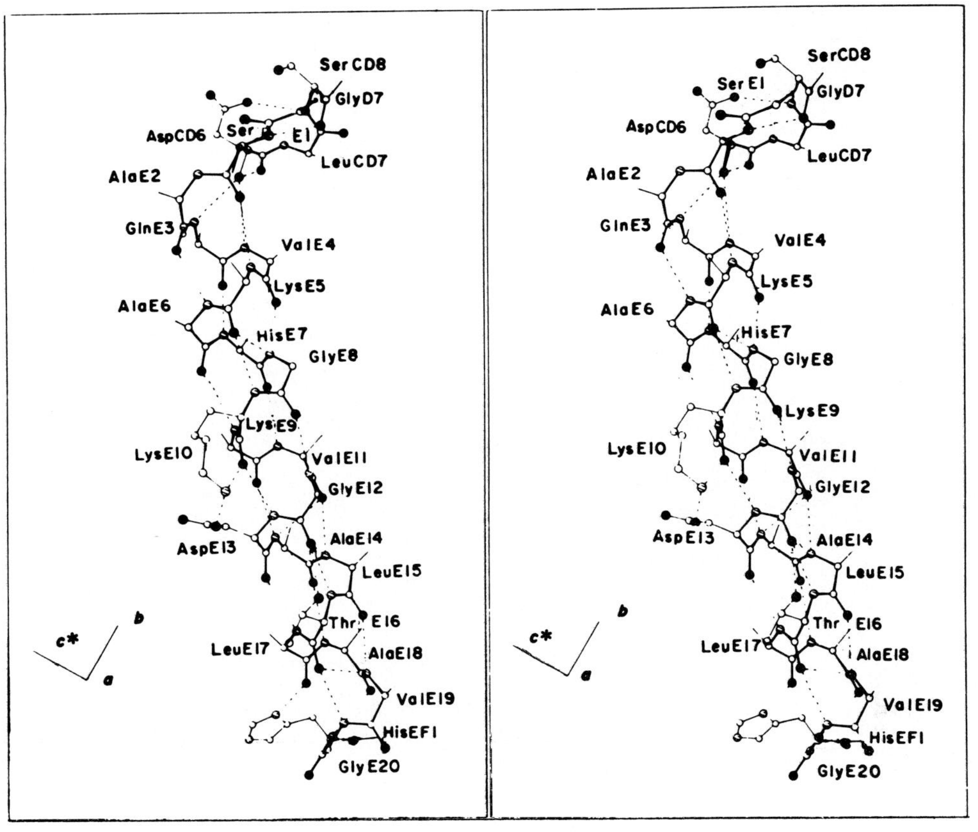

FIGURE 8. Stereo-pair drawing of the CD segment and the E helix in the α subunit of horse methemoglobin. The hydroxyl group of Ser El(52)α accepts protons from the main-chain nitrogens of Gln E3(54)α and Val E4(55)α and donates a proton to the main-chain carbonyl group of Asp CD6(47)α. These hydrogen bonds help stabilize the corner between the CD segment and the E helix. (With permission from Ladner, R. C., Heidner, E. J., and Perutz, M. F., *J. Mol. Biol.*, 114, 385, 1977. Copyright by Academic Press Inc. (London) Ltd.)

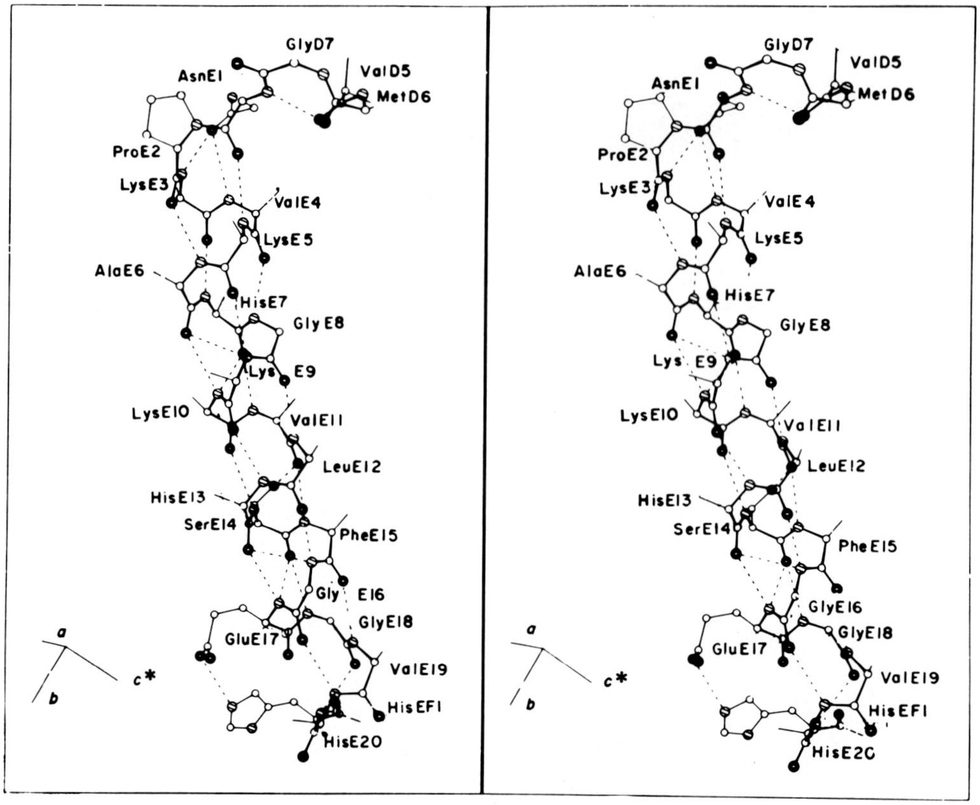

FIGURE 9. Stereo-pair drawing of the E helix in the *β* subunit of horse methemoglobin. The side-chain carbonyl group of Asn El(57)*β* accepts protons from the main-chain nitrogens of Lys E3(59)*β* and Val E4(60)*β*, while the main-chain nitrogen of Asn El(57)*β* donates a proton to the main-chain carbonyl group of Val D5(54)*β*. These hydrogen bonds stabilize the start of the E helix. (With permission from Ladner, R. C., Heidner, E. J., and Perutz, M. F., *J. Mol. Biol.*, 114, 385, 1977. Copyright by Academic Press Inc. (London) Ltd.)

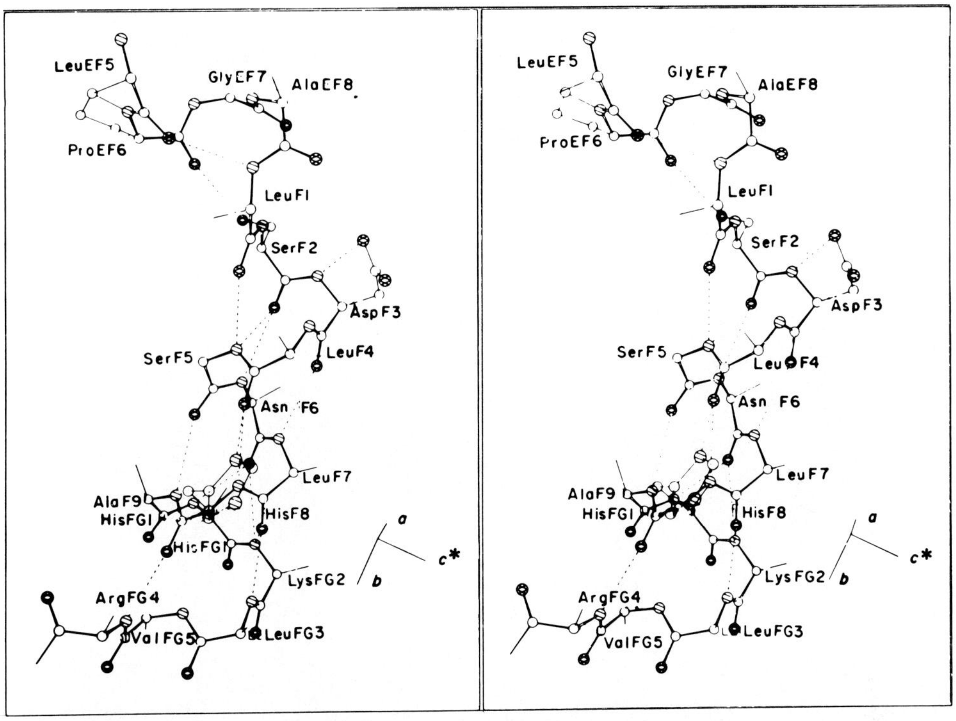

FIGURE 10. Stereo-pair drawing of the F helix in the α subunit of horse methemoglobin. This helix is particularly irregular with several bifurcated hydrogen bonds and with additional hydrogen bonds involving the side chains of Ser F2(81)α, Asp F3(82)α, and His F8(87)α. (With permission from Ladner, R. C., Heidner, E. J., and Perutz, M. F., *J. Mol. Biol.*, 114, 385, 1977. Copyright by Academic Press Inc. (London) Ltd.)

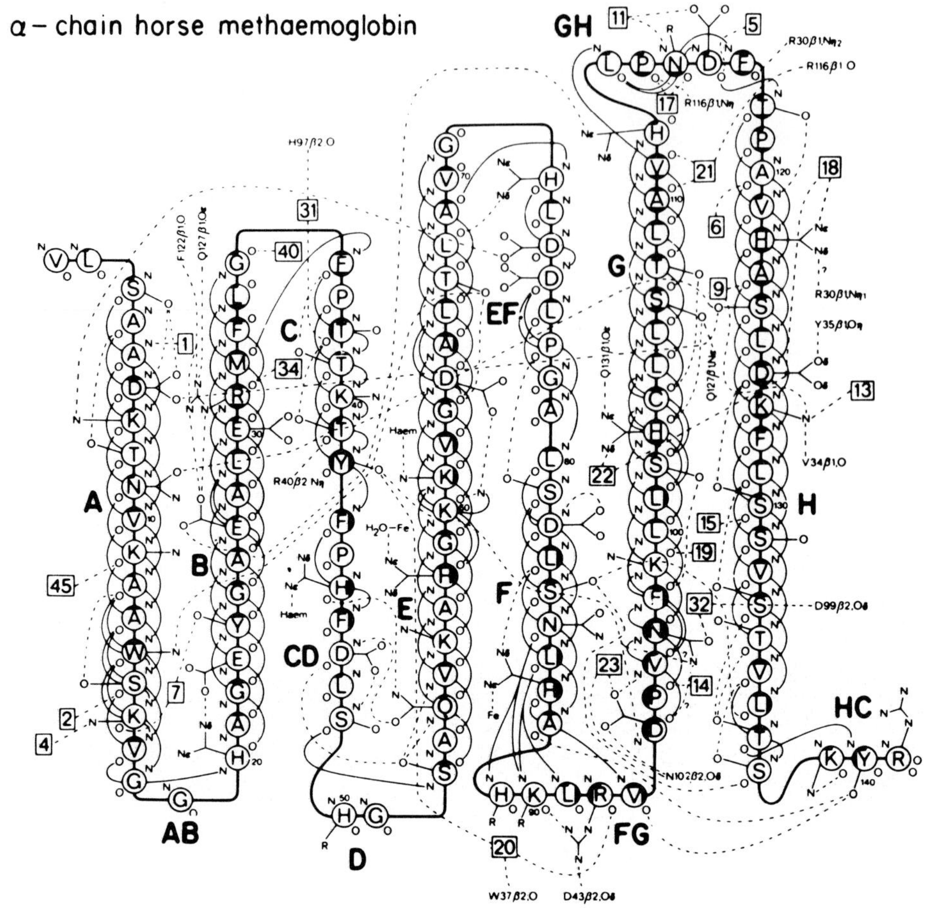

FIGURE 11. Network of hydrogen bonds stabilizing the α-chain of horse methemoglobin. Full lines depict bonds between main-chain atoms and broken lines depict bonds involving side-chain atoms. The marks in the circles mean: ○, external residue; ◓, internal residue; ◔, residue in surface crevice; ◑, heme contact; ◒, $\alpha_1\beta_1$ contact; ◐, $\alpha_1\beta_2$ contact. The letters denote the amino acid residues as noted above. The numbers in squares refer to bound water molecules. Bold capitals denote the segments of secondary structure. (With permission from Ladner, R. C., Heidner, E. J., and Perutz, M. F., *J. Mol. Biol.*, 114, 385, 1977. Copyright by Academic Press Inc. (London) Ltd.)

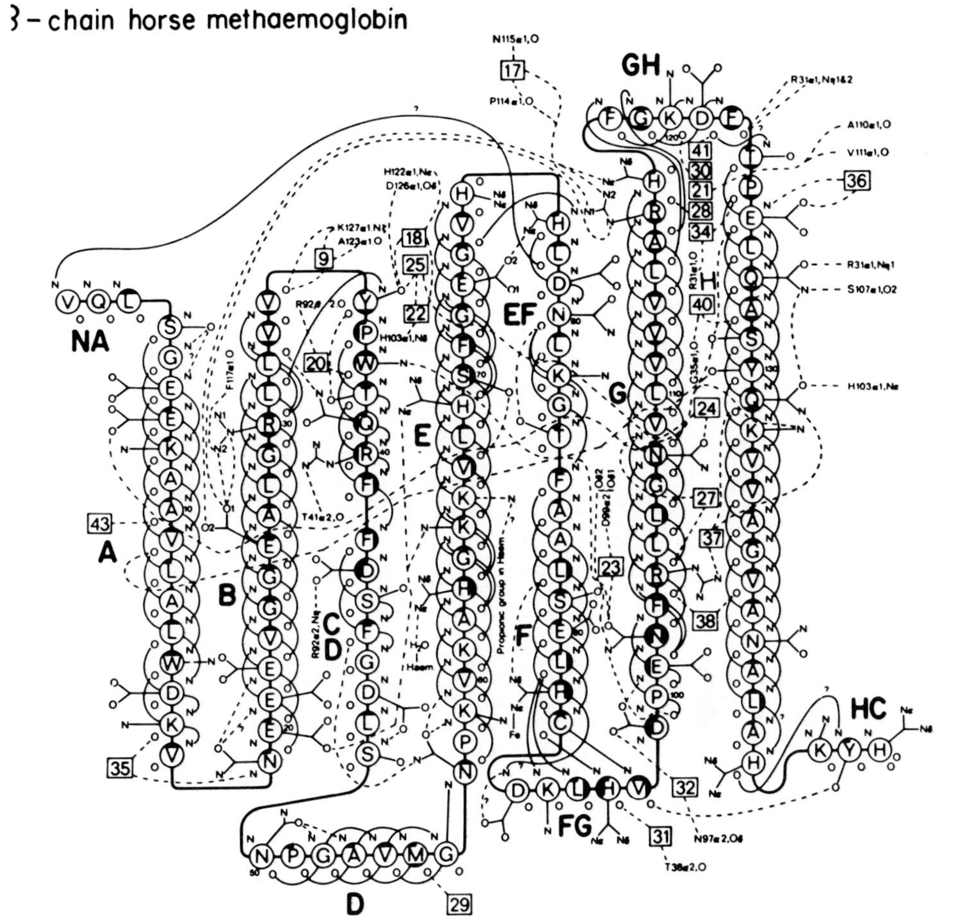

FIGURE 12. Network of hydrogen bonds stabilizing the β-chain of horse methemoglobin. The key is the same as in Figure 11. (With permission from Ladner, R. C., Heidner, E. J., and Perutz, M. F., *J. Mol. Biol.*, 114, 385, 1977. Copyright by Academic Press Inc. (London) Ltd.)

STRUCTURE OF HORSE METHAEMOGLOBIN

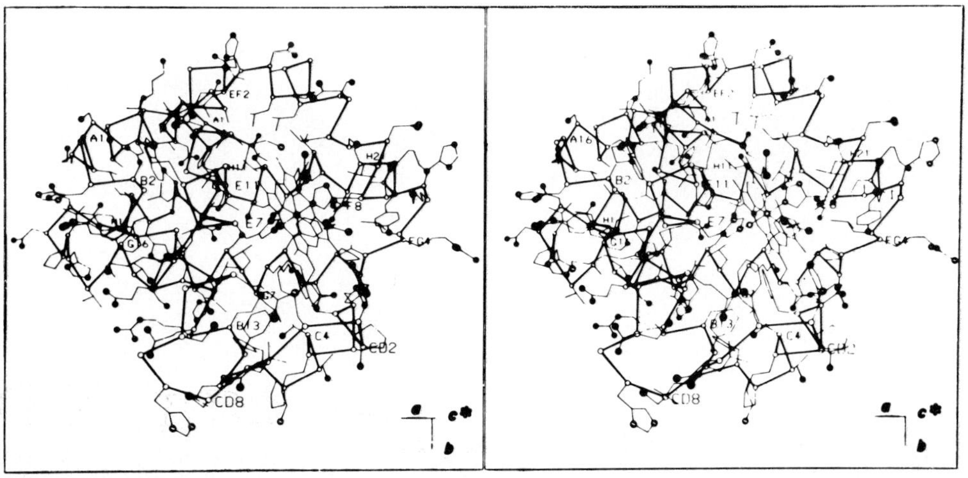

FIGURE 13. Stereo-pair drawing of the α subunit of horse methemoglobin. Only the α carbons and simplified side chains are shown. (With permission from Ladner, R. C., Heidner, E. J., and Perutz, M. F., *J. Mol. Biol.*, 114, 385, 1977. Copyright by Academic Press Inc. (London) Ltd.)

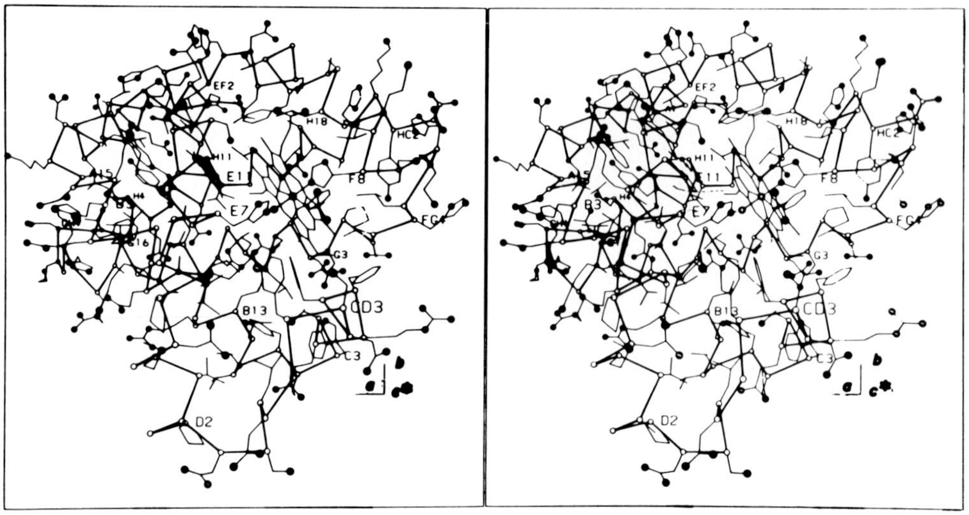

FIGURE 14. Stereo-pair drawing of the β subunit of horse methemoglobin. Only the α carbons and simplified side chains are shown. (With permission from Ladner, R. C., Heidner, E. J., and Perutz, M. F., *J. Mol. Biol.*, 114, 385, 1977. Copyright by Academic Press Inc. (London) Ltd.)

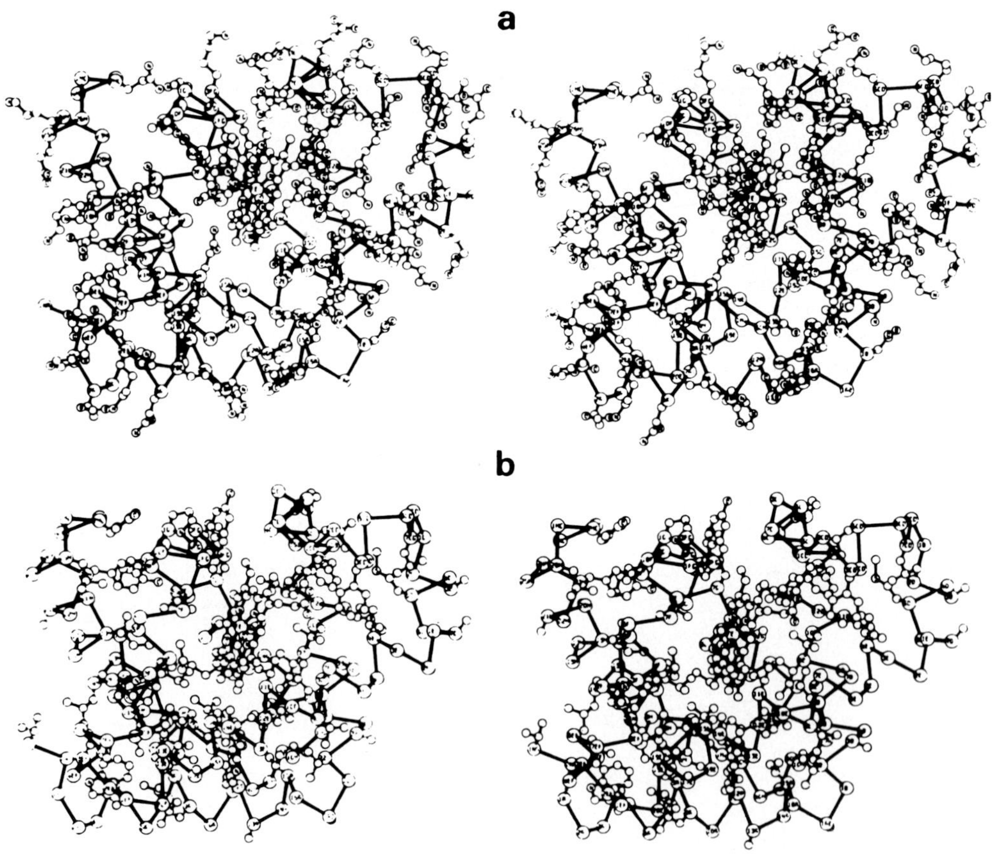

FIGURE 15. Stereo-pair drawing of sperm whale myoglobin. In Figure 15A the hydrophilic side chains are shown. All of these residues are external, except Thr C4, Ser G9, His B5, His E7, and His F8, which are hydrogen bonded internally. Phe CD1 is included by mistake. In Figure 15B the hydrophobic side chains are shown. (With permission from Takano, T., *J. Mol. Biol.*, 110, 569, 1976. Copyright by Academic Press Inc. (London) Ltd.)

Table 6
REPLACEMENTS AMONG THE 33 INTERNAL SITES[a]

Residue	Observed
A 8	Val, Ile
11	Ala, Thr, Ile, Leu, Cys, Ser, Phe, Val, Met
12	Trp, Phe, Val
15	Val, Ile, Ala, Asn
B 6	Gly, Ala
9	Ala, Tyr, Gly, Val, Ile
10	Leu, Val
13	Met, Thr, Leu
14	Phe, Leu
C 4	Thr
CD 1	Phe
4	Phe, Met, Trp, Lys, Ile, Leu
D 5	Val, Ile, Met
E 4	Val, Ile, Leu, Met
8	Gly
11	Val, Ile
12	Ala, Ile, Ser, Met, Leu
15	Leu, Ile, Val, Phe
18	Ala, Gly, Ile
19	Val, Gly, Ala, Ile, Leu, Met
F 1	Leu, Phe, Tyr, Ile, Val
FG 5	Val, Ile
G 5	Phe, Leu
8	Leu, Ile
11	Cys, Ser, Gly, Asn, His, Val, Ile, Met, Ala
12	Leu, Phe, Ile
16	Leu, Ile, Met, Phe
H 8	Leu, Val, Met, Tyr, Phe, Trp, His
11	Phe, Val, Leu, Met, His, Ala
12	Leu, Phe, Val
15	Val, Leu, Phe
19	Leu, Ile, Met, Ala
HC 2	Tyr

[a] The internal sites are the ones listed by Perutz, Kendrew, and Watson.[49] The sequences used include 20 α chains, 22 β-type chains, and 17 myoglobin chains listed in alignments 33, 34, and 35 of Reference 37.

Table 7
REPLACEMENTS AMONG NONPOLAR SURFACE RESIDUES[a]

Residue	Observed
NA 2	Val, Ser, Met, His, Gln, Gly
3	Leu, Phe, Trp
A 3	Ala, Glu, Asp, Lys, Pro, Ser, Gly, Gln
5	Lys, Arg, Ser, Trp
7	Asn, Glu, His, Arg, Ala, Asp, Leu, Gln, Ser, Thr
9	Lys, Thr, Arg, Ser, Leu, Asn, Ala, Ile
13	Gly, Glu, Asp, Ala, Thr, Ser
AB 1	Gly, Ala, Ser, Pro, Glu, Thr
B 2	Ala, Gly, Pro, Glu, Val, Ile, Glu, Leu
3	Gly, Glu, Ala, Asp, Pro, Asn, His, Val
4	Glu, Asp, Ala, Gly, Gln, Lys, Ser
11	Glu, Gly, Gln, Thr, Phe, Asp, Ala, Ile, Met
C 2	Pro, Thr
5	Lys, Arg, Gln, Ser, Leu, Met
CD 7	Leu, Val, Phe
D 3	Asp, Ser, Lys, Asn, Gly, Thr, Glu
7	Gly, Asn, Ser, Asp, Ala, His
E 9	Lys, Ala, Glu, Ser, Asn, Val, Thr, Asp, Ile
14	Ala, Gly, Ser
16	Thr, Gly, Ala, Asp, Ser, Cys
17	Asn, Lys, Thr, Asp, Leu, Asn, Glu, Gly, Ala
EF 3	Asp, Asn, Glu, Gly
7	Gly, Ser, Asn, Ala, Val, Ala
F 3	Ala, Lys, Asp, Thr, Ser, Glu, Gln, Pro, His
4	Leu
5	Ser, Ala
9	Ala, Cys, Ser
G 1	Asp, Pro, Ser, Ala
2	Pro, Ile, Val
4	Asn, Tyr, Phe
7	Leu, Ile, Phe, Lys, Arg
13	Leu, Val, Thr, Ile, Ala
15	Thr, Val, Gly, Cys
GH 2	Pro, Gly, Asn, Lys, Ser, Gln
3	Ala, Ser, Gly, Thr, Asn, Asp, Glu, Pro, Lys, His
5	Phe, Leu
H 1	Thr, Pro, Gly, Ala, Asx, Ser
2	Pro, Tyr, Ile, Ala, Thr
4	Val, Ala, Met, Leu, Thr, Cys
6	Ala, Cys Met, Val, Ser, His, Gly
7	Ser, Ala, Glu, Asx, Ala, Asp
14	Ser, Asn, Ala, Arg, Asp, Val, Gly, Leu
20	Thr, Glu, Asx, Ser, Gly, Ala
21	Ser, Ala, Glu, Gln, His, Arg, Lys, Thr

[a] The nonpolar surface residues are the ones listed by Perutz, Kendrew, and Watson.[49] The sequences used are the same as for Table 6.

Table 8
CONSERVATION OF RESIDUES IN THE GLOBIN FOLD

Conservation of Polar and Nonpolar Residues in Internal and Surface Positions[a]

Structural position	Residue type	Number of residues	Position (%)	Total (%)
Internal	—	33	—	22
	Polar	1	3	1
	Nonpolar	24	73	16
	Either	8	24	5
Surface	—	115	—	78
	Polar	14	12	9
	Nonpolar	6	5	4
	Either	95	83	64

Completely Conserved Positions

Position	Residue	Role
C4	Thr	Unknown
E7	His	Distal histidine
E8	Gly	Unknown
F4	Leu	Heme contact
F8	His	Proximal histidine
HC2	Tyr	Hydrogen bond holds H and F helices together

[a] The positions used to obtain these data are the ones listed by Perutz, Kendrew, and Watson.[49] The sequences used are the same as for Table 6.

Table 9
SOME DERIVATIVES OF HEMOGLOBIN AND THEIR SPINS

Note that each molecule of hemoglobin binds 2 ligands: thus, for example, HbO_2 is an abbreviated version of $Hb(O_2)_4$. The same nomenclature applies to the other derivatives.

	Ligand in sixth position	Spin
Ferrous derivatives		
Oxyhemoglobin (HbO_2)	O_2	0
Carboxyhemoglobin (HbCO)	CO	0
Deoxyhemoglobin (Hb)	None	2
NO-hemoglobin (HbNO)	NO	0
Ferric derivatives		
Acid methemoglobin (HbH_2O) (methemoglobin, ferrihemoglobin)	H_2O	5/2
Alkaline methemoglobin (HbOH) (ferrihemoglobin hydroxide)	OH^-	1/2, 5/2
Ferrihemoglobin fluoride (HbF)	F^-	5/2
Ferrihemoglobin azide (HbN_3)	N_3^-	1/2
Ferrihemoglobin cyanide (HbCN) (cyanomethemoglobin)	CN^-	1/2

From Weissbluth, M., *Hemoglobin: Cooperativity and Electronic Properties,* Springer-Verlag, New York, 1974, 3. With permission.

Table 10
HEME STEREOCHEMISTRY

Distances (Å)	Myoglobin		Hemoglobin α Chain		Hemoglobin β Chain		2-Methylimidazole iron(11)[52] TPP[a]	Picket-fence oxygen adduct[53]
	Aquomet	Deoxy	Aquomet	Deoxy	Aquomet	Deoxy		
Fe to porphyrin plane	0.40	0.55	0.07	0.60	0.21	0.63	0.55	0
His N_ϵ to porphyrin plane	2.5	2.6	2.2	2.6	2.4	2.8	2.68	2.07
Fe to N_ϵ	2.1	2.1	2.1	2.0	2.2	2.2	2.16	2.07
Fe to $N_{pyrrole}$ (average)	2.04	2.06	2.0[b]	2.1	2.0[b]	2.1	—	—
Imidazole angle[c]	19°	19°	21°	20°	15°	25°	—	—

[a] Abbreviation: TPP: tetraphenylporphin.
[b] Constrained to be equidistant.
[c] Angle between plane of imidazole projected on to heme plane and line joining heme center to the nitrogens of pyrroles I and III, as defined in Figures 2 and 3 of Fermi (1975).[25]

From Perutz, M. F., *Br. Med. Bull.*, 32, 195, 1976. Reproduced by permission of the Medical Department, The British Council.

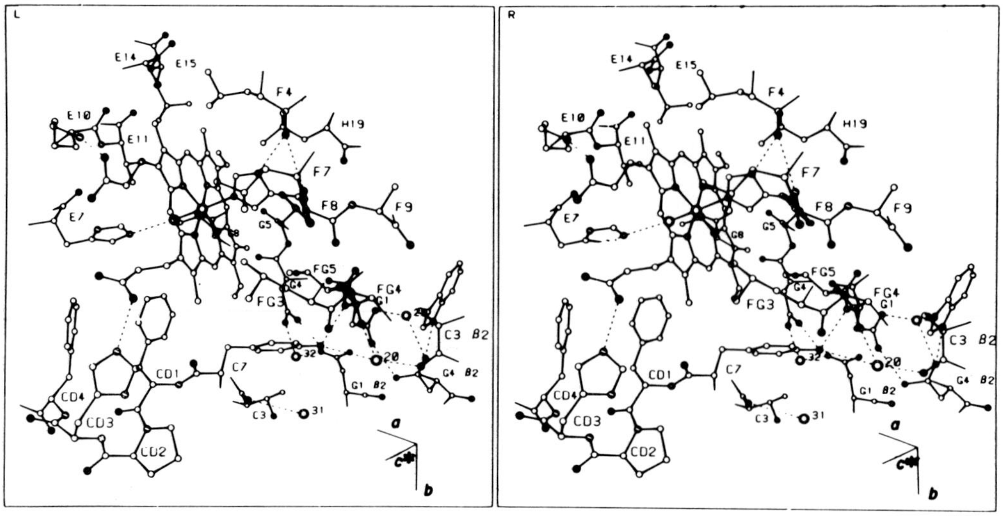

FIGURE 16. Stereo-pair drawing of the heme environment in the α-subunit of horse methemoglobin. (With permission from Ladner, R. C., Heidner, E. J., and Perutz, M. F., *J. Mol. Biol.*, 114, 385, 1977. Copyright by Academic Press Inc. (London) Ltd.)

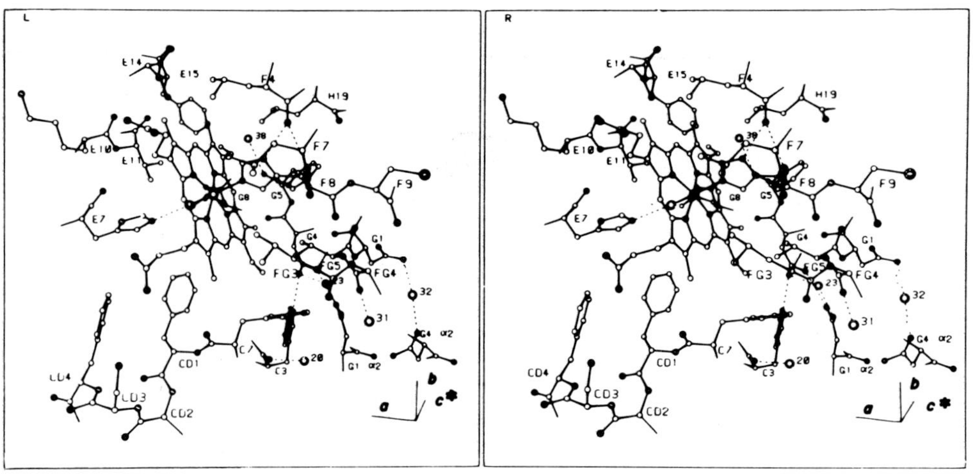

FIGURE 17. Stereo-pair drawing of the heme environment in the β subunit of horse methemoglobin. (With permission from Ladner, R. C., Heidner, E. J., and Perutz, M. F., *J. Mol. Biol.*, 114, 385, 1977. Copyright by Academic Press Inc. (London) Ltd.)

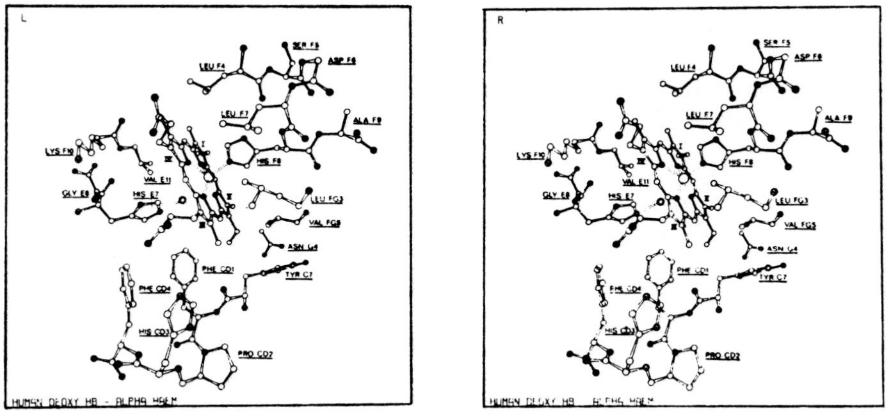

FIGURE 18. Stereo-pair drawing of the heme environment in the α subunit of human deoxyhemoglobin. "Lys F10" should read "Lys E10." There is a solvent molecule present in the heme pocket of the α subunit, but not in that of the β subunit. (With permission from Fermi, G., *J. Mol. Biol.*, 97, 237, 1975. Copyright by Academic Press Inc. (London) Ltd.)

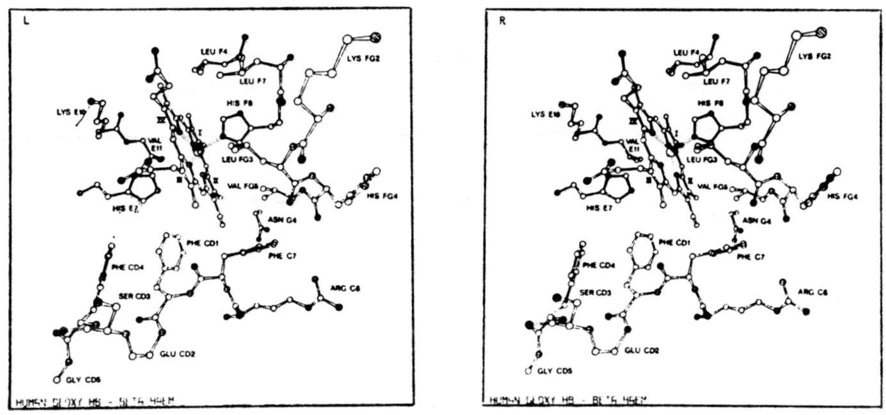

FIGURE 19. Stereo-pair drawing of the heme environment in the β subunit of human deoxyhemoglobin. The position of Val E11 is closer to the iron atom in the β subunit than in the α subunit. (With permission from Fermi, G., *J. Mol. Biol.*, 97, 237, 1975. Copyright by Academic Press Inc. (London) Ltd.)

Table 11
INTERATOMIC CONTACTS OF THE HEME GROUPS AND THEIR SURROUNDING RESIDUES, AND NUMBERS OF ATOMS INVOLVED IN HEME-GLOBIN CONTACTS

Myoglobin			α Heme			β Heme		
	Number of atoms			Number of atoms			Number of atoms	
Residue	Globin	Heme	Residue	Globin	Heme	Residue	Globin	Heme
CDI Phe	4	6	C7 Tyr	2	2	C7 Phe	1	1
CD3 Arg	2	4	CD1 Phe	3	5	CD1 Phe	2	2
E7 His	2	7	CD3 His	1	1	E7 His	3	10
E10 Thr	1	3	CD4 Phe	2	1	E10 Lys	1	1
E11 Val	2	5	E7 His	2	7	E11 Val	4	10
E14 Ala	1	2	E10 Lys	1	1	E14 Ala	1	3
E15 Leu	1	1	E11 Val	1	1	F1 Phe	1	1
F7 Ser	2	2	F4 Leu	3	2	F4 Leu	3	6
F8 His	3	12	F7 Leu	1	2	F7 Leu	1	2
FG2 His	3	7	F8 His	3	7	F8 His	2	6
FG4 Ile	2	2	FG3 Leu	2	5	FG3 Leu	1	3
G4 Tyr	2	1	FG5 Val	3	6	FG5 Val	1	1
G5 Leu	1	1	G4 Asn	3	1	G4 Asn	5	2
G8 Ile	1	1	G5 Phe	4	4	G5 Phe	2	3
			G8 Leu	1	3	G8 Leu	1	1
			H19 Leu	1	4	H19 Leu	1	4
Total	27	54		33	52		30	56

Note: All interatomic distances of 4 Å or less were counted. In metmyoglobin the distal water molecule was taken as part of the heme.

From Perutz, M. F., *Br. Med. Bull.*, 32, 195, 1976. Reproduced by permission of the Medical Department, The British Council.

Table 12
DISTANCES (Å) FROM HEME TO SURROUNDING AMINO ACID SIDE-CHAINS IN HORSE MET- AND HUMAN DEOXYHEMOGLOBIN

Group	Residue	Atom	1 Distance to porphyrin plane[a]		2 Distance to heme axis		3 Distance to porphyrin center		4 Distance to Fe		5 Distance to heme-linked water	
					α							
B10	Leu29	Cδ2	6.3	6.5	2.4	2.5	6.8	7.0	6.9	7.5	5.0	—
		Cδ1	7.7	8.1	0.5	0.6	7.7	8.1	7.8	8.7	5.8	—
B13	Met32	Cε	5.1	5.2	6.2	6.5	8.0	8.3	8.1	8.7	6.9	—
		Sδ	4.6	4.6	7.3	7.5	8.6	8.8	8.7	9.1	7.7	—
CD1	Phe43	Cε2	3.7	3.9	4.7	5.1	6.0	6.4	6.0	6.8	4.9	—
		Cζ	3.4	3.4	4.4	4.6	5.5	5.8	5.6	6.1	4.5	—
		Cε1	3.5	3.3	5.5	5.7	6.5	6.6	6.6	6.9	5.6	—
E7	His58	Nε	3.6	3.8	2.3	1.7	4.3	4.2	4.4	4.7	2.8	—
		Cε	3.3	3.1	3.4	2.4	4.7	4.0	4.8	4.5	3.7	—
E11	Val62	Cγ2	4.3	3.8	2.8	2.5	5.1	4.6	5.2	5.1	3.8	—
		Cγ1	4.7	4.4	4.8	4.3	6.7	6.2	6.8	6.7	5.7	—
F4	Leu83	Cδ2	−3.3	−2.8	7.1	6.9	7.8	7.4	7.8	7.3	8.9	—
		Cδ1	−3.5	−3.8	5.6	5.7	6.6	6.9	6.6	6.6	7.9	—
F7	Leu86	Cδ2	−3.8	−4.3	4.8	5.4	6.1	6.9	6.0	6.6	7.4	—
		Cδ1	−5.3	−6.1	5.7	5.9	7.8	8.5	7.8	8.1	9.2	—
F8	His87	H_2O	1.9	—	0.1	—	1.9	—	2.0[b]	—	—	—
		Fe	−0.1	−0.6	0[b]	0[b]	0.1	0.6	—	—	2.0[b]	—
		Nε	−2.2	−2.6	0.2	0.3	2.2	2.6	2.1	2.0	4.1	—
		Cε	−2.8	−3.1	1.2	1.5	3.1	3.4	3.0	2.9	4.9	—
FG3	Leu91	Cδ2	−3.9	−3.7	7.0	5.8	8.0	6.9	7.9	6.6	9.0	—
		Cδ1	−3.3	−3.5	4.6	3.3	5.6	4.9	5.6	4.5	6.9	—
FG5	Val93	Cγ2	−3.8	−3.0	4.9	5.4	6.3	6.2	6.2	5.9	7.5	—
		Cγ1	−3.3	−2.8	6.3	6.4	7.1	7.0	7.0	6.7	8.0	—

Table 12 (continued)
DISTANCES (Å) FROM HEME TO SURROUNDING AMINO ACID SIDE-CHAINS IN HORSE MET- AND HUMAN DEOXYHEMOGLOBIN

Group	Residue	Atom	1 Distance to porphyrin plane[a]		2 Distance to heme axis		3 Distance to porphyrin center		4 Distance to Fe		5 Distance to heme-linked water	
						α						
G5	Phe98	Cε2	−4.3	−4.4	5.8	5.4	7.2	7.0	7.1	6.6	8.4	—
		Cζ	−4.0	−4.0	4.7	4.4	6.1	6.0	6.1	5.5	7.5	—
		Cε1	−3.2	−3.2	5.0	4.9	5.9	5.8	5.9	5.5	7.1	—
G8	Leu101	Cδ2	3.0	5.3	4.9	6.6	5.8	8.4	5.8	8.8	5.1	—
		Cδ1	5.1	3.2	6.2	5.3	8.0	6.2	8.1	6.5	7.0	—
H19	Leu136	Cδ2	−5.5	−5.1	4.8	5.3	7.3	7.4	7.2	7.0	8.9	—
		Cδ1	−3.5	−3.4	4.5	5.5	5.7	6.4	5.6	6.2	7.1	—
						β						
B10	Leu28	Cδ2	6.8	6.8	3.2	2.7	7.5	7.3	7.7	7.8	5.9	—
		Cδ1	7.6	5.5	1.7	4.6	7.8	7.2	8.0	7.7	6.1	—
B13	Leu31	Cδ2	4.6	3.7	6.3	7.8	7.8	8.6	7.9	8.9	6.8	—
		Cδ1	4.7	3.4	8.4	10.2	9.7	10.7	9.8	10.9	8.8	—
CD1	Phe42	Cε2	3.6	3.2	4.5	7.2	5.8	7.9	5.9	8.1	4.8	—
		Cζ	3.3	3.0	4.4	6.0	5.5	6.7	5.6	7.0	4.5	—
		Cε1	3.6	3.3	5.5	6.0	6.6	6.8	6.7	7.1	5.7	—
E7	His63	Nε	3.3	3.2	2.4	2.4	4.0	4.0	4.2	4.5	2.8	—
		Cε	3.0	2.9	3.5	2.2	4.6	3.6	4.7	4.1	3.8	—
E11	Val67	Cγ2	3.9	3.0	2.3	1.4	4.6	3.3	4.8	3.9	3.3	—
		Cγ1	4.2	3.6	4.2	3.7	5.9	5.2	6.0	5.7	4.8	—
F4	Leu88	Cδ2	−3.6	−3.2	5.7	5.3	6.8	6.2	6.6	5.9	7.9	—
		Cδ1	−3.0	−2.5	6.6	6.3	7.2	6.8	7.1	6.6	8.2	—

F7	Leu91	Cδ2	−4.2	−4.7	4.8	5.4	6.4	7.2	6.3	6.8	7.7	—
		Cδ1	−5.8	−6.4	5.9	6.8	8.3	9.3	8.1	8.9	9.7	—
F8	His92	H_2O	1.8	—	0.1	—	1.8	—	2.0[b]	—	—	—
		Fe	−0.2	−0.6	0[b]	0[b]	0.2	0.6	—	—	2.0[b]	—
		Nε	−2.4	−2.9	0.2	0.3	2.4	2.9	2.2	2.2	4.2	—
		Cε	−3.0	−3.4	1.2	1.5	3.3	3.7	3.1	3.1	5.0	—
FG3	Leu96	Cδ2	−4.2	−4.1	6.6	6.1	7.8	7.3	7.7	7.0	8.8	—
		Cδ1	−3.5	−3.6	4.2	3.6	5.5	5.1	5.3	4.7	6.7	—
FG5	Val98	Cγ2	−3.5	−4.3	5.4	4.7	6.6	6.4	6.4	6.0	7.6	—
		Cγ1	−3.4	−3.9	6.1	5.5	7.0	6.8	6.9	6.4	7.9	—
G5	Phe103	Cε2	−5.7	−5.8	5.3	5.0	7.8	7.6	7.7	7.1	9.1	—
		Cζ	−5.0	−4.9	4.4	4.0	6.7	6.4	6.5	5.2	8.1	—
		Cε1	−3.7	−3.6	4.6	4.3	5.9	5.6	5.8	5.9	7.1	—
G8	Leu106	Cδ2	3.1	2.8	4.9	6.4	5.8	6.9	5.9	7.2	5.0	—
		Cδ1	5.1	4.6	6.3	7.3	8.1	8.6	8.3	9.0	7.1	—
H19	Leu141	Cδ2	−4.8	−4.9	4.8	5.2	6.8	7.1	6.6	6.7	8.2	—
		Cδ1	−3.1	−3.4	5.9	4.9	6.7	6.0	6.6	5.7	7.7	—

Note: In each column met is first and deoxy second. Plus on distal, minus on proximal side; the probable errors of these distances are 0.20 Å for met and 0.32 Å for deoxy.

Angle between plane of imidazole F8 projected onto heme plane and line joining heme center to nitrogens of pyrroles I and III, as defined in Figures 2 and 3 of Fermi (1975):[25]

α, met 21°, deoxy 20°.

β, met 15°, deoxy 25°.

The probable errors are based on the assumption that the positions of side chains surrounding the hemes are as well-defined as those of the hemes, so that the probable error in their positions is 0.57 × the overall error, which is 0.25 Å for this structure and 0.40 for human deoxyhemoglobin. ($0.57 \times 0.25 \times \sqrt{2} = 0.20$; $0.57 \times 0.40 \times \sqrt{2} = 0.32$).

[a] The porphyrin plane is defined as the mean plane of the ring nitrogens and carbons and the first carbons of all the side chains.

[b] Constrained.

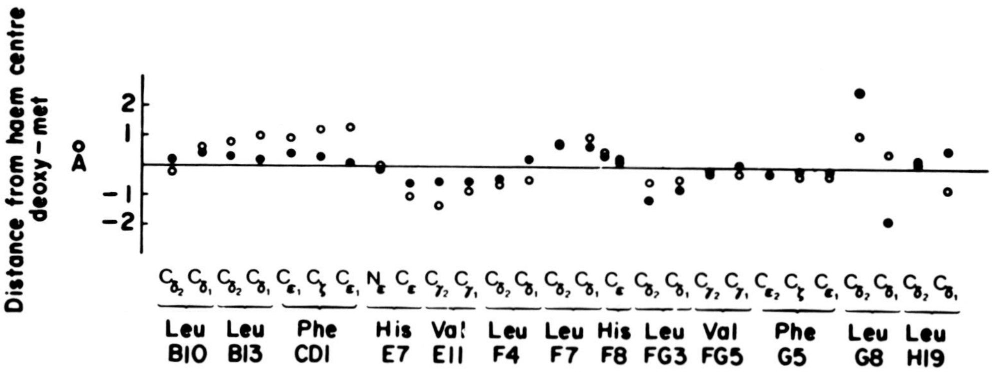

FIGURE 20. Movements of the heme environment relative to the heme center due to the transition from met- to deoxyhemoglobin. (●) α chain; (O) β chain. (With permission from Ladner, R. C., Heidner, E. J., and Perutz, M. F., *J. Mol. Biol.*, 114, 385, 1977. Copyright by Academic Press Inc. (London) Ltd.)

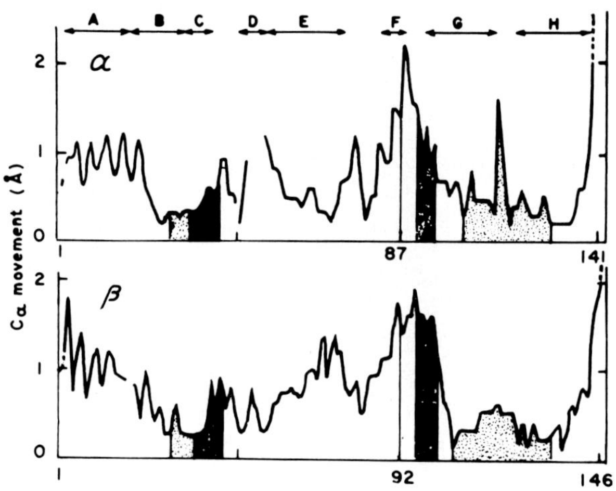

FIGURE 21. Tertiary structure changes during oxygenation. The distance between equivalent alpha carbon atoms in deoxy- and methemoglobin is plotted against residue number. This diagram shows that the movements of the two types of chains are quite similar. The proximal His F8 is residue 87α and 92β. The $\alpha_1\beta_2$ contact residues are lightly shaded; the $\alpha_1\beta_2$ residues are more strongly shaded. The positions of the amino- and carboxyl-terminal residues are shown with dashed lines, because they are not clearly defined in methemoglobin. Random errors in the structures are expected to give distances of 0.4 A in this diagram. Courtesy of Chothia, C., Wodak, S., and Janin, J., *Proc. Natl. Acad. Sci. U.S.A.*, 73, 3793, 1976.

Table 13
COMPARISON OF THE MODEL ATOMIC COORDINATES OF HUMAN AND HORSE DEOXYHEMOGLOBIN BEFORE AND AFTER RIGID-BODY FITTING

	r. m. s. Difference (Å)		Rigid-body motion		
Portion fitted	Before fitting	After fitting	r. m. s. Shift (Å)[a]	Translation (Å)	Rotation (degree)[b]
Overall	1.18	—	—	—	—
α Subunit					
Globin chain	1.06	1.03	0.28	0.24	0.7
A helix	1.10	0.97	0.52	0.50	1.3
B helix	1.10	0.97	0.52	0.38	4.1
C helix	1.42	1.32	0.53	0.35	6.2
E helix	1.13	1.08	0.36	0.33	1.5
F helix	0.74	0.63	0.39	0.35	2.2
G helix	0.97	0.89	0.38	0.23	3.7
H helix	0.68	0.65	0.18	0.16	1.1
Heme	0.53	0.38	0.37	0.31	2.6
β Subunit					
Globin chain	1.30	1.19	0.52	0.38	1.7
A helix	1.85	1.06	1.51	1.28	12.4
B helix	1.27	1.15	0.55	0.49	3.4
C helix	0.76	0.73	0.21	0.16	1.4
D helix	0.96	0.74	0.62	0.58	4.5
E helix	1.38	1.09	0.85	0.58	4.0
F helix	0.62	0.49	0.38	0.28	3.5
G helix	0.80	0.59	0.54	0.30	3.7
H helix	0.89	0.81	0.37	0.33	1.9
Heme	0.70	0.56	0.41	0.28	4.2

[a] Calculated as $\sqrt{(\Delta\chi_b)^2 - (\Delta\chi_a)^2}$, where $\Delta\chi_b$ and $\Delta\chi_a$ are the r.m.s. difference in the coordinates of the two structures before and after fitting. This assumes that the mean inner product between the vector shift due to rotation (about the center mass) and the residual vectors is zero, an assumption that could either overestimate or underestimate the shift during rigid-body motion.

[b] About center of mass.

Fermi, G., *J. Mol. Biol.*, 97, 237, 1975. With permission.

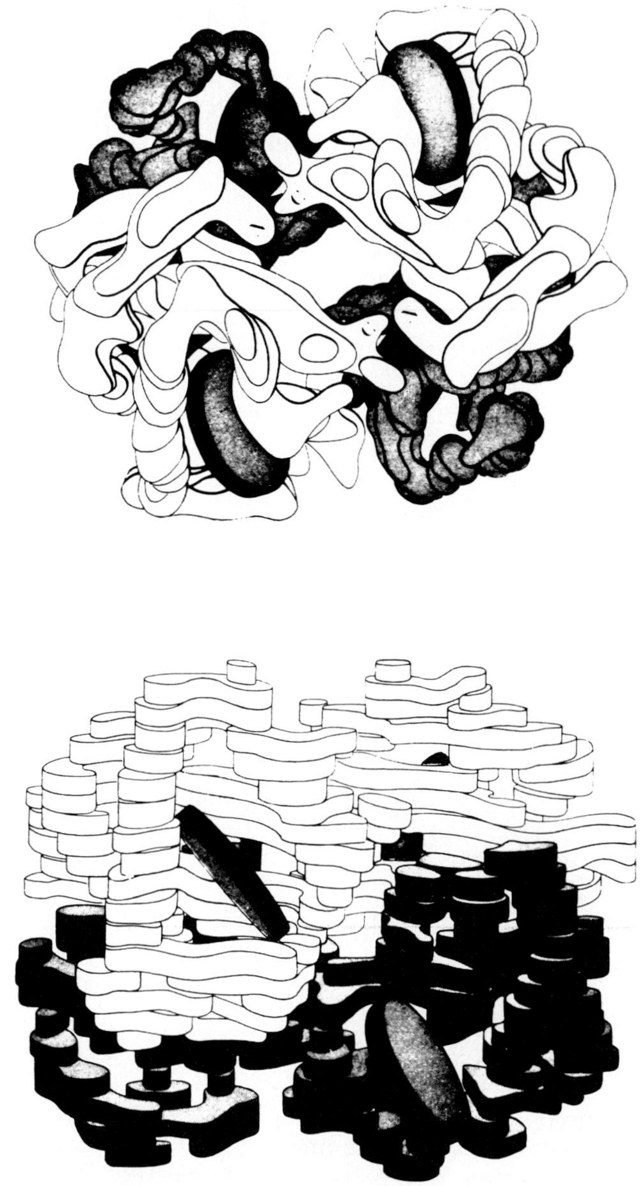

FIGURE 22. Quaternary structure of hemoglobin. The irregular block represents the electron-density pattern of the molecule. The α chains are the light blocks; the β chains are the dark blocks. The disks are the four heme groups. In the top view, the letter "N" denotes the amino termini of the α chains; the letter "C" denotes the carboxyl termini. (From Perutz, M. F., The Hemoglobin Molecule, *Sci. Am.*, 211, 64, 1964. Copyright © 1964 by Scientific American, Inc. All rights reserved.)

Table 14
SURFACE AREA BURIED IN CONTACTS

	Human deoxyhemoglobin		Horse methemoglobin	
	Surface area (Å^2)	Polar fraction (%)[b]	Surface area (Å^2)	Polar fraction (%)
Accessible surface area of subunit[a]				
α	7100	37	6900	37
β	7500	41	7200	40
Surface area buried in contact				
$\alpha_1\beta_1$ or $\alpha_2\beta_2$	1650	37	1750	32
$\alpha_1\beta_2$ or $\alpha_2\beta_1$	1300	40	950	38
$\alpha_1\alpha_2$	500	65	<200[c]	—
$\beta_1\beta_2$	0	—	<200[c]	—
Total buried surface area[d]	6400	40	~5800	35

[a] The accessible surface area of isolated subunits is calculated in the conformation observed in the tetrameric molecules. Values near 7200 A^2 are expected on the basis of the molecular weights. After differences due to amino acid substitutions are subtracted, the values obtained for α chains in the deoxy- and in methemoglobin are the same to within 3%, and to within 2% for the β chains. This yields an estimate of the precision in determining accessible (or buried) surface areas from two independent crystallographic structure determinations.

[b] Fraction of surface area contributed by nitrogen, oxygen, and, marginally, sulfur atoms.

[c] The calculations based on atomic coordinates provided by Ladner give significant values for the surface buried between the subunits in methemoglobin. However, most of this comes from the amino- and carboxyl-terminal residues for which little density is seen in the electron density map, and which are probably free to move in solution.

[d] Contacts between α and β chains occur twice; contacts between like chains, once.

Courtesy of Chothia, C., Wodak, S., and Janin, J., *Proc. Natl. Acad. Sci. U. S. A.*, 73, 3793, 1976.

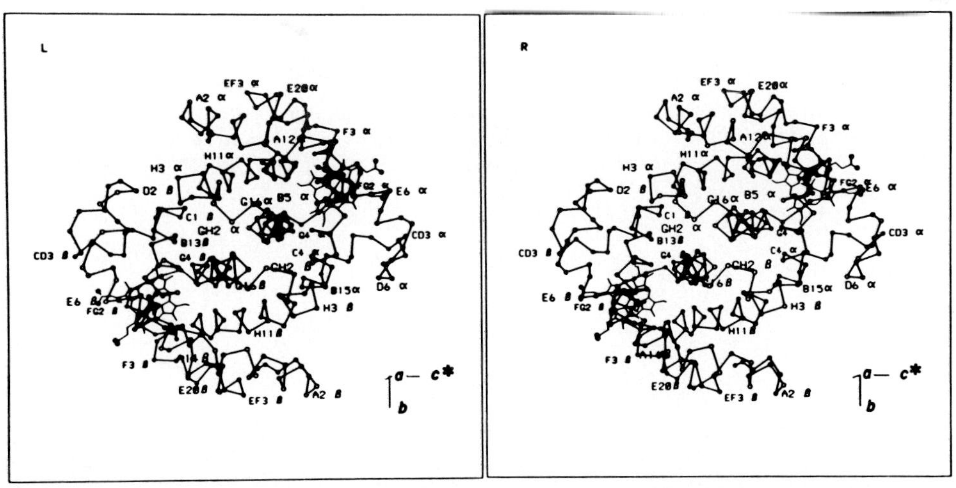

FIGURE 23. Stereo-pair drawing of the $\alpha_1\beta_1$ dimer in horse methemoglobin viewed along the pseudo-dyad symmetry axis between the two G helices. (With permission from Ladner, R. C., Heidner, E. J., and Perutz, M. F., *J. Mol. Biol.*, 114, 385, 1977. Copyright by Academic Press Inc. (London) Ltd.)

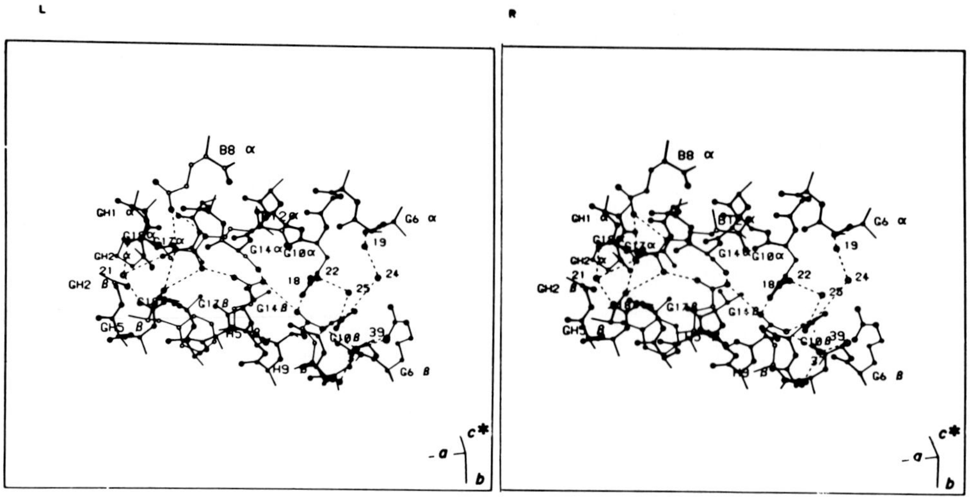

FIGURE 24. Stereo-pair drawing of the hydrogen bonding between the G helices in the $\alpha_1\beta_1$ contact of horse methemoglobin. (With permission from Ladner, R. C., Heidner, E. J., and Perutz, M. F., *J. Mol. Biol.*, 114, 385, 1977. Copyright by Academic Press Inc. (London) Ltd.)

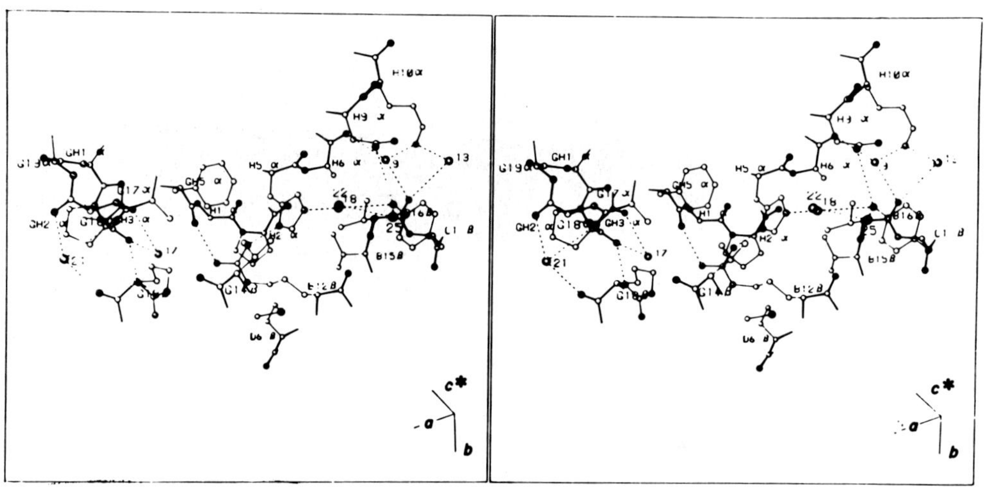

FIGURE 25. Stereo-pair drawing of the hydrogen bonding in the $\alpha_1\beta_1$ contact near the molecular center of horse methemoglobin. Water molecules 18, 22, and 25 are also seen in Figure 24. (With permission from Ladner, R. C., Heidner, E. J., and Perutz, M. F., *J. Mol. Biol.*, 114, 385, 1977. Copyright by Academic Press Inc. (London) Ltd.)

Table 15
SUBUNIT CONTACTS IN HORSE METHEMOGLOBIN

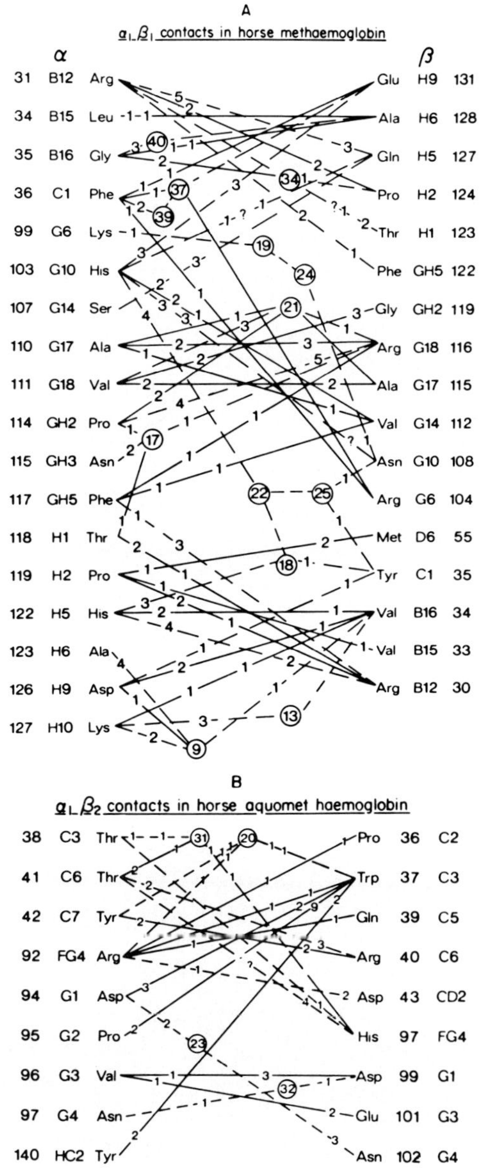

Table 16
SUBUNIT CONTACTS IN HUMAN DEOXYHEMOGLOBIN

(A) The contact $\alpha_1\beta_1$ (32 residues including about 126 atoms in contact)

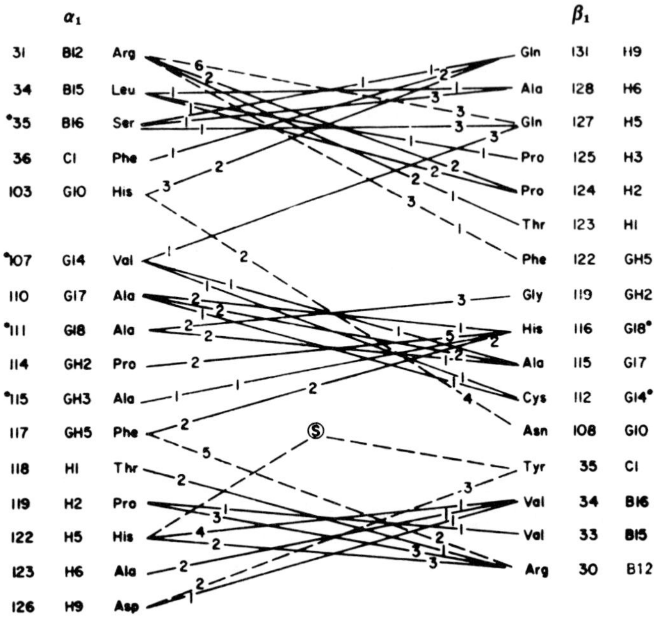

(B) The contact $\alpha_1\beta_2$ (27 residues including about 107 atoms in contact)

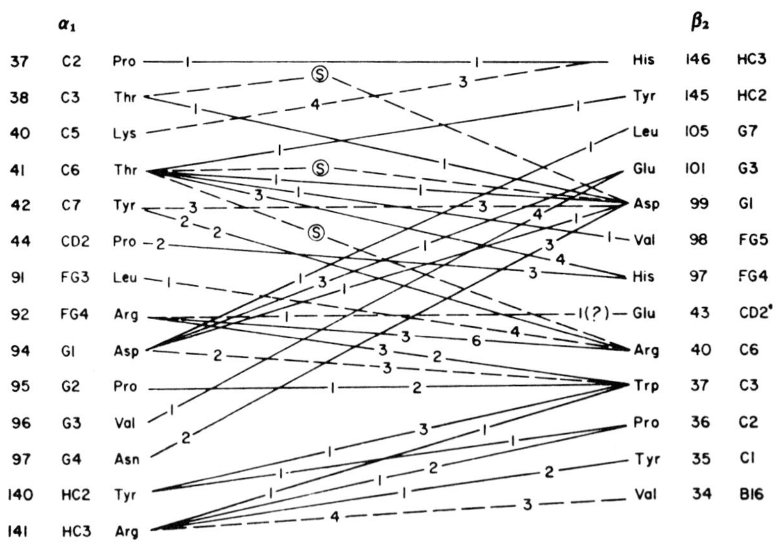

Note: All interatomic distances of 4.0 Å or less were counted as contacts. Plain lines indicate van der Waals' contacts; broken ones indicate that the contact includes a hydrogen bond. The symbol S represents a solvent molecule (identified as a positive peak in a difference map of observed minus calculated structure-factor amplitudes). Numbers on the lines give the number of atoms, contributed to the contact by the residues on each side. For future reference in studies of the differences between oxy- and deoxyhaemoglobin, it is noted that the distance between the imidazole of His H5(122)α_1 and the guanidinium of Arg B12(30)β_1 is 3.2 Å. Residues marked with an asterisk differ in horse and human hemoglobin.

From Fermi, G., *J. Mol. Biol.*, 97, 237, 1975. With permission.

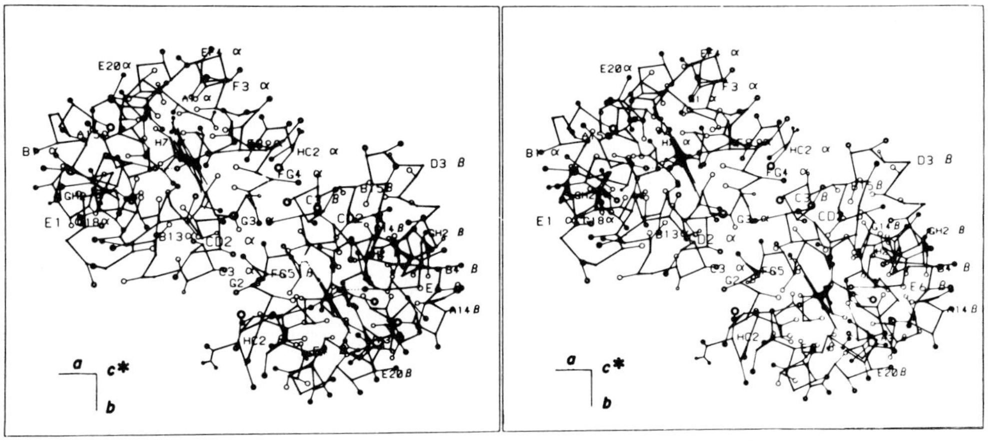

FIGURE 26. Stereo-pair drawing of the $\alpha_1\beta_2$ dimer in horse methemoglobin viewed along the pseudo-dyad that relates the subunits. The alpha carbons and an atom at the center of mass of each side chain are shown. Open circles indicate hydrophobic side chains; cross-hatched circles, acidic ones; striped circles, basic ones; small double circles, neutral hydrophilic ones; large double circles, Tyr and Trp. (With permission from Ladner, R. C., Heidner, E. J., and Perutz, M. F., *J. Mol. Biol.*, 114, 385, 1977. Copyright by Academic Press Inc. (London) Ltd.)

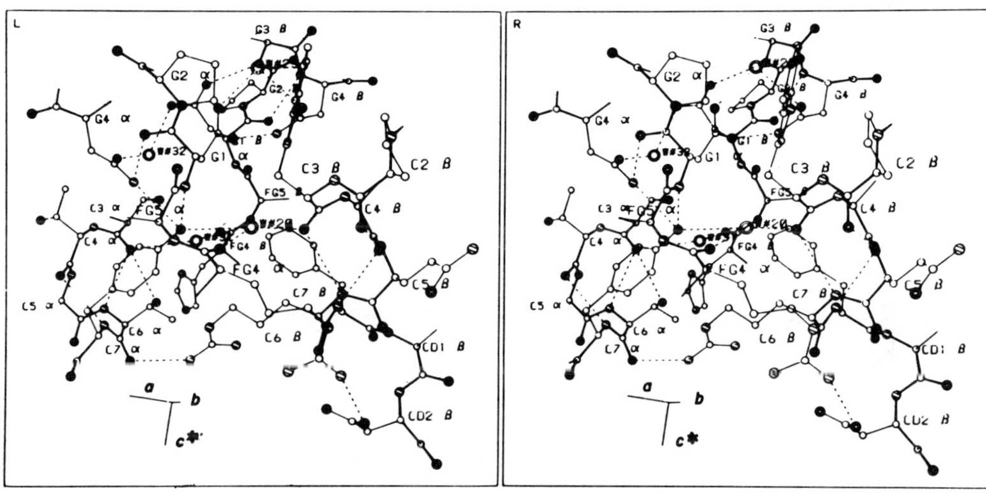

FIGURE 27. Stereo-pair drawing of the $\alpha_1\beta_2$ contact in horse methemoglobin showing the dove-tailing of helix Cβ with FGα at the top and of helix Cα with FGβ underneath. The double circles indicate hydrogen bonded water molecules. (With permission from Ladner, R. C., Heidner, E. J., and Perutz, M. F., *J. Mol. Biol.*, 114, 385, 1977. Copyright by Academic Press Inc. (London) Ltd.)

HUMAN DEOXYHAEMOGLOBIN STRUCTURE

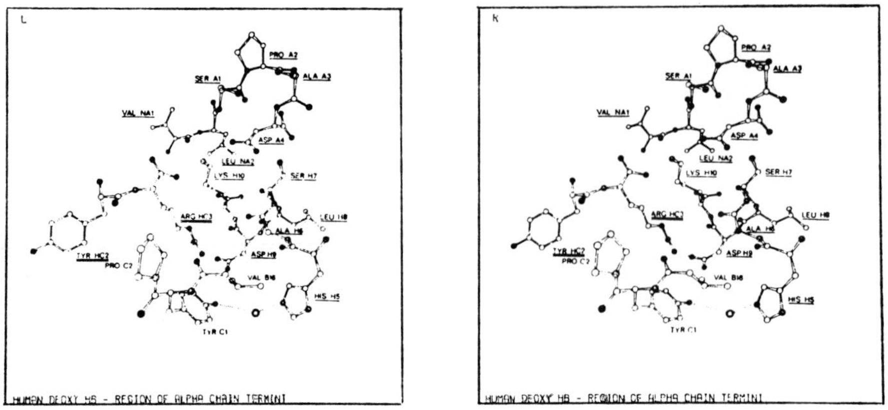

FIGURE 28. Stereo-pair drawing showing parts of segments NA, A, and H of the α_2 chain, segments B and C of the β_2 chains, and segment HC of the α_1 chain in human deoxyhemoglobin. Residue labels of the α_2 chain are underlined once. Those of the α_1 chain are underlined twice. (With permission from Fermi, G., *J. Mol. Biol.*, 97, 237, 1975. Copyright by Academic Press Inc. (London) Ltd.)

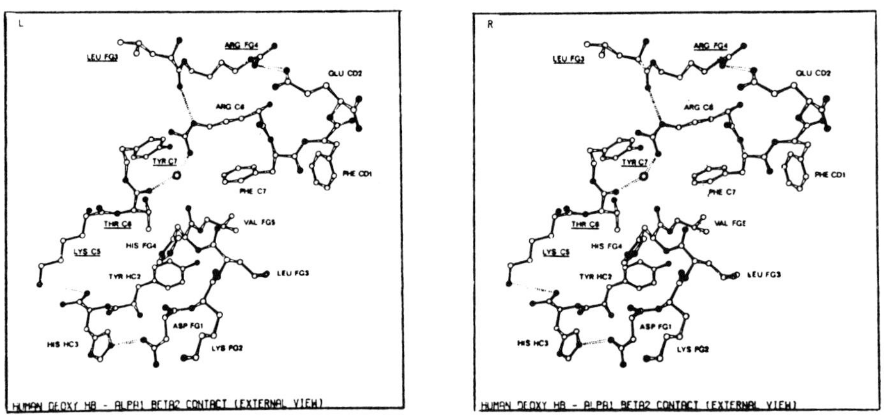

FIGURE 29. Stereo-pair drawing of the external residues of the $\alpha_1\beta_2$ contacts in human deoxyhemoglobin. The salt bridges involving His HC3(146)β are shown. There is a water molecule linking the side-chain of Arg C6(40)β and the carbonyl group of Thr C6(41)α. The hydrogen bond involving the γ carboxyl group of Glu CD2(43)β is questionable, since this group is poorly resolved in the electron density map. (With permission from Fermi, G., *J. Mol. Biol.*, 97, 237, 1975. Copyright by Academic Press Inc. (London) Ltd.)

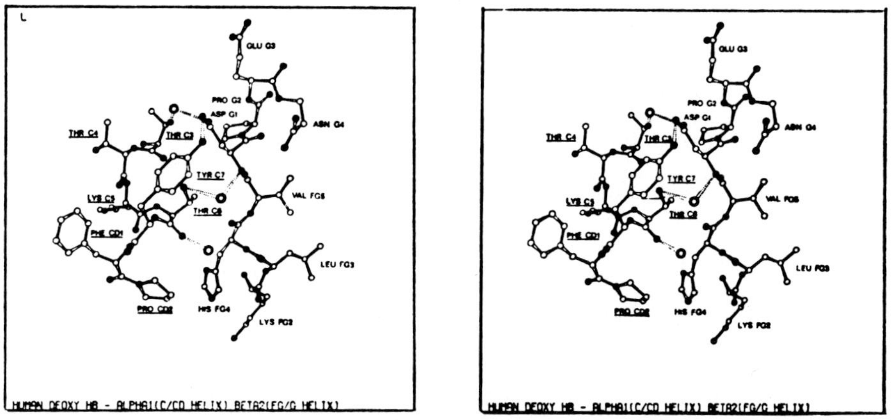

FIGURE 30. Stereo-pair drawing of the dovetailing in the $\alpha_1\beta_2$ contact of human deoxyhemoglobin. Underlined residues are in the α subunit. The side-chain of Thr C6(41)α fits into the groove at the alpha carbon of Val FG5(98)β. (With permission from Fermi, G., *J. Mol. Biol.*, 97, 237, 1975. Copyright by Academic Press Inc. (London) Ltd.

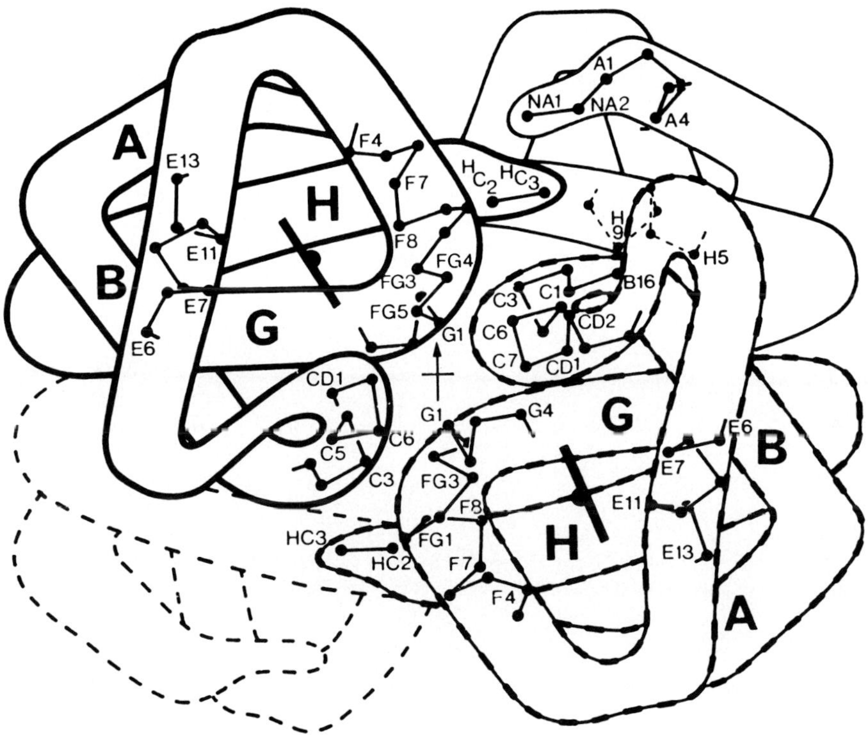

FIGURE 31. The deoxyhemoglobin tetramer. The α subunits are drawn in the solid line; the β subunits, in broken line. The $\alpha_1\beta_2$ dimer is drawn closer to the reader than the $\alpha_2\beta_1$ dimer. The figure is viewed along one of the pseudo-dyads. The molecular two-fold axis is the vertical arrow in the plane of the figure. (With permission from Fermi, G., *J. Mol. Biol.*, 97, 237, 1975. Copyright by Academic Press Inc. (London) Ltd.)

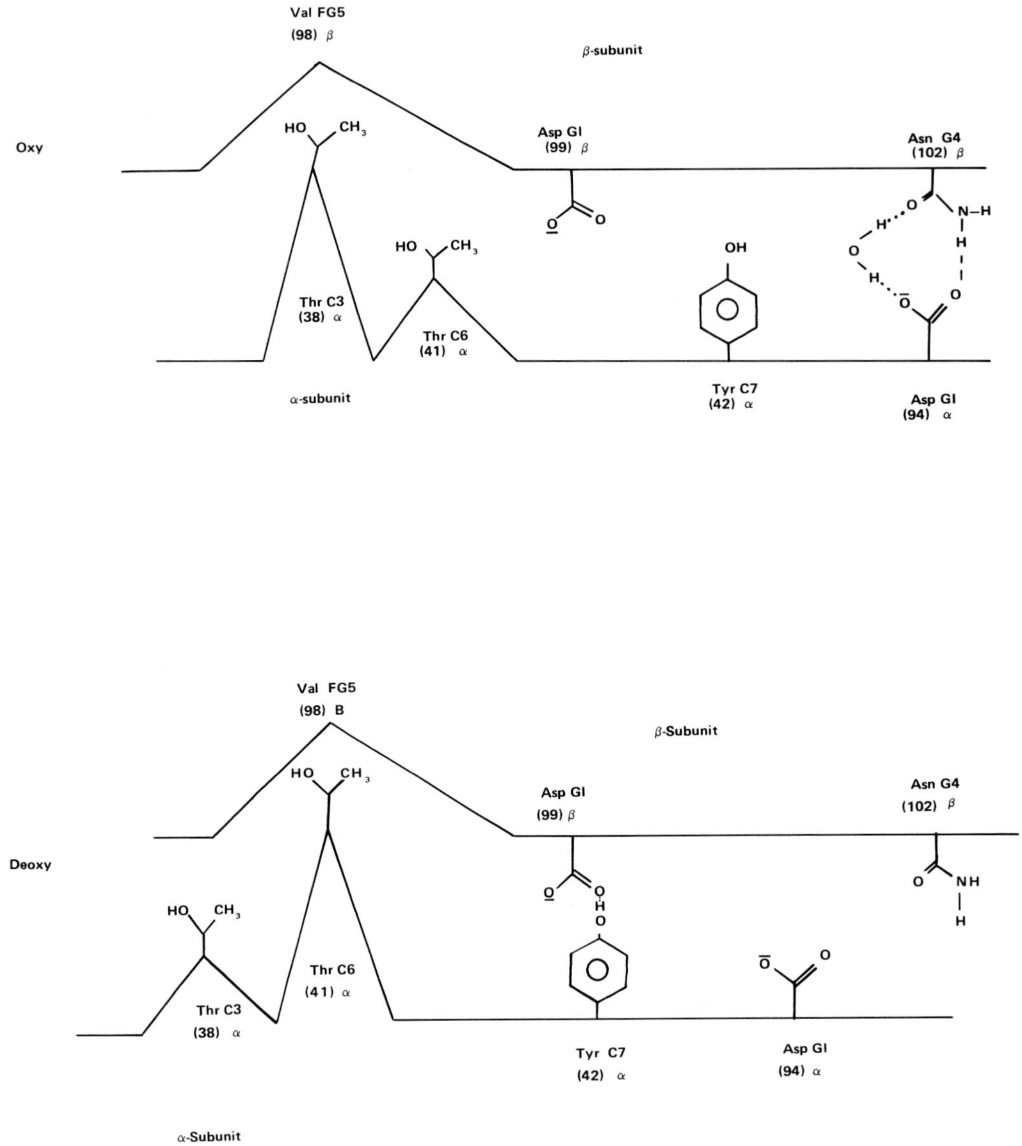

FIGURE 32. Schematic drawing of the changes in the $\alpha_1\beta_2$ contact during oxygenation, showing the two possible interactions between the C helix of the α chain and Val FG5(98)β.

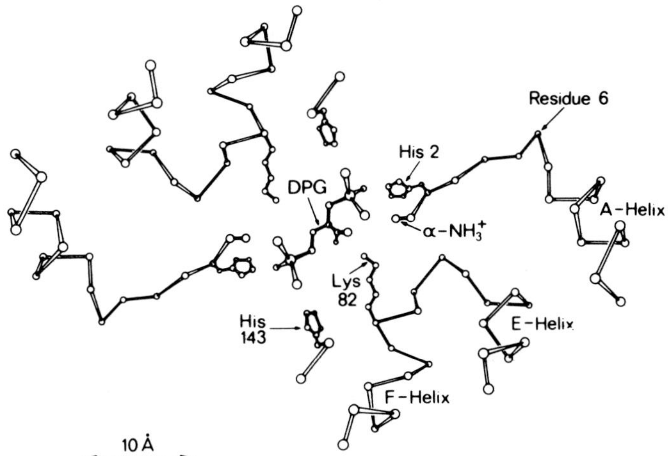

FIGURE 33. Drawing of the binding of diphosphoglycerate to human deoxyhemoglobin. (From Arnone, A., *Nature (London)*, 237, 146, 1972. With permission.)

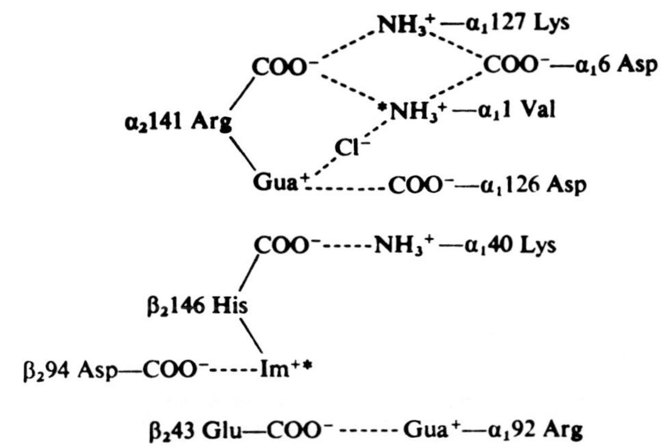

FIGURE 34. Schematic drawing of the salt bridges in deoxyhemoglobin that are not present in oxyhemoglobin. (From Baldwin, J. D., *Br. Med. Bull.*, 32, 213, 1976. Reproduced by permission of the Medical Department, The British Council.)

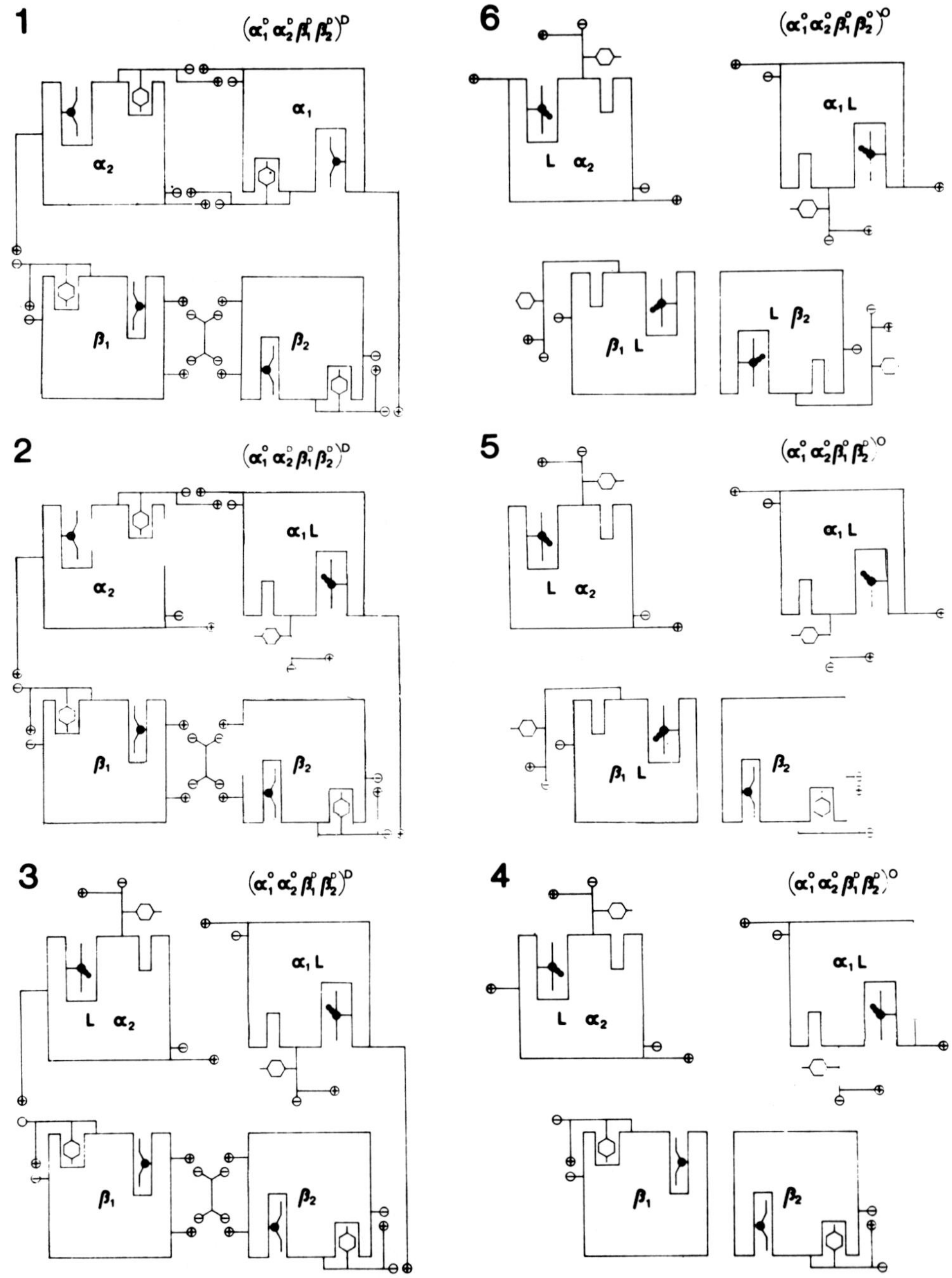

FIGURE 35. Schematic drawing of the proposed sequence of conformational changes that occur during oxygenation. One molecule of DPG is bound between the β subunits in the deoxy quarternary structure. Panel 1 shows deoxyhemoglobin. The α chains are oxygenated between panels 1 and 2 and between panels 2 and 3; while the β chains are oxygenated between panels 4 and 5 and between panels 5 and 6. The quaternary structure changes from deoxy to oxy between panels 3 and 4, accompanied by the expulsion of DPG and the breaking of the salt bridges between subunits α_1 and β_2 and between α_2 and β_1. This change of quaternary structure could occur at any stage of the reaction. More recent work by Perutz and his colleagues has confirmed that the rupture of salt bridges in the quaternary deoxy structure is linked to oxygen uptake, but has shown no evidence that the rupture of any particular salt bridge is linked to uptake of oxygen by any particular heme. Their work has confirmed that the penultimate tyrosines are firmly bonded in their pockets in the quaternary deoxy structure, and that they are loose in the quaternary oxy structure, but it has failed to show evidence of the release of tryosines from their pockets being directly linked to oxygen uptake — it may be linked to the change in quaternary structure instead. (From Perutz, M. F., *Nature (London),* 228, 726, 1970.)

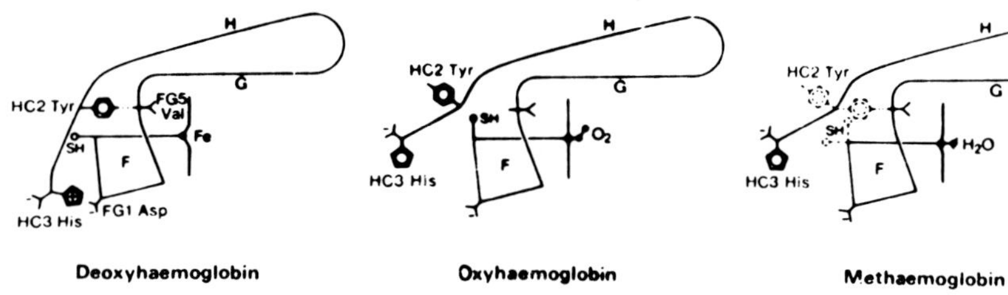

FIGURE 36. Schematic drawing of the conformational changes involving Tyr HC2 and Cys F9 during oxygenation. The Tyr side chain is forced out of its pocket during oxygenation. The Cys side chain faces outward in deoxyhemoglobin, but it is screened from solution by His HC3. In liganded hemoglobin, this screening effect is absent, and there is an equilibrium: Cys in, Tyr out ⇌ Cys out, Tyr in. Low spin ligands, such as oxygen, strongly favor the Cys in, Tyr out position. On the other hand, high spin ligands, as in methemoglobin, shift the equilibrium toward the Cys out, Tyr in position. (From Perutz, M. F., *Br. Med. Bull.*, 32, 195, 1976. Reproduced by permission of the Medical Department, The British Council.)

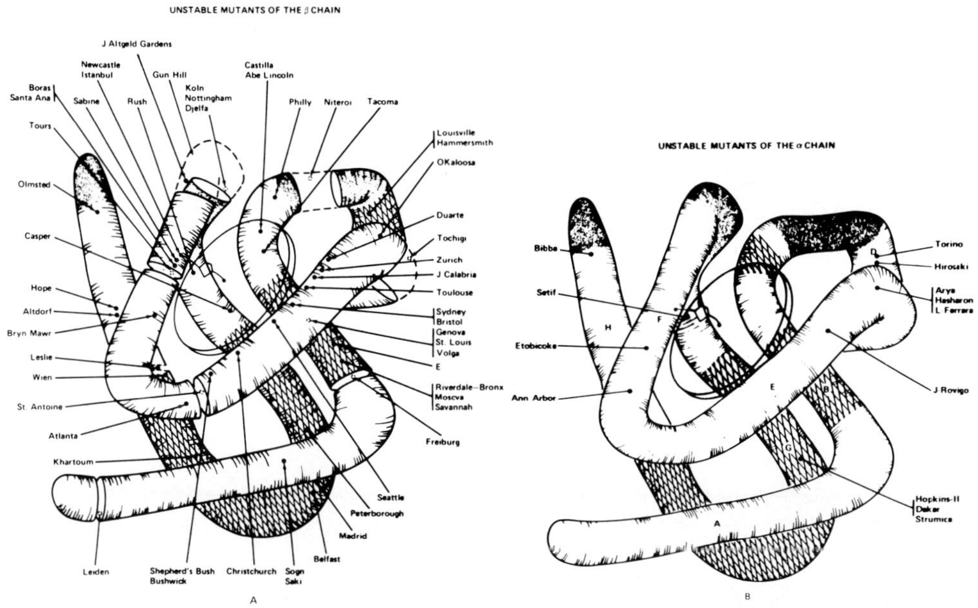

FIGURE 37. Locations of amino acid substitutions in the α (B) and β (A) chains of unstable hemoglobins. The $\alpha_1\beta_1$ contact regions are indicated by the dotted areas. The $\alpha_1\beta_2$ contact regions are indicated by the cross-hatched areas. Deletions, which have been found only in the β chain, are also shown. (From Winslow, R. M. and Anderson, W. F., *The Metabolic Basis of Inherited Disease*, 4th ed., Stanbury, J. B., Wyngaarden, J. B., and Fredrickson, D. S., Eds., McGraw-Hill, 1978, 1465. With permission.

Table 17
RESIDUES IN CONTACT WITH HEME GROUPS

Designation	Residue No.	Residue Position	Replacement From	Replacement To	Variability	Clinical symptoms	Abnormal properties	Structural effects of replacement	Ref.
						α Chain			
Torino	43	CD1	phe	val	I	Inclusion body anemia[a]	Unstable at 50°C	Substitution removes the contact of the heme group with Cδ and Cζ of phe, leaving a gap at the surface of the heme pocket. $C\gamma_2$ of val makes a short contact with Cβ of the phe CD4(46) which would disturb the conformation of the CD segment	75
M Boston	58	E7	his	tyr	I	Cyanosis[b]	Difficult to reduce. α-Chains do not combine with O_2	Phenol group of tyrosine probably forms ionic links with Fe^+, thus stabilizing it in the ferric state	76
M Iwate	87	F8	his	tyr	I	Methmemoglobinemia		In addition to the effects described for Hb Boston, the heme group must be displaced towards helix E. X-ray studies show that Hb Iwate has a conformation similar to normal deoxyhemoglobin in both the reduced and oxidized states. A small conformational change occurs, but does not alter the crystal lattice.	77, 129
Bibba	136	H19	leu	pro	I	Inclusion body anemia	Unstable at 50°C. Separable by electrophoresis at pH 8.6	Substitution removes contact of $C\delta_2$ with the heme group and leads to unfolding of residues 136—8 of helix H. Should inhibit normal function of the α-chains	78
						β-Chain			
Hammersmith	42	CD1	phe	ser	I	Inclusion body anemia: cyanosis	Unstable at 50°C, easily oxidized, then loses heme. Lower oxygen affinity	Substitution removes the contact of the heme group with the Cε and Cζ of phe, leaving a gap at the surface of the heme pocket. The presence of the hydrophilic OH opens the pocket to water	79,80

Table 17 (continued)
RESIDUES IN CONTACT WITH HEME GROUPS

Designation	Residue No.	Residue Position	Replacement From	Replacement To	Variability	Clinical symptoms	Abnormal properties	Structural effects of replacement	Ref.
						α Chain			
M Saskatoon	63	E7	his	tyr	I	Properties similar to Hb Boston			76
Zürich	63	E7	his	arg	I	Hemolytic inclusion body anemia on treatment with sulphonamides	Combines reversibly with O_2 but is more easily oxidized and precipitated	The arginine side chain cannot be accommodated in the heme pocket, but must protrude at the surface leaving a large cavity at the ligand site of the iron atom	81,82
M Milwaukee	67	E11	val	glu	I	Properties similar to Hb Boston		COO^- of glu forms a salt bridge with Fe^+ and pushes the side chain of his E7 out of the heme pocket	76
Sydney	67	E11	val	ala	I	Hemolytic anemia. Inclusion bodies formed on incubation of blood at 37°C	Unstable at 50°C. Easily oxidized; loss of heme on heating	Breaks contact of the heme group with 2 Cγ's of val. Loosens heme group	83
Santa Ana	88	F4	leu	pro	I	Hemolytic anemia. Inclusion bodies in vivo after splenectomy	No heme in *β*-chain	Proline occurs at the amino end of helix F and may not cause any change in the conformation of the main chain, but the replacement removes the contact of the heme group with Cγ and Cδ of leu. This opens a crevice on the proximal side into which water could enter	84,129
M Hyde Park	92	F8	his	tyr	I	Cyanosis. Methemoglobinemia	Difficult to reduce. *β*-Chains do not combine with O_2. Unstable	See Hb M Iwate	89

Table 17 (continued)
RESIDUES IN CONTACT WITH HEME GROUPS

Designation	Residue No.	Residue Position	Replacement From	Replacement To	Variability	Clinical symptoms	Abnormal properties	Structural effects of replacement	Ref.
						α Chain			
Köhn	98	FG5	val	met	I	Hemolytic anemia. Inclusion bodies in vivo after splenectomy	Slightly increased +ve charge at pK 8.6, suggesting a rise in the pK of a histidine. Abnormally high oxygen affinity in red cells	There are two possibilities. (1) The side chain of met could go into an internal position by the heme group. This would displace the heme towards the distal histidine or cause a change in conformation of the FG corner. (2) The side chain of met could be external, which could happen only at the expense of a change in conformation of the FG corner	86,87
Kansas	102	G4	asn	thr	I	Cyanosis	Unstable at 50°C. Decreased oxygen affinity. Decreased Hill's constant.[c] Large Bohr effect.[d] High rate of autoxidation. Oxyhemoglobin dissociates into αβ dimers	Cγ of thr probably makes short contact with vinyl and methyl of pyrrol II. This would displace either the heme or helix G. Also asn G4 of chain β, normally forms a hydrogen bond with asp G1 of chain α. This would be broken by the replacement, which should favor dissociation into αβ dimers	88

[a] Inclusion body anemia: precipitated hemoglobin forms inclusion bodies in the red cell and shortens its life span.
[b] Cyanosis: blue color of skin due to deoxyhemoglobin in the capillaries; can be due to the oxygen affinity of hemoglobin being too low.
[c] Hill's constant: a measure of the interaction between the four heme groups causing the sigmoid shape of the oxygen dissociation curve.
[d] Bohr effect: dependence of the oxygen affinity on pH.

From Perutz, M. F. and Lehmann, H., *Nature (London)*, 219, 902, 1968. With permission.

Table 18
RESIDUES AT CONTACTS BETWEEN SUBUNITS

Designation	Residue No.	Residue Position	Replacement From	Replacement To	Variability	Clinical symptoms	Abnormal properties	Structural effects of replacement in oxyhemoglobin	Contact affected	Ref.
							α-Chain			
G Chinese	30	B11	glu	gln	I	None	None	glu B11α_1 makes contact with pro H2β_1, but replacement of CO by NH_2 should not matter	$\alpha_1\beta_1$	89
J Capetown	92	FG4	arg	gln	I	Possibly mild polycythemia	High oxygen affinity; diminished heme-heme interaction	arg FG4α_1 is in Van der Waals contact with arg C6β_2. In addition, its guanidinium group may make a hydrogen bond with a recipient group in β_2. Replacement may interfere with structural transition between oxy and deoxy forms	$\alpha_1\beta_2$	90,91
Chesapeake	92	FG4	arg	leu	I	Polycythemia[a]	High oxygen affinity; diminished heme-heme interaction; normal Bohr effect	See Hb J Capetown	$\alpha_1\beta_2$	92,93
Chiapas	114	GH2	pro	arg	I	None	None	Would be expected to weaken GH corner and make α-chain and $\alpha_1\beta_1$ contact less stable	$\alpha_1\beta_1$	94

Table 18 (continued)
RESIDUES AT CONTACTS BETWEEN SUBUNITS

Designation	Residue No.	Residue Position	Replacement From	Replacement To	Variability	Clinical symptoms	Abnormal properties	Structural effects of replacement in oxyhemoglobin	Contact affected	Ref.
							β-Chain			
E	26	B8	glu	lys	I	None in heterozygotes. Mild hemolytic anemia in homozygotes	Diminished affinity of normal α-chains for these abnormal β-chains. Diminished oxygen affinity.	Replacement of the glu B8β_1, removes one of the residues designed to neutralize arg B12, introducing instead an extra +ve charge. This would disturb the hydrogen bonding between the arginine and the α_1 chain	$\alpha_1\beta_1$	95,96
Tacoma	30	B12	arg	ser	I	None reported	Increased oxygen affinity. Unstable at 50°C	Removes the hydrogen bond between arg B12β_1 and phe GH5α_1, thus weakening bonds between α_1 and β_1	$\alpha_1\beta_1$	97,130
Philly	35	C1	tyr	phe	I	Mild hemolytic anemia, splenomegaly.[b] Inclusion bodies formed on incubation of blood with brillant cresyl blue	All six cysteines react with PMB. Unstable at 50°C	Removes the hydrogen bond between tyr C1β_1 and asp H9α_1, thus weakening bonds between α_1 and β_1	$\alpha_1\beta_1$	98,131

Table 18 (continued)
RESIDUES AT CONTACTS BETWEEN SUBUNITS

Designation	Residue		Replacement		Variability	Clinical symptoms	Abnormal properties	Structural effects of replacement in oxyhemoglobin	Contact affected	Ref.
	No.	Position	From	To						
Yakima	99	G1	asp	his	I	Polycythemia	Increased oxygen affinity; diminished heme-heme interaction; normal Bohr effect	The carboxyl group of asp $G1\beta_2$ normally forms a hydrogen bond with NH of glu $G3\beta_2$. It also touches $C\gamma$ of val $G3\alpha_1$. The imidazole ring of histidine could still make the same hydrogen bond, though it would be weaker, and touch val $G3\alpha_1$. In addition it would make a new contact with leu $G7\alpha_1$	$\alpha_1\beta_2$	99,100
Kempsey	99	G1	asp	asn	I	Polycythemia; less severe than in Hb Yakima	Increased oxygen affinity; diminished heme-heme interaction; Bohr effect present	Replacement of Co^- by NH_2 would weaken internal hydrogen bond and alter contact with val $G3\alpha_1$	$\alpha_1\beta_2$	101
Kansas	102	G4	asn	thr	I	See Table 17			$\alpha_1\beta_2$	88
New York	113	G15	val	glu	I	None reported	No increased electrophoretic mobility at pH 8.6, despite extra − ve charge	Introduces a −ve charge deep in a surface crevice. Might cause rearrangement of arg B12, glu B8 and his G19. Unchanged electrophoretic mobility might be due to a rise in pK of his G19	$\alpha_1\beta_1$	102

Table 18 (continued)
RESIDUES AT CONTACTS BETWEEN SUBUNITS

	Residue		Replacement							
Designation	No.	Position	From	To	Variability	Clinical symptoms	Abnormal properties	Structural effects of replacement in oxyhemoglobin	Contact affected	Ref.
K Woolwich	132	H10	lys	glu	I	None	None	Lys H10β is in a position to form a hydrogen bond with the α-carboxyl group of histidine H24 of the opposite β chain in oxy, but not in deoxyhemoglobin. In deoxyhemoglobin it may bind diphosphoglycerate. Its replacement by glutamic acid may affect the oxygen dissociation curve	$\beta_1\beta_2$	103

[a] Polycythemia: excess of red blood cells. Can be caused by stimulation of red cell production by shortage of oxygen in the tissues; for example, if the oxygen affinity of hemoglobin is too high.
[b] Splenomegaly: rapid destruction of red cells enlarges the spleen.

From Perutz, M. F. and Lehmann, H., *Nature (London)*, 219, 902, 1968. With permission.

Table 19
RESIDUES IN GENERAL POSITIONS

Designation	Residue No.	Residue Position	Replacement From	Replacement To	Variability	Clinical symptoms	Abnormal properties	Structural effects of replacement	Ref.
α-Chain									
Etobicoke	84	F5	ser	arg	I	None reported	Heat labile	In Hb A the OH of serine F5 probably forms a hydrogen bond with CO of leu H19. Substitution of arg would force a conformational change, either within helix F (short contact between Cγ (arg) and OH (ser F2)), or by prising helices F and G apart	104
Manitoba	102	G9	ser	arg	I	None. Present only in small proportion	Difficult to separate from Hb A by electrophoresis at pH 8.6	In central cavity. May introduce instability through excess of + ve charges in central cavity	105,132
β-Chain									
Tokuchi	2	NA2	his	tyr	V	None reported	Little evidence	The imidazole ring of his 2 is probably external. The phenyl ring of tyrosine is more hydrophobic and is rarely found in external positions. The replacement is likely to lead to a conformational change in the NA segment	106
Sogn	14	A11	leu	arg	Vn	None	Increased rate of denaturation at 58°C. Appearance of free α-chains	Removes contact of $C\delta_1$ of leu A11 with $C\delta$ + $C\varepsilon$ of phe GH5 and of $C\delta_2$ with $C\varepsilon$ of phe GH1. Also of $C\delta_1$ of leu A11 with $C\delta_1$ and $C\delta_2$ of leu H4. Could form salt bridge with asp GH4	107
Freiburg	23	B5	val	—	Vn	Cyanosis[a]	High oxygen affinity	Deletion would draw the carboxyl group of glu 22 (B4) into a crevice about 4 A below the protein surface. It would also remove the last turn of the B helix and disturb the conformation of the AB corner	108

Table 19 (Continued)
RESIDUES IN GENERAL POSITIONS

Designation	Residue No.	Residue Position	Replacement From	Replacement To	Variability	Clinical symptoms	Abnormal properties	Structural effects of replacement	Ref.
Genova	28	B10	leu	pro	I	Inclusion body hemolytic anemia	Heat labile at 50°C	Introduction of proline would disrupt helix B	109
Gun Hill	Deletion of 5 residues between 91 and 97					Hemolytic anemia	No heme in β-chain	Removes section of polypeptide chain which forms essential heme contacts and contacts with α subunits	110
Wien	130	H8	tyr	asp	Vn	Hemolytic anemia	Unstable at 50°C. No increased electrophoretic mobility at pH 8.6 despite extra negative charge	In Hb A the phenyl ring of tyrosine is internal; its hydroxyl emerges in a surface crevice near helix A, probably forming a hydrogen bond with CO of val A8(11)β Its replacement by asp creates an internal −ve charge which would be unstable and draw a + ve charge near it. The absence of an increased electrophoretic mobility at pH 8.6 suggests that a new + ve charge is created by a rise in pK of a previously uncharged group. This could be the imidazole of his NA2 or the α amino group of val NA1. Either of these could be drawn in to neutralize asp H8 at the expense of a displacement of helix A.	111,133
Hope	136	H14	gly	asp	I	None	Difficult to separate from Hb A by electrophoresis at pH 8.6	Could form salt bridge with α amino group of val NA1 and by raising its pK produce a compensating charge	112

Table 19 (Continued)
RESIDUES IN GENERAL POSITIONS

Designation	Residue No.	Residue Position	Replacement From	Replacement To	Variability	Clinical symptoms	Abnormal properties	Structural effects of replacement	Ref.
Rainier	145	HC2	tyr	his	I	Polycythemia[b]	Increased oxygen affinity. Unusual resistance to alkali	Hb A the phenolic OH forms a hydrogen bond with CO of val FG5, and the phenyl ring acts as a spacer between helix H and the FG segment. The imidazole ring is too short to make this bond but could instead form a hydrogen bond with CO of leu H19. While the former hydrogen bond would be broken by alkali, the latter might not	113

[a] Cyanosis: blue color of skin due to deoxyhemoglobin in the capillaries; can be due to the oxygen affinity of hemoglobin being too low.
[b] Polycythemia: excess of red blood cells. Can be caused by stimulation of red cell production by shortage of oxygen in the tissues; for example, if the oxygen affinity of hemoglobin is too high.

From Perutz, M. F. and Lehmann, H., *Nature (London)*, 219, 902, 1968. With permission.

Table 20
RESULTS OF CRYSTALLOGRAPHIC STUDIES OF ABNORMAL HEMOGLOBINS

Name	Mutation	n	O_2 affinity	Bohr effect	Comments	Å	Structural changes	Ref.
M Boston	His E7(58)α → Tyr (Distal His)	1.2	Low	Absent	Hb M Boston is more stable to heat denaturation than HbA; carriers show cyanosis	3.5	The iron atom is on the distal side of the α heme and bonded to the phenolate side chain; thus the changes in the α chain stabilize the deoxy quaternary structure, causing abnormal properties; heat stability is due to strong bond between ferric iron and the phenolate	114
Capetown	Arg FG4(92)α → Gln	2.2	Slightly high	—	See Hb Chesapeake	5.5	Deoxy Hb Capetown showed no significant distortions compared to HbA; the oxy structure has not been determined	115
Chesapeake	Arg FG4(92)α → Leu	1.3	High	—	See Hb Capetown	5.5	Deoxy Hb Chesapeake showed no significant distortions, but the oxy structure did; helices C, B, D, and G of the β chain, which lies across the $\alpha_1\beta_2$ interface, move away from the FG4α position and towards the $\alpha_2\beta_2$ interface	115
Cochin-Port-Royal	His HC3(146)β → Arg	3.0	Normal	Low(73%)	See Hb Hiroshima	3.5	Only the intrasubunit salt bridge between His HC3 (146)β and Asp FG1 (94)β is lost; no other structural changes were detected; deoxy form studied	116

Table 20 (Continued)
RESULTS OF CRYSTALLOGRAPHIC STUDIES OF ABNORMAL HEMOGLOBINS

Name	Mutation	n	O_2 affinity	Bohr effect	Comments	A	Structural changes	Ref.
Hiroshima	His HC3(146) $\beta \rightarrow$ Asp	2.4	Low (log p O_2 = 0.30)	Normal	See Hb Cochin-Port-Royal	3.5	Only the intrasubunit salt bridge between His HC3 (146)β and Asp FG1(94)β is lost; other structural changes are small; deoxy form studied	117
M Hyde Park	His F8(92)$\beta \rightarrow$ Tyr (Proximal His)	1.3	Normal	Normal	See Hb M Iwate	3.5	Approximately 25% of the β chains have lost their hemes; the resulting distortions are restricted to the heme pocket and are not significant in the rest of the molecule	118
M Iwate	His F8(87)$\beta \rightarrow$ Tyr (Proximal His)	1.1	Low	Very low	See Hb M Hyde Park	5.5	Two crystal forms were observed: α chains were in the met state in both but the β chains are deoxy in one and met in the other; in both forms the α hemes are bound to both the distal His E7(58)α and the proximal Tyr F8(87)α; both forms are in the deoxy quaternary structure, although the β chain does undergo some conformational changes when it is liganded	

Table 20 (Continued)
RESULTS OF CRYSTALLOGRAPHIC STUDIES OF ABNORMAL HEMOGLOBINS

Name	Mutation	n	O_2 affinity	Bohr effect	Comments	A	Structural changes	Ref.
Kansas	Asn G4(102)$\beta \rightarrow$ Thr	1.3	Low	Large	Dissociates to dimers more easily than HbA; inositol hexaphosphate keeps it in the deoxy quarternary structure, even when it is liganded	3.5 5.5	In deoxy Hb Kansas, Asp (99)β moves towards the hole caused by a smaller residue at residue G4, provoking a series of small movements across the $\alpha_1\beta_2$ interface, and in the α subunit; in carbomonoxy Hb Kansas, there are marked changes in the tertiary structure similar to oxidation of HbA, but the salt bridges are not broken and the penultimate Tyr HC2(140)α and (145)β are not displaced	119, 120
M Milwaukee	Val E11(67)$\beta \rightarrow$ Glu	1.4	Low	Large	—	3.5	The introduction of the Glu into the heme pocket of the β chains leads to a link between the α carboxyl group and the ferric iron; in the crystal structures, the quarternary conformation is controlled by the state of ligation of the ferrous α subunits; if the abnormal β chain favors the deoxy tertiary and quaternary structures in solution, the abnormal properties can be explained	121

Table 20 (Continued)
RESULTS OF CRYSTALLOGRAPHIC STUDIES OF ABNORMAL HEMOGLOBINS

Name	Mutation	n	O_2 affinity	Bohr effect	Comments	A	Structural changes	Ref.
Nancy	Tyr HC2(145)β → Asp	1.1	Very high	Low (50%)	Inositol hexaphosphate increases the Hill constant to 2, but this effect is less than with HbA	3.5	The C-terminal tetrapeptide is severely disordered, resulting in the rupture of the salt bridges; the decreased inositol hexaphosphate is due to the movement of His HC3(143)β, which forms part of its binding site	116
Rainier	Tyr HC2(145)β → Cys	1.5	High	Low (68%)	—	3.5	Structure of deoxy Hb Rainier shows that a disulfide bridge is formed between the new Cys and Cys F9(93)β; the resulting distortions of the C-terminus break the salt bridges associated with His HC3(146)β, as well as the hydrogen bond between Tyr HC2(145)β and Val FG5(98)β, thereby inhibiting the Bohr effect and cooperativity	122
Richmond	Asn G4(102)β → Lys	2.5	Normal	Normal	Dissociates into dimers more easily than Hb A, but not as easily as Hb Kansas	4.0	The deoxy structure shows small changes surrounding the mutated residue, but the heme group is not perturbed, except for a small rotation of a vinyl group	120

Table 20 (Continued)
RESULTS OF CRYSTALLOGRAPHIC STUDIES OF ABNORMAL HEMOGLOBINS

Name	Mutation	n	O_2 affinity	Bohr effect	Comments	A	Structural changes	Ref.
San Diego	Val G11(109)β → Met	2.1	High	Normal		3.5	The side chain at G11β acts as a spacer between the β-G helix and the β-G and α-H helices; this substitution allows β-G to move closer, while α-H is pushed away; the movements in the $\alpha_1\beta_1$ contact weaken the hydrogen bond between Tyr C1(35)β and Asp H9(126)α, and allow the formation of an intrachain hydrogen bond between Asp H9(126)α and His H5(122)α; these changes destabilize the deoxy form and, thus, increase oxygen affinity	123
Seattle	Ala E14(70)β → Asp		Low	Normal	Hb Seattle shows an increased rate of met-hemoglobin formation in vitro and an increased heat lability	3.5	This mutation introduces a negatively charged carboxy group into the heme binding pocket, which may lower the oxygen affinity by polarizing the β-hemes; in addition, the tilt of the heme has changed	124
Sickle Cell (HbS)	Glu A3(6)β → Val	—	—	—	Deoxy HbS is much less soluble than HbA and forms rods inside erythrocytes and in cell-free solution	5.0	There are no large conformational differences between HbS and HbA; in the crystal, the molecules form double strands running parallel to one of the	125

Table 20 (Continued)
RESULTS OF CRYSTALLOGRAPHIC STUDIES OF ABNORMAL HEMOGLOBINS

Name	Mutation	n	O_2 affinity	Bohr effect	Comments	A	Structural changes	Ref.
							crystallographic axes; Val A3(6)β is involved in side-to-side contacts between adjacent strands, these contacts must stabilize the strands, which are likely to be very similar to the fibers seen in electron micrographs of sickle cells	
St. Louis	Leu B10(28)β → Gln	2.2	High	Normal	Hb St. Louis is a valency hybrid, $\alpha_2\beta_2^+$; diphosphoglycerate effect is decreased	3.5	Gln B10(28)β and the distal His E7(63)β swing towards each other and stabilize a water molecule between them with hydrogen bonds; the introduction of this water into the normally hydrophobic heme pocket causes the oxidation of the β hemes to the met-state; since these two met-state chains would closely resemble oxygenated subunits, the molecule always appears to be at least half saturated, which accounts for the low cooperativity and high oxygen affinity; in the deoxy structure reported, there are no additional changes other than a small increase in the tilt of the heme	126

Table 20 (Continued)
RESULTS OF CRYSTALLOGRAPHIC STUDIES OF ABNORMAL HEMOGLOBINS

Name	Mutation	n	O_2 affinity	Bohr effect	Comments	A	Structural changes	Ref.
Tacoma	Arg B12(30)$\beta \rightarrow$ Ser	Low	Low	Low	In spite of the loss of two arginines per tetramer, Hb Tacoma has the same electrophoretic mobility as HbA	3.5	The carboxylate of Glu B8(26)β, which forms a salt bridge with the guanidinium group of Arg B12(30)β in HbA, swings round its α-β carbon bond towards the imidazoles of His G18(116) and G19(117)β in Hb Tacoma; this interaction raises the pK values of the histidines, and their increased positive charge may compensate for the loss of the arginine on the electrophoretic mobility; the loss of the hydrogen bonds across the $\alpha_1\beta_1$ interface made by Arg B12(30)β would loosen the deoxy structure, explaining the decreases in the allosterism and stability, but not in the Bohr effect	127

Table 20 (Continued)
RESULTS OF CRYSTALLOGRAPHIC STUDIES OF ABNORMAL HEMOGLOBINS

Name	Mutation	n	O_2 affinity	Bohr effect	Comments	A	Structural changes	Ref.
Yakima	Asp G1(99)$\beta \rightarrow$ His	Low	High	Normal	—	3.5	The His G1(99)β_2 does not form a hydrogen bond to Tyr C7(42)α_1; since His is bulkier than Asp, it makes additional contacts with Pro G2(100)β_2, Glu G3(101)β_2, Thr C3 (38)α_1, which causes rearrangements in the contact; the subunits slide past each other so that deoxy Hb Yakima is partially in the oxy conformation, which lowers the cooperativity and raises the oxygen affinity; since the salt bridges are not broken, the Bohr effect is normal	128

REFERENCES

1. Perutz, M. F., Structure and mechanism of haemoglobin, *Br. Med. Bull.*, 32, 195, 1976.
2. Baldwin, J. M., Structure and function of haemoglobin, *Prog. Biophys. Mol. Biol.*, 29, 225, 1975.
3. Weissbluth, M., *Hemoglobin: Cooperativity and Electronic Properties*, Springer-Verlag, New York, 1974, 1.
4. Perutz, M. F., The haemoglobin molecule, *Proc. R. Soc. London Ser. B.*, 173, 113, 1969.
5. Perutz, M. F., The hemoglobin molecule, *Sci. Am.*, 211, 64, 1964.
6. Stryer, L., *Biochemistry*, W. H. Freeman, San Francisco, 1975, 46.
7. Lehninger, A., *Biochemistry; the Molecular Basis of Cell Structure and Function*, 2nd ed., Worth, New York, 1975, 145.
8. Metzler, D. E., *Biochemistry: The Chemical Reactions of Living Cells*, Academic Press, New York, 1977, 226.
9. Orten, J. M. and Neuhaus, O. W., *Human Biochemistry*, 9th ed., C. V. Mosby, St. Louis, 1975, 776.
10. White, A., Handler, P., and Smith, E. L., *Principles of Biochemistry*, 5th ed., McGraw-Hill, New York, 1973, 1971.
11. Kendrew, J. C., Dickerson, R. E., Strandberg, B. E., Hart, R. G., Davies, D. R., Phillips, D. C., and Shore, V. C., Structure of myoglobin, *Nature (London)*, 185, 422, 1960.
12. Takano, T., Structure of myoglobin refined at 2.0 Å resolution. I. Crystallographic refinement of metmyoglobin from sperm whale, *J. Mol. Biol.*, 110, 537, 1976.
13. Takano, T., Structure of myoglobin refined at 2.0 Å resolution. II. Structure of deoxymyoglobin from sperm whale, *J. Mol. Biol.*, 110, 569, 1976.
14. Stryer, L., Kendrew, J. C., and Watson, H. C., The mode of attachment of the azide ion to sperm whale metmyoglobin, *J. Mol. Biol.*, 8, 96, 1964.
15. Bretscher, P. A., The X-ray Analysis of Cyanide and Carboxymethylated Metmyoglobin, Ph.D. thesis, University of Cambridge, 1968, 1.
16. Norvell, J. C., Nunes, A. C., and Schoenborn, B. P., Neutron diffraction analysis of myoglobin: structure of the carbon monoxide derivative, *Science*, 190, 568, 1975.
17. Scouloudi, H., X-ray crystallographic studies of seal myoglobin: the molecule at 6 Å and 5 Å resolution, *J. Mol. Biol.*, 40, 353, 1969.
18. Lattman, E. E., Nockolds, C. E., Kretsinger, R. H., and Love, W. E., Structure of yellow fin tuna metmyoglobin at 6 Å resolution, *J. Mol. Biol.*, 60, 271, 1971.
19. Huber, R., Epp, O., Steigemann, W., and Formanek, G., The atomic structure of erythrocruorin in the light of the chemical sequence and its comparison with myoglobin, *Eur. J. Biochem.*, 19, 42, 1971.
20. Huber, R., Epp, O., and Formanek, H., Structures of deoxy- and carbomonoxy-erythrocruorin, *J. Mol. Biol.*, 52, 349, 1970.
21. Padlan, E. A. and Love, W. E., Structure of the haemoglobin of the marine annelid worm, *Glycera dibranchiata*, at 5.5 Å resolution, *Nature (London)*, 220, 376, 1968.
22. Padlan, E. A. and Love, W. E., Three-dimensional structure of hemoglobin from the polychaete annelid, *Glycera dibranchiata*, at 2.5 A resolution, *J. Biol. Chem.*, 249, 4067, 1974.
23. Hendrickson, W. A. and Love, W. E., Structure of lamprey haemoglobin, *Nature (London) New Biol.*, 232, 197, 1971.
24. Vainshtein, B. K., Harutyunyan, E. H., Kuranova, I. P., Borisov, V. V., Sosfenov, N. I., Pavlovsky, A. G., Grebenko, A. I., and Konareva, N. V., Structure of leghaemoglobin from lupin root nodules at 5 Å resolution, *Nature (London)*, 254, 163, 1975.
25. Fermi, G., Three-dimensional Fourier synthesis of human deoxyhaemoglobin at 2.5 Å resolution: refinement of the atomic model, *J. Mol. Biol.*, 97, 237, 1975.
26. Ten Eyck, L. F. and Arnone, A., Three-dimensional Fourier synthesis of human deoxyhemoglobin at 2.5 Å resolution. I. X-ray analysis, *J. Mol. Biol.*, 100, 3, 1976.
27. Baldwin, J. M., in preparation.
28. Frier, J. A. and Perutz, M. F., Structure of human foetal deoxyhaemoglobin, *J. Mol. Biol.*, 112, 97, 1977.
29. Ladner, R. C., Heidner, E. J., and Perutz, M. F., The structure of horse methaemoglobin at 2.0 Å resolution, *J. Mol. Biol.*, 114, 385, 1977.
30. Bolton, W. and Perutz, M. F., Three-dimensional Fourier synthesis of horse deoxyhaemoglobin at 2.8 Å resolution, *Nature (London)*, 228, 551, 1970.
31. Heidner, E. J., Ladner, R. C., and Perutz, M. F., Structure of horse carbonmonoxyhaemoglobin, *J. Mol. Biol.*, 104, 707, 1976.
32. Perutz, M. F. and Mathews, F. S., An X-ray study of azide methaemoglobin, *J. Mol. Biol.*, 21, 199, 1966.
33. Deatherage, J. F., Loe, R. S., Anderson, C. M., and Moffat, K., Structure of cyanide methemoglobin, *J. Mol. Biol.*, 104, 687, 1976.

34. **Deatherage, J. F., Loe, R. S., and Moffat, K.**, Structure of fluoride methemoglobin, *J. Mol. Biol.*, 104, 723, 1976.
35. **Seybert, D. W. and Moffat, K.**, The structure of hemoglobin reconstituted with deuteroheme, *J. Mol. Biol.*, 106, 895, 1976.
36. **Moffat, K., Loe, R. S., and Hoffman, B. M.**, The structure of metmanganoglobin, *J. Mol. Biol.*, 104, 669, 1976.
37. **Dayhoff, M. O.**, Atlas of protein sequence and structure, *Natl. Biomed. Res. Found.*, 5 (Supp. 2), 191, 1976.
38. **Hill, R. L., Harris, C. M., Naylor, J. T., and Sams, W. M.**, The partial amino acid sequence of human myoglobin, *J. Biol. Chem.*, 244, 2182, 1969.
39. **Hill, R. J. and Konigsberg, W.**, The structure of human hemoglobin, *J. Biol. Chem.*, 237, 3151, 1962.
40. **Braunitzer, G., Gehring-Muller, R., Hilschmann, N., Helse, K., Halom, G., Rudloff, V., and Wittmann-Liebold, B.**, Die Konstitution des normalen adulten Humanhämoglobins, *Hoppe-Seyler's Z. Physiol. Chem.*, 325, 283, 1961.
41. **Schroeder, W. A., Shelton, J. R., Shelton, J. B., Cormick, J., and Jones, R. T.**, The amino acid sequence of the γ chain of human fetal hemoglobin, *Biochemistry*, 2, 992, 1963.
42. **Jones, R. T.**, Structural studies of aminoethylated hemoglobins by automatic peptide chromatography, *Cold Spring Harbor Symp. Quant. Biol.*, 29, 297, 1964.
43. **Pauling, L., Corey, R. B., and Branson, H. R.**, The structure of proteins: two hydrogen bonded helical configurations of the polypeptide chain, *Proc. Natl. Acad. Sci. U.S.A.*, 37, 205, 1951.
44. **Donohue, J.**, Hydrogen bonded helical configurations of the polypeptide chain, *Proc. Natl. Acad. Sci. U.S.A.*, 39, 470, 1953.
45. **Low, B. W. and Grenville-Wells, H. J.**, Generalized mathematical relationships for polypeptide chain helices. The coordinates of the II helix, *Proc. Natl. Acad. Sci. U.S.A.*, 39, 785, 1953.
46. **Ramachandran, G. N. and Sasisekharan, V.**, Conformation of polypeptides and proteins, *Adv. Protein Chem.*, 23, 283, 1968.
47. **Kauzmann, W.**, Some factors in the interpretation of protein denaturation, *Adv. Protein Chem.*, 14, 1, 1959.
48. **Tanford, C.**, Contribution of hydrophobic interactions to the stability of the globular conformation of proteins, *J. Am. Chem. Soc.*, 84, 4240, 1962.
49. **Perutz, M. F., Kendrew, J. C., and Watson, H. C.**, Structure and function of haemoglobin II. Some relations between polypeptide chain configuration and amino acid sequence, *J. Mol. Biol.*, 13, 669, 1965.
50. **Olsen, K. W.**, Relationships of Sequence and Three-dimensional Structure in Proteins, 10th International Congress of Biochemistry, Hamburg, 1976.
51. **Perutz, M. F. and Lehmann, H.**, Molecular pathology of human haemoglobin, *Nature (London)*, 219, 902, 1968.
52. **Hoard, J. L. and Scheidt, W. R.**, Stereochemical trigger for initiating cooperative interaction of the subunits during the oxygenation of cobalthemoglobin, *Proc. Natl. Acad. Sci. U.S.A.*, 70, 3919, 1973.
53. **Collman, J. P., Gagne, R. R., Reed, C. A., Robinson, W. F., and Rodley, G. A.**, Structure of an iron (II) dioxygen complex; a model for oxygen carrying hemeproteins, *Proc. Natl. Acad. Sci. U.S.A.*, 71, 1326, 1974.
54. **Chothia, C., Wodak, S., and Janin, J.**, Role of subunit interfaces in the allosteric mechanism of hemoglobin, *Proc. Natl. Acad. Sci. U.S.A.*, 73, 3793, 1976.
55. **Perutz, M. F.**, Stereochemistry of cooperative effects in haemoglobin, *Nature (London)*, 228, 726, 1970.
56. **Perutz, M. F. and Ten Eyck, L. F.**, Stereochemistry of cooperative effects in hemoglobin, *Cold Spring Harbor Symp. Quant. Biol.*, 36, 295, 1971.
57. **Perutz, M. F., Muirhead, H., Cox, J. M., Goaman, L. C. G., Mathews, F. S., McGandy, E. L., and Webb, L. E.**, Three-dimensional Fourier synthesis of horse oxyhaemoglobin at 2.8 A resolution: (1) X-ray analysis, *Nature (London)*, 219, 29, 1968.
58. **Perutz, M. F., Muirhead, H., Cox, J. M., and Goaman, L. C. G.**, Three-dimensional Fourier synthesis of horse oxyhaemoglobin at 2.8 Å resolution: the atomic model, *Nature (London)*, 219, 131, 1968.
59. **Muirhead, H., Cox, J. M., Mazzarella, L., and Perutz, M. F.**, Structure and function of haemoglobin III. A three-dimensional Fourier synthesis of human deoxyhaemoglobin at 5.5 Å resolution, *J. Mol. Biol.*, 28, 117, 1967.
60. **Arnone, A.**, X-ray diffraction study of binding of 2,3-diphosphoglycerate to human deoxyhaemoglobin, *Nature (London)*, 237, 146, 1972.
61. **Arnone, A. and Perutz, M. F.**, Structure of inositol hexaphosphate-human deoxyhaemoglobin complex, *Nature (London)*, 249, 34, 1974.
62. **Fermi, G. and Perutz, M. F.**, Structure of human fluoromethaemoglobin with inositol hexaphosphate, *J. Mol. Biol.*, 114, 421, 1977.

63. **Kilmartin, J. V. and Rossi-Bernardi, L.**, Inhibition of CO_2 combination and reduction of the Bohr effect in haemoglobin chemically modified at its α-amino group, *Nature (London)*, 222, 1243, 1969.
64. **Arnone, A., O'Donnell, S., and Schuster, T.**, X-ray diffraction studies of carbamylated human deoxyhemoglobin, *Fed. Proc.*, 35, 1604, 1976.
65. **Garner, M. H., Bogardt, R. A., Jr., and Gurd, F. R. N.**, Determination of the pK values for the α amino groups of human hemoglobin, *J. Biol. Chem.*, 250, 4398, 1975.
66. **Kibmartin, J. V.**, Interaction of haemoglobin with protons, CO_2 and 2,3-diphosphoglycerate, *Br. Med. Bull.*, 32, 209, 1976.
67. **Roughton, F. J. W.**, Some recent work on the interactions of oxygen, carbon dioxide, and haemoglobin. The Seventh Hopkins Memorial Lecture, *Biochem. J.*, 117, 801, 1970.
68. **Arnone, A.**, X-ray studies of the interaction of CO_2 with human deoxyhaemoglobin, *Nature (London)*, 247, 143, 1974.
69. **Monod, J., Wyman, J., and Changeux, J.-B.**, On the nature of allosteric transitions: a plausible model, *J. Mol. Biol.*, 12, 88, 1965.
70. **Koshland, D. E., Jr., Nemethy, G., and Filmer, D.**, Comparison of experimental binding data and theoretical models in proteins containing subunits, *Biochemistry*, 5, 365, 1966.
71. **Perutz, M. F.**, Nature of haem-haem interaction, *Nature (London)*, 237, 495, 1972.
72. **Lindstrom, T. R. and Ho, C.**, Functional nonequivalence of α and β hemes in human adult hemoglobin, *Proc. Natl. Acad. Sci. U.S.A.*, 69, 1707, 1972.
73. **Winslow, R. M. and Anderson, W. F.**, The Hemoglobinopathies, in *The Metabolic Basis of Inherited Disease*, 4th ed., Stanbury, J. B., Wyngaarden, J. B., and Fredrickson, D. S., Eds., McGraw-Hill, New York, 1978, 1465.
74. **Morimoto, H., Lehmann, H., and Perutz, M. F.**, Molecular pathology of human haemoglobin: Stereochemical interpretation of abnormal oxygen affinities, *Nature (London)*, 232, 408, 1971.
75. **Beretta, A., Prato, V., Gallo, E., and Lehmann, H.**, Haemoglobin Torino- α 43 (CDI) phenylalanine → valine, *Nature (London)*, 217, 1016, 1968.
76. **Gerald, P. S. and Efron, M. L.**, Chemical studies of several varieties of HbM, *Proc. Natl. Acad. Sci. U.S.A.*, 47, 1758, 1958.
77. **Miyaji, T., Iuchi, I., Shibata, S., Takeda, I., and Tamura, A.**, Possible amino acid substitution in the alpha chain (alpha-87Tyr) of Hb M-lwate, *Acta Haematol. Jpn.*, 26, 538, 1963.
78. **Kleihauer, E. F., Reynolds, C. A., Dozy, A. M., Wilson, J. B., Moores, R. R., Berenson, M. P., Wright, C. S., and Huisman, T. H. J.**, Hemoglobin$_{Bibba}$ or α_2^{136} Pro β_2, an unstable α chain abnormal hemoglobin, *Biochim. Biophys. Acta*, 154, 220, 1968.
79. **Dacie, J. V., Shinton, N. K., Gaffney, P. J., Jr., Carrell, R. W., and Lehmann, H.**, Haemoglobin Hammersmith (β42 (CD1)Phe → Ser), *Nature (London)*, 216, 663, 1967.
80. **Jacob, H. S., Brain, M. C., Dacie, J. V., Carrell, R. W., and Lehmann, H.**, Abnormal haem binding and globin SH group blockade in unstable haemoglobins, *Nature (London)*, 218, 1214, 1968.
81. **Muller, C. J. and Kingma, A.**, Haemoglobin Zurich: $\alpha_2{}^A\beta_2{}^{63Arg}$, *Biochim. Biophys. Acta*, 50, 595, 1961.
82. **Hitzig, W. H., Frick, P. G., Betke, K., and Huisman, T. H. J.**, Hemoglobin Zuerich: a new hemoglobin anomaly with sulfonamide-induced inclusion body anemia, *Helv. Paediatr. Acta*, 15, 499, 1960.
83. **Carrell, R. W., Lehmann, H., Lorkin, P. A., Raik, E., and Hunter, E.**, Haemoglobin Sydney: β67 (E11) Valine → Alanine: an emerging pattern of unstable haemoglobins, *Nature (London)*, 215, 626, 1967.
84. **Opfell, R. W., Lorkin, P. A., and Lehmann, H.**, Hereditary non-spherocytic haemolytic anaemia with post-splenectomy inclusion bodies and pigmenturia caused by an unstable haemoglobin Santa Ana β88 (F4) Leucine → Proline, *J. Med. Genet.*, 5, 292, 1968.
85. **Heller, P., Coleman, R. D., and Yakulis, J.**, Structural Studies of Hemoglobin M Hyde Park, *Proc. Eleventh Cong. Intl. Soc. Haematol.*, 1966, 427.
86. **Carrell, R. W., Lehmann, H., and Hutchison, H. E.**, Haemoglobin Koln (β-98 valine → methionine): an unstable protein causing inclusion-body anaemia, *Nature (London)*, 210, 915, 1966.
87. **Vaughan-Jones, R., Grimes, A. J., Carrell, R. W., and Lehmann, H.**, Koln haemoglobinopathy, further data and a comparison with other hereditary Heinz body anaemias, *Br. J. Haematol.*, 13, 394, 1976.
88. **Bonaventura, J. and Riggs, A.**, Hemoglobin Kansas, a human hemoglobin with a neutral amino acid substitution and an abnormal oxygen equilibrium, *J. Biol. Chem.*, 243, 980, 1968.
89. **Swenson, R. T., Hill, R. L., Lehmann, H., and Jim, R. T. S.**, A chemical abnormality in hemoglobin G from Chinese individuals, *J. Biol. Chem.*, 237, 1517, 1962.
90. **Botha, M. C., Beale, D., Isaacs, W. A., and Lehmann, H.**, Haemoglobin J-Cape Town — α_2 92 Arginine → Glutamine, *Nature (London)*, 212, 792, 1966.
91. **Lines, J. G. and McIntosh, R.**, Oxygen binding by haemoglobin J-Cape Town (α_2 92 Arg → Gln), *Nature (London)*, 215, 297, 1967.

92. **Clegg, J. B., Naughton, M. A., and Weatherall, D. J.**, Abnormal human haemoglobins separation and characterization of the α and β chains by chromatography, and the determination of two new variants, Hb Chesapeake and HbJ (Bangkok), *J. Mol. Biol.*, 19, 91, 1966.
93. **Nagel, R. L., Gibson, Q. H., and Charache, S.**, Relation between structure and function in hemoglobin Chesapeake, *Biochemistry*, 6, 2395, 1967.
94. **Jones, R. T., Brimhall, B., and Lisker, R.**, Chemical characterization of Haemoglobin Mexico and Haemoglobin Chiapas, *Biochim. Biophys. Acta*, 154, 488, 1968.
95. **Hunt, J. A. and Ingram, V. M.**, Abnormal human haemoglobins: human haemoglobin E: the chemical effect of gene mutation, *Nature (London)*, 184, 870, 1959.
96. **Bellingham, A. J. and Huehns, E. R.**, Compensation in haemolytic anaemias caused by abnormal haemoglobins, *Nature (London)*, 218, 924, 1968.
97. **Baur, E. W. and Motulsky, A. G.**, Hemoglobin Tacoma — A β-chain variant associated with increased HbA_2, *Humangenetik*, 1, 621, 1965.
98. **Rieder, R. F., Oski, F. A., and Clegg, J. B.**, Hemoglobin Philly. (β35 tyrosine → phenylalanine): studies in the molecular pathology of hemoglobin, *J. Clin. Invest.*, 48, 1627, 1969.
99. **Jones, R. T., Osgood, E. E., Brimhall, B., and Koler, R. D.**, Hemoglobin Yakima. I. Clinical and biochemical studies, *J. Clin. Invest.*, 46, 1840, 1967.
100. **Miles, J. N., Miles, J. E., and Metcalfe, J.**, Hemoglobin Yakima. II. High blood oxygen affinity associated with compensatory erythrocytosis and normal hemodynamics, *J. Clin. Invest.*, 46, 1848, 1967.
101. **Reed, C. S., Hanpson, R., Gordon, S., Jones, R. T., Navy, M. J., Brimhall, B., Edwards, M. J., and Koler, R. D.**, Erythrocytosis secondary to increased oxygen affinity of a mutant hemoglobin, hemoglobin Kenpsey, *Blood*, 31, 623, 1968.
102. **Ranney, H. M., Jacobs, A. S., and Nagel, L. L.**, Haemoglobin New York, *Nature (London)*, 213, 876, 1976.
103. **Allan, N., Beale, D., Irvine, D., and Lehmann, H.**, Three haemoglobins K: Woolwich, an abnormal, Cameroon and Ibadan, two unusual variants of human haemoglobin A, *Nature (London)*, 208, 658, 1965.
104. **Crookston, J. H., Farquarson, H. A., Beale, D., and Lehmann, H.**, Hemoglobin Etobicoke: alpha-84(F5) serine replaced by arginine, *Can. J. Biochem.*, 47, 143, 1969.
105. **Crookston, J. H., Goldstein, J., Lehmann, H., and Beale, D.**, unpublished results.
106. **Shibata, S., Iuchi, I., Miyaji, T., and Takeda, I.**, Spectrophotometric determination of Hb M-Iwate in the hemolysate of hereditary Nigremia, *Bull. Yamaguchi Med. Sch.*, 10, 31, 1963.
107. **Monn, E., Gaffney, P. J., and Lehmann, H.**, Haemoglobin Sogn (beta 14 arginine) a new haemoglobin variant, *Scand. J. Haematol.*, 5, 353, 1968.
108. **Jones, R. T., Brimhall, B., Huisman, J. H. J., Kleihaver, E. F., and Betke, K.**, Hemoglobin Freiburg: abnormal hemoglobin due to deletion of a single amino acid residue, *Science*, 154, 1024, 1976.
109. **Sansone, G., Carrell, R. W., and Lehmann, H.**, Haemoglobin Genova: β28 (B10) leucine → proline, *Nature (London)*, 214, 877, 1967.
110. **Bradley, T. B., Wohl, R. C., and Rieder, R. F.**, Hemoglobin Gun Hill: deletion of five amino acid residues and impaired heme-globin binding, *Science*, 157, 1581, 1967.
111. **Lorkin, P. A., Pietschmann, H., Braunsteiner, H., and Lehmann, H.**, Structure of Haemoglobin Wien β130(H8) tyrosine → aspartic acid: an unstable haemoglobin variant, *Acta Haematol.*, 51, 351, 1974.
112. **Minnich, V., Hill, R. L., Khuri, P. D., and Anderson, M. E.**, Hemoglobin hope: a beta chain variant, *Blood*, 25, 830, 1965.
113. **Stanmatoyannopoulos, G., Adamson, J., Yoshida, A., and Heinenberg, S.**, Hemoglobin Rainier: an adult alkali resistant hemoglobin associated with erythrocytosis, *Blood*, 30, 879, 1967.
114. **Pulsinelli, P. D., Perutz, M. F., and Nagel, R. L.**, Structure of hemoglobin M Boston, a variant with a five-coordinated ferric heme, *Proc. Natl. Acad. Sci. U.S.A.*, 70, 3870, 1973.
115. **Greer, J.**, Three-dimensional structure of abnormal haemoglobins Chesapeake and J. Capetown, *J. Mol. Biol.*, 62, 241, 1971.
116. **Arnone, A., Gacon, G., and Wajcman, H.**, X-ray and functional studies of hemoglobins Nancy and Cochin-Port-Royal, *J. Biol. Chem.*, 251, 5875, 1976.
117. **Perutz, M. F., Pulsinelli, P. D., Ten Eyck, L., Kilmartin, J. V., Shibata, S., Iuchi, I., Miyaji, T., and Hamilton, H. B.**, Haemoglobin Hiroshima and the mechanism of the alkaline Bohr effect, *Nature (London) New Biol.*, 232, 147, 1971.
118. **Greer, J.**, Three-dimensional structure of abnormal human haemoglobins M Hyde Park and M Iwate, *J. Mol. Biol.*, 59, 107, 1971.
119. **Anderson, L.**, Structures of deoxy and carbonmonoxy haemoglobin Kansas in the deoxy quaternary conformation, *J. Mol. Biol.*, 94, 33, 1975.
120. **Greer, J.**, Three-dimensional structure of abnormal human haemoglobin Kansas and Richmond, *J. Mol. Biol.*, 59, 99, 1971.

121. **Perutz, M. F., Pulsinelli, P. D., and Ranney, A. M.,** Structure and subunit interaction of haemoglobin M Milwaukee, *Nature (London) New Biol.*, 237, 259, 1972.
122. **Greer, J. and Perutz, M. F.,** Three-dimensional structure of haemoglobin Rainier, *Nature (London) New Biol.*, 230, 261, 1971.
123. **Anderson, N. L.,** Hemoglobin San Diego (β109 (G 11) Val → Met) crystal structure of the deoxy form, *J. Clin. Invest.*, 53, 329, 1974.
124. **Anderson, N. L., Perutz, M. F., and Stamatoyannopoulos, G.,** Site of the amino acid substitution in haemoglobin Seattle ($\alpha_2^A\ \beta_2^{70Asp}$), *Nature (London), New Biol.*, 243, 274, 1973.
125. **Wishner, B. C., Ward, K. B., Lattman, E. E., and Love, W. E.,** Crystal structure of sickle-cell deoxyhemoglobin at 5 Å resolution, *J. Mol. Biol.*, 98, 179, 1975.
126. **Anderson, N. L.,** Hemoglobin St. Louis β28(B10) Leu → Gln) crystal structure of the fully reduced (deoxy) form, *J. Clin. Invest.*, 58, 1107, 1976.
127. **Tucker, P. W. and Perutz, M. F.,** Mechanism of charge compensation and impairment of cooperative functions in haemoglobin Tacoma (Arg B12(30 β) → Ser), *J. Mol. Biol.*, 114, 415, 1977.
128. **Pulsinelli, P. D.,** Structure of deoxyhaemoglobin Yakima: A high-affinity mutant form exhibiting oxy-like $\alpha_1\ \beta_2$ subunit interactions, *J. Mol. Biol.*, 74, 57, 1973.
129. **Green, J.,** personal communication.
130. **Jones, R. T.,** personal communications.
131. **Rieder, R. F., Oski, F. A., and Clegg, J. B.,** personal communication.
132. **Crookston, J. H., Goldstein, J., Lehmann, H., and Beale, O.,** unpublished results.
133. **Pietschmann, H., Lorkin, P. A., Lehman, H., and Braunsteiner, H.,** unpublished results.

HEMOGLOBINOPATHIES

Ruth N. Wrightstone

Introduction

The following tables of hemoglobin variants are arranged according to the specific polypeptide chain, i.e., α, β, γ, δ, in which the abnormality is found and according to the type of change, i.e., substitution, deletion. The first four tables list the hemoglobin variants resulting from a change(s) in a nucleotide of the mRNA triplet codon. A second group of variants results from deletion of one to five mRNA triplet codons. These variants are generally unstable because the deletion of a codon shortens the chain and disrupts the conformation of the molecule, breaking or changing normal bonding sites. All deleted hemoglobins are found in the β chain. They are Hbs Leiden, Lyon, Freiburg, Niteroi, Tochigi, St. Antoine, Tours, Gun Hill, Deaconess (Leslie), and Coventry. No α chain variants have been reported that are the result of deleted residues.

The extended chains form another group of variants. These hemoglobins are formed when there is a substitution or frameshift in the mRNA strand that fails to terminate the synthesis of the polypeptide chain at the normal terminating codon. As many as 31 additional amino acids have been added to a polypeptide chain before the next terminating codon is reached. The hemoglobins with extended α chains are Hbs Constant Spring, Icaria, Koya Dora, and Wayne. Hemoglobins with extensions of the β chain are Hb Tak and Hb Cranston. One hemoglobin, Hb Grady, is the result of an insertion of three amino acids in the α chain, probably due to a tandem duplication of base pairs which may have arisen by a process of mismatched intragenic crossing-over.

The fusion group of hemoglobins is the result of nonhomologous crossing-over of genetic material during meiosis. Fusion chains have been formed between $\delta\beta$ chains in which the N-terminal part of the chain is from the δ polypeptide chain, and the C-terminal part is from the β polypeptide chain. The crossovers may exist anywhere in the two chains but still retain the normal number of amino acids per chain. These are known as Lepore hemoglobins. They are Lepore Hollandia, Lepore Baltimore, and Lepore Washington-Boston. There are also anti-Lepore hemoglobins. These have, as the N-terminal, amino acids found in the β polypeptide chain, whereas the C-terminal has the sequence of the δ chain. These are Hbs Miyada, P Congo, and P Nilotic. One fusion hemoglobin (Hb Kenya) is the result of a crossover between the γ and β polypeptide chains; the N-terminal follows the sequence of the γ chain, and the C-terminal follows that of the β chain.

The hemoglobin variants are also grouped according to their functional properties. Substitutions in certain areas of the molecule may cause either an increase or decrease in affinity for oxygen. These may occur in either the α or β chain and may cause a polycythemia or anemia.

Five hemoglobin variants are known in which there is a change in two different mRNA triplet codons appearing in two different areas of the same chain. This results in the substitution of two amino acids in a single polypeptide chain. These are Hbs C Harlem, Arlington Park, J Singapore, C Ziguinchor, and Travis.

Included in the major tables are the contacts that each individual amino acid makes within the quaternary structure. Each of the hemoglobins are listed with appropriate reference(s).

Since hemoglobin variants are continually reported in the literature, these tables will be out-of-date by the time this volume is published. An addendum listing hemoglobins reported from the time of proofreading to just before the final publishing date is therefore included. A current list of hemoglobin variants is maintained by the director of the International Hemoglobin Information Center. Anyone desiring additional information on any hemoglobinopathy or a current list of hemoglobin variants may write to Ruth N. Wrightstone, Director, International Hemoglobin Information Center, Medical College of Georgia, Augusta, Georgia, 30901.

Table 1
VARIANTS OF THE ALPHA CHAIN

Residue	Substitution	Name	Major abnormal property	Contacts	Ref.
1(NA1)	Val	—	—	α-α	—
2(NA2)	Leu	—	—	Central	—
3(A1)	Ser	—	—	External	—
4(A2)	Pro	—	—	External	—
5(A3)	Ala → Asp	Hb J Toronto	—	External	1
6(A4)	Asp → Ala	Hb Sawara	—	External	2
7(A5)	Lys	—	—	External	—
8(A6)	Thr	—	—	External	—
9(A7)	Asn	—	—	External	—
10(A8)	Val	—	—	Internal	—
11(A9)	Lys → Glu	Hb Anantharaj	—	External	3
12(A10)	Ala → Asp	Hb J Paris-I	—	External	4
		J Aljezur	—		5
13(A11)	Ala	—	—	Internal	—
14(A12)	Trp	—	—	Internal	—
15(A13)	Gly → Asp	Hb I Interlaken	—	External	6
		J Oxford	—		7
		N Cosenza	—		8
	Gly → Arg	Hb Ottawa	—		9
		Siam	—		10
16(A14)	Lys → Glu	Hb I	—	External	11
		I Philadelphia	—		12
		I Texas	—		13
		I Burlington	—		14
		I Skamania	—		15
17(A15)	Val	—	—	Internal	—
18(A16)	Gly → Arg	Hb Handsworth	—	External	16
19(AB1)	Ala → Asp	Hb J Kurosh	—	External	17
20(B1)	His	—	—	External	—
21(B2)	Ala → Asp	Hb J Nyanza	—	External	18
22(B3)	Gly → Asp	Hb J Medellin	—	External	19
23(B4)	Glu → Gln	Hb Memphis	—	External	20
	Glu → Lys	Hb Chad	—		21
	Glu → Val	Hb G Audhali	—		22
24(B5)	Tyr	—	—	OH external, ring internal	—
25(B6)	Gly	—	—	Internal	—
26(B7)	Ala	—	—	External	—
27(B8)	Glu → Gly	Hb Ft. Worth	—	External	23
	Glu → Val	Hb Spanish Town	—		24
28(B9)	Ala	—	—	Internal	—
29(B10)	Leu	—	—	Internal	—
30(B11)	Glu → Lys	Hb O Padova	—	α_1-β_1	25
	Glu → Gln	Hb G Honolulu	—		26
		G Singapore	—		27
		G Chinese	—		28
		G Hong Kong	—		28
31(B12)	Arg	—	—	α_1-β_1	—
32(B13)	Met	—	—	Heme	—
33(B14)	Phe	—	—	Internal	—
34(B15)	Leu	—	—	α_1-β_1	—

Table 1 (continued)
VARIANTS OF THE ALPHA CHAIN

Residue	Substitution	Name	Major abnormal property	Contacts	Ref.
35(B16)	Ser	—	—	α_1-β_1	—
36(C1)	Phe	—	—	α_1-β_1	—
37(C2)	Pro	—	—	α_1-β_2	—
38(C3)	Thr	—	—	α_1-β_2	—
39(C4)	Thr	—	—	Heme	—
40(C5)	Lys	—	—	Deoxy: α_1-β_2	—
41(C6)	Thr	—	—	α_1-β_2	—
42(C7)	Tyr	—	—	α_1-β_2; heme	—
43(CE1)	Phe → Val	Hb Torino	Unstable, $\downarrow O_2$ affinity	Heme	29
	Phe → Leu	Hb Hirosaki	—		30
44(CE2)	Pro	—	—	α_1-β_2	—
45(CE3)	His → Arg	Hb Fort de France	$\uparrow O_2$ Affinity	Heme	393
46(CE4)	Phe	—	—	Heme	—
47(CE5)	Asp → Gly	Hb Umi	—	External	31
		Kokura	—		31
		Michigan-I	—		—
		Michigan-II	—		—
		Yukuhashi-II	—		31
		L Gaslini	—		—
		Tagawa-II	—		31,32
		Beilinson	—		33
		Mugino	—		31
	Asp → His	Hb Hasharon	Unstable		34
		Sinai	—		35
		Sealy	—		36
		L Ferrara	—		37,38
	Asp → Asn	Hb Arya	Slightly unstable		39
48(CE6)	Leu → Arg	Hb Montgomery	—	Surface	40
49(CE7)	Ser	—	—	External	—
50(CE8)	His → Asp	Hb J Sardegna	—	External	41
51(CE9)	Gly → Asp	Hb J Abidjan	—	External	42
	Gly → Arg	Hb Russ	—		43
52(E1)	Ser	—	—	External	—
53(E2)	Ala → Asp	Hb J Rovigo	Unstable	External	44
54(E3)	Gln → Arg	Hb Shimonoseki	—	External	45
		Hikoshima	—		—
	Gln → Glu	Hb Mexico	—		46
		J Paris-II	—		47
		Uppsala	—		48
55(E4)	Val	—	—	Internal	—
56(E5)	Lys	—	—	External	—
57(E6)	Gly → Arg	Hb L Persian Gulf	—	External	49
	Gly → Asp	Hb J Norfolk	—		50
		Kagoshima	—		51
		Nishik-I, II, III	—		—
58(E7)	His → Tyr	Hb M Boston	$\downarrow O_2$ Affinity, "n" = 1.2	Heme, "distal"	52
		M Osaka			53
		Gothenburg	—		54
		M Kiskunhalas	—		55
59(E8)	Gly	—	—	Internal	—
60(E9)	Lys → Asn	Hb Zambia	—	External	56
61(E10)	Lys → Asn	Hb J Buda	—	External	57
62(E11)	Val	—	—	Heme	—
63(E12)	Ala → Asp	Hb Pontoise	—	Surface	390
64(E13)	Asp → Asn	Hb G Waimanalo	—	External	58
		Aida	—		59
	Asp → His	Hb Q India	—		60
	Asp → Tyr	Hb Perspolis	—		17
65(E14)	Ala	—	—	External	—
66(E15)	Leu	—	—	Internal	—
67(E16)	Thr	—	—	External	—
68(E17)	Asn → Asp	Hb Ube-2	—	External	61

Table 1 (continued)
VARIANTS OF THE ALPHA CHAIN

Residue	Substitution	Name	Major abnormal property	Contacts	Ref.
	Asn → Lys	Hb G-Philadelphia	—		62
		G Knoxville-I	—		63
		Stanleyville-I	—		64
		D Washington	—		63
		D St. Louis	—		65
		G Bristol	—		66
		G Azakuoli	—		63
		D Baltimore	—		63
69(E18)	Ala	—	—	Internal	—
70(E19)	Val	—	—	Surface	—
71(E20)	Ala → Glu	Hb J Habana	—	External	67
72(EF1)	His → Arg	Hb Daneskgah-Tehran	—	External	68
73(EF2)	Val	—	—	Surface	—
74(EF3)	Asp → His	Hb Mahidol	—	External	69
		G Taichung	—		70
		Q Thailand	—		71
	Asp → Asn	Hb G Pest	—		57
	Asp → Gly	Hb Chapel Hill	—		72
75(EF4)	Asp → His	Hb Q Iran	—	External	71
	Asp → Tyr	Hb Winnipeg	—		73
	Asp → Asn	Hb Matsue-Oki	—		74
76(EF5)	Met	—	—	Internal	—
77(EF6)	Pro	—	—	External	—
78(EF7)	Asn → Lys	Hb Stanleyville-II	—	External	75
79(EF8)	Ala	—	—	External	—
80(F1)	Leu → Arg	Hb Ann Arbor	Unstable	Surface	76,77
81(F2)	Ser	—	—	External	—
82(F3)	Ala → Asp	Hb Garden State	—	External	78
83(F4)	Leu	—	—	Heme	—
84(F5)	Ser → Arg	Hb Etobicoke	↑O_2 Affinity	Internal	79,385
85(F6)	Asp → Asn	Hb G Norfolk	(?)↑O_2 Affinity, "n" = 2.6	External	80,81
	Asp → Tyr	Hb Atago	—		82
	Asp → Val	Hb Inkster	—		83
86(F7)	Leu	—	—	Heme	—
87(F8)	His → Tyr	Hb M Iwate	Ferri Hb,	Heme	84
		M Kankakee	↓O_2 Affinity, "n" = 1.0	"proximal"	85
		M Oldenburg	—		86
88(F9)	Ala	—	—	Surface	—
89(FG1)	His	—	—	External	—
90(FG2)	Lys → Asn	Hb J Broussais	—	External	87,88
		Tagawa-I	—		89
	Lys → Thr	Hb J Rajappen	—		90
91(FG3)	Leu	—	—	α_1-β_2	—
92(FG4)	Arg → Gln	Hb J Cape Town	↑O_2 Affinity, "n" = 2.2	α_1-β_2	91,92
	Arg → Leu	Hb Chesapeake	↑O_2 Affinity, "n" = 2.2		93,94
93(FG5)	Val	—	—	Heme; α_1-β_2	—
94(G1)	Asp → Tyr	Hb Setif	Unstable	α_1-β_2	95
	Asp → Asn	Hb Titusville	↓O_2 Affinity, ↑dissociation, "n" = 1.06		96
95(G2)	Pro → Leu	Hb G Georgia	↑Dissociation	α_1-β_2	97
	Pro → Ser	Hb Rampa	↑Dissociation		98,99
	Pro → Ala	Hb Denmark Hill	↑O_2 Affinity, "n" = 1.8—2.4		100
	Pro → Arg	Hb St. Lukes	↑Dissociation		101
96(G3)	Val	—	—	α_1-β_2	—
97(G4)	Asn	—	—	Heme	—
98(G5)	Phe	—	—	Heme	—
99(G6)	Lys	—	—	Central	—
100(G7)	Leu	—	—	Surface	—
101(G8)	Leu	—	—	Heme	—

Table 1 (continued)
VARIANTS OF THE ALPHA CHAIN

Residue	Substitution	Name	Major abnormal property	Contacts	Ref.
102(G9)	Ser → Arg	Hb Manitoba	—	Central	102
103(G10)	His	—	—	α_1-β_1	—
104(G 11)	Cys	—	—	α_1-β_1	—
105(G12)	Leu	—	—	Internal	—
106(G13)	Leu	—	—	α_1-β_1	—
107(G14)	Val	—	—	α_1-β_1	—
108(G15)	Thr	—	—	Internal	—
109(G16)	Leu	—	—	Internal	—
110(G17)	Ala	—	—	Internal	—
111(G18)	Ala	—	—	α_1-β_1	—
112(G19)	His → Asp	Hb Hopkins-II	Unstable, ↑O_2 Affinity, "n" = 2.2	External	103
	His → Arg	Hb Strumica	—		104
		Serbia	—		105
113(GH1)	Leu	—	—	Surface	—
114(GH2)	Pro → Arg	Hb Chiapas	—	α_1-β_1	46
115(GH3)	Ala → Asp	Hb J Tongariki	—	External	106
116(GH4)	Glu → Lys	Hb O Indonesia	—	External	107
		Buginese-X	—		108
		Oliviere	—		109
117(GH5)	Phe	—	—	α_1-β_1	—
118(H1)	Thr → Gly	Hb Hopkins-2-II	—	External	110
119(H2)	Pro	—	—	α_1-β_1	—
120(H3)	Ala → Glu	Hb J Meerut	—	External	111
		J Birmingham	—		111a
121(H4)	Val	—	—	Surface	—
122(H5)	His	—	—	α_1-β_1	—
123(H6)	Ala	—	—	α_1-β_1	—
124(H7)	Ser	—	—	Surface	—
125(H8)	Leu	—	—	Internal	—
126(H9)	Asp → Asn	Hb Tarrant	↑O_2 Affinity, "n" = 1.8	α_1-β_1	112
127(H10)	Lys → Thr	Hb St. Claude	—	Central	113
	Lys → Asn	Hb Jackson	—		114
128(H11)	Phe	—	—	Internal	—
129(H12)	Leu	—	—	Heme	—
130(H13)	Ala	—	—	Central	—
131(H14)	Ser	—	—	Central	
132(H15)	Val	—	—	Heme	—
133(H16)	Ser	—	—	Central	—
134(H17)	Thr	—	—	Central	—
135(H18)	Val	—	—	Surface	—
136(H19)	Leu → Pro	Hb Bibba	Unstable, ↑dissociation	Heme	115
137(H20)	Thr	—	—	Central	—
138(H21)	Ser	—	—	Central	—
139(HC1)	Lys	—	—	External	—
140(HC2)	Tyr	—	—	Deoxy: HB to FG5 same α chain oxy: mobile, cooperativity	—
141(HC3)	Arg → Pro	Hb Singapore	—	External, deoxy, salt bonds to H9, H10, NA1 other α chain, oxy: mobile, Bohr	116
	Arg → His	Hb Suresnes	↑O_2 Affinity, "n" = 2.06		117

Table 2
VARIANTS OF THE BETA CHAIN

Residue	Substitution	Name	Major abnormal property	Contacts	Ref.
1(NA1)	Val → Ac-ala	Hb Raleigh	—	DPG binding	118
2(NA2)	His → Arg	Hb Deer Lodge	—	DPG binding	119
3(NA3)	Leu	—	—	Surface	—
4(A1)	Thr	—	—	External	—
5(A2)	Pro	—	—	External	—
6(A3)	Glu → Val	Hb S	Sickling	External	120
	Glu → Lys	Hb C	—		121
	Glu → Ala	Hb G Makassar	—		122
7(A4)	Glu → Gly	Hb G San José	—	External	123
	Glu → Lys	Hb Siriraj	—		124
8(A5)	Lys	—	—	External	—
9(A6)	Ser → Cys	Hb Porto Alegre	Polymerization	External	125
10(A7)	Ala → Asp	Hb Ankara	—	External	126
11(A8)	Val	—	—	Internal	—
12(A9)	Thr	—	—	Surface	—
13(A10)	Ala	—	—	External	—
14(A11)	Leu → Arg	Hb Sögn	—	Surface	127
	Leu → Pro	Hb Saki	Unstable		128,129
15(A12)	Trp → Arg	Hb Belfast	Unstable, ↑O_2 Affinity, "n" diminished	Internal	130,131
16(A13)	Gly → Asp	Hb J Baltimore	—	External	132
		J Trinidad	—		133
		J Ireland	—		133
		N New Haven	—		134
		J Georgia	—		135
	Gly → Arg	Hb D Bushman	—		136
17(A14)	Lys → Glu	Hb Nagasaki	—	External	137
18(A15)	Val	—	—	Internal	—
19(B1)	Asn → Lys	Hb D Ouled Rabah	—	External	138
	Asn → Asp	Hb Alamo	—		326
20(B2)	Val → Met	Hb Olympia	↑O_2 Affinity, "n" = 2.5—2.7	External	139
	Val → Asp	Hb Strasbourg	Unstable (slight)		140
21(B3)	Asp	—	—	External	—
22(B4)	Glu → Lys	Hb E Saskatoon	—	External	141
	Glu → Gly	Hb G Taipei	—		142
	Glu → Ala	Hb G Saskatoon	—		143
		Hsin Chu	—		144
		G Coushatta	—		145
		G Taegu	—		146
	Glu → Gln	Hb D Iran	—		147
23(B5)	Val	—	—	Internal	—
24(B6)	Gly → Arg	Hb Riverdale-Bronx	Unstable	Internal	148
	Gly → Val	Hb Savannah	Unstable		149
	Gly → Asp	Hb Moscva	Unstable, ↓O_2 Affinity "n" = near normal		150
25(B7)	Gly → Arg	Hb G Taiwan Ami	—	External	151
26(B8)	Glu → Lys	Hb E	—	External	152
	Glu → Val	Hb Henri Mondor	Unstable (slight)		153
27(B9)	Ala → Asp	Hb Volga	Unstable	Internal	154
		Drenthe	—		155
28(B10)	Leu → Gln	Hb St. Louis	Unstable, ferri Hb, ↑O_2 Affinity, "n" = 2.2	Internal	156,157
	Leu → Pro	Hb Genova	Unstable, ↑O_2 Affinity, "n" = 1.0		158
29(B11)	Gly → Asp	Hb Lufkin	—	Internal	159
30(B12)	Arg → Ser	Hb Tacoma	Unstable, ↓ Bohr and heme-heme, normal O_2, affinity, "n" = 2.8	α_1-β_1	160
31(B13)	Leu	—	—	Heme	—
32(B14)	Leu → Pro	Hb Perth	Unstable	Internal	161
		Abraham Lincoln	—		162
	Leu → Arg	Hb Castilla	Unstable		163
33(B15)	Val	—	—	α_1-β_1	—
34(B16)	Val	—	—	α_1-β_1	—

Table 2 (continued)
VARIANTS OF THE BETA CHAIN

Residue	Substitution	Name	Major abnormal property	Contacts	Ref.
35(C1)	Tyr → Phe	Hb Philly	Unstable, ↑O_2 Affinity, "n" = 1.3	α_1-β_1	164
36(C2)	Pro	—	—	α_1-β_1	—
37(C3)	Trp → Ser	Hb Hirose	↑O_2 Affinity, "n" = 1.5	α_1-β_1	165
38(C4)	Thr	—	—	Heme	—
39(C5)	Gln → Lys	Hb Alabama	—	α_1-β_2	166
	Gln → Glu	Hb Vaasa	—		167
40(C6)	Arg → Lys	Hb Athens-Ga	↑O_2 Affinity, "n" = 2.8	α_1-β_2	168
		Waco	—		169
	Arg → Ser	Hb Austin	↑O_2 Affinity, ↑ dissociation, "n" reduced		169
41(C7)	Phe → Tyr	Hb Mequon	—	Heme	170
42(CD1)	Phe → Ser	Hb Hammersmith	Unstable, ↓O_2 affinity,	Heme	171
		Chiba	"n" = 2.25		172
	Phe → Leu	Hb Louisville	Unstable, ↓O_2 Affinity,		173
		Bucuresti	"n" = 1.85		174
43(CD2)	Glu → Ala	Hb G Galveston	—	External	175
		G Port Arthur	—		175
		G Texas	—		175
44(CD3)	Ser	—	—	Heme	—
45(CD4)	Phe	—	—	Heme	—
46(CD5)	Gly → Glu	Hb K Ibadan	—	External	176
47(CD6)	Asp → Asn	Hb G Copenhagen	—	External	177
48(CD7)	Leu → Arg	Hb Okaloosa	Unstable, ↓O_2 Affinity, "n" = 2.85	Surface	178
49(CD8)	Ser	—	—	External	—
50(D1)	Thr → Lys	Hb Edmonton	—	External	179
51(D2)	Pro → Arg	Hb Willamette	↑O_2 Affinity, "n" = 2.9	α_1-β_1	180
52(D3)	Asp → Asn	Hb Osu Christiansborg	—	External	181
	Asp → Ala	Hb Ocho Rios	—		182
53(D4)	Ala	—	—	External	—
54(D5)	Val	—	—	Internal	—
55(D6)	Met	—	—	α_1-β_1	—
56(D7)	Gly → Asp	Hb J Bangkok	—	External	183
		J Meinung	—		184
		J Korat	—		184
		J Manado	—		185
	Gly → Arg	Hb Hamadan	—		186
57(E1)	Asn → Lys	Hb G Ferrara	—	External	187
58(E2)	Pro → Arg	Hb Yukuhashi	—	External	188
		Dhofar	—		189
59(E3)	Lys → Glu	Hb I High Wycombe	—	External	190
	Lys → Thr	Hb J Kaohsiung	—		191
		J Honolulu	—		192
60(E4)	Val	—	—	Internal	—
61(E5)	Lys → Glu	Hb N Seattle	—	External	193
	Lys → Asn	Hb Hikari	—		194
62(E6)	Ala → Pro	Hb Duarte	Unstable, ↑O_2 Affinity, "n" = 2.9	External	195
63(E7)	His → Arg	Hb Zürich	Unstable, ↑O_2 Affinity, "n" = 1.8	Heme "distal"	196
	His → Tyr	Hb M Saskatoon	Ferri-Hb, ↑O_2 Affinity, "n" = 2.1—2.3		197
		M Emory	—		197
		M Kurume	—		198
		M Hida	—		—
		M Radom	—		199
		M Arhus	—		200
		M Chicago	—		201
		Leipzig	—		202
		Hörlein-Weber	—		203
		Novi Sad	—		204
		M Erlangen	—		205
	His → Pro	Hb Bicêtre	Unstable, autoxidizing		206

Table 2 (continued)
VARIANTS OF THE BETA CHAIN

Residue	Substitution	Name	Major abnormal property	Contacts	Ref.
64(E8)	Gly → Asp	Hb J Calabria	Unstable	Internal	207
		J Bari	—		—
		J Cosenza	—		—
65(E9)	Lys → Asn	Hb J Sicilia	—	External	208
	Lys → Gln	Hb J Cairo	—		209
66(E10)	Lys → Glu	Hb I Toulouse	Unstable, Ferri-Hb	External, ? heme	210
67(E11)	Val → Asp	Hb Bristol	Unstable	Heme	211
	Val → Glu	Hb M Milwaukee-I	Ferri-Hb, ↓O_2 Affinity, "n" = 1.2		197
	Val → Ala	Hb Sydney	Unstable		212
68(E12)	Leu → Pro	Hb Mizuho	Unstable	Internal	213
69(E13)	Gly → Asp	Hb J Cambridge	—	External	177
		J Rambam	—		214
70(E14)	Ala → Asp	Hb Seattle	↓O_2 Affinity, "n" = 2.6	Heme	215
71(E15)	Phe → Ser	Hb Christchurch	Unstable	Heme	216
72(E16)	Ser	—	—	External	—
73(E17)	Asp → Tyr	Hb Vancouver	↓O_2 Affinity, "n" = 2.7	External	217
	Asp → Asn	Hb Korle Bu	—		218
		G Accra	—		219
	Asp → Val	Hb Mobile	↓O_2 Affinity, "n" = 2.7		220
74(E18)	Gly → Val	Hb Bushwick	—	External	221
	Gly → Asp	Hb Shepherds Bush	Unstable, ↑O_2 Affinity, "n" = 2.2—2.4		222
75(E19)	Leu → Pro	Hb Atlanta	Unstable	Internal	223
76(E20)	Ala → Asp	Hb J Chicago	—	External	224
77(EF1)	His → Asp	Hb J Iran	—	External	225
78(EF2)	Leu	—	—	Internal	—
79(EF3)	Asp → Gly	Hb G Hsi-Tsou	↑O_2 Affinity	External	226,386
80(EF4)	Asn → Lys	Hb G Szuhu	—	External	227
		Gifu	—		228
81(EF5)	Leu → Arg	Hb Baylor	↑O_2 Affinity, "n" = 2.0	Internal	229
82(EF6)	Lys → Asn → Asp	Hb Providence	↓O_2 Affinity, "n" = 2.5—2.7	DPG binding	230,231
	Lys → Thr	Hb Rahere	↑O_2 Affinity, "n" = normal		232
	Lys → Met	Hb Helsinki	↑O_2 Affinity, "n" = 2.3		233
83(EF7)	Gly → Cys	Hb Ta-li	—	External	234
	Gly → Asp	Hb Pyrgos	—		235,236
84(EF8)	Thr	—	—	External	—
85(F1)	Phe → Ser	Hb Bryn Mawr	Unstable, ↑ O_2 Affinity	Internal	237
		Buenos Aires			238
86(F2)	Ala	—	—	External	—
87(F3)	Thr → Lys	Hb D Ibadan	—	External	239
88(F4)	Leu → Arg	Hb Böras	Unstable	Heme	240
	Leu → Pro	Hb Santa Ana	Unstable		241
89(F5)	Ser → Asn	Hb Creteil	↑O_2 Affinity, "n" = 1.2	Internal	242
	Ser → Arg	Hb Vanderbilt	—		243,384
90(F6)	Glu → Lys	Hb Agenogi	↓O_2 Affinity, "n" = normal	External	244
91(F7)	Leu → Pro	Hb Sabine	Unstable	Heme	245
	Leu → Arg	Hb Caribbean	Unstable, ↓O_2 Affinity		246
92(F8)	His → Tyr	Hb M Hyde Park	Normal O_2 Affinity,	Heme	247
		M Akita	ferri-Hb	"Proximal"	248
	His → Gln	Hb St. Etienne	Unstable, ↑O_2 Affinity, ↑		249
		Istanbul	dissociation, "n" = 1.8		250
	His → Asp	Hb J Altgeld Gardens	Normal O_2 Affinity		251
	His → Pro	Hb Newcastle	—		252
93(F9)	Cys	—	—	External	—
94(FG1)	Asp	—	—	External	—
95(FG2)	Lys → Glu	Hb N Baltimore	—	External	253
		Hopkins-I	—		254
		Jenkins	—		255
		N Memphis	—		256

Table 2 (continued)
VARIANTS OF THE BETA CHAIN

Residue	Substitution	Name	Major abnormal property	Contacts	Ref.
		Kenwood	—		257
96(FG3)	Leu	—	—	Heme	—
97(FG4)	His → Gln	Hb Malmö	↑O_2 Affinity, "n" = 1.87	α_1-β_2	258
	His → Leu	Hb Wood	↑O_2 Affinity, "n" = 1.5		259,260
98(FG5)	Val → Met	H Köln	Unstable	Heme	261
		San Francisco (Pacific)	↑O_2 Affinity, "n" = 1.46	α_1-β_2	262
		Ube I	—		263
	Val → Gly	Hb Nottingham	Unstable, ↑O_2 Affinity, "n" = "impaired"		264
	Val → Ala	Hb Djelfa	Unstable, ↑O_2 Affinity, "n" = 1.0—2.3		265
99(G1)	Asp → Asn	Hb Kempsey	↑O_2 Affinity, "n" = 1.0	α_1-β_2	266
	Asp → His	Hb Yakima	↑O_2 Affinity, "n" = 1.1		267
	Asp → Ala	Hb Radcliffe	↑O_2 Affinity, "n" = 1.1		268
	Asp → Tyr	Hb Ypsilanti	↑O_2 Affinity		269
100(G2)	Pro → Leu	Hb Brigham	↑O_2 Affinity	α_1-β_2	270
101(G3)	Glu → Lys	Hb British Columbia	↑O_2 Affinity, "n" = 1.6	α_1-β_2	271
	Glu → Gln	Hb Rush	Unstable		272
	Glu → Gly	Hb Alberta	↑O_2 Affinity, "n" = 1.0		273
	Glu → Asp	Hb Potomac	↑O_2 Affinity		274
102(G4)	Asn → Lys	Hb Richmond	Asymmetric hybrids	Heme, α_1-β_2	275
	Asn → Thr	Hb Kansas	↓O_2 Affinity, ↑ dissociation, "n" = 1.3		276
	Asn → Ser	Hb Beth Israel	↓O_2 Affinity, "n" = 1.0—1.8		277
103(G5)	Phe → Leu	Hb Heathrow	↑O_2 Affinity, "n" = 1.2	Heme	278
104(G4)	Arg → Ser	Hb Camperdown	Slightly unstable	Central cavity	279
105(G7)	Leu	—	—	Internal	—
106(G8)	Leu → Pro	Hb Southampton	↑O_2 Affinity, "n" = 1.5		280
		Casper	—		281
	Leu → Gln	Hb Tubingen	Unstable, ↑O_2 affinity, "n" = 2.15		282,283
107(G9)	Gly → Arg	Hb Burke	↓O_2 Affinity, "n" = 2.1	Internal	284
108(G10)	Asn → Asp	Hb Yoshizuka	↓O_2 Affinity, "n" = 2.3—3.0	α_1-β_1	285
109(G11)	Val → Met	Hb San Diego	↑O_2 Affinity, "n" = 2.02-2.24	Internal	286
110(G12)	Leu	—	—	Internal	—
111(G13)	Val → Phe	Hb Peterborough	Unstable, ↓O_2 Affinity, "n" = near normal	Internal	287
112(G14)	Cys	—	—	α_1-β_1	—
113(G15)	Val → Glu	Hb New York	—	Internal	288
114(G16)	Leu	—	—	Internal	—
115(G17)	Ala → Pro	Hb Madrid	Unstable	α_1-β_1	289
116(G18)	His	—	—	α_1-β_1	—
117(G19)	His → Arg	Hb P Galveston	—	External	290
118(GH1)	Phe	—	—	Surface	—
119(GH2)	Gly → Asp	Hb Fannin-Lubbock	Unstable (slightly)	α_1-β_1	291,292
120(GH3)	Lys → Glu	Hb Hijiyama	—	External	293
	Lys → Asn	Hb Riyadh, Karatsu	—	External	294,388
121(GH4)	Glu → Gln	D Los Angeles	↑O_2 Affinity	External	295
		D Punjab	—		296,387
		D North Carolina	—		297
		D Portugal	—		298
		Oak Ridge	—		299
		D Chicago	—		300
	Glu → Lys	Hb O Arab	—		301
		Egypt	—		302
	Glu → Val	Hb Beograd	—		303
122(GH5)	Phe	—	—	α_1-β_1	—
123(H1)	Thr	—	—	α_1-β_1	—
124(H2)	Pro → Arg	Hb Khartoum	Unstable	α_1-β_1	304

Table 2 (continued)
VARIANTS OF THE BETA CHAIN

Residue	Substitution	Name	Major abnormal property	Contacts	Ref.
125(H3)	Pro	—	—	α_1-β_1	—
126(H4)	Val → Glu	Hb Hofu	—	Surface	305
127(H5)	Gln → Glu	Hb Hacettepe	—	α_1-β_1	306
128(H6)	Ala → Asp	Hb J Guantanamo	Unstable	α_1-β_1	391
129(H7)	Ala → Asp	Hb J Taichung	—	Surface	307
	Ala → Glu or Asp	Hb K Cameroon	—		176
130(H8)	Tyr → Asp	Hb Wien	Unstable	Internal	308
131(H9)	Gln → Glu	Hb Camden	—	α_1-β_1	309
		Tokuchi	—		310
132(H10)	Lys → Gln	Hb K Woolwich	—	Surface	176
133(H11)	Val	—	—	Internal	—
134(H12)	Val → Glu	Hb North Shore	Unstable	Internal	311
135(H13)	Ala → Pro	Hb Altdorf	Unstable, ↑O_2 Affinity, "n" = 1.0	Central	312
136(H14)	Gly → Asp	Hb Hope	Unstable	Central	313
137(H15)	Val	—	—	Heme	—
138(H16)	Ala	—	—	Central	—
139(H17)	Asn	—	—	Central	—
140(H18)	Ala	—	—	Central	—
141(H19)	Leu → Arg	Hb Olmsted	—	Heme	258
142(H20)	Ala	—	—	Central	—
143(H21)	His → Arg	Hb Abruzzo	↑O_2 Affinity, "n" = 2.7	DPG binding	314
	His → Gln	Hb Little Rock	↑O_2 Affinity, "n" = 2.5—3.0	—	315
	His → Pro	Hb Syracuse	↑O_2 Affinity, "n" = 1.1		316
144(HC1)	Lys → Asn	Hb Andrew-Minneapolis	↑O_2 Affinity, "n" = 2.4	External	317
145(HC2)	Tyr → His	Hb Bethesda	↑O_2 Affinity,"n" = 1.1	Hydrogen bond to Val FG5 same β chain in deoxy form	318
	Tyr → Cys	Hb Rainier	↑O_2 Affinity, alkali resistant, "n" = 1.5		318
	Tyr → Asp	Hb Ft. Gordon	↑O_2 Affinity, "n" = 1.0		319
		Osler			320
		Nancy			321
	Tyr → Term	Hb McKees Rocks	↑↑O_2 Affinity, "n" = 1.0		322
146(HC3)	His → Asp	Hb Hiroshima	↑O_2 Affinity, "n" = 2.4	α_1-β_2	323
	His → Pro	Hb York	↑O_2 Affinity, "n" = 1.8		324
	His → Arg	Hb Cochin-Port Royal	Normal oxygen Affinity, "n" = 3.0		325

Table 3
VARIANTS OF THE δ CHAIN

Residue	Substitution	Name	Ref.
2(NA2)	His → Arg	Hb A_2 Sphakia	327
12(A9)	Asn → Lys	Hb A_2 NYU	328
16(A13)	Gly → Arg	Hb A_2' (B_2)	329
20(B2)	Val → Glu	Hb A_2 Roosevelt	330
22(B4)	Ala → Glu	Hb A_2 Flatbush	331
43(CD2)	Glu → Lys	Hb A_2 Melbourne	332
51(D2)	Pro → Arg	Hb A_2 Adria	392
69(E13)	Gly → Arg	Hb A_2 Indonesia	333
116(G18)	Arg → His	Hb A_2 Coburg	334
136(H14)	Gly → Asp	Hb A_2 Babinga	335

Table 4
GAMMA CHAINS

Residue	Substitution	Name	Ref.
1(NA1)	Gly → Cys (136Gly)	Hb F Malaysia	336
5(A2)	Glu → Lys (136Ala)	Hb F Texas-I	337,338
6(A3)	Glu → Lys	Hb F Texas-II	339
7(A4)	Asp → Asn (136Gly)	Hb F Auckland	340
12(A9)	Thr → Lys	Hb Alexandra	341
16(A13)	Gly → Arg (136Gly)	Hb F Melbourne	342
22(B4)	Asp → Gly (136Ala)	Hb F Kuala Lumpur	343
61(E5)	Lys → Glu (136Ala)	Hb F Jamaica	344
80(EF4)	Asp → Tyr (136Ala)	Hb F Victoria Jubilee	345
97(FG4)	His → Arg (136Ala)	Hb F Dickinson	346
117(G19)	His → Arg (136Gly)	Hb F Malta-I	347
121(GH4)	Glu → Lys (136Ala)	Hb F Hull	348
121(GH4)	Glu → Lys (136Gly)	Hb F Carlton	342
125(H3)	Glu → Ala (136Gly)	Hb F Port Royal	349
130(H8)	Trp → Gly (136Gly)	Hb F Poole	350

Table 5
FUSION HEMOGLOBINS

											Ref.
	A6	A9	B4	D1	F2	F3	G18	G19	H2	H4	
	9	12	22	50	86	87	116	117	124	126	
δ Chain →→→→	Thr	Asn	Ala	Ser	Ser	Gln	Arg	Asn	Gln	Met	
β Chain →→→	Ser	Thr	Glu	Thr	Ala	Thr	His	His	Pro	Val	
Lepore-Hollandia			δ	β							351
Lepore-Baltimore				δ	β						352
Lepore-Washington-Boston						δ	β				353
Miyada		β	δ								188
P Congo			β				δ				354
P Nilotic			β	δ							355
	NA1		EF4	EF5	F2	F3				HC3	
	1		80	81	86	87				146	
γ Chain →→→→	Gly		Asp	Leu	Ala	Gln				His	
β Chain →→→→	Val		Asn	Leu	Ala	Thr				His	
Kenya				γ	β						356

Table 6
EXTENDED CHAINS

	Residue	Name	Ref.
α141	140 150 (31 Additional residues) Tyr-Arg-Gln-Ala-Gly- Ala-Ser-Val-Ala-Val- Pro-Pro-Ala- 160 170 Arg-Trp-Ala-Ser-Gln-Arg-Ala-Leu-Leu-Pro-Ser-Leu-His-Arg-Pro-Phe-Leu-Val- Phe-Glu	Hb Constant Spring	357
α141	31 Additional residues — identical to Hb Constant Spring except for residue 142 which is lysine instead of glutamine	Hb Icaria	358
α141	140 150 (16 or 17 Additional residues Tyr-Arg(Ser,Ala,Gly,Ala,Ser,Val,Ala,Val,Pro,Pro,Ala) -Arg(?,Ala,Ser,Gln)-Arg-COOH	Hb koya Dora	359
β146	150 (11 Additional residues)Thr-Lys-Leu-Ala-Phe-Leu-Leu-Ser-Asn-Phe-Try	Hb Tak ↑O_2 affinity	360,361,362
α139—141	140 Thr-Ser-Asn-Thr-Val-Lys-Leu-Glu-Pro-Arg(Frameshift)	Hb Wayne	363
β145	144 150 155 Lys-Ser-Ile-Thr-Lys-Leu-Ala-Phe-Leu-Leu-Ser-Asn-Phe-Tyr-COOH	Hb Cranston, unstable	364
α115—118	115 116 117 118 118 Ala-Glu-Phe-Thr-*Glu-Phe-Thr*-Pro(insertion)	Hb Grady, Dakar	365,366,389

Table 7
DELETED RESIDUES

Residue	Substitution	Name	Major abnormal property	Ref.
β6 or 7	Glu → 0	Hb Leiden	Unstable, slightly ↑O_2 affinity	367
β17—18	(Lys-Val) → O	Hb Lyon	↑O_2 Affinity	368
β23	Val → O	Hb Freiburg	↑O_2 Affinity	369
β42—44 or 43—45	(Phe-Glu-Ser) → O or (Glu-Ser-Phe) → O	Hb Niteroi	↓O_2 Affinity, unstable	370
β56—59	(Gly-Asn-Pro-Lys) → O	Hb Tochigi	Unstable, O_2 affinity not known	371
β74—75	(Gly-Leu) → O	Hb St. Antoine	Unstable, normal O_2 Affinity	372
β87	Thr → O	Hb Tours	↑O_2 Affinity, unstable	372
β91—95	(Leu-His-Cys-Asp-Lys) → O	Hb Gun Hill	Unstable, ↑O_2 Affinity	373
β131	Gln → O	Hb Leslie, Deaconess	Unstable, normal O_2 affinity	374,383,375
β141	Leu → O	Hb Coventry		376

Table 8
MORE THAN ONE POINT MUTATION IN THE SAME POLYPEPTIDE CHAIN

Residue	Substitution	Name	Major abnormal property	Ref.
β6(A3)	Glu → Val, 73Asp → Asn	Hb C Harlem, C Georgetown	Normal O_2 Affinity	377,378
	Glu → Lys 95Lys → Glu	Hb Arlington Park	Not done	379
α78—79	Asn → Asp Ala → Gly	Hb J Singapore	Not done	380
β6(A3)	Glu → Val 58Pro → Arg	Hb C Ziguinchor	—	381
β6(A3)	Glu → Val 142Ala → Val	Hb S Travis	—	382

Table 9
ALPHA CHAIN VARIANTS WITH HIGH OXYGEN AFFINITY

Residue	Substitution	Name	Contact
45(CE3)	His → Arg	Hb Fort de France	Heme
84(F5)	Ser → Arg	Hb Etobicoke	Internal
85(F6)	Asp → Asn	Hb G Norfolk	External
92(FG4)	Arg → Gln	Hb J Cape Town	α_1-β_2
	Arg → Leu	Hb Chesapeake	
95(G2)	Pro → Ala	Hb Denmark Hill	α_1-β_2
112(G19)	His → Asp	Hb Hopkins-II	External
126(H9)	Asp → Asn	Hb Tarrant	α_1-β_1
141(HC3)	Arg → His	Hb Suresnes	External, deoxy, salt bonds to H9, H10, NA1 other α chain, oxy: Mobile, Bohr

Table 10
ALPHA CHAIN VARIANTS WITH LOW OXYGEN AFFINITY

Residue	Substitution	Name	Contact
43(CE1)	Phe → Val	Hb Torino	Heme
58(E7)	His → Tyr	Hb M Boston, M Osaka, Gothenburg, M Kiskunhalas	Heme, "distal"
87(F8)	His → Tyr	Hb M Iwate, M Kankakee, M Oldenburg	Heme, "proximal"
94(G1)	Asp → Asn	Hb Titusville	α_1-β_2

Table 11
ALPHA CHAINS (UNSTABLE)

Residue	Substitution	Name	Contact
43(CE1)	Phe → Val	Hb Torino	Heme
47(CE5)	Asp → Gly	Hb Hasharon, Sinai, Sealy, L Ferrara	External
	Asp → Asn	Hb Arya	
53(E2)	Ala → Asp	Hb J Rovigo	External
80(F1)	Leu → Arg	Hb Ann Arbor	Surface
94(G1)	Asp → Tyr	Hb Setif	α_1-β_2
112(G19)	His → Asp	Hb Hopkins-II	External
137(H19)	Leu → Pro	Hb Bibba	Heme

Table 12
BETA CHAIN VARIANTS WITH LOW OXYGEN AFFINITY

Residue	Substitution	Name	Contact
24(B6)	Gly → Asp	Hb Moscva	Internal
42(CD1)	Phe → Ser	Hb Hammersmith, Chiba	Heme
	Phe → Leu	Hb Louisville, Bucuresti,	
48(CD7)	Leu → Arg	Hb Okaloosa	Surface
67(E11)	Val → Glu	Hb M Milwaukee-I	Heme
70(E14)	Ala → Asp	Hb Seattle	Heme
73 (E17)	Asp → Tyr	Hb Vancouver	External
	Asp → Val	Hb Mobile	
82(EF6)	Lys → Asn → Asp	Hb Providence	DPG binding
90(F6)	Glu → Lys	Hb Agenogi	External
91(F7)	Leu → Arg	Hb Carribean	Heme
102(G4)	Asn → Thr	Hb Kansas	Heme, α_1-β_2
	Asn → Ser	Hb Beth Israel	
107(G9)	Gly → Arg	Hb Burke	Internal
108(G10)	Asn → Asp	Hb Yoshizuka	α_1-β_1
111(G13)	Val → Phe	Hb Peterborough	Internal

Table 13
BETA CHAIN VARIANTS WITH HIGH OXYGEN AFFINITY

Residue	Substitution	Name	Contact
15(A12)	Trp → Arg	Hb Belfast	Internal
20(B2)	Val → Met	Hb Olympia	External
28(B10)	Leu → Gln	Hb St. Louis	Internal
	Leu → Pro	Hb Genova	
35(C1)	Tyr → Phe	Hb Philly	α_1-β_1
37(C3)	Trp → Ser	Hb Hirose	α_1-β_2
40(C6)	Arg → Lys	Hb Athens-Ga., Waco	α_1-β_2
	Arg → Ser	Hb Austin	
57(D2)	Pro → Arg	Hb Willamette	α_1-β_1
62(E6)	Ala → Pro	Hb Duarte	External
63(E7)	His → Arg	Hb Zürich	Heme "distal"
	His → Tyr	Hb M Saskatoon, M Emory, M Kurume, M Hida, M Radom, M Arhus, M Chicago, Leipzig, Hörlein-Weber Novi Sad, M Erlangen	
78(E18)	Gly → Asp	Hb Shepherds Bush	Internal
79(EF3)	Asp → Gly	Hb G Hsi-Tsou	External
81(EF5)	Leu → Arg	Hb Baylor	Internal
82(EF6)	Lys → Thr	Hb Rahere	DPG binding
	Lys → Met	Hb Helsinki	
85(F1)	Phe → Ser	Hb Bryn Mawr, Buenos Aires	Internal
89(F5)	Ser → Asn	Hb Creteil	Internal
92(F8)	His → Gln	Hb St. Etienne, Istanbul	Heme, "proximal"

Table 13 (continued)
BETA CHAIN VARIANTS WITH HIGH OXYGEN AFFINITY

Residue	Substitution	Name	Contact
97(FG4)	His → Gln	Hb Malmö	α_1-β_2
	His → Leu	Hb Wood	
98(FG5)	Val → Met	Hb Köln, San Francisco (Pacific)	Heme, α_1-β_2
	Val → Gly	Hb Nottingham	
	Val → Ala	Hb Djelfa	
99(G1)	Asp → Asn	Hb Kempsey	α_1-β_2
	Asp → His	Hb Yakima	
	Asp → Tyr	Hb Ypsilanti	
	Asp → Ala	Hb Radcliffe	
100(G2)	Pro → Leu	Hb Brigham	α_1-β_2
101(G3)	Glu → Lys	Hb British Columbia, Hb Alberta, Hb Potomac	α_1-β_2
103(G5)	Phe → Leu	Hb Heathrow	Heme
106(G8)	Leu → Pro	Hb Southampton, Hb Casper	Heme
	Leu → Gln	Hb Tübingen	
109(G11)	Val → Met	Hb San Diego	Internal
121(GH4)	Glu → Gln	Hb D Los Angeles, Hb D, D Chicago, D Punjab, D North Carolina, D Portugal, Oak Ridge	External
135(H13)	Ala → Pro	Hb Altdorf	Central
143(H21)	His → Arg	Hb Abruzzo	DPG binding
	His → Gln	Hb Little Rock	
	His → Pro	Hb Syracuse	
144(HC1)	Lys → Asn	Hb Andrew-Minneapolis	External
145(HC2)	Tyr → His	Hb Bethesda	Hydrogen bond to Val FG5 same β chain in deoxy form
	Tyr → Cys	Hb Rainier	
	Tyr → Asp	Hb Ft. Gordon, Osler, Nancy	
	Tyr → Term	Hb McKees Rocks	
146(HC3)	His → Asp	Hb Hiroshima	α_1-β_2
	His → Pro	Hb York	

Table 14
BETA CHAINS (UNSTABLE)

Residue	Substitution	Name	Contact
14(A 11)	Leu → Pro	Hb Saki	Surface
15(A12)	Trp → Arg	Hb Belfast	Internal
20(B2)	Val → Asp	Hb Strasbourg	External
24(B6)	Gly → Arg	Hb Riverdale-Bronx	Internal
	Gly → Val	Hb Savannah	
	Gly → Asp	Hb Moscva	
26(B8)	Glu → Val	Hb Henri Mondor	External
27(B9)	Ala → Asp	Hb Volga, Drenthe	Internal
28(B10)	Leu → Gln	Hb St. Louis	Internal
	Leu → Pro	Hb Genova	
30(B12)	Arg → Ser	Hb Tacoma	α_1-β_1

Table 14 (Continued)
BETA CHAINS (UNSTABLE)

Residue	Substitution	Name	Contact
32(B14)	Leu → Pro	Hb Perth, Abraham Lincoln	Internal
	Leu → Arg	Hb Castilla	
35(C1)	Tyr → Phe	Hb Philly	α_1-β_1
42(CD1)	Phe → Ser	Hb Hammersmith, Chiba	Heme
	Phe → Leu	Hb Louisville, Bucuresti	
48(CD7)	Leu → Arg	Hb Okaloosa	Surface
62(E6)	Ala → Pro	Hb Duarte	External
63(E7)	His → Arg	Hb Zürich	Heme "distal"
	His → Pro	Hb Bicêtre	
64(E8)	Gly → Asp	Hb J Calabria, J Bari, J Cosenza	Internal

Table 15
BETA CHAIN VARIANTS (UNSTABLE)

Residue	Substitution	Name	Contacts
66(E10)	Lys → Glu	Hb I Toulouse	External, ? heme
67(E11)	Val → Asn	Hb Bristol	Heme
	Val → Ala	Hb Sydney	
68(E12)	Leu → Pro	Hb Mizuho	Internal
71(E15)	Phe → Ser	Hb Christchurch	Heme
74(E18)	Gly → Asp	Hb Shepherds Bush	External
75(E19)	Leu → Pro	Hb Atlanta	Internal
85(F1)	Phe → Ser	Hb Bryn Mawr, Buenos Aires	Internal
88(F4)	Leu → Arg	Hb Böras	Heme
	Leu → Pro	Hb Santa Ana	
91(F7)	Leu → Pro	Hb Sabine	Heme
	Leu → Arg	Hb Caribbean	
92(F8)	His → Gln	Hb St. Etienne Istanbul Ube I	Heme, "proximal"
98(FG5)	Val → Met	Hb Köln, San Francisco (Pacific)	Heme, α_1-β_2
	Val → Gly	Hb Nottingham	
	Val → Ala	Hb Djelfa	
101(G3)	Glu → Lys	Hb Rush	α_1-β_2
104(G6)	Arg → Ser	Hb Camperdown	Central cavity
106(G8)	Leu → Gln	Hb Tübingen	Heme
111(G3)	Val → Phe	Hb Peterborough	Internal
115(G17)	Ala → Pro	Hb Madrid	α_1-β_1
119(GH2)	Gly → Asp	Hb Fannin-Lubbock	α_1-β_1

Table 16
BETA CHAINS (UNSTABLE)

Residue	Substitution	Name	Contact
124(H2)	Pro → Arg	Hb Khartoum	α_1-β_1
128(H6)	Ala → Asp	Hb Guantanamo	α_1-β_1
130(H8)	Tyr → Asp	Hb Wien	Internal
134(H12)	Val → Glu	Hb North Shore	Internal
135(H13)	Ala → Pro	Hb Altdorf	Central
136(H14)	Gly → Asp	Hb Hope	Central

ADDENDUM[a]

Residue	Substitution	Name	Major abnormal property	Contacts	Ref.
		Variants of the Alpha Chain			
56 (E5)	Lys → Thr	Hb Thailand	—	External	1
91 (FG3)	Leu → Pro	Hb Port Phillip	Unstable	α_1-β_2	2
116 (GH4)	Glu → Ala	Hb Ube-4	—	External	3
141 (HC3)	Arg → Ser	Hb J Cubujuqui	—	External, deoxy, salt bonds to H9, H10, NA1 other α chain, oxy: mobile, Bohr	4
	Arg → Leu	Hb Legnano	↑O_2 Affinity		5
	Arg → Gly	Hb J Camagüey	—		6
		Variants of the Beta Chain			
37 (C3)	Trp → Arg	Hb Rothchild	—	α_1-β_1	7
47 (CD6)	Asp → Gly	Hb Gavello	—	External	8
59 (E3)	Lys → Asn	Hb J Lome	—	External	9
104 (G6)	Arg → Thr	Hb Sherwood Forest	—	Central cavity	10

[a] The addendum goes through March 1, 1978.

REFERENCES

1. Pootrakul, S., Boonyarat, D., Kematorn, B., Suanpan, S., and Wasi, P., Hemoglobin Thailand [α56 (E5) Lys → Thr]: a new abnormal human hemoglobin, *Hemoglobin*, 1, 781, 1977.
2. Brennan, S. P., Tauro, G. P., Melrose, W., and Carrell , R. W., Haemoglobin Port Phillip α91 (FG3) Leu → Pro. A new unstable haemoglobin, *FEBS Lett.*, 81, 115, 1977.
3. Ohba, Y., Miyaji, T., Matsouka, M., Morito, M., and Iuchi, I., Characterization of Hb Ube-4: alpha 116 (GH4) Glu → Ala, *Hemoglobin*, 2, 181, 1978.
4. Saenz, G. F., Elizondo, J., Alvarado, M. A., Atmetlla, F., Arroyo, G., Martinez, G., Lima, F., and Colombo, B., Chemical characterization of a new haemoglobin variant. Haemoglobin J Cubujuqui [α_2 141 (HC3) Arg → Ser β_2], *Biochim. Biophys. Acta*, 494, 48, 1977.
5. Mavilio, F., Marinucci, M., Tentori, L., Fontanarosa, P. P., Rossi, U., and Biagiotti, S., Hemoglobin Legnano [α_2 141 (HC3) Arg → Leu β_2]: a new abnormal human hemoglobin with high oxygen affinity, *Hemoglobin*, 2, 249, 1978.
6. Martinez, G., Lima, F., Residenti, C., and Colombo, B., Hb J Camagüey α_2 141 (HC3) Arg → Gly β_2, *Hemoglobin*, 2, 47, 1978.
7. Gacon, G., Belkhodja, O., Wajcman, H., and Labie, D., Structural and functional studies of Hb Rothchild β37 (C3) Trp → Arg. A new variant of the $\alpha_1\beta_2$ contact, *FEBS Lett.*, 82, 243, 1977.
8. Marinucci, M., Mavilio, F., Tentori, L., and Alberti, R., Hemoglobin Gavello $\alpha_2\beta_2$ 47 (CD6) Asp → Gly. A new hemoglobin variant from Polesine (Italy), *Hemoglobin*, 1, 771, 1977.
9. Wajcman, H., Amegnizin, K. P. E., Belkhodja, O., and Labie, D., Hemoglobin J Lome [β59 (E3) Lys → Asn]. A new fast moving variant found in a Togolese, *FEBS Lett.*, 84, 372, 1977.
10. Ryrie, D. R., Plowman, D., and Lehmann, H., Haemoglobin Sherwood Forest β104 (G6) Arg → Thr, *FEBS Lett.*, 83, 260, 1977.

REFERENCES

1. **Crookston, J. H., Beale, D., Irvine, D., and Lehmann, H.,** A new haemoglobin, J Toronto (α5 alanine → aspartic acid), *Nature (London),* 208, 1059, 1965.
2. **Sumida, I., Ohta, Y., Imamura, T., and Yanase, T.,** Hemoglobin Sawara: α6 (A4) aspartic acid → alanine, *Biochim. Biophys. Acta,* 322, 23, 1973.
3. **Pootrakul, S., Kematorn, B., Na-Nakorn, S., and Suanpan, S.,** A new haemoglobin variant: Haemoglobin Anantharaj alpha 11 (A9) lysine → glutamic acid, *Biochim. Biophys. Acta,* 405, 161, 1975.
4. Rosa, J., Maleknia, N., Vergoz, D., and Dunet, R., Une nouvelle hémoglobine anormale: l'hémoglobin Jα Paris 12 Ala → Asp, *Nouv. Rev. Fr. Hematol.,* 6, 423, 1965.
5. **Trincao, C., Martins De Melo, J., Lorkin, P. A., and Lehmann, H.,** Haemoglobin J Paris in the south of Portugal (Algarve), *Acta Haematol.,* 39, 291, 1968.
6. **Marti, H. R., Pik, C., and Mosimann, P.,** Eine Neue Hämoglobin I-variante: Hb I Interlaken, *Acta Haematol.,* 32, 9, 1964.
7. **Liddell, J., Brown, D., Beale, D., Lehmann, H., and Huntsman, R. G.,** A new haemoglobin — Jα Oxford found during a survey of an English population, *Nature (London),* 204, 269, 1964.
8. **Silvestroni, E., Bianco, I., Tentori, L., Vivaldi, G., Carta, S., Sorcini, M., and Brancati, C.,** *Proc. 10th Congr. Eur. Soc. Haematol. Strasbourg 1965, Part II,* Karger, Basel, New York, 1967, 232.
9. **Vella, F., Casey, R., Lehmann, H., Labossiere, A., and Jones, T. G.,** Haemoglobin Ottawa: α2 15(A13) Gly → Arg β2, *Biochim. Biophys. Acta,* 336, 25, 1974.
10. **Pootrakul, S., Srichiyanont, S., Wasi, P., and Suanpan, S.,** Hemoglobin Siam (α2 15 Arg β2): a new α chain variant, *Humangenetik,* 23, 199, 1974.
11. **Beale, D. and Lehmann, H.,** Abnormal haemoglobins and the genetic code, *Nature (London),* 207, 259, 1965.
12. **Schneider, R. G., Alperin, J. B., Beale, D., and Lehmann, H.,** Hemoglobin I in an American black family: structural and hematologic studies, *J. Lab. Clin. Med.,* 68, 940, 1966.
13. **Bowman, B. H. and Barnett, D. R.,** Amino acid substitution in Haemoglobin I (Texas variant), *Nature (London),* 214, 499, 1967.
14. **O'Brien, C., Gray, M. J., and Jacobs, A. S.,** A survey of cord bloods for abnormal hemoglobin with further observations on Hemoglobin I, *Am. J. Obstet. Gynecol.,* 88, 816, 1964.
15. **Baur, E. W.,** Hb $\alpha_2{}^{glu}\beta_2$ (Hb I) in a Caucasian family: independent mutation or common origin? *Humangenetik,* 6, 368, 1968.
16. **Griffiths, K. D., Lang, A., Lehmann, H., Mann, J. R., Plowman, D., and Raine, D. N.,** Haemoglobin Handsworth α18 (A16) glycine → arginine, *FEBS Lett.,* 75, 93, 1977.
17. **Rahbar, S., Ala, F., Akhavan, E., Nowzari, G., Shoa'i, I., and Zamanianpoor, M. H.,** Two new haemoglobins: Haemoglobin Perspolis [α64 (E13) Asp → Tyr] and Haemoglobin J-Kurosh [α19 (AB) Ala → Asp], *Biochim. Biophys. Acta,* 427, 119, 1976.
18. **Kendall, A. G., Barr, R. D., Lang, A., and Lehmann, H.,** Haemoglobin J Nyanza: α21 (B2) Ala → Asp, *Biochim. Biophys. Acta,* 310, 357, 1973.
19. **Gottlieb, A. J., Restrepo, A., and Itano, H. A.,** Hemoglobin J Medellin. Chemical and genetic study, *Fed. Proc.,* 23, 172, 1964.
20. **Kraus, A. P., Miyaji, T., Iuchi, I., and Kraus, L. M.,** Memphis. A new variety of sickle cell anemia with clinically mild symptoms due to an α-chain variant of hemoglobin (α23 Glu NH2), *J. Lab. Clin. Med.,* 66, 886, 1965.
21. **Boyer, S. H., Crosby, E. F., Fuller, G. F., Ulenurm, L., and Buck, A. A.,** A survey of hemoglobins in the Republic of Chad and characterization of Hemoglobin Chad: α2 23 Glu → Lys β2, *Am. J. Hum. Genet.,* 20, 570, 1968.
22. **Marengo-Rowe, A. J., Beale, D., and Lehmann, H.,** New human haemoglobin variant from southern Arabia: G-Audhali [α23 (B4) glutamic acid → valine] and the variability of B4 in human haemoglobin, *Nature (London),* 219, 1164, 1968.
23. **Schneider, R. G., Brimhall, B., Jones, R. T., Bryant, R., Mitchell, C. B., and Goldberg, A. I.,** Hb Fort Worth: α27 Glu → Gly (B8) a variant present in unusually low concentration, *Biochim. Biophys. Acta,* 243, 164, 1971.
24. **Ahern, E., Ahern, V., Holder, W., Palomino, E., Serjeant, G. R., Serjeant, B. E., Forbes, M., Brimhall, B., and Jones, R. T.,** Haemoglobin Spanish Town α27 Glu → Val (B8), *Biochim. Biophys. Acta,* 427, 530, 1976.
25. **Vettore, L., DeSandre, G., Dilorio, E. E., Winterhalter, K. H., Lang, A., and Lehmann, H.,** A new abnormal Hemoglobin O Padova, α30 (B11) Glu → Lys and a dyserythropoietic anemia with erythroblastic multinuclearity coexisting in the same patient, *Blood,* 44, 869, 1974.
26. **Schneider, R. G. and Jim, R. T. S.,** A new haemoglobin variant (the "Honolulu Type") in a Chinese, *Nature (London),* 190, 454, 1961.

27. **Vella, F., Ager, J. A. M., and Lehmann, H.**, An abnormal haemoglobin in a Chinese: Haemoglobin G, *Nature (London)*, 182, 460, 1958.
28. **Swenson, R. T., Hill, R. L., Lehmann, H., and Jim, R. T. S.**, A chemical abnormality in Hemoglobin G from Chinese individuals, *J. Biol. Chem.*, 237, 1517, 1962.
29. **Beretta, A., Prato, V., Gallo, E., and Lehmann, H.**, Haemoglobin Torino — α43 (CDI) phenylalanine → valine, *Nature (London)*, 217, 1016, 1968.
30. **Ohba, Y., Miyaji, T., Matsuoka, M., Yokoyama, M., Numakura, H., Nagata, K., Takebe, Y., Izumi, Y., and Shibata, S.**, Hemoglobin Hirosaki [α43 (CE 1) Phe → Leu], a new unstable variant, *Biochim. Biophys. Acta*, 405, 155, 1975.
31. **Sumida, I.**, Studies of abnormal hemoglobins in western Japan. Frequency of visible hemoglobin variants, and chemical characterization of Hemoglobin Sawara ($\alpha_2{}^{6Ala}\beta_2$) and Hemoglobin Mugino (Hb L Ferrara; $\alpha_2{}^{47Gly}\beta_2$, *Jpn. J. Hum. Genet.*, 19, 343, 1975.
32. **Fujimura, T., Kawasaki, K., Imamura, T., Ohta, Y., Hanada, M., and Yamaoka, K.**, Two kindreds of abnormal hemoglobin; Hb Tagawa I and Hb Tagawa II, *Jpn. J. Clin Hematol.*, 6, 71, 1964.
33. **DeVries, A., Joshua, H., Lehmann, H., Hill, R. L., and Fellows, R. E.**, The first observation of an abnormal haemoglobin in a Jewish family: Haemoglobin Beilinson, *Br. J. Haematol.*, 9, 484, 1963.
34. **Halbrecht, I., Isaacs, W. A., Lehmann, H., and Ben-Porat, F.**, Hemoglobin Hasharon (α47 aspartic acid → histidine), *Isr. J. Med. Sci.*, 3, 827, 1967.
35. **Ostertag, W. and Smith, E. W.**, Hb Sinai; a new α chain mutant α47 His, *Humangenetik*, 6, 377, 1968.
36. **Schneider, R. G., Ueda, S., Alperin, J. B., Brimhall, B., and Jones, R. T.**, Hemoglobin Sealy ($\alpha_2{}^{47His}\beta_2$): a new variant in a Jewish family, *Am. J. Hum. Genet.*, 20, 151, 1968.
37. **Bianco, J., Modiano, G., Bottini, E., and Lucci, R.**, Alteration in the α-chain of Haemoglobin L Ferrara, *Nature (London)*, 198, 395, 1963.
38. **Tentori, L.**, Hemoglobin L Ferrara = Hemoglobin Hasharon, *Hemoglobin*, 1(6), 602, 1977.
39. **Rahbar, S., Mahdavi, N., Nowzari, G., and Mostafavi, I.**, Hemoglobin Arya: α_2 47 (CD5) aspartic acid → asparagine, *Biochim. Biophys. Acta*, 386, 525, 1975.
40. **Brimhall, B., Jones, R. T., Schneider, R. G., Hosty, T. S., Tomlin, G., and Atkins, R.**, Two new hemoglobins: Hemoglobin Alabama [β39 (C5) Gln → Lys] and Hemoglobin Montgomery [α48 (CD6) Leu → Arg], *Biochim. Biophys. Acta*, 379, 28, 1975.
41. **Tangheroni, W., Zorcolo, G., Gallo, E., and Lehmann, H.**, Haemoglobin J Sardegna: α50 (CD8) histidine → aspartic acid, *Nature (London)*, 218, 470, 1968.
42. **Cabannes, R., Renaud, R., Mauran, A., Pennors, H., Charlesworth, D., Price, B. G., and Lehmann, H.**, Deux hémoglobines rapides an Côte-D' Ivoire: l'Hb K Woolwich et une nouvelle hémoglobine, l'Hb J Abidjan (α51 Gly → Asp), *Nouv. Rev. Fr. Hematol.*, 12, 289, 1972.
43. **Reynolds, C. A. and Huisman, T. H. J.**, Hemoglobin Russ or α2 51 Arg β2, *Biochim. Biophys. Acta*, 130, 541, 1966.
44. **Alberti, R., Mariuzzi, G. M., Artibani, L., Bruni, E., and Tentori, L.**, A new haemoglobin variant: J-Rovigo alpha 53 (E-2) alanine → aspartic acid, *Biochim. Biophys. Acta*, 342, 1, 1974.
45. **Miyaji, T., Iuchi, I., Takeda, I., and Shibata, S.**, Hemoglobin Shimonoseki (α2 54Arg β2A), a slow-moving hemoglobin found in a Japanese family, with special reference to its chemistry, *Acta Haematol.*, 26, 531, 1963.
46. **Jones, R. T., Brimhall, B., and Lisker, R.**, Chemical characterization of Hemoglobin Mexico and Hemoglobin Chiapas, *Biochim. Biophys. Acta*, 154, 488, 1968.
47. **Rosa, J., Labie, D., Maleknia, N., and Blum, N.**, Sur quelques Hémoglobines Anormales Nouvelles Recemment Isolées en France, *Int. Symp. Comp. Hemoglobin Struct.*, Thessalaniki, April 11—13, 1966, 140.
48. **Fessas, Ph., Kaltsoya A., Loukopoulos, D., and Nilsson, L.-O.**, On the chemical structure of Haemoglobin Uppsala, *Hum. Hered.*, 19, 152, 1969.
49. **Rahbar, S., Kinderlerer, J. L., and Lehmann, H.**, Haemoglobin L Persian Gulf: α 57 (E6) glycine → arginine, *Acta Haematol.*, 42, 169, 1969.
50. **Baglioni, C.**, A chemical study of Hemoglobin Norfolk, *J. Biol. Chem.*, 237, 69, 1962.
51. **Imamura, T.**, Hemoglobin Kagoshima: an example of Hemoglobin Norfolk in a Japanese family, *Am. J. Hum. Genet.*, 18, 584, 1966.
52. **Gerald, P. S. and Efron, M. L.**, Chemical studies of several varieties of Hb M, *Proc. Natl. Acad. Sci. U.S.A.*, 47, 1758, 1961.
53. **Shimizu, A., Hayashi, A., and Yamamura, Y.**, The structural study on a new hemoglobin variant, Hb M Osaka, *Biochim. Biophys. Acta*, 97, 472, 1965.
54. **Hansen, H. A., Jagenburg, O. R., and Johansson, B. G.**, Studies on an abnormal hemoglobin causing hereditary congenital cyanosis, *Acta Paediatr.*, 49, 503, 1960.
55. **Hollán, S. R., Szelényi, J. G., Lehmann, H., and Beale, D.**, A Boston-type haemoglobin M in Hungary: Haemoglobin M Kiskunhalas, *Haematologia*, 1, 11, 1967.

56. **Barclay, G. P. T., Charlesworth, D., and Lehmann, H.**, Abnormal haemoglobins in Zambia. A new Haemoglobin Zambia α60 (E9) lysine → asparagine, *Br. Med. J.*, 4, 595, 1969.
57. **Brimhall, B., Duerst, M., Hollán, S. R., Stenzel, P., Szelényi, J., and Jones, R. T.**, Structural characterizations of Hemoglobins J Buda [α61 (E10) Lys → Asn] and G Pest [α74 (EF3) Asp → Asn], *Biochim. Biophys. Acta*, 336, 344, 1974.
58. **Blackwell, R. Q., Jim, R. T. S., Tan, T. G. H., Weng, M. I., Liu, C. S., and Wang, C. L.**, Hemoglobin G Waimanalo: α64 Asp → Asn, *Biochim. Biophys. Acta*, 322, 27, 1973.
59. **Ramot, B., Kinderlerer, J. B., and Lehmann, H.**, *as cited in WHO Tech. Rep. Ser. No. 509, Annex I, Geneva*, 1972.
60. **Sukumaran, P. K., Merchant, S. M., Desai, M. P., Wiltshire, B. G., and Lehmann, H.**, Haemoglobin Q [α64 (E13) aspartic acid → histidine] associated with β-thalassemia in three Sindhi families, *J. Med. Genet.*, 9, 436, 1972.
61. **Miyaji, T., Iuchi I., Yamamoto, K., Ohba Y., and Shibata, S.**, Amino acid substitution of Hemoglobin Ube 2 (α2 68 Asp β2): an example of successful application of partial hydrolysis of peptide with 5% acetic acid, *Clin. Chim. Acta*, 16, 347, 1967.
62. **Baglioni, C. and Ingram, V. M.**, Abnormal human haemoglobins. V. Chemical investigation of Haemoglobins A, G, C, X from one individual, *Biochim. Biophys. Acta*, 48, 253, 1961.
63. **Chernoff, A. I. and Pettit, N., Jr.**, The amino acid composition of hemoglobin. VI. Separation of the tryptic peptides of Hemoglobin Knoxville No. 1 on Dowex-1 X-2® and Sephadex®, *Biochim. Biophys. Acta*, 97, 47, 1965.
64. **Bowman, B., Barnett, D. R., Hodgkinson, K. T., and Schneider, R. G.**, Chemical characterization of Haemoglobin G St-1, *Nature (London)*, 211, 1305, 1966.
65. **Minnich, V., Cordonnier, J. K., Williams, W. J., and Moore, C. V.**, Alpha, beta and gamma hemoglobin polypeptide chains during the neonatal period with description of a fetal form of Hemoglobin D St. Louis, *Blood*, 19, 137, 1962.
66. **Dance, N., Huehns, E. R., and Shooter, E. M.**, The chemical investigation of Haemoglobins G Bristol and G Bristol C, *Biochim. Biophys. Acta*, 86, 144, 1964.
67. **Colombo, B., Vidal, G., Kamuzora, H., and Lehmann, H.**, A new haemoglobin J-Habana α71 (E20) alanine → glutamic acid, *Biochim. Biophys. Acta*, 351, 1, 1974.
68. **Rahbar, S., Nowzari, G., and Danêshmand, P.**, Hemoglobin-Tehran α2 72 (EF1) histidine → arginine β2A, *Nature New Biol.*, 245, 268, 1973.
69. **Pootrakul, S. and Dixon, G. H.**, Hemoglobin Mahidol: a new hemoglobin α-chain mutant, *Can. J. Biochem.*, 48, 1066, 1970.
70. **Blackwell, R. Q. and Liu, C.-S.**, Hemoglobin G Taichung: α74 Asp → His, *Biochim. Biophys. Acta*, 200, 70, 1970.
71. **Lorkin, P. A., Charlesworth, D., Lehmann, H., Rahbar, S., Tuchinda, S., and Lie-Injo, L. E.**, Two Haemoglobins Q, α74 (EF3) and α75 (EF4) aspartic acid → histidine, *Br. J. Haematol.*, 19, 117, 1970.
72. **Orringer, E. P., Wilson, J. B., and Huisman, T. H. J.**, Hemoglobin Chapel Hill or α_2 74Asp → Gly β_2, *FEBS Lett.*, 65, 297, 1976.
73. **Vella, F., Wiltshire, B. G., Lehmann, H., and Galbraith, P.**, Hemoglobin Winnipeg α2 75 Asp → Tyr β2, *Clin. Biochem.*, 6, 66, 1973.
74. **Ohba, Y., Miyaji, T., Matsuoka, M., Takeda, I., Fukuba, Y., Shibata, S., and Ohkura, K.**, Hemoglobin Matsue-Oki: alpha 75 (EF4) aspartic acid → asparagine, *Hemoglobin*, 1, 383, 1977.
75. **Van Ros, G., Beale, D., and Lehmann, H.**, Haemoglobin Stanleyville-II (α78 asparagine → lysine), *Br. Med. J.*, 4, 92, 1968.
76. **Rucknagel, D. L., Brandt, N. J., and Spencer, H. H.**, α-chain mutants of human hemoglobin contributing to the genetics of the α-chain locus, *Proc. First Inter-Am. Symp. Hemoglobins, Caracas*, 1969.
77. **Adams, J. G., III, Winter, W. P., Rucknagel, D. L., and Spencer, H. H.**, Biosynthesis of hemoglobin Ann Arbor: evidence for catabolic and feedback regulation, *Science*, 176, 1427, 1972.
78. **Winter, W. P., Rucknagel, D. L., and Fielding, J.**, Identification of several rare hemoglobin variants discovered in a population survey including a new variant Hb Garden State α82 Ala → Asp, *Clin. Res.*, 26, 22A, 1978.
79. **Crookston, J. H., Farquharson, H. A., Beale, D., and Lehmann, H.**, Hemoglobin Etobicoke. α84 (F5) serine replaced by arginine, *Can. J. Biochem.*, 47, 143, 1969.
80. **Lorkin, P. A., Huntsman, R. G., Ager, J. A. M., Lehman, H., Vella, F., and Darbre, P. D.**, Haemoglobin G Norfolk: α85 (F6) Asp → Asn, *Biochim. Biophys. Acta*, 379, 22, 1975.
81. **Cohen-Solal, M., Manesse, B., Thillet, J., and Rosa, J.**, Haemoglobin G Norfolk α85 (F6) Asp → Asn. Structural characterization by sequenator analysis and functional properties of a new variant with high oxygen affinity, *FEBS Lett.*, 50, 163, 1975.
82. **Fujiwara, N., Maekawa, T., and Matsuda, G.**, Hemoglobin Atago (α2 85 Tyr β2) a new abnormal human hemoglobin found in Nagasaki, *Int. J. Protein Res.*, 3, 35, 1971.

83. **Reed, R. E., Winter, W. P., and Rucknagel, D. L.**, Hemoglobin Inkster (α2 85 aspartic acid → valine β2) coexisting with β-thalassemia in a Caucasian family, *Br. J. Haematol.*, 26, 475, 1974.
84. **Miyaji, T., Iuchi, I., Shibata, S., Takeda, I., and Tamura, A.**, Possible amino acid substitution in the α-chain (α87 Tyr) of Hb M Iwate, *Acta Haematol. Jpn.*, 26, 538, 1963.
85. **Heller, P., Weinstein, H. G., Yakulis, V. J., and Rosenthal, I. M.**, Hemoglobin M Kankakee, a new variant of Hemoglobin M, *Blood*, 20, 287, 1962.
86. **Pik, C. and Tönz, O.**, Nature of Haemoglobin M Oldenburg, *Nature (London)*, 210, 1182, 1966.
87. **De Traverse, P. M., Lehmann, H., Coquelet, M. L., Beale, D., and Isaacs, W. A.**, Etude d'une hémoglobine J α non encore décrite, dans une famille Francais, *C. R. Seances Soc. Biol.*, 160, 2270, 1966.
88. **Vella, F., Charlesworth, D., Lorkin, P. A., and Lehmann, H.**, Hemoglobin Broussais $\alpha^{90\ Lys \rightarrow Asn}$, *Can. J. Biochem.*, 48, 908, 1970.
89. **Braconnier, F., Cohen-Solal, M., Schlegel, N., Blouquit, Y., Thillet, J., Cassius De Linval, J., and Rosa, J.**, Hémoglobine J. Broussais α2 90 Lys → Asn $\beta 2^A$ (FG2), decouverte dans une famille Martiniquaise, *Nouv. Rev. Fr. Hematol.*, 3, 333, 1975.
90. **Hyde, R. D., Kinderlerer, J. L., Lehmann, H., and Hall, M. D.**, Haemoglobin J Rajappen: α90 (FG2) Lys → Thr, *Biochim. Biophys. Acta*, 243, 515, 1971.
91. **Botha, M. C., Beale, D., Isaacs, W. A., and Lehmann, H.**, Haemoglobin J Cape Town α2 92 arginine → glutamine β2, *Nature (London)*, 212, 792, 1966.
92. **Lines, J. G. and McIntosh, R.**, Oxygen binding by Haemoglobin J Cape Town. (α2 92 Arg → Gln), *Nature (London)*, 215, 297, 1967.
93. **Clegg, J. B., Naughton, M. A., and Weatherall, D. J.**, Abnormal human haemoglobins. Separation and characterization of the α and β chains by chromatography, and the determination of two new variants, Hb Chesapeake and Hb J (Bangkok), *J. Mol. Biol.*, 19, 91, 1966.
94. **Charache, S., Weatherall, D. J., and Clegg, J. B.**, Polycythemia associated with a hemoglobinopathy, *J. Clin. Invest.*, 45, 813, 1966.
95. **Wajcman, H., Belkhodja, O., and Labie, D.**, Hb Setif: G1(94) α Asp → Tyr. A new α chain hemoglobin variant with substitution of the residue involved in a hydrogen bond between unlike subunits, *FEBS Lett.*, 27, 298, 1972.
96. **Schneider, R. G., Atkins, R. J., Hosty, T. S., Tomlin, G., Casey, R., Lehmann, H., Lorkin, P. A., and Nagai, K.**, Haemoglobin Titusville: α94 Asp → Asn, a new haemoglobin with a lowered affinity for oxygen, *Biochim. Biophys. Acta*, 400, 365, 1975.
97. **Huisman, T. H. J., Adams, H. R., Wilson, J. B., Efremov, G. D., Reynolds, C. A., and Wrightstone, R. N.**, Hemoglobin G Georgia or α2 95 Leu (G2) β2, *Biochim. Biophys. Acta*, 200, 578, 1970.
98. **Smith, L. L., Plese, C. L., Barton, B. P., Charache, S., Wilson, J. B., and Huisman, T. H. J.**, Subunit dissociation of the abnormal hemoglobins G Georgia [α2 95 Leu (G2) β2] and Rampa [α2 95 Ser (G2) β2], *J. Biol. Chem.*, 247, 1433, 1972.
99. **De Jong, W. W. W., Bernini, L. F., and Khan, P. M.**, Haemoglobin Rampa: 95 Pro → Ser, *Biochim. Biophys. Acta*, 236, 197, 1971.
100. **Wiltshire, B. G., Clark, K. G. A., Lorkin, P. A., and Lehmann, H.**, Haemoglobin Denmark Hill α95 (G2) Pro → Ala, a variant with unusual electrophoretic and oxygen binding properties, *Biochim. Biophys. Acta*, 278, 459, 1972.
101. **Bannister, W. H., Grech, J. L., Plese, C. F., Smith, L. L., Barton, B. P., Wilson, J. B., Reynolds, C. A., and Huisman, T. H. J.**, Hemoglobin St. Luke's or α2 95 Arg (G2) β2, *Eur. J. Biochem.*, 29, 301, 1972.
102. **Crookston, J. H., Farquharson, H., Kinderlerer, J., and Lehmann, H.**, Hemoglobin Manitoba: α102 (G9) serine replaced by arginine, *Can. J. Biochim.*, 48, 911, 1970.
103. **Charache, S. and Ostertag, W.**, Hemoglobin Hopkins-2 [(α112 Asp) 2 β2]: "low output" protects from potentially harmful effects, *Blood*, 36, 852, 1970.
104. **Niazi, G. A., Efremov, G. D., Nikolov, N., Hunter, E., Jr., and Huisman, T. H. J.**, Hemoglobin Strumica or α_2^{112} (G19) His → Arg β_2. (With an addendum: Hemoglobin J Paris-I, α_2^{12} (A10) Ala → Asp β_2 in the same population.) *Biochim. Biophys. Acta*, 412, 181, 1975.
105. **Beksedic, D., Rajevska, T., Lorkin, P. A., and Lehmann, H.**, Hb Serbia, [α^{112} (G19) His → Arg], a new haemoglobin variant from Yugoslavia, *FEBS Lett.*, 58, 226, 1975.
106. **Gajdusek, D. C., Guiart, J., Kirk, R. L., Carrell, R. W., Irvine, D., Kynoch, P. A. M., and Lehmann, H.**, Haemoglobin J Tongariki (α115 alanine → aspartic acid): the first new haemoglobin variant found in a Pacific (Melanesian) population, *J. Med. Genet.*, 4, 1, 1967.
107. **Baglioni, C. and Lehmann, H.**, Chemical heterogeneity of Haemoglobin O, *Nature (London)*, 196, 229, 1962.
108. **Lie-Injo, L. E., and Sadono, M. D.**, Haemoglobin O (Buginese X) in Sulawesi, *Br. Med. J.*, i, 1461, 1958.
109. **Sansone, G., Centa, A., Sciarratta, V., Gallo, E., and Lehmann, H.**, Haemoglobin O Indonesia (α 116 Glu → Lys) in an Italian family, *Acta Haematol.*, 43, 40, 1970.

110. **Ostertag, W., von Ehrenstein, G., and Charache, S.**, Duplicated α-chain genes in Hopkins-2 Haemoglobin of man and evidence for unequal crossing over between them, *Nature New Biol.*, 237, 90, 1972.

111. **Blackwell, R. Q., Wong, H. B., Wang, C. L., Weng, M. L., and Liu, C.-S.**, Hemoglobin J Meerut: α 120 Ala → Glu, *Biochim. Biophys. Acta*, 351, 7, 1974.

111a. **Kamuzora, H., Lehmann, H., Griffiths, K. D., Mann, J. R., and Raine, D. N.**, A new haemoglobin variant Hemoglobin J Birmingham α 120 (H3) Ala → Glu, *Ann. Clin. Biochem.*, 11, 53, 1974.

112. **Moo-Penn, W. F., Jue, D. L., Johnson, M. H., Wilson, S. M., Therrel, B., Jr., and Schmidt, R. M.**, Hemoglobin Tarrant: α126 (H9) Asp → Asn. A new hemoglobin variant in the $\alpha_1\beta_1$ contact region showing high oxygen affinity and reduced cooperativity, *Biochim. Biophys. Acta*, 490, 443, 1977.

113. **Vella, F., Galbraith, P., Wilson, J. B., Wong, S. C., Folger, G. C., and Huisman, T. H. J.**, Hemoglobin St. Claude or α2 127 (H10) Lys → Thr β2, *Biochim. Biophys. Acta*, 365, 318, 1974.

114. **Moo-Penn, W. F., Bechtel, K. C., Johnson, M. H., Jue, D. L., Holland, S., Huff, C., and Schmidt, R. M.**, Hemoglobin Jackson, α127 (H10) Lys → Asn, *Am. J. Clin. Pathol.*, 66, 453, 1976.

115. **Kleihauer, E. F., Reynolds, C. A., Dozy, A. M., Wilson, J. B., Moores, R. R., Berenson, M. P., Wright, C.-S., and Huisman, T. H. J.**, Hemoglobin Bibba or α2 136 Pro β2, an unstable α-chain abnormal hemoglobin, *Biochim. Biophys. Acta*, 154, 220, 1968.

116. **Clegg, J. B., Weatherall, D. J., Wong Hock Boon, and Mustafa, D.**, Two new haemoglobin variants involving proline substitutions, *Nature (London)*, 222, 379, 1969.

117. **Poyart, C., Krishnamoorthy, R., Bursaux, E., Gacon, G., and Labie, D.**, Structural and functional studies of Haemoglobin Suresnes or α_2 141 (HC3) Arg → His β_2, a new high oxygen affinity mutant, *FEBS Lett.*, 69, 103, 1976.

118. **Moo-Penn, W. F., Bechtel, K. C., Schmidt, R. M., Johnson, M. H., Jue, D. L., Schmidt, D. E., Jr., Dunlap, W. M., Opella, S. J., Bonaventura, J., and Bonaventura, C.**, Hemoglobin Raleigh (β1 Valine → Acetylalanine. Structural and Functional Characterization, *Biochemistry*, 16, 4872, 1977.

119. **Labossiere, A., Vella, F., Hiebert, J., and Galbraith, P.**, Hemoglobin Deer Lodge: α2β2 2 His → Arg, *Clin. Biochem.*, 5, 46, 1972.

120. **Ingram, V. M.**, Abnormal human haemoglobins. III. The chemical difference between normal and sickle cell hemoglobins, *Biochim. Biophys. Acta*, 36, 402, 1959.

121. **Hunt, J. A. and Ingram, V. M.**, Abnormal human haemoglobins. IV. The chemical difference between normal human haemoglobin and haemoglobin C, *Biochim. Biophys. Acta*, 42, 409, 1960.

122. **Blackwell, R. Q., Oemijati, S., Pribadi, W., Weng, M.-I., and Liu, C.-S.** Hemoglobin G Makassar: β6 Glu → Ala, *Biochim. Biophys. Acta*, 214, 396, 1970.

123. **Hill, R. I., Swenson, R. T., and Schwartz, H. C.**, Characterization of a chemical abnormality in Hemoglobin G, *J. Biol. Chem.*, 235, 3182, 1960.

124. **Tuchinda, S., Beale, D., and Lehmann, H.**, A new haemoglobin in a Thai family. A case of Haemoglobin Siriraj-β Thalassemia, *Br. Med. J.*, 1, 1583, 1965.

125. **Bonaventura, J. and Riggs, A.**, Polymerization of hemoglobins of mouse and man. Structural basis, *Science*, 158, 800, 1967.

126. **Arcasoy, A., Casey, R., Lehmann, H., Cavdar, A. O., and Berki, A.**, A new haemoglobin J from Turkey — Hb Ankara [β10 (A7) Ala → Asp], *FEBS Lett.*, 42, 121, 1974.

127. **Monn, E., Gaffney, P. J., and Lehmann, H.**, Hemoglobin Sögn (β14 arginine). A new haemoglobin variant, *Scand. J. Haematol.*, 5, 353, 1968.

128. **Beuzard, Y., Basset, P., Braconnier, F., El Gammal, H., Martin, L., Oudard, J. L., and Thillet, J.**, Haemoglobin Saki α2β2 141 Leu → Pro (A ll) structure and function, *Biochim. Biophys. Acta*, 393, 182, 1975.

129. **Milner, P. F., Corley, C. C., Pomeroy, W. L., Wilson, J. B., Gravely, M., and Huisman, T. H. J.**, Thalassemia intermedia caused by heterozygosity for both β-Thalassemia and Hemoglobin Saki [β14 (A ll) Leu→ Pro], *Am. J. Hematol.*, 1, 283, 1976.

130. **Kennedy, C. C., Blundell, G., Lorkin, P. A., Lang, A., and Lehmann, H.**, Haemoglobin Belfast 15(A12) tryptophan → arginine: a new unstable haemoglobin variant, *Br. Med. J.*, 4, 324, 1974.

131. **Gacon, G., Wajcman, H., Labie, D., Varet, B., and Christoforov, B.**, A second case of haemoglobin Belfast [β^{15} (A12) Trp → Arg] observed in a French patient, *Acta Haematol.*, 55, 313, 1976.

132. **Baglioni, C. and Weatherall, D. J.**, Abnormal human hemoglobins. IX. Chemistry of Hemoglobin J Baltimore, *Biochim. Biophys. Acta*, 78, 637, 1963.

133. **Weatherall, D. J.**, Hemoglobin J (Baltimore) coexisting in a family with Hemoglobin S, *Johns Hopkins Hosp. Bull.*, 114, 1, 1964.

134. **Chernoff, A. I. and Perillie, P. E.**, The amino acid composition of HGB New Haven No. 2 (HGB N New Haven), *Biochim. Biophys. Res. Comm.*, 16, 368, 1964.

135. **Wong, S. C., Bouver, N., Wilson, J. B., and Huisman, T. H. J.**, Hb J Georgia = Hb J Baltimore = $\alpha_2\beta_2$ 16 Gly → Asp, *Clin. Chim. Acta*, 35, 521, 1971.

136. Wade, P. T., Jenkins, T., and Huehns, E. R., Haemoglobin variant in a Bushman: Haemoglobin D β Bushman $\alpha2\beta2$ 16 Gly → Arg, *Nature (London),* 216, 688, 1967.
137. Maekawa, M., Maekawa, T., Fujiwara, N., Tabara, K., and Matsuda, G., Hemoglobin Nagasaki: $\alpha2\beta2$ 17 Glu. A new abnormal human hemoglobin found in one family in Nagasaki, *Int. J. Protein Res.,* 1(11), 147, 1970.
138. Elion, J., Belkhodja, O., Wajcman, H., and Labie, D., Two variants of Hemoglobin D in the Algerian population: Hemoglobin D Ouled Rabah β19 (B1) Asn → Lys and Hemoglobin D Iran β22(B4) Glu → Gln, *Biochim. Biophys. Acta,* 310, 360, 1973.
139. Stamatoyannopoulos, G., Nute, P. E., Adamson, J. W., Bellingham, A. J., Funk, D., and Hornung, S., Hemoglobin Olympia (β20 valine → methionine): an electrophoretically silent variant associated with high oxygen affinity and erythrocytosis, *J. Clin. Invest.,* 52, 342, 1973.
140. Garel, M. C., Blouquit, Y., Arous, N., and Rosa, J., Hb Strasbourg $\alpha_2\beta_2$ 20(B2) Val → Asp: a variant at the same locus as Hb Olympia β^{20} Val → Met, *FEBS Lett.,* 72, 1, 1976.
141. Vella, F., Lorkin, P. A., Carrell, R. W., and Lehmann, H., A new hemoglobin variant resembling Hemoglobin E. Hemoglobin E Saskatoon: β22 Glu → Lys, *Can. J. Biochem.,* 45, 1385, 1967.
142. Blackwell, R. Q., Yang, H. J., and Wang, C. C., Hemoglobin G Taipei: $\alpha2\beta2$ 22 Glu → Gly, *Biochim. Biophys. Acta,* 175, 237, 1969.
143. Vella, F., Isaacs, W. A., and Lehmann, H., Hemoglobin G Saskatoon: β22 Glu → Ala, *Can. J. Biochem.,* 45, 351, 1967.
144. Blackwell, R. Q., Liu, C. S., Yang, H. J., Wang, C. C., Huang, J. T. H., Hemoglobin variant common to Chinese and North American Indians: $\alpha2\beta2$ 22 Glu → Ala., *Science,* 161, 381, 1968.
145. Bowman, B. H., Barnett, D. R., and Hite, R., Hemoglobin G Coushatta: a beta variant with a delta-like substitution, *Biochim. Biophys. Acta,* 26, 466, 1967.
146. Blackwell, R. Q., Ro, I. H., Liu, C. S., Yang, H. J., Wang, C. C., and Huang, J. T. H., Hemoglobin variant found in Koreans, Chinese, and North American Indians: $\alpha2\beta2$ 22 Glu → Ala, *Am. J. Phys. Anthropol.,* 30, 389, 1967.
147. Rahbar, S., Haemoglobin D Iran: β2 22 glutamic acid → glutamine (B4) *Br. J. Haematol.,* 24, 31, 1973.
148. Ranney, H. M., Jacobs, A. S., Udem, L., and Zalusky, R., Hemoglobin Riverdale-Bronx, an unstable hemoglobin resulting from the substitution of arginine for glycine at helical residue B6 of the β polypeptide chain, *Biochim. Biophys. Acta,* 33, 1004, 1968.
149. Huisman, T. H. J., Brown, A. K., Efremov, G. D., Wilson, J. B., Reynolds, C. A., Uy, R., and Smith, L. L., Hemoglobin Savannah [B6 (24) β-glycine → valine]: an unstable variant causing anemia with inclusion bodies, *J. Clin. Invest.,* 50, 650, 1971.
150. Idelson, L. I., Didkowsky, N. A., Casey, R., Lorkin, P. A., and Lehmann, H., New unstable haemoglobin [Hb Moscva, β24(B6) Gly → Asp] found in the U.S.S.R., *Nature (London),* 249, 768, 1974.
151. Blackwell, R. Q. and Liu, C.-S., Hemoglobin G Taiwan-Ami $\alpha2\beta2$ 25 Gly → Arg, *Biochim. Biophys. Res. Comm.,* 30, 690, 1968.
152. Hunt, J. A. and Ingram, V. M., Abnormal human haemoglobin. VI. The chemical difference between haemoglobins A and E., *Biochim. Biophys. Acta,* 49, 520, 1961.
153. Blouquit, Y., Arous, N., Machado, P. E. A., and Garel, M. C., Hb Henri Mondor: β^{26} (B8) Glu → Val: a variant with a substitution localized at the same position as that of Hb E β^{26} Glu → Lys, *FEBS Lett.,* 72, 5, 1977.
154. Idelson, L. I., Didkovsky, N. A., Filippova, A. V., Casey, R., Kynoch, P. A. M., and Lehmann, H. , Haemoglobin Volga, β27 (B9) Ala → Asp, a new highly unstable haemoglobin with a suppressed charge, *FEBS Lett.,* 58, 122, 1975.
155. Kuis-Reerink, J. D., Jonxis, J. H. P., Niazi, G. A., Wilson, J. B., Bolch, K. C., Gravely, M., and Huisman, T. H. J., Hb Volga or $\alpha2\beta2$ 27(B9) Ala → Asp: an unstable hemoglobin variant in three generations of a Dutch family, *Biochim. Biophys. Acta,* 439, 63, 1976.
156. Cohen-Solal, M., Seligmann, M., Thillet, J., and Rosa, J., Haemoglobin Saint Louis β28(B10) leucine → glutamine. A new unstable haemoglobin only present in a ferri form, *FEBS Lett.,* 33 (Abstr. 408), 37, 1973.
157. Thillet, J., Cohen-Solal, M., Seligmann, M., and Rosa, J., Functional and physicochemical studies of Hemoglobin St. Louis β^{28} (B10) Leu → Gln, *J. Clin. Invest.,* 58, 1098, 1976.
158. Sansone, G., Carrell, R. W., and Lehmann, H., Haemoglobin Genova: β28 (B10) leucine → proline, *Nature (London),* 214, 877, 1967.
159. Schmidt, R. M., Bechtel, K. C., Johnson, M. H., Therrell, B. L., Jr., Moo-Penn, W. F., Hemoglobin Lufkin: β29 (B11) Gly → Asp. An unstable hemoglobin variant involving an internal amino acid residue, *Hemoglobin,* 1, 799, 1977.
160. Brimhall, B., Jones, R. T., Baur, E. W., and Motulsky, A. G., Structural characterization of Hemoglobin Tacoma, *Biochemistry,* 8, 2125, 1969.
161. Jackson, J. M., Yates, A., and Huehns, E. R., Haemoglobin Perth: β32 (B14) Leu → Pro. An unstable haemoglobin causing haemolysis, *Br. J. Haematol.,* 25, 607, 1973.

162. **Honig, G. R., Green, D., Shamsuddin, M., Vida, L. N., Mason, R. G., Gnarra, D. J., and Maurer, H. S.,** Hemoglobin Abraham Lincoln, β32 (B14) leucine → proline. An unstable variant producing severe hemolytic disease, *J. Clin. Invest.*, 52, 1746, 1973.
163. **Garel, M. C., Blouquit, Y., and Rosa, J.,** Hemoglobin Castilla β32 (B14) Leu → Arg: a new unstable variant producing severe hemolytic disease, *FEBS Lett.*, 58, 145, 1975.
164. **Rieder, R. F., Oski, F. A., and Clegg, J. B.,** Hemoglobin Philly (β35 tyrosine → phenylalanine): studies in the molecular pathology of hemoglobin, *J. Clin Invest.*, 48, 1627, 1969.
165. **Yamaoka, K.,** Hemoglobin Hirose; α2β2 37(C3) tryptophan yielding serine, *Blood*, 38, 730, 1971.
166. **Brimhall, B., Jones, R. T., Schneider, R. G., Hosty, T. S., Tomlin, G., and Atkins, R.,** Two new hemoglobins: Hemoglobin Alabama [β39 (C5) Gln → Lys] and Hemoglobin Montgomery [α48(CD6) Leu → Arg], *Biochim. Biophys. Acta*, 379, 28, 1975.
167. **Kendall, A. G., Wilson, J. B., Cope, N., Bolch, K., and Huisman, T. H. J.,** Hb Vaasa or α2β2 [39(C5) Gln → Glu], a mildly unstable variant found in a Finnish family, *Hemoglobin*, 1, 292, 1977.
168. **Brown, W. J., Niazi, G. A., Jayalakshmi, M., Abraham, E. C., and Huisman, T. H. J.,** Hemoglobin Athens-Georgia, or α2β2 40(C6) Arg → Lys, a hemoglobin variant with an increased oxygen affinity, *Biochim. Biophys. Acta*, 439, 70, 1976.
169. **Moo-Penn, W. F., Johnson, M. H., Bechtel, K. C., Jue, D. L., Therrel, B. L., and Schmidt, R. M.,** Hemoglobin Austin and Waco: two hemoglobins with substitutions in the $\alpha_1\beta_2$ contact region, *Arch. Biochem. Biophys.*, 179, 86, 1977.
170. **Buckett, L. B., Sharma, V. S., Piscotta, A. V., Ranney, H., and Bruckheimer, P.,** Hemoglobin Mequon β41 (C7) phenylalanine → tyrosine, *Clin. Res.*, 22 (Abstr.), 176, 1974.
171. **Dacie, J. V., Shinton, N. K., Gaffney, P. J., Jr., Carrell, R. W., and Lehmann, H.,** Haemoglobin Hammersmith [β42 (CD1) Phe → Ser], *Nature (London)*, 216, 663, 1967.
172. **Ohba, Y., Miyaji, T., Matsuoka, M., Yamaguchi, K., Yonemitsu, H., Ishii, T., and Shibata, S.,** Hemoglobin Chiba: Hb Hammersmith in a Japanese girl, *Acta Haematol. Jpn.*, 38, 53, 1975.
173. **Keeling, M. M., Ogdon, L. L., Wrightstone, R. N., Wilson, J. B., Reynolds, C. A., Kitchens, J. L., and Huisman, T. H. J.,** Hemoglobin Louisville [β42 (CD1) Phe → Leu]: an unstable variant causing mild hemolytic anemia, *J. Clin. Invest.*, 50, 2395, 1971.
174. **Bratu, V., Lorkin, P. A., Lehmann, H., and Predescu, C.,** Haemoglobin Bucuresti β42 (CD1) Phe → Leu, a cause of unstable haemoglobin haemolytic anemia, *Biochim. Biophys. Acta*, 251, 1, 1971.
175. **Bowman, B. H., Oliver, C. P., Barnett, D. R., Cunningham, J. R., and Schneider, R. G.,** Chemical characterization of three hemoglobins G, *Blood*, 23, 193, 1964.
176. **Allan, N., Beale, D., Irvine, D., and Lehmann, H.,** Three haemoglobins K: Woolwich, an abnormal, Cameroon and Ibadan, two unusual variants of human haemoglobin A, *Nature (London)*, 208, 658, 1965.
177. **Sick, K., Beale, D., Irvine, D., Lehmann, H., Goodall, P. T., and MacDougall, S.,** Haemoglobin G Copenhagen and Haemoglobin J Cambridge. Two new β-chain variants of Haemoglobin A, *Biochim. Biophys. Acta*, 140, 231, 1967.
178. **Charache, S., Brimhall, B., Milner, P., and Cobb, L.,** Hemoglobin Okaloosa [β48 (CD7) Leu → Arg]: an unstable hemoglobin with decreased oxygen affinity, *J. Clin. Invest.*, 52, 2858, 1973.
179. **Labossiere, A., Hill, J. R., and Vella, F.,** A new βTp V Hemoglobin variant: Hb Edmonton, *Clin. Biochem.*, 4, 114, 1971.
180. **Jones, R. T., Koler, R. D., Duerst, M. L., and Dhindsa, S.,** Hemoglobin Willamette [α2β2 51Pro → Arg (D2)] — a new abnormal human hemoglobin, *Hemoglobin*, 1, 45, 1976.
181. **Konotey-Ahulu, F. I. D., Kinderlerer, J. L., Lehmann, H., and Ringelhann, B.,** Haemoglobin Osu-Christiansborg: a new β-chain variant of haemoglobin A [β52 (D3) aspartic acid → asparagine] in combination with Haemoglobin S, *J. Med. Genet.*, 8, 302, 1971.
182. **Beresford, C. H., Clegg, J. B., and Weatherall, D. J.,** Haemoglobin Ocho Rios [β52 (D3) aspartic acid → alanine]; a new β-chain variant of Haemoglobin A found in combination with Haemoglobin S, *J. Med. Genet.*, 9, 151, 1972.
183. **Clegg, J. B., Naughton, M. A., and Weatherall, D. J.,** Abnormal human haemoglobins. Separation and characterization of the α and β chains by chromatography, and the determination of two new variants, *J. Mol. Biol.*, 19, 91, 1966.
184. **Blackwell, R. Q. and Liu, C.-S.,** The identical structural anomalies of Hemoglobins J Meinung and J Korat, *Biochem. Biophys. Res. Comm.*, 24, 732, 1966.
185. **Blackwell, R. Q., Liu, C.-S., Lie-Injo, L. E., and Pribadi, W.,** Fast hemoglobin variant in Minahassan people of Sulawesi, Chinese and Thais: α2β2 56 Gly → Asp, *Am J. Phys. Anthropol.*, 32, 147, 1970.
186. **Rahbar, S., Nowzari, G., Haydari, H., and Daneshmand, P.,** Haemoglobin Hamadan αA2β2 56 glycine → arginine (D7), *Biochim. Biophys. Acta*, 379, 645, 1975.
187. **Vullo, C., Christofori, G., Salsini, G., Tentori, L., Marinucci, M., and Bruni, E.,** Haemoglobin G Ferrara; β2 57 (E1) Asn → Lys, *Int. Res. Comm. Syst.*

188. **Yanase, T., Hanada, M., Seita, M., Obya, I., Ohta, Y., Imamura, T., Fijimura, T., Kawasaki, K., and Yamaoka, K.**, Molecular basis of morbidity — from a series of studies of hemoglobinopathies in Western Japan, *Jpn. J. Hum. Genet.*, 13, 40, 1968.
189. **Marengo-Rowe, A. J., Lorkin, P. A., Gallo, E., and Lehmann, H.**, Haemoglobin Dhofar — a new variant from Southern Arabia, *Biochim. Biophys. Acta*, 168, 58, 1968.
190. **Boulton, F. E., Huntsman, R. G., Lehmann, H., Lorkin, P., and Romero Herrera, A.**, Myoglobin variants, *Br. J. Haematol.*, 20, 671, 1971.
191. **Blackwell, R. Q., Liu, C.-S., and Shih, T.-B.**, Hemoglobin J Kaohsiung: β59 Lys → Thr, *Biochim. Biophys. Acta*, 229, 343, 1971.
192. **Blackwell, R. Q., Jim, R. T. S., Liu, C.-S., Weng, M.-I., Wang, C.-L., and Shih, T.-B.**, Fast haemoglobin variant found in Hawaiian-Chinese-Caucasian family in Hawaii and a Chinese subject in Taiwan, *Vox Sang.*, 22, 469, 1972.
193. **Jones, R. T., Brimhall, B., Huehns, E. R., and Motulsky, A. G.**, Structural characterization of Hemoglobin N Seattle: α2Aβ2 61 Lys → Glu, *Biochim. Biophys. Acta*, 154, 278, 1968.
194. **Shibata, S., Miyaji, T., Iuchi, I., Ueda, S., and Takeda, I.**, Hemoglobin Hikari (α2Aβ2 61 AspNH2); a fast moving hemoglobin found in two unrelated Japanese families, *Clin. Chim. Acta*, 10, 101, 1964.
195. **Beutler, E., Lang, A., and Lehmann, H.**, Hemoglobin Duarte: α2β2 62(E6) Ala → Pro: a new unstable hemoglobin with increased oxygen affinity, *Blood*, 43, 527, 1974.
196. **Muller, C. J. and Kingma, S.**, Haemoglobin Zürich α2β2 63 Arg, *Biochim. Biophys. Acta*, 50, 595, 1961.
197. **Gerald, P. S. and Efron, M. L.**, Chemical studies of several varieties of Hb M. *Proc. Natl. Acad. Sci. U.S.A.*, 47, 1758, 1961.
198. **Shibata, S., Miyaji, T., Iuchi, I., and Ueda, S.**, A comparative study of Hemoglobin M Iwate and Hemoglobin M Kurume by means of electrophoresis, chromatography and analysis of peptide chains, *Acta Haematol. Jpn.*, 24, 486, 1961.
199. **Murawski, K., Szymanowska, Z., and Kozlowska, J.**, A new variant of abnormal methaemoglobin: Hb M Radom, *Biochim. Biophys. Acta*, 69, 442, 1963.
200. **Hobolth, N.**, Haemoglobin M Arhus. I. Clinical family study, *Acta Paediatr. Scand.*, 54, 357, 1965.
201. **Josephson, A. M., Weinstein, H. G., Yakulis, V. J., Singer, L., and Heller, P.**, A new variant of Hemoglobin M disease: Hemoglobin M Chicago, *J. Lab. Clin. Med.*, 59, 918, 1962.
202. **Betke, K., Groschner, E., and Bock, K.**, Properties of a further variant of Haemoglobin M, *Nature (London)*, 188, 864, 1960.
203. **Hörlein, H. and Weber, G.**, Uber chronishe familiäre Methämoglobinämie und eine neue Modifikation des Methämoglobins, *Dtsch. Med. Wochenschr.*, 73, 476, 1948.
204. **Efremov, G. D., Huisman, T. H. J., Stanulovic M., Zurovec, M., Duma, H., Wilson, J. B., and Jeremic, V.**, Haemoglobin M Saskatoon and Haemoglobin M Hyde Park in two Yugoslavian families, *Scand. J. Haematol.*, 13, 48, 1974.
205. **Kohne, E., Grosse, H. P., Versmold, H., Kley, H. P., and Kleihauer, E.**, Hb M Erlangen: α2β2 63 (E7) Tyr, *Z. Kinderheilkd.*, 120, 69, 1975.
206. **Wajcman, H., Krishnamoorthy, R., Gacon, G., Elion, J., Allard, C., and Labie, D.**, A new hemoglobin variant involving the distal histidine: Hb Bicêtre [β 63 (E7) His → Pro], *J. Mol. Med.*, 1, 187, 1976.
207. **Tentori, L., Bruni, E., and Marinucci**, Three examples of double heterozygosis beta-thalassemia and rare hemoglobin variant, in *International Istanbul Symposium on Abnormal Hemoglobins and Thalassemia*, Aksoy, M., Ed., Istanbul, 1974, 53.
208. **Ricco, G., Pich, P. G., Mazza, U., Rossi, G., Ajmar, F., Arese, P., and Gallo, E.**, Hb J Sicilia: β65 (E9) Lys → Asn, a beta homologue of Hb Zambia, *FEBS Lett.*, 39, 200, 1974.
209. **Garel, M. C., Hassan, W., Coquelet, M. T., Gosens, M., and Rosa, J.**, Hemoglobin J Cairo: β65 (E9) Lys → Gln, a new hemoglobin variant discovered in an Egyptian family, *Biochim. Biophys. Acta*, 420, 97, 1976.
210. **Rosa, J., Labie, D., Wajcman, H., Boigne, J. M., Cabannes, R., Bierme, R., and Ruffie, J.**, Haemoglobin I Toulouse: β66 (E10) Lys → Glu: a new abnormal hemoglobin with a mutation localized on the E10 porphyrin surrounding zone, *Nature (London)*, 223, 190, 1969.
211. **Steadman, J. H., Yates, A., and Huehns, E. R.**, Idiopathic Heinz Body Anaemia: Hb-Bristol [β67 (E11) Val → Asp], *Br. J. Haematol.*, 18, 435, 1970.
212. **Carrell, R. W., Lehmann, H., Lorkin, P. A., Raik, E., and Hunter, E.**, Haemoglobin Sydney: β67 (E11) valine → alanine: an emerging pattern of unstable haemoglobins, *Nature (London)*, 215, 626, 1967.
213. **Ohba, Y., Miyaji, T., Matsuoka, M., Sugiyama, K., Suzuki, T., and Sugiura, T.**, Hemoglobin Mizuho or beta 68 (E12) leucine → proline, a new unstable variant associated with severe hemolytic anemia, *Hemoglobin*, 1(5), 467, 1977.

214. **Salomon, H., Tatarski, I., Dance, N., Huehns, E. R., and Shooter, E. M.**, A new hemoglobin variant found in a Beduin tribe: Hemoglobin "Rambam," *Isr. J. Med. Sci.*, 1, 836, 1965.
215. **Kurachi, S., Hermodson, M., Hornung, S., and Stamatoyannopoulos, G.**, Structure of Haemoglobin Seattle, *Nature New Biol.*, 243, 275, 1973.
216. **Carrell, R. W. and Owen, M. C.**, A new approach to haemoglobin variant identification. Haemoglobin Christchurch β71 (E15) phenylalanine → serine, *Biochim. Biophys. Acta*, 236, 507, 1971.
217. **Jones, R. T., Brimhall, B., Pootrakul, S., and Gray, G.**, Hemoglobin Vancouver [$\alpha_2\beta_2$ 73 (E17) Asp → Tyr]: its structure and function, *J. Mol. Evol.*, 9, 37, 1976.
218. **Konotey-Ahulu, F. I. D., Gallo, E., Lehmann, H., and Ringelhann, B.**, Haemoglobin Korle-Bu (β73 aspartic acid → asparagine) showing one of the two amino acid substitutions of Haemoglobin C Harlem, *J. Med. Genet.*, 5, 107, 1968.
219. **Bio-Doku, F. S., Kinderlerer, J., and Lehmann, H.**, *submitted to Atlas of Protein Sequence and Structure*, 5, 73, 1972.
220. **Schneider, R. G., Hosty, T. S., Tomlin, G., Atkins, R., Brimhall, B., and Jones, R. T.**, Hb Mobile [α2β2 73 (E17) Asp → Val]; a new variant, *Biochem. Genet.*, 13, 411, 1975.
221. **Rieder, R. F., Wolf, D. J., Clegg, J. B., and Lee, S. L.**, Rapid post-synthetic destruction of unstable Haemoglobin Bushwick, *Nature (London)*, 254, 725, 1975.
222. **White, J. M., Brain, M. C., Lorkin, P. A., Lehmann, H., and Smith, M.**, Mild "Unstable Haemoglobin Haemolytic Anaemia" caused by Haemoglobin Shepherds Bush [β74 (E18) Gly → Asp], *Nature (London)*, 225, 939, 1970.
223. **Hubbard, M., Winton, E., Lindeman, J. G., Dessauer, P. L., Wilson, J. B., Wrightstone, R. N., and Huisman, T. H. J.**, Hemoglobin Atlanta or α2β2 75 Leu → Pro (E19): an unstable variant found in several members of a Caucasian family, *Biochim. Biophys. Acta*, 386, 538, 1975.
224. **Romain, P. L., Schwartz, A. D., Shamsuddin, M., Adams, J. G., III, Mason, R. G., Vida, L. N., and Honig, G. R.**, Hemoglobin J Chicago [β76 (E20) Ala → Asp]; a new hemoglobin variant resulting from substitution of an external residue, *Blood*, 45, 387, 1975.
225. **Rahbar, S., Beale, D., Isaacs, W. A., and Lehmann, H.**, Abnormal haemoglobins in Iran. Observations of a new variant — Haemoglobin J Iran (α2β2 77 His → Arg), *Br. Med. J.*, 1, 674, 1967.
226. **Blackwell, R. Q., Shih, T.-B., Wang, C.-L., and Liu, C.-S.**, Hemoglobin G-Hsi-Tsou: β79 Asp → Gly, *Biochim. Biophys. Acta*, 257, 49, 1972.
227. **Blackwell, R. Q., Yang, H. T., and Wang, C. C.**, Hemoglobin G Szuhu: β80 Asn → Lys, *Biochim. Biophys. Acta*, 188, 59, 1969.
228. **Imai, K., Morimoto, H., Kotani, M., Shibata, S., Miyaji, T., and Masutomo, K.**, Studies on the function of abnormal hemoglobins. II. Oxygen equilibrium of abnormal hemoglobins: Shimonoseki, Ube II, Hikari, Gifu, and Agenogi, *Biochim. Biophys. Acta*, 200, 197, 1970.
229. **Schneider, R. G., Hettig, R. A., Bilunos, M., and Brimhall, B.**, Hemoglobin Baylor [α2β2 81 (EF5) Leu → Arg] — an unstable mutant with high oxygen affinity, *Hemoglobin*, 1, 85, 1976.
230. **Moo-Penn, W. F., Jue, D. L., Bechtel, K. C., Johnson, M. H., Schmidt, R. M., McCurdy, P. R., Fox, J., Bonaventura, J., Sullivan, B., and Bonaventura, C.**, Hemoglobin Providence. A human hemoglobin variant occurring in two forms *in vivo*, *J. Biol. Chem.*, 251, 7557, 1976.
231. **Bonaventura, J., Bonaventura, C., Sullivan, B., Ferruzzi, G., McCurdy, P. R., Fox, J., and Moo-Penn, W. F.**, Hemoglobin Providence. Functional consequences of two alterations of the 2, 3-diphosphoglycerate binding site at position β82, *J. Biol. Chem.*, 251, 7563, 1976.
232. **Lorkin, P. A., Stephens, A. D., Beard, M. E. J., Wrigley, P. F. M., Adams, L., and Lehmann, H.**, Haemoglobin Rahere (β82 Lys → Thr): a new high affinity haemoglobin associated with decreased 2, 3-diphosphoglycerate binding and relative polycythaemia, *Br. Med. J.*, 4, 200, 1975.
233. **Ikkala, E., Koskela, J., Pikkarainen, P., and Rahiala, E.**, Hb Helsinki: a variant with a high oxygen affinity and a substitution at a 2, 3-DPG binding site [β^{82} (EF6) Lys → Met], *Acta Haematol.*, 56, 257, 1976.
234. **Blackwell, R. Q., Liu, C.-S., and Wang, C.-L.**, Hemoglobin Ta-Li: β83 Gly → Cys, *Biochim. Biophys. Acta*, 243, 467, 1971.
235. **Tatsis, B., Sofroniadou, K., and Stergiopoulos, C. I.**, Hemoglobin Pyrgos [α2β2 83 (EF7) Gly → Asp]. A new hemoglobin (Hb) variant, *Annu. Meet. Am. Soc. Hematol. Miami, Abstr.*, 168, 1972.
236. **Tatsis, B., Sofroniadou, K., and Stergiopoulos, C. I.**, Hemoglobin Pyrgos α2β2 83 (EF7) Gly → Asp: a new hemoglobin variant in double heterozygosity with Hemoglobin S, *Blood*, 47, 827, 1976.
237. **Bradley, T. B., Wohl, R. C., Murphy, S. B., Oski, F. A., and Bunn, H. F.**, Properties of Hemoglobin Bryn Mawr, β85 Phe → Ser, a new spontaneous mutation producing an unstable hemoglobin with high oxygen affinity, *Annu. Meet. Am. Soc. Hematol.* Abstr. 67, 1972.
238. **de Weinstein, B. I., White, J. M., Wiltshire, B. G., and Lehmann, H.**, A new unstable haemoglobin: Hb Buenos Aires, β85 (F1) Phe → Ser, *Acta Haematol.*, 50, 357, 1973.
239. **Watson-Williams, E. J., Beale, D., Irvine, D., and Lehmann, H.**, A new haemoglobin, D Ibadan (β87 threonine → lysine), producing no sickle cell haemoglobin D disease with haemoglobin S, *Nature (London)*, 205, 1273, 1965.

240. **Hollender, A., Lorkin, P. A., Lehmann, H., and Svensson, B.**, New unstable Haemoglobin Böras: β88 (F4) leucine → arginine, *Nature (London)*, 222, 953, 1969.
241. **Opfell, R. W., Lorkin, P. A., and Lehmann, H.**, Hereditary non-spherocytic haemolytic anaemia with post-splenectomy inclusion bodies and pigmenturia caused by an unstable haemoglobin Santa Ana — β88 (F4) leucine → proline, *J. Med. Genet.*, 5, 292, 1968.
242. **Thillet, J., Blouquit, Y., Garel, M. C., Dreyfus, B., Reyes, F., Cohen-Solal, M., Beuzard, Y., and Rosa, J.**, Hemoglobin Creteil β89 (F5) Ser → Asn: high oxygen affinity variant of hemoglobin frozen in a quarternary R-structure, *J. Mol. Med.*, 1, 135, 1976.
243. **Puett, D., Paniker, N. V., Lin, K. D., Flexner, J. M., Wasserman, B. K., and Krantz, S. B.**, Hemoglobin Vanderbilt (β89 Ser → Arg). A new hemoglobin with increased oxygen affinity and lowered response to 2,3-diphosphoglycerate, *Clin. Res.*, 25, 53A, 1977.
244. **Miyaji, T., Suzuki, H., Ohba, Y., and Shibata, S.**, Hemoglobin Agenogi (α2β2 90 Lys), a slow moving hemoglobin of a Japanese family resembling Hb-E, *Clin. Chim. Acta*, 14, 624, 1966.
245. **Schneider, R. G., Satoshi, U., Alperin, J. B., Brimhall, B., and Jones, R. T.**, Hemoglobin Sabine, β91 (F7) Leu → Pro. An unstable variant causing severe anemia with inclusion bodies, *N. Engl. J. Med.*, 280, 739, 1969.
246. **Ahern, E , Ahern, V., Hilton, T., Serjeant, G. R., Serjeant, B. E., Seakins, M., Lang, A., Middleton, A., and Lehmann, H.**, Haemoglobin Caribbean β91 (F7) Leu → Arg: a mildly unstable haemoglobin with a low oxygen affinity, *FEBS Lett.*, 69, 99, 1976.
247. **Heller, P., Coleman, R. D., and Yakulis, V.**, Hemoglobin M Hyde Park: a new variant of abnormal methemoglobin, *J. Clin. Invest.*, 45, 1021, 1966.
248. **Shibata, S., Yamamoto, K., Ohba, Y., Miyaji, T., Karita, K., and Iuchi, I.**, Hemoglobin M Akita disease, *Acta Haematol. Jpn.*, 32, 311, 1969.
249. **Beuzard, Y., Courvalin, J. C., Cohen-Solal, M., Carel, M. C., Rosa, J., Brizard, C. P., and Gibaud, A.**, Structural studies of Hemoglobin Saint Etienne β92 (F8) His → Gln: a new abnormal hemoglobin with loss of β proximal histidine and absence of heme on the β chains, *FEBS Lett.*, 27, 76, 1972.
250. **Aksoy, M., Erden, S., Efremov, G. D., Wilson, J. B., Huisman, T. H. J., Schroeder, W. A., Shelton, J. R., Shelton, J. B., Ulitin, O. N., and Müftüglu, A.**, Hemoglobin Istanbul: substitution of glutamine for histidine in a proximal histidine [F8 (92) β], *J. Clin. Invest.*, 51, 2380, 1972.
251. **Adams, J. G., III, Przywara, K. P., Shamsuddin, M., and Heller, P.**, Hemoglobin J Altgeld Gardens [β92 (F8) His → Asp]: A New Hemoglobin Variant Involving a Substitution of the Proximal Histidine, Am. Soc. Hematol. 18th Ann. Meet., Dallas, 1975.
252. **Finney, R., Casey, R., Lehmann, H., and Walker, W.**, Hb Newcastle: β92 (F8) His → Pro, *FEBS Lett.*, 60, 435, 1975.
253. **Clegg, J. B., Naughton, M. A., and Weatherall, D. J.**, An improved method for the characterization of human haemoglobin mutants: identification of α2β2 95 Glu, Haemoglobin N (Baltimore), *Nature (London)*, 207, 945, 1965.
254. **Gottlieb, A. J., Robinson, E. A., and Itano, H. A.**, Primary structure of Hopkins-I Haemoglobin, *Nature (London)*, 214, 189, 1967.
255. **Dobbs, N. B., Jr., Simmons, J. W., Wilson, J. B., and Huisman, T. H. J.**, Hemoglobin Jenkins or Hemoglobin-N-Baltimore or α2β2 95 Glu, *Biochim. Biophys. Acta*, 117, 492, 1966.
256. **Bayrakci, C., Josephson, A., Singer, L., Heller, P., and Coleman, R. D.**, A New Fast Hemoglobin, Xth Congr. Int. Soc. Haematol., Stockholm, Sweden, 1964.
257. **Heller, P.**, personal communication; as cited in **Hamilton, H. B., Iuchi, I, Miyaji, T., and Shibata, S.**, Hemoglobin Hiroshima (β^{143} Histidine → Aspartic Acid): a newly identified fast moving Beta chain variant associated with increased oxygen affinity and compensatory erythremia, *J. Clin. Invest.*, 48, 525, 1969.
258. **Lorkin, P. A., Lehmann, H., Fairbanks, V. F., Berglund, G., and Leonhardt, T.**, Two new pathological haemoglobins: Olmsted β141 (H19) Leu → Arg and Malmö: β97 (FG4) His → Gln, *Biochem. J.* 119, 68, 1970.
259. **Taketa, F., Huang, Y. P., Libnoch, J. A., and Dessel, B. H.**, Hemoglobin Wood β97 (FG4) His → Leu; a new high-oxygen-affinity hemoglobin associated with familial erythrocytosis, *Biochim. Biophys. Acta*, 400, 348, 1975.
260. **Taketa, F., Antholine, W. E., Mauk, A. G., and Libnoch, J. A.**, Nitrosylhemoglobin Wood: effects of inositol hexaphosphate on thiol reactivity and electron paramagnetic resonance spectrum, *Biochemistry*, 14, 3229, 1975.
261. **Carrell, R. W., Lehmann, H., and Hutchison, H. E.**, Haemoglobin Köln β 98 valine → methionine): an unstable protein causing inclusion-body anaemia, *Nature (London)*, 210, 915, 1966.
262. **Woodson, R. D., Heywood, J. D., and Lenfant, C.**, Oxygen transport in Hemoglobin San Francisco, *Clin. Res.*, 18, 134, 1970.
263. **Ohba, Y., Miyaji, T., and Shibata, S.**, Identical substitution in Hb Ube-1 and Hb Köln, *Nature New Biol.*, 243, 205, 1973.

264. **Gordon-Smith, E. C., Dacie, J. V., Blecher, T. E., French, E. A., Wiltshire, B. G., and Lehmann, H.**, Haemoglobin Nottingham, β98 (FG5) Val → Gly: a new unstable haemoglobin producing severe haemolysis, *Proc. R. Soc. Med.*, 66, 507, 1973.
265. **Gacon, G., Wajcman, H., and Labie, D.**, A new unstable hemoglobin mutated in β98 (FG5) Val → Ala: Hb Djelfa, *FEBS Lett.*, 58, 238, 1975.
266. **Reed, C. S., Hampson, R., Gordon, S., Jones, R. T., Novy, M. J., Brimhall, B., Edwards, M. J., and Koler, R. D.**, Erythrocytosis secondary to increased oxygen affinity of a mutant hemoglobin, Hemoglobin Kempsey, *Blood*, 31, 623, 1968.
267. **Jones, R. T., Osgood, E. E., Brimhall, B., and Koler, R. D.**, Hemoglobin Yakima. I. Clinical and biochemical studies, *J. Clin. Invest.*, 46, 1840, 1967.
268. **Weatherall, D. J., Clegg, J. B., Callender, S. T., Wells, R. M. G., Gale, R. E., Huehns, E. R., Perutz, M. F., Viggiano, G., and Ho, C .**, Haemoglobin Radcliffe [$\alpha_2\beta_2$ 99 (G1) Ala]: a high oxygen-affinity variant causing familial polycythaemia, *Br. J. Haematol.*, 35, 177, 1977.
269. **Rucknagel, D. L., Glynn, K. P., and Smith, J. R.**, Hemoglobin Ypsilanti characterized by increased oxygen affinity, abnormal polymerization and erythremia, *Clin. Res.*, 15, 270, 1967.
270. **Lokich, J. J., Mahoney, C., Bunn, H. F., Bruckheimer, S. M., and Ranney, H.**, Hemoglobin Brigham (α2Aβ2 100 Pro → Leu). Hemoglobin variant associated with familial erythrocytosis, *J. Clin. Invest.*, 52, 2060, 1973.
271. **Jones, R. T., Brimhall, B., and Gray, G.**, Hemoglobin British Columbia [$\alpha2\beta2$ 101 (G3) Glu → Lys]: a new variant with high oxygen affinity, *Hemoglobin*, 1, 171, 1976.
272. **Adams, J. B., Winter, W. P., Tausk, K., and Heller, P.**, Hemoglobin Rush [(β-101 (G3) glutamine)]: a new unstable hemoglobin causing mild hemolytic anemia, *Blood*, 43, 261, 1974.
273. **Mant, M. J., Salkie, M. L., Cope, N., Appling, F., Bolch, K., Jayalakshmi, M., Gravely, M., Wilson, J. B., and Huisman, T. H. J.**, Hb Alberta or $\alpha2\beta2$ [101 (G3) Glu → Gly], a new high-oxygen-affinity hemoglobin variant causing erythrocytosis, *Hemoglobin*, 1, 183, 1977.
274. **Charache, S., Jacobson, R., Brimhall, B., Murphy, E. A., Hathaway, P., Winslow, R., Jones, R., Rath, C., and Simkovich, J.**, Hb Potomac (β101 Glu → Asp): speculations on placental oxygen transport in carriers of high-affinity hemoglobins, *Blood*, 51, 331, 1978.
275. **Efremov, G. D., Huisman, T. H. J., Smith, L. L., Wilson, J. B., Kitchens, J. L., Wrightstone, R. N., and Adams, H. R.**, Hemoglobin Richmond, a human hemoglobin which forms asymmetric hybrids with other hemoglobins, *J. Biol. Chem.*, 244, 6105, 1969.
276. **Bonaventura, J. and Riggs, A.**, Hemoglobin Kansas, a human hemoglobin with a neutral amino acid substitution and an abnormal oxygen equilibrium, *J. Biol. Chem.*, 243, 980, 1968.
277. **Nagel, R. L., Joshua, L., Johnson, J., Landau, L., Bookchin, R. M., and Harris, M. B.**, Hemoglobin Beth Israel: a mutant causing clinically apparent cyanosis, *N. Eng. J. Med.*, 295, 125, 1976.
278. **White, J. M., Szur, L., Gillies, I. D. S., Lorkin, P. A., and Lehmann, H.**, Familical polycythaemia caused by a new haemoglobin variant. Hb Heathrow β103 (G5) Phe → Leu, *Br. Med. J.*, 3, 665, 1973.
279. **Wilkinson, T., Ching Geh Chua, Carrell, R. W., Robin, H., Exner, T., Kit Ming Lee, and Kronenberg, H.**, A new haemoglobin variant, Haemoglobin Camperdown β104 (G6) arginine → serine, which has normal physiological function, *Biochim. Biophys. Acta*, 393, 195, 1975.
280. **Hyde, R. D., Hall, M. D., Wiltshire, B. G., and Lehmann, H.**, Haemoglobin Southampton, β106 (G8) Leu → Pro: an unstable variant producing severe haemolysis, *Lancet*, 2.12.72, 1170, 1972.
281. **Koler, R. D., Jones, R. T., Bigley, R. H., Litt, M., Lovrien, E., Brooks, R., Lahey, M. E., and Fowler, R.**, Hemoglobin Casper: β106 (G8) Leu → Pro, a contemporary mutation, *Am. J. Med.*, 55, 549, 1973.
282. **Kleihauer, E., Waller, H. D., Benöhr, H. C., Kohne, E., and Gelinsky, P.**, Hb Tübingen Eine neue β-Kettenvariante (βTp 10-12) mit erhöhter Spontanoxydation, *Klin. Wochenschr.*, 48, 651, 1971.
283. **Kohne, E., Kley, H. P., and Kleihauer, E.**, Structural and functional characteristics of the Hb Tubingen: β^{106} (G8) Leu → Gln, *FEBS Lett.*, 64, 443, 1976.
284. **Jones, R. T. and Koler, R. D.**, Functional Studies of Seven New Abnormal Hemoglobins, *16th Int. Congr. Hematol., Abstr. 1-21, September 1976.*
285. **Imamura, T., Fujita, S., Ohta , Y., Hanada, M., and Yanase, T.**, Hemoglobin Yoshizuka [G10 (108) β asparagine → aspartic acid]: a new variant with a reduced oxygen affinity from a Japanese family, *J. Clin. Invest.*, 48, 2341, 1969.
286. **Nute, P. E., Stamatoyannopoulos, G., Hermodson, M. A., Roth, D., and Hornung, S.**, Hemoglobinopathic erythrocytosis due to a new electrophoretically silent variant, Hemoglobin San Diego [β109 (G11) Val → Met], *J. Clin. Invest.*, 53, 320, 1974.
287. **King, M. A. R., Wiltshire, B. G., Lehmann, H., and Morimoto, H.**, An unstable haemoglobin with reduced oxygen affinity: Haemoglobin Peterborough, β111 (G13) valine → phenylalanine, its interaction with normal haemoglobin and with Haemoglobin Lepore, *Br. J. Haematol.*, 22, 125, 1972.
288. **Ranney, H. M., Jacobs, A. S., and Nagel, R. L.**, Haemoglobin New York, *Nature (London)*, 213, 876, 1967.

289. **Outeirino, J., Casey, R., White, J. M., and Lehmann, H.**, Haemoglobin Madrid, β115 (G17) alanine → proline: an unstable variant associated with haemolytic anaemia, *Acta Haematol.*, 52, 53, 1974.
290. **Schneider, R. G., Alperin, J. B., Brimhall, B., and Jones, R. T.**, Hemoglobin P ($\alpha 2\beta 2$ 117 Arg): structure and properties , *J. Lab. Clin. Med.*, 73, 616, 1969.
291. **Schneider, R. G., Berkman, N. L., Brimhall, B., and Jones, R. T.**, Hemoglobin Fannin-Lubbock [$\alpha_2\beta_2{}^{119}$ (GH2) Gly → Asp]: a slightly unstable mutant, *Biochim. Biophys. Acta*, 453, 478, 1976.
292. **Moo-Penn, W. F., Bechtel, K. C., Johnson, M. H., Jue, D. L., Therrell, B. L., Jr., Morrison, B. Y., and Schmidt, R. M.**, Hemoglobin Fannin-Lubbock [$\alpha_2\beta_2{}^{119}$ (GH2) Gly → Asp]: a new hemoglobin variant at the $\alpha_1\beta_1$ contact, *Biochim. Biophys. Acta*, 453, 472, 1976.
293. **Miyaji, T., Ohba, Y., Yamamoto, K., Shibata, S., Iuchi, I., and Hamilton, H. B.**, Hemoglobin Hijiyama: a new fast-moving hemoglobin in a Japanese family, *Science*, 159, 204, 1968.
294. **El-Hazmi, M. A. F. and Lehmann, H.**, Hemoglobin Riyadh [$\alpha 2\beta 2$ 120 (GH3) Lys → Asn] — a new variant found in association with α-thalassemia and iron deficiency, *Hemoglobin*, 1, 59, 1976.
295. **Baglioni, C.**, Abnormal human haemoglobins. VIII. Chemical studies on Haemoglobin D, *Biochim. Biophys. Acta*, 59, 437, 1962.
296. **Özsoylo, S.**, Homozygous Hemoglobin D Punjab, *Acta Haematol.*, 43, 353, 1970.
297. **Smith, E. W. and Conley, C. L.**, Sickle cell-hemoglobin D disease, *Ann. Intern. Med.*, 50, 94, 1959.
298. **Wasi, P., Pootrakul, S., Na-Nakorn, S., Beale, D., and Lehmann, H.**, Haemoglobin D β Los Angeles (D Punjab, $\alpha_2\beta_2$ 121 Glu NH_2) in a Thai family, *Acta Haematol.*, 39, 151, 1968.
299. **Imamura, T. and Riggs, A.**, Identification of Hemoglobin Oak Ridge with Hemoglobin D Punjab (Los Angeles), *Biochem. Genet.*, 7, 127, 1972.
300. **Bowman, B. and Ingram, V. M.**, Abnormal human haemoglobins. VII. The comparison of normal human haemoglobin and haemoglobin D Chicago, *Biochim. Biophys. Acta*, 53, 569, 1961.
301. **Baglioni, C. and Lehmann, H.**, Chemical heterogeneity of Haemoglobin O, *Nature (London)*, 196, 229, 1962.
302. **Kamel, K., Hoerman, K., and Awny, A.**, Ethnological significance of Hemoglobin $\alpha 2\beta 2$ 121 Lys, *Am. J. Phys. Anthropol.*, 26, 107, 1970.
303. **Efremov, G. D., Duma, H., Ruvidic, R., Rolovic, Z., Wilson, J. B., and Huisman, T. H. J.**, Hemoglobin Beograd or $\alpha 2\beta 2$ 121 Glu → Val (GH4), *Biochim. Biophys. Acta*, 328, 81, 1973.
304. **Clegg, J. B., Weatherall, D. J., Wong Hock Boon, and Mustafa, D.**, Two new haemoglobin variants involving proline substitutions, *Nature (London)*, 22, 379, 1969.
305. **Miyagi, T., Ohba, Y., Yamamoto, K., Shibata, S., Iuchi, I., and Takenaka, H.**, Japanese haemoglobin variant, *Nature (London)*, 217, 89, 1968.
306. **Altay, C., Altinöz, N., Wilson, J. B., Bolch, K. C., and Huisman, T. H. J.**, Hemoglobin Hacettepe or $\alpha 2\beta 2$ 127 (H5) Gln → Glu, *Biochim. Biophys. Acta*, 434, 1, 1976.
307. **Blackwell, R. Q., Yang, Y.-J., and Wang, C.-C.**, Hemoglobin J Taichung: β129 Ala → Asp, *Biochim. Biophys. Acta*, 194, 1, 1969.
308. **Lorkin, P. A., Pietschmann, H., Braunsteiner, H., and Lehmann, H.**, Structure of Haemoglobin Wien β130 (H8) Tyrosine → Aspartic acid: an unstable haemoglobin variant, *Acta Haematol.*, 51, 351, 1974.
309. **Wade Cohen, P. T., Yates, A., Bellingham, A. J., and Huehns, E. R.**, Amino-acid substitution on the $\alpha 1\beta 1$ intersubunit contact of Haemoglobin Camden β131 (H9) Gln → Glu, *Nature New Biol.*, 243, 467, 1973.
310. **Ohba Y., Miyaji, T., Matsuoka, M., Ueda, S., Iuchi, I., and Shibata, S.**, Hemoglobin Tokuchi: β131 glutamine → glutamic acid, an example of Hb Camden in Japan, *Acta Haematol. Jpn.*, 38, 1, 1975.
311. **Brennan, S. O., Arnold, B., Fleming, P., and Carrell, R. W.**, A new unstable Haemoglobin, β134 Val → Glu, *Proc. N. Z. Med. J.*, 85, 398, 1977.
312. **Marti, H. R., Winterhalter, K. H., Di Iorio, E. E., Lorkin, P. A., and Lehmann, H.**, Hb Altdorf $\alpha 2\beta 2$ 135(H13) Ala → Pro: a new electrophoretically silent unstable haemoglobin variant from Switzerland, *FEBS Lett.*, 63, 193, 1976.
313. **Minnich, V., Hill, R. J., Khuri, P. D., and Anderson, M. E.**, Hemoglobin Hope: a beta chain variant, *Blood*, 25, 830, 1965.
314. **Tentori, L., Carta Sorcini, M., and Bucella, C.**, Hemoglobin Abruzzo: Beta 143 (H21) His → Arg, *Clin. Chim. Acta*, 38, 258, 1972.
315. **Bromberg, P. A., Alben, J. O., Bare, G. H., Balcerzak, S. P., Jones, R. T., Brimhall, B., and Padilla, F.**, Hemoglobin Little Rock [β143 His → Gln; (H21)]. A high oxygen affinity haemoglobin variant with unique properties, *Nature New Biol.*, 243, 177, 1973.
316. **Jensen, M., Oski, F. A., Nathan, D. G., and Bunn, H. F.**, Hemoglobin Syracuse [$\alpha 2\beta 2$ 143 (H21) His → Pro], a new high-affinity variant detected by special electrophoretic methods, *J. Clin. Invest.*, 55, 469, 1975.
317. **Zak, S. J., Brimhall, B., Jones, R. T., and Kaplan, M. E.**, Hemoglobin Andrew-Minneapolis $\alpha 2A\beta 2$ 144 Lys → Asn: a new high-oxygen-affinity mutant human hemoglobin, *Blood*, 44, 543, 1974.

318. Hayashim, A., Stamatoyannopoulos, G., Yoshida, A., and Adamson, J., Haemoglobin Rainier: β145 (HC2) tyrosine → cysteine and Haemoglobin Bethesda: β145 (HC2) Tyrosine → Histidine, *Nature New Biol.*, 230, 264, 1971.
319. Kleckner, H. B., Wilson, J. B., Lindeman, J. G., Stevens, P. D., Niazi G., Hunter, E., Chen, C. J., and Huisman, T. H. J., Hemoglobin Fort Gordon or α2β2 145 Tyr → Asp, a new high-oxygen-affinity-hemoglobin variant, *Biochim. Biophys. Acta*, 400, 343, 1975.
320. Charache, S., Brimhall, B., and Jones, R. T., Polycythemia produced by Hemoglobin Osler [β145 (HC2) Tyr → Asp], *Johns Hopkins Med. J.*, 136, 132, 1975.
321. Gacon, G., Wajcman, H., and Labie, D., Structural and functional study of Hb Nancy β145 (HC2) Tyr → Asp: a high oxygen affinity hemoglobin, *FEBS Lett.*, 56, 39, 1975.
322. Winslow, R. M., Swenberg, M.-L., Gross, E., Chervenick, P. A., Buchman, R. R., and Anderson, W. F., Hemoglobin McKees Rocks (α2β2 145 Tyr → Term): a human "nonsense" mutation leading to a shortened β-chain, *J. Clin. Invest.*, 57, 772, 1976.
323. Perutz, M. F., del Pulsinelli, P., Ten Eyck, L., Kilmartin, J. V., Shibata, S., Iuchi, I., Miyaji, T., and Hamilton, H. B., Haemoglobin Hiroshima and the mechanisms of the alkaline Bohr effect, *Nature New Biol.*, 232, 147, 1971.
324. Barem, G. H., Bromberg, P. A., Alben, J. O., Brimhall, B., Jones, R. T., Mints, S., and Rother, I., Altered C-terminal salt bridges in Haemoglobin York cause high oxygen affinity, *Nature (London)*, 259, 155, 1976.
325. Wajcman, H., Kilmartin, J. V., Najman, A., and Labie, D., Hemoglobin Cochin-Port-Royal consequences of the replacement of the β chain C-terminal by an arginine, *Biochim. Biophys. Acta*, 400, 354, 1975.
326. Lam, H., Wilson, J. B., Harris, H., Gravely, M., and Huisman, T. H. J., Hemoglobin Alamo [$\alpha_2\beta_2$ 19 (B1) Asn → Asp] *Hemoglobin*, 1, 703, 1977.
327. Jones, R. T., Brimhall, B., Huehns, E. R., and Barnicot, N. A., Hemoglobin Sphakiã: a delta chain variant of hemoglobin A_2 from Crete, *Science*, 151, 1406, 1966.
328. Ranney, H. M., Jacobs, A. S., Ramot, B., and Bradley, T. B., Jr., Hemoglobin NYU, a delta chain variant, α2δ2 12 Lys, *J. Clin. Invest.*, 48, 2057, 1969.
329. Ball, E. W., Meynell, M. J., Beale, D., Kynoch, P., Lehmann, H., and Stretton, A. O. W., Haemoglobin A_2'; α2δ2 16 glycine → arginine, *Nature (London)*, 209, 1217, 1968.
330. Rieder, R. F., Clegg, J. B., Weiss, H. J., Christy, N. P., and Rabinowitz, R., Hemoglobin A_2-Roosevelt: α2δ2 20 Val → Glu, *Biochim. Biophys. Acta*, 439, 501, 1976.
331. Jones, R. T. and Brimhall, B., Structural characterization of two δ chain variants, *J. Biol. Chem.*, 242, 5141, 1967.
332. Sharma, R. S., Harding, D. L., Wong, S. C., Wilson, J. B., Gravely, M. E., and Huisman, T. H. J., A new δ chain variant, Haemoglobin A_2-Melbourne or α2δ2 43 Glu → Lys (CD2), *Biochim. Biophys. Acta*, 359, 233, 1974.
333. Lie-Injo, L. E., Pribada, W., Boerma, F. W., Efremov, G. D., Wilson, J. B., Reynolds, C. A., and Huisman, T. H. J., Hemoglobin A_2-Indonesia or α2δ2 69 (E13) Gly → Arg, *Biochim. Biophys. Acta*, 229, 335, 1971.
334. Sharma, R. S., Williams, L., Wilson, J. B., and Huisman, T. H. J., Hemoglobin A_2-Coburg or α2δ2 116 Arg → His (G18), *Biochim. Biophys. Acta*, 393, 379, 1975.
335. DeJong, W. W. W. and Bernini, L. F., Haemoglobin Babinga (δ136 glycine → aspartic acid): a new delta chain variant, *Nature (London)*, 219, 1360, 1968.
336. Lie-Injo, L. E., Kamuzora, H., and Lehmann, H., Haemoglobin F Malaysia: α2γ2 1 (NA1) glycine → cysteine: 136 Glycine, *J. Med. Genet.*, 11, 25, 1974.
337. Jenkins, G. C., Beale, D., Black, A. J., Huntsman, G. R., and Lehmann, H., Haemoglobin F Texas I (α2γ2 5 Glu → Lys): a variant of Haemoglobin F, *Br. J. Hematol.*, 13, 252, 1967.
338. Ahern, E. J., Wiltshire, B. G., and Lehmann, H., Further characterization of Haemoglobin F Texas I γ5 glutamic acid → lysine; γ136 alanine, *Biochim. Biophys. Acta*, 271, 61, 1972.
339. Larkin, I. L. M., Baker, T., Lorkin, P. A., Lehmann, H., Black, A. J., and Huntsman, R. G., Haemoglobin F Texas II (α2γ2 6 Glu → Lys). The second of the Haemoglobin F Texas variants, *Br. J. Haematol.*, 14, 233, 1968.
340. Carrell, R. W., Owen, M. C., Anderson, R., and Berry, E., Haemoglobin F Auckland Gγ7 Asp → Asn — further evidence for multiple genes for the gamma chain, *Biochim. Biophys. Acta*, 365, 323, 1974.
341. Loukopoulos, D., Kaltsoya, A., and Fessas, Ph., On the chemical abnormality of Hb "Alexandra" a fetal hemoglobin variant, *Blood*, 33, 114, 1969.
342. Brennan, S. O., Smith, Merran B., and Carrell, R. W., Haemoglobin F Melbourne $^G\gamma$ 16 Gly → Arg and Haemoglobin F Carlton $^G\gamma$ 121 Glu → Lys, *Biochim. Biophys. Acta*, 490, 452, 1977.
343. Lie-Injo, L. E., Wiltshire, B. G., and Lehmann, H., Structural identification of Haemoglobin F Kuala Lumpur [α2γ2 22 (B4) Asp → Gly: (136Ala)], *Biochim. Biophys. Acta*, 322, 224, 1973.

344. Ahern, E. J., Jones, R. T., Brimhall, B., and Gray, R. H., Haemoglobin F Jamaica ($\alpha 2\gamma 2$ 61 Lys → Glu; 136Ala), *Br. J. Haematol.*, 18, 369, 1970.
345. Ahern, E., Holder, W., Ahern, V., Serjeant, G. R., Serjeant, B. E., Forbes, M., Brimhall, B., and Jones, R. T., Haemoglobin F Victoria Jubilee ($\alpha 2 A\gamma 2$ 80 Asp → Tyr), *Biochim. Biophys. Acta*, 393, 188, 1975.
346. Schneider, R. G., Haggard, M. E., Gustavson, L. P., Brimhall, B., and Jones, R. T., Genetic haemoglobin abnormalities in about 9000 black and 7000 white newborns: Haemoglobin F Dickinson ($A\gamma 97$ His → Arg), a new variant, *Br. J. Haematol.*, 28, 515, 1974.
347. Cauchi, M. N., Clegg, J. B., and Weatherall, D. J., Haemoglobin F (Malta) a new foetal haemoglobin variant with a high incidence in Maltese infants, *Nature (London)*, 223, 311, 1969.
348. Sacker, L. S., Beale, D., Black, A. J., Huntsman, R. G., Lehmann, H., and Lorkin, P. A., Haemoglobin F Hull ($\gamma 121$ glutamic acid → lysine), homologous with Haemoglobins O and O Indonesia, *Br. Med. J.*, 3, 531, 1967.
349. Brimhall, B., Vedvick, T. S., Jones, R. T., Ahern, E., Palomino, E., and Ahern, V., Haemoglobin F Port Royal ($\alpha 2 G\gamma$ 125 Glu → Ala), *Br. J. Haematol.*, 27, 313, 1973.
350. Lee-Potter, J. P., Deacon-Smith, R. A., Simpkiss, M. J., Kamuzora, H., and Lehmann, H., A new cause of haemolytic anemia in the newborn. A description of an unstable fetal haemoglobin: F Poole, $\alpha 2 G\gamma 2$ 130 tryptophan → glycine, *J. Clin. Pathol.*, 28, 317, 1975.
351. Barnabas, J. and Muller, C. J., Haemoglobin Lepore Hollandia, *Nature (London)*, 194, 931, 1962.
352. Ostertag, W. and Smith, E. W., Hemoglobin-Lepore Baltimore, a third type of a $\delta\beta$ crossover ($\delta 50$, $\beta 86$),*Eur. J. Biochem.*, 10, 371, 1969.
353. Baglioni, C., The fusion of two peptide chains in Hemoglobin Lepore and its interpretation as a genetic deletion, *Proc. Natl. Acad. Sci. U.S.A.*, 48, 1880, 1962.
354. Lehmann, H. and Charlesworth, D., Observation on Haemoglobin P (Congo type), *Biochem. J.*, 119, 43, 1970.
355. Badr, F. M., Lorkin, P. A., and Lehmann, H., Haemoglobin P-Nilotic; containing a β-δ chain, *Nature New Biol.*, 242, 107, 1973.
356. Huisman, T. H. J., Wrightstone, R. N., Wilson, J. B., Schroeder, W. A., and Kendall, A. G., Hemoglobin Kenya, the product of fusion of γ and β polypeptide chains, *Arch. Biochem. Biophys.*, 153, 850, 1972.
357. Clegg, J. B., Weatherall, D. J., and Milner, P. F., Haemoglobin Constant Spring — a chain termination mutant, *Nature (London)*, 234, 337, 1971.
358. Clegg, J. B., Weatherall, D. J., Contopolou-Griva, I., Caroutsos, K., Poungouras, P., and Tsevrenis, H., Haemoglobin Icaria, a new chain-termination mutant which causes α thalassemia, *Nature (London)*, 251, 245, 1974.
359. DeJong, W. W. W., Meera Khan, P., and Bernini, L. F., Hemoglobin Koya Dora: high frequency of a chain termination mutant, *Am. J. Hum. Genet.*, 27, 81, 1975.
360. Flatz, G., Kinderlerer, J. L., Kilmartin, J. V., and Lehmann, H., Haemoglobin Tak: a variant with additional residues at the end of the β-chains, *Lancet*, 10, 732, 1971.
361. Imai, K. and Lehmann, H., The oxygen affinity of Haemoglobin Tak, a variant with an elongated β chain, *Biochim. Biophys. Acta*, 412, 288, 1975.
362. Lehmann, H., Casey, R., Lang, A., Stathopoulou, R., Imai, K., Tuchinda, S., Vinai, P., and Flatz, G., Haemoglobin Tak: a β-chain elongation, *Br. J. Haematol.*, Suppl. 31, 119, 1975.
363. Seid-Akhavan, M., Winter, W. P., Abramson, R. K., and Rucknagel, D. L., Hemoglobin Wayne: a frameshift mutation detected in human hemoglobin alpha chains, *Proc. Natl. Acad. Sci. U.S.A.*, 73, 882, 1976.
364. Bunn, H. F., Schmidt, G. J., Haney, D. N., and Dluhy, R. G., Hemoglobin Cranston, an unstable variant having an elongated β chain due to nonhomologous crossover between two normal β chain genes, *Proc. Natl. Acad. Sci. U.S.A.*, 72, 3609, 1975.
365. Huisman, T. H. J., Wilson, J. B., Gravely, M., and Hubbard, M., Hemoglobin Grady: the first example of a variant with elongated chains due to an insertion of residues, *Proc. Natl. Acad. Sci. U.S.A.*, 71, 3270, 1974.
366. Tentori, L., personal communication, Int. Comm. Stand. Hematol., Kyoto, 1976.
367. Dejong, W. W. W., Went, L. N., and Bernini, L. F., Haemoglobin Leiden: deletion of $\beta 6$ or 7 glutamic acid, *Nature (London)*, 220, 788, 1968.
368. Cohen-Solal, M., Blouquit, Y., Garel, M. C., Thillet, J., Gaillard, L., Creyssel, R., Gibaud, A., and Rosa, J., Haemoglobin Lyon [β17-18(A14-15) Lys-Val → O] determination by sequenator analysis, *Biochim. Biophys. Acta*, 351, 306, 1974.
369. Jones, R. T., Brimhall, B., Huisman, T. H. J., Kleihauer, E., and Betke, K., Hemoglobin Freiburg: abnormal hemoglobin due to deletion of a single amino acid residue *Science*, 154, 1024, 1966.
370. Praxedes, H. and Lehmann, H., Haemoglobin Niteroi — A New Unstable Variant, Proc. 14th Int. Congr. Hematol., Sao Paulo, Brazil, 1972.

371. **Shibata, S., Miyaji, T., Ueda, S., Matsuoka, M., Iuchi, I., Yamada, K., and Shinkai, N.,** Hemoglobin Tochigi (Beta 56-59 deleted). A new unstable hemoglobin discovered in a Japanese family, *Proc. Jpn. Acad.,* 46, 440, 1970.
372. **Wajcman, H., Labie, D., and Schapira, G.,** Two new hemoglobin variants with deletion. Hemoglobin Tours: Thr β87 (F3) deleted and Hemoglobin St. Antoine: Gly-Leu β74-75 (E18-19) deleted. Consequences for oxygen affinity and protein stability, *Biochim. Biophys. Acta,* 295, 495, 1973.
373. **Bradley, T. B., Wohl, R. C., and Rieder, R. F.,** Hemoglobin Gun Hill: deletion of five amino acid residues and impaired heme-globin binding, *Science,* 157, 1581, 1967.
374. **Lutcher, C. L., Wilson, J. B., Gravely, M. E., Stevens, P. D., Chen, C. J., Lindeman, J. G., Wong, S. C., Miller, A., Gottleib, M., and Huisman, T. H. J.,** Hb Leslie, an unstable hemoglobin due to deletion of glutaminyl residue β131 (H9) occurring in association with β^0-thalassemia, Hb C, and Hb S, *Blood,* 47, 99, 1976.
375. **Moo-Penn, W. F., Jue, D. L., Bechtel, K. C., Johnson, M. H., Bemis, E., Brosious, E., and Schmidt, R. M.,** Hemoglobin Deaconess, a new deletion mutant: β131 (H9) glutamine deleted, *Biochem. Biophys. Res. Comm.,* 65, 8, 1975.
376. **Casey, R., Lang, A., Lehmann, H., and Shinton, N. K.,** Double Heterozygosity for two unstable haemoglobins; Hb Sydney [β67 E11 (Val → Ala)] and Hb Coventry [β141 (H19) Leu Deleted], *Br. J. Haematol.,* 33, 143, 1976.
377. **Bookchin, R. M., Nagel, R. L., and Ranney, H. M.,** Structure and properties of Hemoglobin C Harlem, a human hemoglobin variant with amino acid substitutions in 2 residues of the β-polypeptide chain, *J. Biol. Chem.,* 242, 248, 1967.
378. **Lang, A., Lehmann, H., McCurdy, P. R., and Pierce, L.,** Identification of Haemoglobin C Georgetown, *Biochim. Biophys. Acta,* 278, 57, 1972.
379. **Adams, J. G. and Heller, P.,** Hemoglobin Arlington Park (β6 Glu → Lys, 95 Lys → Glu): electrophoretically "Silent" hemoglobin variant with two amino acid substitutions in the same polypeptide chain, *Blood,* 42, 990, 1973.
380. **Blackwell, R. Q., Wong Hock Boon, Liu, C.-S., and Weng, M. I.,** Hemoglobin J Singapore: α78 Asn → Asp; α79 Ala → Gly, *Biochim. Biophys. Acta,* 278, 482, 1972.
381. **Goossens, M., Garel, M. C., Auvinet, J., Basset, P., Gomes, P. F., and Rosa, J.,** Hemoglobin C Ziguinchor $\alpha_2A\beta_26$ (A3) Glu → Val, β58 (E2) Pro → Arg: the second sickling variant with amino acid substitutions in 2 residues of the β polypeptide chain, *FEBS Lett.,* 58, 149 , 1975.
382. **Moo-Penn, W. F., Schmidt, R. M., Jue, D. L., Bechtel, K. C., Wright, J. M., Horne, M. K., III, Haycraft, G. L., Roth, E. F., and Nagel, R. L.,** Hemoglobin S Travis. A Sickling Hemoglobin with two amino acid substitutions [β6 (A3) glutamic acid → valine and β142 (H20) alanine → valine], *Eur. J. Biochem.,* 77, 561, 1977.
383. **Lutcher, C. L., Wilson, J. B., Gravely, M. E., Stevens, P. D., Chen, C. J., Linderman, J. G., Wong, S. C., Miller, A., Gottleib, M., and Huisman, T. H. J.,** Hb Leslie, an unstable hemoglobin due to deletion of Glutaminyl residue β131 (H9) occurring in association with β^0-thalassemia, Hb C, and Hb S, *Blood,* 47, 99, 1976.
384. **Puett, D., Paniker, N. V., Lin, K. D., Flexner, J. M., Wasserman, B. K., and Krantz, S. B.,** Hemoglobin Vanderbilt [β 89 (F5) Ser → Arg]: a new hemoglobin mutant with increased oxygen affinity and lowered response to 2, 3-diphosphoglycerate, *Clin. Res.,* 25, 53(Abstr.), 1977.
385. **Huehns, E. R.,** The unstable hemoglobins, *Bull. Soc. Chim. Bio.,* 52, 1131, 1970.
386. **Benesch, R., Edilji, R., and Benesch, R. E.,** Oxygenation properties of hemoglobin variants with substitutions near the polyphosphate binding site, *Biochim. Biophys. Acta,* 393, 368, 1975.
387. **Ramot, B., Rotem, J., Rahbar, S., Jacobs, A. S., Uden, L., and Ranney, H. M.,** Hemoglobin D Punjab in a Bulgarian Jewish family, *Isr. J. Med. Sci.,* 5, 1066, 1969.
388. **Miyaji, T., Ohba, Y., Matsuoka, M., Kudoh, H., Asano, M., Yamamoto, K., and Satoh, T.,** Hemoglobin Karatsu; Beta 120 (GH3) lysine → asparagine. An example of Hb Riyadh in Japan, *Hemoglobin,* 1, 461, 1977.
389. **Garel, M. C., Goossens, M., Oudart, J. L., Blouquit, Y., Thillet, J., and Rosa, J.,** Hemoglobin Dakar = Hb Grady; demonstration by a new approach to the analysis of the tryptic core region of the α chain and oxygen equilibrium properties, *Biochim. Biophys. Acta,* 453, 459, 1976.
390. **Thillet, J., Blouquit, Y., Perrone, F., and Rosa, J.,** Hemoglobin Pontoise α63 Ala → Asp (E12). A new fast moving variant, *Biochim. Biophys. Acta,* 491, 16, 1977.
391. **Martinez, G., Lima, F., and Colombo, B.,** Haemoglobin J Guantanamo [$\alpha_2\beta_2$ 128 (H6) Ala → Asp]. A new fast unstable haemoglobin found in a Cuban family, *Biochim. Biophys. Acta,* 491, 1, 1977.
392. **Alberti, R., Tentori, L., Marinucci, M., Borghesi, V.,** Hb A_2-Adria [δ 51 Pro → Arg (D2)]: a new δ-chain variant found in association with β-thalassemia, *Hemoglobin,* 2, 171, 1978.
393. **Braconnier, F., Gacon, G., Thillet, J., Wajcman, H., Soria, J., Maigret, P., Labie, D., and Rosa, J.,** Hemoglobin Fort de France [α_2^{45} (CD3) His → Arg β_2] a new variant with increasing oxygen affinity, *Biochim. Biophys. Acta,* 493, 228, 1977.

HEMOGLOBINOMETRY

O. W. van Assendelft

Introduction

"Although the determination of the amount of haemoglobin is one of the most important of all chemical tests of the blood, yet as a rule it is one which is determined with less care and by methods more inaccurate than those in use for any other constituent of the body."[1]

A great many more or less inaccurate methods have indeed been used to determine the total hemoglobin concentration (c_{Hb}) in blood. A summary is given in Table 1.

Reviews of the literature on the methods given in Table 1 were published in 1953, 1964, and 1970.[18-20] Errors ascribed to some of the more widely used methods are summarized in Table 2.

Measurement of c_{Hb} after Conversion of Hemoglobins to HiCN

In 1958, the Panel on the Establishment of a Hemoglobin Standard, Division of Medical Sciences, National Research Council—National Academy of Sciences, reviewed several photometric methods in current use for the determination of c_{Hb} and concluded, for several reasons, that c_{Hb} was best determined as HiCN. "The HiCN method involves dilution with a single reagent. All forms of hemoglobin likely to occur in circulatory blood, with the exception of sulfhemoglobin, are determined. The color is suitable for measurement in filter as well as in narrow-band spectrophotometers, because its absorption band at λ = 540 nm is broad and relatively flat. Standards prepared from either crystalline hemoglobin or washed erythrocytes, and stored in a brown glass container and in sterile condition are stable for at least 9 months (change 2%)."[20]

A value of 11.5 was adopted for the quarter millimolar extinction coefficient of HiCN at λ = 540 nm (ε^{540}_{HiCN}). After extensive investigations, a value of 11.0 was established during the IX European Congress of Haematology, by the Standardizing

Table 1
PROPERTIES OF BLOOD, AND METHODS UPON WHICH THE DETERMINATION OF C_{Hb} HAS BEEN BASED

Property	Measurement of	Ref.
Physical	Specific gravity	2
	Refractive index	3
Chemical composition	Hemoglobin iron	4
Reversible gas-binding capacity	Oxygen	5
	Carbon monoxide	6
Spectral characteristics	Hemoglobin (Hb)	7
	Oxyhemoglobin (HbO_2)	8,9,10
	Carboxyhemoglobin (HbCo)	11
	Hemiglobin (Hi, methemoglobin)	12
	Hemiglobin azide (HiN_3)	13
	Hemiglobin cyanide (HiCN, cyanmethemoglobin)	14
	Alkaline hematin	15
	Acid hematin	16
	Pyridine hemochromogens	17

Table 2
ERRORS ASCRIBED TO VARIOUS METHODS USED FOR THE DETERMINATION OF HEMOGLOBIN CONCENTRATION

Method	Inaccuracy (%)	Ref.
O_2-binding capacity	3	21
CO-binding capacity	2	22
Hemoglobin Fe using atomic absorption photometry	Up to 15	23
Spectrophotometry, as Hb	Up to 10	24
Spectrophotometry, as HbO_2	2—4	25
Acid hematin method	Up to 40	20

Committee of the European Society of Haematology, in 1963.[26] This value has since been confirmed by a number of investigators using not only Fe analysis but also N analysis and, as shown by Itano,[27] by C analysis (Table 3).

In 1964, the International Committee for Standardization of Hematology (ICSH) adopted the HiCN method for the determination of c_{Hb}. An international Expert Panel on Hemoglobinometry was established with the task of drawing up recommendations for hemoglobinometry and controlling the HiCN reference solutions (prepared by the Dutch Institute of Public Health on behalf of ICSH) to be used as the international HiCN reference solution. The recommendations for hemoglobinometry, with the HiCN method, were finally adopted at the XI International Congress of Haematology in 1966.[38] The international HiCN reference solution was established by the World Health Organization as the WHO International HiCN Reference Preparation, in 1968.[39]

The Standardized HiCN Method

In the HiCN method, 0.02 mℓ of blood is mixed with 5.0 mℓ of a reagent containing $K_3Fe(CN)_6$, KCN, KH_2PO_4, and Sterox® SE.[40] Hemoglobin is first oxidized to hemiglobin (Hi) by the action of the $K_3Fe(CN)_6$, after which CN^- is taken up to form HiCN. KH_2PO_4 is added to allow these reactions to take place at a pH at which the conversion time is sufficiently short. A nonionic detergent has been added to suppress turbidity, as well as to facilitate hemolysis. The absorbance of the resulting solution is then measured at $\lambda = 540$ nm with a filter photometer or a spectrophotometer, and the hemoglobin concentration is read from a calibration graph or calculated.

The sequence in the standardized HiCN method is

1. Pipette 5.0 mℓ of reagent into tube.
2. Add 0.02 mℓ blood.
3. Mix well and wait 5 min.
4. Measure at 540 nm with (spectro)photometer.
5. Read or calculate hemoglobin content.

The Reagent

The reagent[40] is made up as follows: dissolve 200 mg $K_3Fe(CN)_6$, 50 mg KCN, 140 mg KH_2PO_4, and 0.5 mℓ Sterox® SE* in distilled or deionized water and make up to 1000 mℓ. When $KH_2PO_4nH_2O$ is used, the amount must be increased accordingly. The

* Hartman-Leddon Co., Philadelphia.

Table 3
ε^{540}_{HiCN} VALUES AS REPORTED BY DIFFERENT AUTHORS. BASED ON IRON, NITROGEN, OR CARBON DETERMINATIONS[a]

Author	Material	ε^{540}_{HiCN}	$s/(n)^{1/2}$	n	Method
Meyer-Wilmes and	Horse Hb	11.0	0.04	12	Fe; o-phenanthroline
Remmer(28)	Horse Hb	11.0	0.04	12	Fe; $TiCl_3$
Remmer (29)	Human whole blood	11.09	0.03	11	Fe; $TiCl_3$
	Human whole blood	11.19	0.065	4	Fe; complexon
Minkowski and Swierczewski (30)	Fetal whole blood	*11.15*[b]	—	5	Fe; o-phenanthroline
Zijlstra and van Kampen (31)	Human Hb, toluene hemolysis	10.99	0.01	123	Fe; α, α′-dipyridyl
		10.94	0.03	35	Fe; α, α′-dipyridyl
		11.05	0.02	101	Fe; $TiCl_3$
Wootton and Blevin (32)	Human Hb, toluene hemolysis	*10.68*[c]	0.04	14	Fe; ferric perchlorate
van Oudheusden et al.	Human whole blood	10.99	0.05	10	Fe; α, α′-dipyridyl
(33)	Human whole blood	11.06	0.08	8	Fe; α, α′-dipyridyl
Salvati et al. (34)	Human Hb purified on CMC column	10.95	0.03	46	Fe; α, α′-dipyridyl
Tentori et al. (35)	Human Hb purified on CMC column	10.90	0.05	55	N analysis
Morningstar et al. (36)	Human whole blood	11.02	0.03	10	Fe; X-ray emission spectrography
	Human washed cells	10.97	0.07	6	
Stigbrand (37)	Human Hb purified on CMC or Sephadex column or by dialysis against Na_2-EDTA	11.00	0.02	55	Fe; sulfosalicylic acid
Itano (27)	Human Hb A purified by chromatography	10.88	0.04	16	C analysis

[a] $s/(n)^{1/2}$ = standard error of the mean; n = number of determinations. Overall mean value for ε^{540}_{HiCN} = 10.99, calculated using the equation

$$\bar{x}_g = \frac{1}{n_{tot}} \cdot \sum_i n_i \cdot \bar{x}_i$$

Standard error of the overall mean $S_{\bar{x}_g}$ = 0.01, calculated using the equation

$$S_{\bar{x}_g} = \left[\sum_{i=1}^{15} n_i \cdot s_i^2\right]^{1/2} \div n_{tot}$$

where n_i = number of determinations in the ith series; n_{tot} = total number of determinations; s_i = standard error of the ith series of determinations.

[b] Excluded from calculation of $\bar{x}_g$ and $s_{\bar{x}_g}$ because $s/(n)^{1/2}$ value was not published.

[c] Excluded from calculation of $\bar{x}_g$ and $s_{\bar{x}_g}$ because the series differs more than three times the standard error of the mean from the total mean value.

reagent must be clear and pale yellow, and the pH must lie between 7.0 and 7.4. When measured in a spectrophotometer at λ = 540 nm against water as blank, A^{540} must be zero. When kept in a well-stoppered bottle of brown borosilicate glass, the reagent will keep for several months.

Quality grade, dry chemicals should be used in preparing the reagent. Although toxic, KCN in the reagent is used in such amount that approximately 4 ℓ of reagent would have to be consumed for cyanide poisoning to occur. Sterox® SE, a nonionic detergent, is added to enhance hemolysis and to prevent turbidity by plasma protein precipitation. Should Sterox® SE not be available, Nonidet P40* may be used (1 mℓ/ℓ reagent).

In Sweden, good results have been obtained with Berol L-048.[41] At present, two

* Shell Int. Chem. Co., The Hague, the Netherlands.

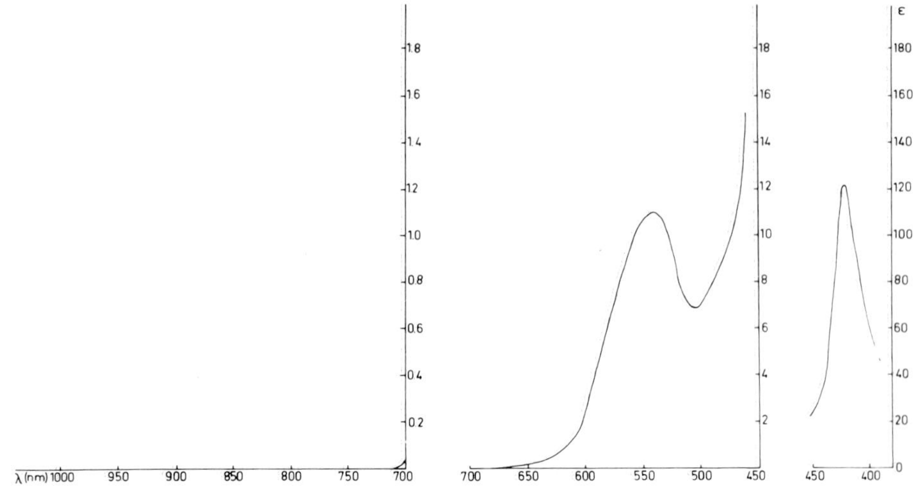

FIGURE 1. Absorption spectrum of International Haemiglobincyanide Reference Solution, based on data obtained with three different spectrophotometers. ICSH purity requirements state no absorption of light at wave-length > 710 nm (A^{750}_{HiCN} ≤ 0.002 per cm light path length) and 1.59 ≤ A^{540}/ ≤ 1.63.

more detergents are available that are suitable to replace Sterox® SE: Saponic 218* and Triton X-100. Both have been tested with samples of normal blood, as well as with samples containing increased amounts of α-globulins. They have been shown to suppress turbidity of the resulting HiCN solutions to the same degree as Sterox® SE.[20] However, in some cases (e.g., with paraproteins having a high α-globulin content) the resulting HiCN solutions will be so turbid that values will be erroneously high.[42] In such cases the solutions may become clear with the addition of a few drops of NH_4OH 1 n. Filtration through a membrane filter (e.g., Millipore®,** mean pore size 0.22 μ [type GSWP]) is also quite effective.

It has been reported that the addition of NaCl to the reagent may prevent development of turbidity when blood samples contain increased amounts of plasma proteins.[43]

To ensure complete conversion of hemoglobins to HiCN at pH 7.0 to 7.4, 3 min must be allowed between mixing the sample with the reagent and measuring. The conversion of HbCO to HiCN takes longer, about 30 min.[44,45] However, even when the samples contain up to 25% HbCO, errors made when measuring after 3 min are slight, certainly not over 7%.[42]

Instead of the reagent described, "Drabkin's solution", containing 200 mg $K_3Fe(CN)_6$, 50 mg KCN, and 1000 mg Na_2CO_3 per liter of distilled water, is still often used. This solution is not recommended because the pH is rather high (8.5), and as a result, conversion of hemoglobins takes about 20 min; conversion of HbCO to HiCN at least 90 min. Moreover, HiCN solutions are turbid far more often with this solution than with the reagent described.

Hemiglobin Cyanide Reference Solutions

In 1962, Zijlstra and van Kampen[46] described the preparation of a HiCN reference solution. The hemoglobin content (c_{Hb}) of this reference solution is calculated from spectrophotometric measurements, and is based on a value of 11.0 for the millimolar extinction coefficient of HiCN at λ = 540 nm ($\varepsilon^{540}_{HiCN} = 11.0$).[31,47] Preliminary studies showed that properly ampoulated HiCN solutions stored at 4°C remain stable for at least 3 years.[48,49]

Figure 1 shows the absorption spectrum of a pure HiCN solution.

* ALCOAC INC., Baltimore, Md., 21226

** Millipore Filter Corp., Bedford, Mass., 01730

In 1964, the Dutch National Institute of Public Health (RIV) started preparing HiCN reference solutions[50] on behalf of the International Committee for Standardization in Haematology (ICSH), to be issued as international HiCN reference solutions.[38] Such a solution was accepted in 1968 by the World Health Organization (WHO) as International HiCN Reference Preparation.[39] RIV has been designated holder of this preparation by WHO and issues international HiCN reference solutions, available on request.[51] A new batch of such reference solutions is made yearly. Content and purity[38] are determined and checked by ICSH-appointed reference laboratories in Germany, Great Britain, Italy, Japan, the Netherlands, and the U.S. The solutions are issued some 9 months after preparation and, at present, are valid for 2 years; thus, two batches are available simultaneously.

Stability of HiCN Reference Solutions

All batches of international HiCN reference solutions issued have been stored at 4°C and have been checked regularly. Measurements have been performed with an Optica CF_4 grating spectrophotometer at λ = 750, 540, and 504 nm (total bandwidth 0.5, 0.13, and 0.13 nm, respectively) in a layer thickness of 1.000 cm against water as blank. Wavelength of the instrument was calibrated regularly with the mercury emission spectrum, and optical density with a certified (Natl. Bureau of Standards) Carbon Yellow filter.[52] The results obtained for HiCN solutions followed for more than 3 years after the date of preparation are shown in Table 4. Because no values greater than 0.002 have been encountered for A^{750}_{HiCN},[38] these measurements have not been included. The results (Table 4) show that, when stored in the dark at 4°C, properly prepared and ampoulated HiCN reference solutions seem to be stable for at least 10 years.

Evaluation of c_{Hb} from Spectrophotometric Absorbance Reading

When a spectrophotometer is used to measure the absorbance of HiCN solutions, the c_{Hb} is calculated from:

$$c_{Hb}\ (g/\ell) = \frac{A^{540}_{HiCN}}{\epsilon^{540}_{HiCN}} \frac{\times F \times M}{\times 1 \times 1000}$$

where A^{540}_{HiCN} = absorbance of the solution at λ = 540 nm, F = dilution factor, M = relative molecular mass of hemoglobin monomere: 64 458/4,[38] ε^{540}_{HiCN} = millimolar extinction coefficient of HiCN (one heme group) at λ = 540 nm: 11.0, l = light path length in cm (usually 1,000), and 1000 = conversion factor mg to g. For a dilution factor of 251 (0.02 mℓ blood plus 5.0 mℓ reagent):

$$\frac{F \times M}{\epsilon^{540}_{HiCN} \times 1 \times 1000} = \frac{251 \times \frac{64458}{4}}{11.0 \times 1.000 \times 1000}$$

$$\approx 368 \quad \text{and}$$

$$c_{Hb}\ (g/\ell) = A^{540}_{HiCN} \times 368$$

Error Possibility in the HiCN Method

1. Errors in measurement:
   Use of noncalibrated instruments

Table 4
STABILITY MEASUREMENTS OF INTERNATIONAL HiCN REFERENCE SOLUTIONS

Time		40400		60400		70400		80400		90400		00400		10400		20400		30400	
Years	Months	A^{540}	A^{540}/A^{504}	A^{540}	A^{540}/A^{504}	A^{540}	A^{540}/A^{504}	A^{540}	A^{540}/A^{504}	A^{540}	A^{540}/A^{504}	A^{540}	A^{540}/A^{504}	A^{540}	A^{540}/A^{504}	A^{540}	A^{540}/A^{504}	A^{540}	A^{540}/A^{504}
0	0	0.391	1.61	0.386	1.61	0.405	1.62	0.383	1.60	0.389	1.61	0.395	1.61	0.413	1.61	0.408	1.61	0.403	1.61
	3	—	—	0.387	1.61	—	—	0.381	1.60	0.389	1.61	0.395	1.61	0.413	1.60	0.408	1.61	0.402	1.61
0	6	—	—	0.387	1.61	0.404	1.62	0.386	1.61^5	0.388	1.62	0.396	1.61	0.415	1.61^5	0.408	1.61	0.403	1.62
	9	—	—	0.387	1.61	—	—	0.383	1.61	—	—	—	—	—	—	—	—	—	—
1	0	0.389	1.61	0.388	1.61	0.405	1.59^5	—	—	0.388	1.60	0.400	1.62	—	—	0.408	1.62	0.402	1.61
	3	—	—	—	—	0.403	1.61	—	—	—	—	—	—	0.414	1.61	—	—	0.401	1.61
1	6	0.391	1.61	—	—	0.407	1.62	0.386	1.61^5	0.389	1.62	0.398	1.62	0.414	1.60^5	—	—	0.403	1.60
	9	—	—	—	—	0.405	1.62	0.385	1.61	0.389	1.61	0.397	1.61	0.415	1.61	0.406	1.61	—	—
2	0	0.391	1.61	—	—	0.405	1.62	—	—	—	—	—	—	0.413	1.61	—	—	0.401	1.61
	3	—	—	—	—	0.406	1.62	—	—	0.390	1.61	0.396	1.62	—	—	—	—	—	—
2	6	0.390	1.61	0.387	1.61	0.404	1.62	0.386	1.61	—	—	0.393	1.60	0.412	1.61	0.404	1.61	0.400	1.61
	9	—	—	—	—	—	—	—	—	0.390	1.60^5	—	—	—	—	—	—	—	—
3	0	0.391	1.62	—	—	0.404	1.61	0.386	1.61	—	—	0.393	1.60	0.411	1.61	0.407	1.60	0.403	1.60
3	6	—	—	0.388	1.61	—	—	—	—	0.387	1.61	0.393	1.61	0.412	1.61	—	—	—	—
4	0	0.389	1.61	0.387	1.61	0.405	1.61	0.388	1.62	0.387	1.61	0.393	1.61	0.412	1.60	0.405	1.60	—	—
4	6	—	—	—	—	0.406	1.60^5	—	—	—	—	—	—	—	—	—	—	—	—
5	0	0.393	1.61	0.386	1.61	—	—	0.384	1.61	0.387	1.60	0.393	1.60	0.412	1.60	—	—	—	—
5	6	—	—	—	—	0.404	1.62	—	—	—	—	—	—	—	—	—	—	—	—
6	0	0.390	1.62	—	—	—	—	0.382	1.60	0.386	1.60	0.393	1.60	—	—	—	—	—	—
7	0	—	—	—	—	0.402	1.61	0.383	1.60	0.386	1.60	—	—	—	—	—	—	—	—
8	0	0.394	1.61	0.386	1.61	0.405	1.60	0.383	1.61	—	—	—	—	—	—	—	—	—	—
9	0	0.390	1.60	—	—	0.404	1.61	—	—	—	—	—	—	—	—	—	—	—	—
10	0	0.389	1.60	0.387	1.61	—	—	—	—	—	—	—	—	—	—	—	—	—	—
11	0	0.390	1.60	—	—	—	—	—	—	—	—	—	—	—	—	—	—	—	—
12	0	0.389	1.60	—	—	—	—	—	—	—	—	—	—	—	—	—	—	—	—

From van Assendelft, O. W., Buursma, A., Holtz, A. H., van Kampen, E. J., and Zijlstra, W. G., *Clin. Chim. Acta,* 70, 161, 1976. With permission.

Use of unclean or unmatched cuvettes
Diluted samples turbid

2. Errors in the conversion to HiCN:
   Use of aged or faultily prepared reagent
   Time lapse to measurement too short
3. Errors in diluting:
   Use of noncalibrated pipettes (5.0 $m\ell$)
   Failure to wipe off excess blood
   Failure to rinse with reagent
   Insufficient cleaning of pipettes
4. Errors in sampling:
   Use of noncalibrated pipettes (0.2 $m\ell$)
   Nonfree-bleeding capillary puncture

The reagent must not be frozen,[53-55] since in that case $K_3Fe(CN)_6$ is converted to $K_4Fe(CN)_6$,[56] and oxidation of the samples to Hi does not take place. When the reagent is kept in polyethylene bottles, loss of CN^- has occurred, resulting in the formation of Hi only, with c_{Hb} values measured up to 50% too low.

REFERENCES

1. **Campbell, R. D.**, Haemoglobinometry, *Br. Med. J.*, 2, 747, 1941.
2. **Barbour, H. G. and Hamilton, W. F.**, The falling drop method for determining specific gravity, *J. Biol. Chem.*, 69, 625, 1926.
3. **Howard, F. H.**, The determination of refractivity of hemoglobin in solution, *J. Biol. Chem.*, 41, 537, 1920.
4. **Herrmann, E., Lang, W., and Stamm, D.**, Hämoglobinbestimmung durch absorptionsflammenspektrophotometrische Eisenanalyse (Atomabsorption) im Gesamtblut, *Blut*, 11, 135, 1965.
5. **van Slyke, D. D. and Neill, J. M.**, The determination of gases in blood and other solutions by vacuum extraction and manometric measurement, *J. Biol. Chem.*, 61, 523, 1924.
6. **van Slyke, D. D. and Salvesen, H. A.**, The determination of carbon monoxide in blood, *J. Biol. Chem.*, 40, 103, 1919.
7. **Bürker, K.**, Ein neuer Hämoglobinometer, *Pfluegers Arch. Gesamte Physiol.*, 203, 274, 1924.
8. **Gowers**, Meeting clinical society of London, *Lancet*, II, 882, 1878.
9. **Tallqvist, T. W.**, Ein einfaches Verfahren zur directen Schätzung der Farbestarke des Blutes, *Z. Klin. Med.*, 40, 137, 1900.
10. **Ray, G. B., Blair, H. A., and Thomas, C. I.**, The spectrophotometric determination of certain blood pigments, *J. Biol. Chem.*, 98, 63, 1932.
11. **Haldane, J.**, The colorimetric determination of haemoglobin, *J. Physiol. (London)*, 26, 497, 1901.
12. **Havemann, R.**, Die Bestimmung von Hämoglobin mit den lichtelektrischen Kolorimeter, *Klin. Wochenschr.*, 19, 503, 1940.
13. **Vanzetti, G.**, An Azide-methemoglobin determination in blood, *J. Lab. Clin. Med.*, 67, 116, 1966.
14. **Stadie, W. C.**, A method for the determination of methemoglobin in blood, *J. Biol. Chem.*, 41, 237, 1920.
15. **Donaldson, R., Sisson, R. B., King, E. J., Wootton, I. D. P., and McFarlane, R. G.**, Determination of haemoglobin. VII. Standardized optical data for absolute estimations, *Lancet*, I, 874, 1951.
16. **Sahli, H.**, Bestimmung des Hämoglobingehaltes des Blutes, in *Lehrbuch der Klininschen Untersuchungsmethoden*, Vol. 2, Deuticke, Leipzig, 1931, 361.
17. **Rimington, C.**, Haemoglobinometry, *Br. Med. J.*, I, 177, 1942.
18. **Sunderman, F. W., MacFabe, R. P., MacFayden, D. A., Stevenson, G. F., and Copeland, B. E.**, Symposium on clinical hemoglobinometry, *Am. J. Clin. Pathol.*, 23, 519, 1953.
19. **Henry, R. G.**, *Clinical Chemistry, Principles, and Techniques*, Harper & Row, New York, 1964.
20. **van Assendelft, O. W.**, The determination of the haemoglobin content of a blood sample, in *Spectrophotometry of Haemoglobin Derivatives*, Van Gorcum, Assen, the Netherlands, 1970, 86.

21. **Ammundsen, E.**, The presence of non-oxygen combining (inactive) hemoglobin in the blood of normal individuals, *Science,* 90, 372, 1939.
22. **van Slyke, D. D., Hiller, A., Weistger, J. R., and Cruz, W. O.**, Determination of carbon monoxide in blood and of total and active hemoglobin by carbon monoxide capacity. Inactive hemoglobin and methemoglobin contents of normal human blood, *J. Biol. Chem.*, 166, 121, 1946.
23. **van Assendelft, O. W., Zijlstra, W. G., Buursma, A., van Kampen, E. J., and Hoek, W.**, The use of atomic absorption spectrophotometry for the measurement of haemoglobin iron, with special reference to the determination of ε_{HiCN}^{540}, *Clin. Chim. Acta,* 22, 281, 1968.
24. **van Kampen, E. J. and Klouwen, H.**, Spectro-photometric determination of carboxyhemoglobin, *Rec. Trav. Chim. Pays-Bas.*, 73, 119, 1954.
25. **Bell, G. H., Chambers, J. W., and Waddel, M. B. R.**, The routine estimation of haemoglobin and oxyhaemoglobin, *Biochem. J.*, 39, 60, 1945.
26. **de Boroviczeny, C. G.**, Decision of the standardizing committee of the European Society of Haematology concerning haemoglobinometry, *Bibl. Haematol. (Basel),* 18, 110, 1964.
27. **Itano, H. A.**, Molar extinction coefficients of cyanmet hemoglobin (hemiglobincyanide) at 540 and 281 nm, in *Modern Concepts in Hematology,* Izak, G. and Lewis, S. M., Eds., Academic Press, New York, 1972, 26.
28. **Meyer-Wilmes, J. and Remmer, H.**, Die Standardisierung des roten Blutfarbstoffes durch Hämiglobincyanid. I. Mitteilung. Bestimmung der spezifischen Extinction von Hämiglobincyanid, *Arch. Exp. Pathol. Pharmakol.*, 229, 441, 1956.
29. **Remmer, H.**, Die Standardisierung des roten Blutfarbstoffes durch Hämiglobincyanid, *Arch. Exp. Pathol. Pharmakol.*, 229, 450, 1956.
30. **Minkowski, A. and Swierczewski, E.**, The oxygen capacity of human foetal blood, in *Oxygen Supply to the Foetus,* Walker, J. and Turnbull, A., Eds., Blackwell Scientific, Oxford, 1959.
31. **Zijlstra, W. G. and van Kampen, E. J.**, Standardization of hemoglobinometry. I. The extinction coefficient of hemiglobincyanide at λ = 540 nm: ε_{HiCN}^{540}, *Clin. Chim. Acta,* 5, 719, 1960.
32. **Wootton, I. D. P. and Blevin, W. R.**, The extinction coefficient of cyanmethemoglobin, *Lancet,* II, 434, 1964.
33. **van Oudheusden, A. P. M., van de Heuvel, J. H., van Stekelenburg, G. J., Siertsema, L. H., and Wadman, S. K.**, De ijking van de haemoglobine bepaling op basis van ijzer (calibration of the haemoglobin determination based on iron), *Ned. Tijdschri. Geneeskd.*, 108, 265, 1964.
34. **Salvati, A. M., Tentori, L., and Vivaldi, G.**, The extinction coefficient of human hemiglobincyanide, *Clin. Chim. Acta,* 2, 477, 1965.
35. **Tentori, L., Vivaldi, G., and Salvati, A. M.**, The extinction coefficient of human haemiglobincyanide as determined by nitrogen analysis, *Clin. Chim. Acta,* 14, 276, 1966.
36. **Morningstar, D. A., Williams, G. Z., and Suutarinen, P.**, The millimolar extinction coefficient of cyanmethemoglobin from direct measurement of iron by X-ray emission spectroscopy, *Am. J. Clin. Pathol.*, 46, 603, 1966.
37. **Stigbrand, T.**, Molar absorbancy of cyanmethaemoglobin, *Scand. J. Clin. Lab. Invest.*, 20, 252, 1967.
38. **International Committee for Standardization in Haematology**, Recommendations for haemoglobinometry in human blood, *Br. J. Haematol.*, 13 (Suppl. 71), 1967; *J. Clin. Pathol.*, 31, 139, 1978.
39. **World Health Organization**, International biological standards and international biological reference preparations 1968, *WHO Tech. Rep. Ser.*, 384, 85, 1968.
40. **van Kampen, E. J. and Zijlstra, W. G.**, Standardization of hemoglobincyanide method, *Clin. Chim. Acta,* 6, 538, 1961.
41. **Haglund, H.**, personal communication, 1966.
42. **van Assendelft, O. W., Zijlstra, W. G., and van Kampen, E. J.**, Haemoglobinometry. Challenges and pitfalls, *Proc. K. Ned. Akad. Wet.*, C73, 104, 1970.
43. **Matsubara, T., Okuzono, H., and Tamagawa, S.**, Proposals for an improved reagent in the hemiglobincyanide method, in *Modern Concepts in Hematology,* Izak, G. and Lewis, S. M., Eds., Academic Press, New York, 1972, 29.
44. **van Kampen, E. J., Zijlstra, W. G., van Assendelft, O. W., and Reinkingh, W. A.**, Determination of haemoglobin and its derivatives, in *Advances in Clinical Chemistry,* Vol. 8, Sobotka, H. and Stewart, C. P., Eds., 141, 1965.
45. **Taylor, J. D. and Miller, J. D. M.**, A source of error in the cyanmethemoglobin method of determination of hemoglobin concentration in blood containing carbon monoxide, *Am. J. Clin. Pathol.*, 43, 265, 1965.
46. **Zijlstra, W. G. and van Kampen, E. J.**, Standardization of hemoglobinometry. III. Preparation and use of a stable hemiglobincyanide standard, *Clin. Chim. Acta,* 7, 96, 1962.
47. **Zijlstra, W. G., van Kampen, E. J., and van Assendelft, O. W.**, Standardization of haemoglobinometry. Establishing the reference point, *Proc. K. Ned. Akad. Wet. Ser.*, C72, 231, 1969.

48. **van Assendelft, O. W., Zijlstra, W. G., van Kampen, E. J., and Holtz, A. H.,** Stability of haemiglobincyanide reference solutions, *Clin. Chim. Acta,* 13, 521, 1966.
49. **van Assendelft, O. W., Holtz, A. H., van Kampen, E. J., and Zijlstra, W. G.,** Control data of international haemiglobincyanide reference solutions, *Clin. Chim. Acta,* 18, 78, 1967.
50. **Holtz, A. H.,** Some experience with a cyanhaemiglobin solution, *Bibl. Haematol. (Basel),* 21, 75, 1965.
51. **International Committee for Standardization in Hematology,** Announcement of availability of International Haemiglobincyanide Reference Standard, *Br. J. Haematol.,* 23, 123, 1972.
52. **National Bureau of Standards,** Standards for checking the calibration of spectrophotometers (200-1000mμ), Letter circular LC929, National Bureau of Standards, U.S. Department of Commerce, Washington, D.C., 1948.
53. **Weatherburn, M. W. and Logan, J. E.,** The effect of freezing on potassium ferricyanidepotassium cyanide reagent used in the cyanmethemoglobin procedure, *Clin. Chim. Acta,* 9, 581, 1964.
54. **Michelsen, O., Woolard, H., and Ness, A. T.,** Decolorization on freezing of ferricyanide solution used for hemoglobin determination, *Clin. Chem.,* 10, 610, 1964.
55. **Rice, E. W. and Lapara, C. Z.,** Reliability of hemoglobin values obtained from ferri-cyanide reagents subjected to freezing temperatures, *Clin. Chem.,* 2, 531, 1965.
56. **von Klein-Wisenberg, A.,** Physicochemical requirements regarding solutions for the determination of haemoglobin as haemiglobincyanide, *Bibl. Haematol. (Basel),* 24, 150, 1966.

IRON METABOLISM

Ch. Hershko and G. Izak

Iron is one of the most abundant elements in nature, but its solubility at a neutral pH is low, and iron deficiency is one of the most common causes of anemia. In order to facilitate the storage and internal transport of this important element, living organisms have developed highly specialized molecules to fulfill these functions. The surprising similarity in amino acid composition of the iron storage molecule ferritin, obtained from plants, fungi, and mammals, indicates its early evolution and widespread functional importance.[1,2]

In man, iron metabolism is characterized by a limited external exchange and an efficient reutilization of iron from internal sources. Normally, about two thirds of the total body iron, or 2100 to 2500 mg, are bound to hemoglobin in circulating red blood cells, 30%, or 800 to 1500 mg, are in iron stores, 3 to 5% in myoglobin, and trace amounts in iron-containing enzymes (Table 1). Only 3 mg of iron is bound to transferrin in the circulation, but this small proportion of body iron is an extremely active one which is normally replaced and lost ten times daily. Most of the daily plasma iron turnover is utilized for erythropoiesis, and erythrocytes are reprocessed at the end of their life span by reticuloendothelial (RE) cells in the spleen, liver, and bone marrow. The sojourn of erythrocyte iron through the RE cells is unidirectional, since RE cells can release iron derived from hemoglobin into the plasma, but cannot take up iron directly from transferrin (Figure 1). A second and less active cycle of internal iron exchange is between transferrin and parenchymal cells represented mainly by the liver. The latter exchange is bidirectional and is determined largely by the level of transferrin iron saturation.[3]

Intestinal Absorption of Iron

The Mechanism of Iron Absorption

The observations available to date suggest a common mechanism for the absorption of iron ingested as iron salts, iron in vegetables, in eggs, and in ferritin; it is different from the absorption process operative in heme, hemoglobin, and, probably, muscle iron absorption. The main difference between these two absorption mechanisms is that in the latter, iron absorption is unaffected by blocking substances in food, reducing agents, ascorbic acid, hydrochloric acid, and synthetic chelating agents which bind ionic iron.[4-10] This difference will be discussed in greater detail later in this chapter.

The process of absorption starts with mastication. In the stomach, iron is split from nonheme complexes by peptic digestion and liberated into a pool of miscible iron, where it may become reduced or, alternatively, chelated and rendered insoluble. Some of the iron-binding compounds such as ascorbic acid, fructose, amino acids, and mucoprotein of the gastric juice may act as carriers, while others may act as blocking substances by forming insoluble compounds with iron, such as phosphates and phytates. Protein has a potentiating effect on iron absorption, probably as a result of the formation of low molecular, weight-digestive products, which form soluble compounds with iron.[11]

Iron is absorbed through the jejunal mucosa in two phases: a rapid phase starting within seconds of reaching the brush borders and rising to a peak in 30 to 60 min and a slow phase extending over about 24 hr.[12-14] Once iron is absorbed into the epithelial cell, it has to pass through its cytoplasm, after which it is released into the circulating plasma where it is bound and carried away by transferrin. These are active processes that are dependent upon oxidative metabolism.[15,16]

Table 1
APPROXIMATE COMPOSITION OF IRON-CONTAINING COMPOUNDS IN THE ADULT MALE

Compound	Iron (mg)	Percentage of total
Hemoglobin	2100—2500	65
Myoglobin	130	3—5
Iron-containing enzymes	8	0.2
Transferrin	4	0.1
Ferritin and hemosiderin	800—1500	30
Total body iron	3000—4000	100

Modified from Bothwell, T. M. and Finch, C. A., *Iron Metabolism,* Little, Brown, Boston, 1962, 4. With permission.

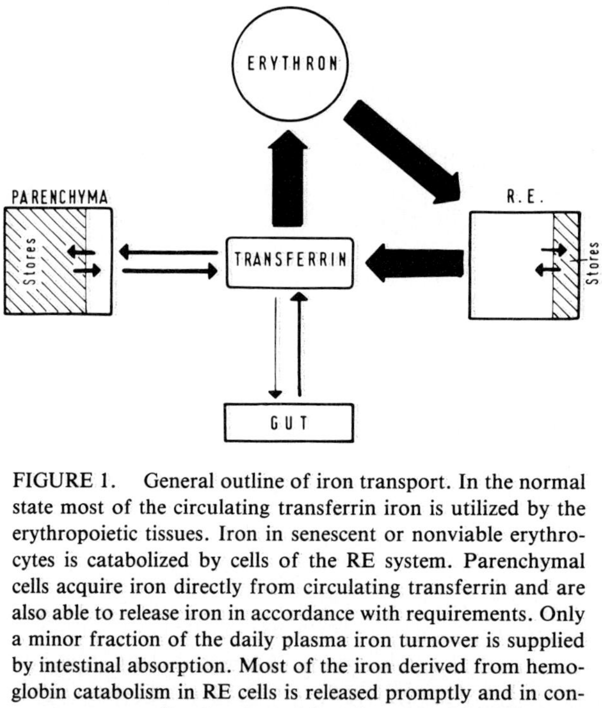

FIGURE 1. General outline of iron transport. In the normal state most of the circulating transferrin iron is utilized by the erythropoietic tissues. Iron in senescent or nonviable erythrocytes is catabolized by cells of the RE system. Parenchymal cells acquire iron directly from circulating transferrin and are also able to release iron in accordance with requirements. Only a minor fraction of the daily plasma iron turnover is supplied by intestinal absorption. Most of the iron derived from hemoglobin catabolism in RE cells is released promptly and in consequence; a smaller fraction of iron is retained in RE stores than in parenchymal stores. (From Hershko, C., *Progress in Hematology,* Vol. 10, Brown, E. B., Ed., Grune & Stratton, 1977, 105. With permission.)

Evidence has been presented to show that there are specific iron receptors on the surface of mucosal cells. Brush borders isolated from jejunal epithelial cells bind more iron than those from ileal cells. This binding is much more pronounced for iron than for other metals.[17,18] It has been further demonstrated that brush borders isolated from iron-loaded animals bind substantially less iron than those isolated from normal or iron-deficient animals.[17] It has also been observed that brush borders derived from ileal epithelium, which bind small quantities of iron in normal animals, increase their uptake significantly in iron deficiency.[17] Once the iron enters the epithelial cell, it is found either in metabolically active cell components or bound to intracellular ligands. After homogenization and differential centrifugation of rat jejunal epithelium, the mitochondrial fraction contains the largest iron concentration[19] in normal, iron-deficient, and iron-loaded animals. A substantial amount of iron is also found in the particle-free soluble fraction in the normal and iron-loaded animals, but not in the iron-deficient animals, where the absolute amount of iron in the epithelial cells is greatly reduced.

Iron can penetrate the epithelial cell not only from the intestinal lumen, but also from the circulating plasma;[20] much of this latter iron can be recovered in the mitochondria,[21] where it remains throughout the life span of the epithelial cell. Iron entering the mucosal cell from the intestinal lumen is mostly concentrated in the soluble cell fraction with the major portion of iron bound to ferritin in the normal animal, while very little of the freshly absorbed iron in the soluble fraction is ferritin bound in the iron-deficient animal.[21-26] This makes it unlikely that ferritin is an important component of the absorptive mechanism of iron in conditions with enhanced iron absorption. Several iron-binding fractions have been isolated from the soluble mucosal cell supernatant;[27-29] however, there is still no agreement concerning the number of these fractions and their nature. Several investigators have reported an iron-binding protein in the soluble cell fraction of the mucosal cell of iron-deficient animals which closely resembled transferrin.[26,28,30,31]

The role of intestinal epithelial ferritin in the regulation of iron absorption was first suggested in 1946. It was proposed that ferritin synthesized in the mucosal cell in response to iron acted as a block to further absorption.[32] This theory was supported by several investigators.[20,25,33-35] However, a number of observations made the mucosal block theory untenable. Thus it was shown that mucosal ferritin synthesis is stimulated by iron in both normal and iron-deficient rats, and absorption of a subsequent dose of iron is greater than normal in iron-deficient rats, although their mucosal cells have accumulated a normal amount of ferritin.[36,37] In rats with turpentine abscesses, the incorporation percentage of absorbed iron into mucosal ferritin is the same as in control animals, indicating that the reduction in absorption in inflammation is not due to diversion of iron into ferritin.[38] Finally, the rate of release of iron from ferritin is far too slow for ferritin to function as a transcellular carrier during the rapid phase of absorption.[39] The most plausible interpretation of the data available to date is that iron entering the mucosa in excess of what can be bound by the "carrier system" becomes bound to ferritin. Some of this iron is absorbed during the slow phase of absorption, while the remainder is lost into the intestinal lumen with the desquamating epithelial cells.

The mechanism of iron uptake by the intestinal epithelium from heme differs from that described above in several respects. Heme iron enters the mucosal cell without being released from the porphyrin ring; in the guinea pig, the absorbed heme passes into the circulating blood to be taken up by the liver.[7] In man, heme is broken down in the mucosa,[9,40] and the absorbed iron is recovered in the plasma bound to transferrin.[5,41,42] The breakdown of absorbed heme is faster in iron deficiency, and the amount absorbed appears to be limited by the transfer capacity of the cell rather than by the uptake of heme into the cell.[9] After iron is liberated from the porphyrin ring, it enters the same pool as absorbed ionic iron and is probably transferred by the same carrier. The liberation of iron from the porphyrin ring is accomplished by xanthine oxidase.[43]

Regulation of Iron Absorption

It has been universally accepted that iron absorption responds to even small changes in storage iron and to the demands of tissues, particularly of the erythroid marrow. It is also well known that the control over the amount of iron absorbed is exercised by the epithelial cell in the jejunum. The unsolved problem is how these cells receive the message of need for iron and how they react to this need. Several mechanisms have been suggested.

The binding of variable amounts of iron to components of gastric juice has been suggested to have a role in the regulation of iron absorption, but this possibility has been discarded in the light of accumulating evidence to the contrary.[44-46] Similarly, the possible role of changes in pancreatic secretion has been shown to be an unlikely factor.[47] On the other hand, exposure of the jejunal mucosa to substances present in gastric and intestinal secretions was shown to affect absorption of iron by the exposed mucosal cells. Thus gastric and intestinal juices of iron-deficient rats or from human subjects after venesections markedly augmented iron uptake by the mucosal cells of the normal rat.[48-51]

The role of mucosal cell iron in the regulation of iron absorption has been the subject of continuous interest during the past 25 years since Conrad et al.[20,52] proposed that the absorptive capacity of the mucosal cell is determined by its iron content, which is derived partly from the diet and partly from the plasma. According to the concept put forward by these workers, mucosal iron is decreased in iron deficiency and increased in iron overload. Strong support for this hypothesis was furnished by the inverse correlation between the amount of iron absorbed and the fraction of intravenous transferrin-bound iron taken up by the duodenal mucosal cells.[53,54] Bleeding was found to augment iron absorption, prior iron loading notwithstanding,[53] and the delay observed under the latter experimental conditions was attributed to the time required for the iron-containing epithelial cells to be replaced by new iron-depleted cells.[55,56] These observations were confirmed by several investigators.[57-59] Other workers reached the conclusion that the changes in iron absorption may not be related to the nonheme iron content of the mucosal cells themselves, but rather to the amount of iron in the subepithelial layer of the jejunum.[60] In still other studies performed in guinea pigs, no correlation was found between iron absorption and the iron content of the mucosal epithelium.[61]

Recently, several groups of workers studied the total nonheme iron content in the epithelial cells and its distribution among different protein fractions, some of them functionally defined such as succinic dehydrogenase, cytochrome oxidase, ferritin, and mitochondrial iron. A marked reduction in the iron content of these fractions was associated with iron depletion, but no increase was produced by iron overload.[62] It has been suggested that the mitochondrial iron in the intestinal epithelium is a true reflection of the body iron status, and it might be a factor in determining the uptake of iron from the intestinal lumen. In accordance with this theory, increased iron uptake was noted in animals with decreased mitochondrial iron and diminished iron-containing enzyme activity.[63] It was also confirmed that the epithelial cell obtains its iron at least partly from the plasma and is taken up largely by mitochondria.[63,64] The mitochondria have shown increased avidity for both parenterally or orally administered iron; it appears to be bound to this fraction within 30 min after it is administered.[65] There seems to be an inverse correlation between the transferrin saturation of plasma and the mitochondrial iron content of the intestinal epithelium;[66] however, increase in absorption can also be seen in patients with diminished iron stores in whom the hemoglobin concentration and plasma iron and iron-binding capacity are normal.[67-69] Furthermore, iron absorption may be decreased in patients with increased iron stores, although their plasma iron is normal.[67] Absorption of iron correlates well with the amount of stainable iron in the bone marrow reticuloendothelial cells,[70,71] presumably because the latter value varies in proportion to total storage iron. It is plausible that this correlates with a similar pool in the mitochondria of the mucosal cells, but this assumption has to be investigated.

The increased iron absorption associated with enhanced marrow activity, such as that observed in thalassemia,[72,73] in hemolytic anemia,[74] and in sideroblastic anemia,[75] cannot be explained on the basis of information available today. A tentative hypothesis has been put forward to account for this phenomenon;[76] one assumes that one of the binding sites of transferrin is more oriented to uptake of iron from the mucosa and its delivery to the marrow, while the other is more oriented to the delivery of iron to stores. Accordingly, the mucosal cell may receive a message of the need for iron without an obvious abnormality in the plasma iron or transferrin saturation. This hypothesis is built on experimental observations suggesting the existence of functional differences between the two iron-binding sites of the transferrin molecule.[76] No clinical or experimental evidence has been presented to support the conccept, and it has been challenged by some subsequent studies.[77]

Attempts were made in the past to search for humoral factors affecting iron absorption, most of which were unsuccessful.[78,79] Erythropoietin was found to augment the intestinal absorption of iron through its stimulating effect on the bone marrow.[80] A similar mechanism was probably operative in cases of hypoxia-associated increase in iron absorption.[81] A plasma factor was isolated from pregnant women that increased iron uptake by the epithelial cells when introduced into the lumen, but was ineffective when given parenterally.[82] There is no solid evidence to support the existence of humoral factors stimulating intestinal iron absorption.

Food Iron Absorption

The accurate estimation of food iron absorption became possible recently, when it was shown that suitable iron salts in tracer quantities are absorbed in a similar fashion to food iron. By using such extrinsic tags, it was demonstrated that assimilation of dietary iron occurs from two independent pools, namely heme and nonheme iron.[83,84] Dietary iron must be converted into one of these two forms in order to be absorbed. Heme iron is derived from hemoglobin, myoglobin, and other heme proteins in foodstuffs of animal origin. Nonheme iron is supplied mainly by vegetables and fruit.

The amount of iron absorbed daily from food in a normal man and in nonmenstruating women is about 1.0 mg (0.6 to 1.6 mg),[85] whereas about twice this amount is absorbed by menstruating women.[86,97] In pregnant women the "iron loss" is about 3½ times that of a normal man, and the absorption of iron from food increases accordingly. The average amount of iron ingested daily in a normal balanced diet is about 6 mg/1000 calories or between 10 to 30 mg of iron daily.[88] About 5 to 10% of this iron is absorbed daily under physiological conditions. The amount of iron absorbed rises fourfold to sixfold in iron deficiency and is diminished in cases of iron overload.[89-91] While the values given here are correct for developed countries, marked variations exist in various parts of the world in the dietary iron intake both below and above the values given here.[92]

Almost all of the mucosal iron destined for absorption enters the portal blood, while less than 5% enters the lymphatics.[93,94] The unsaturated iron-binding capacity of the plasma is probably the single most important factor that determines the rate of release of intraepithelial iron into the circulation.[95-97] Iron entering the circulation is immediately taken up by the iron-carrying protein transferrin.

Transferrin Metabolism

The following discussion deals with the transport of iron in the circulating plasma. This function is performed under physiological circumstances by the specific iron-binding protein transferrin. A brief summary of its structure, physicochemical properties, kinetics, and functions will be followed by the description of methods for its quantitative estimation in the plasma and/or serum.

Transferrin Structure

Despite the large effort invested in characterizing transferrin since it was first isolated and recognized in 1947,[98] there are still differences of opinion on many points. Thus while it is generally accepted that transferrin is a β_1-globulin, various authors have suggested a rather wide range for its molecular weight ranging from 68.000 to 88.000.[98-102,106] Transferrin is a glycoprotein with a single polypeptide chain, which contains one N-terminal amino acid residue per molecule (valine).[103] It has no free sulphydryl groups.[104] Its total carbohydrate content is 5.3%, which is arranged in the form of two identical branched side chains, each branch ending in a sialic acid molecule. Hence, four sialic acid molecules are present per molecule of transferrin.[105] Its sedimentation constant (S_{20}, W) is 5.1 ± 0.2,[107] and its isoelectric point is at pH 5.8.[108]

The amino acid sequence of the transferrin molecule is still unknown. Among the numerous unresolved questions regarding this protein, one of the most important concerns the composition and nature of its iron-binding sites, of which there are two per transferrin molecule. Whether these sites are structurally and functionally identical, whether they bind Fe^{2+} in addition to Fe^{3+}, and whether there is or is not an interaction between these binding sites are some of the unanswered questions.[99,109] Two regions of internal homology were recently identified in the transferrin molecule, supporting the gene duplication-fusion hypothesis for its evolution, which suggested that the structure of the specific binding sites may depend on the three-dimensional configuration of the transferrin molecule contributing to the ligands involved in metal binding. The two sites may then have similar structures despite the absence of internal homology in the molecule.[110]

A more extensive discussion of the accumulated and often conflicting data concerning the many unknown properties of the transferrin molecule exceeds the scope of the present discussion. The reader is referred to the numerous detailed reviews devoted to this subject that have been published recently.[99,109] It should be noted, however, that the binding of iron to transferrin produces several changes in the properties of the protein which are relevant to the following discussion.

The first of these is the acquisition of a pink color by the apotransferrin-iron complex at the time of iron attachment to the protein. The net charge of the molecule is changed by −1 for each iron atom bound with a consequent change in electrophoretic mobility[111] and behavior on ion exchange chromatography.[112,113] Iron binding does not induce a significant change in the molecular weight of transferrin,[114] but it causes the molecule to become more compact and more spherical in shape.[115] Iron-transferrin binding makes the transferrin molecule more stable than apoferritin, and this is manifested by its increased resistance to heat, urea, organic solvents, disulphide-breaking reagents, iodination, and resistance to proteolytic enzymes.[116-120] The conformational change in the transferrin molecule consequent to iron binding may be responsible for making certain antigenic sites on the molecule inaccessible;[121] this change of the antigenic reactivity of transferrin, however, does not significantly affect its quantitative estimation by radial immunodiffusion.[122]

Synthesis

A large variety of tissues have been shown to synthesize transferrin. The methods employed in these studies consisted mostly of culturing cells from various tissues and demonstrating the incorporation of labeled amino acids into transferrin by immunoelectrophoresis and autoradiography. Although this method is useful in proving the ability of cells to produce transferrin, it does not allow for its quantitative estimation or for the assessment of the rate of its elaboration; neither does it answer the question of whether the transferrin synthesized by the cells is secreted by them or not.

The accumulated evidence suggests that in adult animals, only the liver — and in rabbits and rats, the lactating mammary gland — synthesize and secrete quantitatively important amounts of transferrin.[123-128] In human subjects, transferrin synthesis has been demonstrated in the liver and in peripheral blood lymphocytes,[129] the latter source being quantitatively unimportant. Transferrin synthesis has recently been found in the yolk sac of early human and rat fetuses.[130,131] Increased production of transferrin was found in childhood, during pregnancy, and in iron-deficiency anemia. Estrogen administration was also found to stimulate transferrin synthesis.[132-133] On the other hand, fasting and protein depletion lead to markedly diminished rates of transferrin synthesis.[134] The diminished transferrin levels seen in kwashiorkor are probably due to a diminished synthetic rate, which rapidly returns to normal on an adequate diet.[135-136]

Distribution, Turnover, and Catabolism

Transferrin, like many other plasma proteins, is distributed throughout most of the extracellular fluid of the body with continuous circulation from the plasma to the interstitial space and back into the circulation via the lymph vessels. Its presence has been demonstrated in the interstitial fluid,[137] lymph,[138] edema fluid,[139] cerebrospinal fluid,[140-141] and in the urine.[142] The rate of exchange of transferrin between the plasma and extravascular space is similar to that of albumin. In humans, 50 to 60% of the total body transferrin is in the extravascular compartments, while 60 to 70% of this protein is extravascular in rats and rabbits.[143-144] Between 70 to 100% of the plasma transferrin pool passes through the extravascular compartments daily both in man and rabbits.[145-146] The rate of extravascular circulation varies between the different tissues, dependent largely upon the structure of the capillaries determining the permeability of the capillary walls. As a result of structural differences in the capillary network of various tissues, plasma transferrin has an almost unrestricted access to liver cells, spleen, and bone marrow. In contrast, transferrin circulates much more slowly through the interstitial fluid surrounding muscle and skin.[147,148] The functional significance of these differences in the availability of transferrin to the different tissues of the body is obvious.

About 15 to 16% of the total body transferrin pool is catabolized daily. The rate of catabolism in rabbits and rats is much higher (about 70%). The site of transferrin catabolism has not been established with certainty, although evidence has been presented to show that a substantial portion of the daily breakdown of transferrin is accomplished by the liver.[149] Transferrin may also be lost into the stomach and intestines,[150] and insignificant quantities are excreted in the urine.[151] The mechanism of degradation of transferrin has not been elucidated, but this protein seems to be taken up by cells via pinocytosis and broken down within the cells.[150] Increased transferrin catabolism was noted in patients with hemolytic anemia, infection, and nephrosis.[137,152-154] An inverse relationship was found between the fractional catabolic rate of transferrin on the one hand and the plasma transferrin concentration on the other hand. This finding would indicate that the amount of transferrin catabolized daily remains constant, irrespective of the plasma transferrin concentration; it follows that if the fractional catabolic rate increases, plasma transferrin concentration falls.[155]

Quantitative Estimation of Circulating Transferrin

Numerous methods have been published and are employed in various laboratories for the estimation of the concentrations of the saturated serum iron (SI) and unsaturated (UIBC) circulating transferrin. We shall describe the method recommended by the Iron Panel of International Committee for Standardization in Hematology (I.C.S.H.) as a reference method. Other available procedures will be mentioned briefly.

Measurement of Serum Iron[156-158]

The reagents include:

1. Protein precipitant: aqueous solution containing 0.6 mol trichloroacetic acid, 0.3 mol thioglycollic acid, and 1 mol hydrochloric acid per liter (stored in dark).
2. Chromogen solution: sodium acetate (1.6 mol/ℓ) containing disodium 4, 7-diphenyl-l, 10-phenantroline disulphonate (0.5 nmol/ℓ).
3. Iron standard solution containing 40 μmol/ℓ (2.24 μg/mℓ). Iron-free glassware must be used throughout.

The procedure is as follows:

1. Two milliliters of the protein precipitating solution is added to 2 mℓ serum mixed thoroughly for 60 sec, then heated at 56°C for 15 min, followed by centrifugation to obtain an optically clear supernatant.
2. Two milliliters of the iron standard solution is mixed with the protein precipitant solution.
3. A reagent blank is prepared by substituting the iron-free water for the iron standard used above.
4. Two milliliters of the supernatant solution are mixed each with 2 mℓ of chromogen, mixed thoroughly, and allowed to stand for 5 min.
5. The absorbance of the chromogen-treated solutions is measured against a blank of distilled water in a spectrophotometer at a wavelength of 535 nm.
6. The iron concentration of the serum specimen is calculated from the formula:

$$\text{serum iron in } \mu\text{mol}/\ell$$

$$\frac{\text{absorbance serum specimen} - \text{absorbance blank}}{\text{absorbance standard iron} - \text{absorbance blank}} \times 40$$

The absorbance of the blank should not exceed 0.015, read against distilled water in a l-cm pathway.

Measurement of Serum-unsaturated Iron-binding Capacity (UIBC)[146-148]

Iron-free water and glassware are to be used throughout.

The reagents include:

1. Stock ferric chloride solution 1 mmol/ℓ in HCl, 50 nmol/ℓ. Weigh 0.27 g ferric chloride ($FeCl_3 \cdot 6\ H_2O$ AR), dissolve immediately in 50 mℓ HCl, 1 mol/ℓ and dilute with iron-free distilled water to 1 liter in 1 volumetric flask.
2. Saturating iron solution for total iron binding capacity (TIBC), 100 μmol/ℓ in HCl, 5 nmol/ℓ. Into a 250-mℓ volumetric flask, pipette one tenth of its volume of stock ferric chloride solution and dilute to volume with iron-free distilled water.
3. Saturating radioiron solution for UIBC, 100 μmol/ℓ containing sufficient $^{59}FeCl_3$ to give about 100.000 counts/min/μmol Fe. Into a 250-mℓ volumetric flask, pipette one tenth of its volume of stock ferric chloride solution, add a volume of $^{59}FeCl_3$ solution sufficient to give about 10.000 counts/min/mℓ in the final solution, and dilute to volume with iron-free distilled water.
4. Light magnesium carbonate reagent grade, approximate formula $3\ MgCO_3(OH)_2 \cdot 3\ H_2O$.
5. Standard iron solution 40 μmol/ℓ (see above).

The procedure is as follows:

1. To 2 mℓ serum in an iron-free tube add 2 mℓ saturating radioiron solution, mix well, and incubate for 15 min at room temperature.
2. Add 0.4 g of light magnesium carbonate, close tube with parafilm, and place on an angled turntable; rotate for 30 min.

3. Centrifuge for 30 min at 1000 × g, remove supernatant carefully, centrifuge supernatant again as above.
4. Pipette 2 mℓ of supernatant into an iron-free tube.
5. Prepare counting standard — 1 mℓ of saturating radioiron solution and 1 mℓ of water — in another tube.
6. Count each specimen in a gamma counter. The counting time should be such that the total counts recorded for each radioiron-containing specimen exceeds 10.000 after subtraction of background.
7. Estimate iron content of saturating radioiron solution as described above.
8. Calculate UIBC according to the formula:

$$\text{UIBC } \mu\text{mol}/\ell \text{ Fe} = \frac{\text{counts/min (serum specimen)}}{\text{counts/min (counting standard)}} \times \frac{\text{absorbance (counting standard)}}{\text{absorbance (Fe standard)}} \times 80$$

Other methods for the quantitative estimation of serum transferrin include wet digestion,[157] atomic absorption spectroscopy,[157] immunodiffusion, and, more recently, spectrofluorometry.[159]

Storage Iron

Storage Iron Regulation

Oxidation and reduction of iron are essential steps in its storage and mobilization. It was proposed by Mazur et al.[160] that xanthine oxidase is responsible for ferritin iron reduction, but this theory was abandoned when it was shown that allopurinol, the potent xanthine oxidase inhibitor, does not affect iron metabolism.[161,162] An alternative enzyme system, which is more likely to be involved in ferritin iron mobilization, is ferrireductase,[163] which is capable of catalyzing the anaerobic reduction of ferritin iron by the following sequence of reactions:

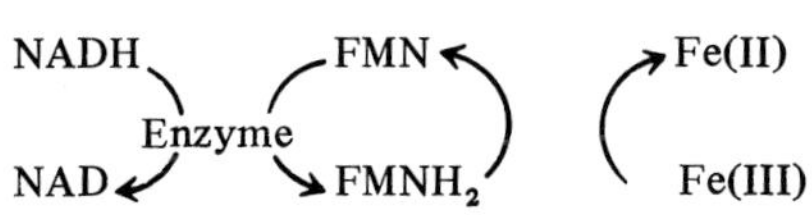

Oxidation of ferrous iron is catalyzed by apoferritin[164] and is followed by the production of microcrystalline particles within the interior of the apoferritin shell through the formation of hydroxyl and oxo bridges.[1]

The capacity of tissues to store iron is increased by their ability to enhance ferritin synthesis in response to increasing rates of iron deposition.[165] This effect cannot be inhibited by actinomycin D; it can be demonstrated in cell-free systems derived entirely from cytoplasmic components[166] indicating its posttranscriptional nature. It has been proposed that iron may promote the aggregation of subunits into ferritin, thus releasing adhering ferritin subunits from mRNA, which in turn becomes available for translation.[167] An alternative explanation for increased ferritin synthesis following iron administration is a posttranslational effect on subunit release, stabilization, or assembly into the multimeric protein shell.[166]

At the cellular level, iron release is facilitated by ceruloplasmin, which by virtue of its extracellular ferroxidase activity produces a steep concentration gradient between intra- and extracellular ferrous iron.[163] The role of ceruloplasmin in iron release is permissive and not regulatory, since its effect is maximal at serum levels corresponding to 10% of normal.[168] Ascorbic acid deficiency interferes with iron release from RE cells but does not affect parenchymal release.[169,170] This difference in ascorbic acid dependence of iron release may be explained by the apparent absence of ferrireductase from RE cells and its presence in parenchymal cells,[163] which provides an alternative mechanism for iron reduction. Other factors involved in the control of iron release from cells are the rate of plasma iron turnover and the amount of cellular exchangeable iron available for binding by transferrin (Figure 2).

As mentioned above, RE cells acquire iron from senescent erythrocytes and the wastage iron of erythropoiesis. Their ferritin stores are relatively small and the turnover rate of storage iron is consequently fast.[171-177] In contrast, parenchymal cells acquire iron mainly from plasma transferrin and are able to incorporate the iron contained in

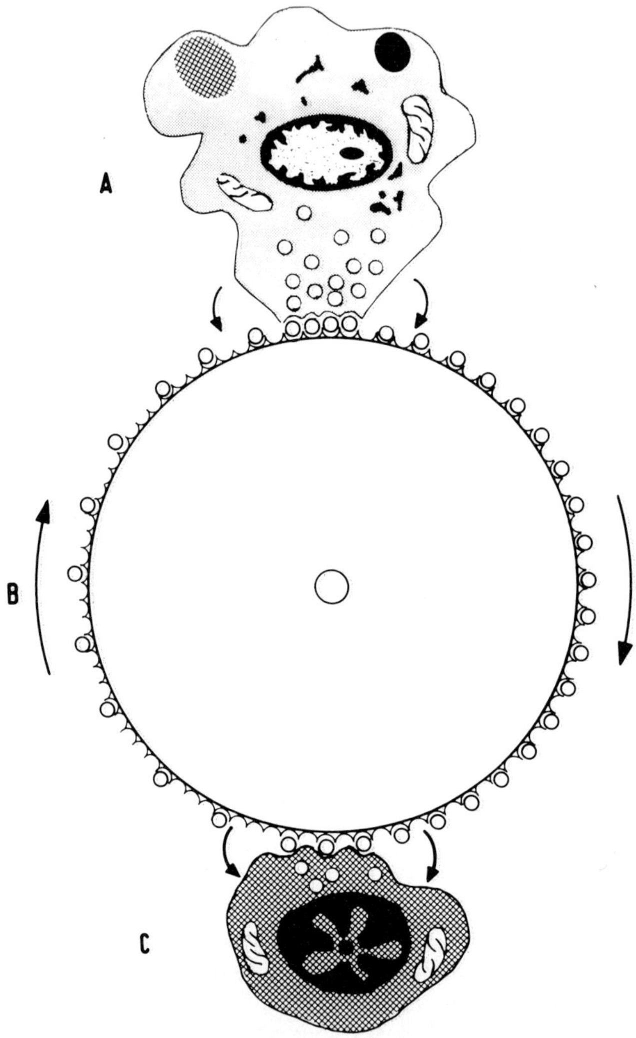

FIGURE 2. Regulation of RE iron release. Plasma iron turnover is described here as a wheel with a constant number of binding sites (B). It is driven by the active uptake of transferrin iron by erythroid precursor cells (C). The clearance of iron by erythroid precursors provides additional free binding sites which become available for interaction with RE iron (A). The amount of exchangeable RE iron is determined by the magnitude of its "pre-release" iron pool derived from RBC catabolism, or ferritin mobilization, and the number of transferrin binding sites on the cell membrane. Exchangeable iron from other cell types (intestinal mucosa, hepatocyte) may compete for available binding sites of transferrin and limit RE iron release. (From Hershko, C., *Progress in Hematology,* Vol. 10, Brown, E. B., Ed. Grune & Stratton, 1977, 105. With permission.)

circulating hemoglobin-haptoglobin, heme-hemopexin, and ferritin by pinocytosis.[174,178-181] Parenchymal ferritin stores are relatively large, and their rates of turnover are slow.[176,177] The known differences in the handling of iron by RE and parenchymal cells are summarized in Table 2.

Clinical Evaluation of Iron Stores

Most of the iron in the body is bound to hemoglobin, but iron stores of ferritin and hemosiderin exist in addition in the liver, spleen, and bone marrow. In conditions characterized by a negative balance between body requirements and food iron absorption, the storage compartment is depleted in order to maintain normal levels of functional iron in hemoglobin, myoglobin, and iron-containing enzymes. Conversely, when dietary iron absorption exceeds body requirements, iron stores increase. Thus the size of iron stores provides an important indicator of the balance between iron absorption and body iron requirements. Several clinical methods for assessing iron stores are in common use.

Examination of bone marrow fragments for stainable iron is one of the most commonly used procedures.[182] The slides are fixed in methyl alcohol and treated with a mixture of freshly prepared 2% potassium ferrocyanide and 2% hydrochloric acid.[183] Hemosiderin granules are stained blue, and the preparations are scored arbitrarily from 0 to 6. A composite figure of reported hemosiderin scorings summarized by Bothwell and Finch[28] is given in Table 3. As a rule, scores are low in iron deficiency and

Table 2
COMPARISON OF RE AND PARENCHYMAL CELL FUNCTION IN STORAGE IRON METABOLISM

	Reticuloendothelial cells	Parenchymal cells	Ref.
Source of iron	Wastage iron of erythropoiesis	Transferrin	174,178—181
	Senescent erythrocytes	Hemoglobin-haptoglobin	191,214
	Colloidal iron preparations	Heme-hemopexin	
^{59}Fe turnover	Rapid	Slow	171—175
Ferritin pool	Small	Large	176,177
Dependence on ascorbic acid	Pronounced	Questionable	169
Ferrireductase activity	Absent	Present	163

From Mershko, C., *Progress in Hematology,* Vol. 10, Brown, E. B., Ed., Grune & Stratton, 1977, 105. With permission.

Table 3
COMPOSITE FIGURE OF REPORTED RESULTS OF STAINABLE MARROW IRON

	Amount of iron			
Condition	0	1—2	3—4	5—6
Normal	6	57	19	0
Infection	6	13	31	11
Iron-deficiency anemia	132	38	0	0
Pernicious anemia	6	20	69	7
Idiopathic hemochromatosis	0	0	11	13
Transfusional hemosiderosis	0	0	0	13

From Bothwell, T. M. and Finch, C. A., *Iron Metabolism,* Little, Brown, Boston, 1962, 287. With permission.

high in iron overload because of idiopathic hemochromatosis or transfusional hemosiderosis. A shift of iron from the red cell mass to reticuloendothelial cells may be found in conditions characterized by ineffective erythropoiesis, such as in pernicious anemia, or in inflammation where the release of hemoglobin iron from RE cells is blocked. In general, stainable marrow iron reflects the amount of total body iron stores. However, there are some exceptions to this rule. Since marrow iron is a reflection of RE iron deposits, in clinical states with predominantly parenchymal iron overload, such as idiopathic hemochromatosis, marrow iron may not reflect the true magnitude of iron overload. Conversely, in patients receiving parenteral iron complexes or blood transfusions, stainable iron in the marrow may be increased in the face of iron deficiency.[184]

Chelating agents such as desferrioxamine (DF) or diethylene-triamine pentaacetic acid (DTPA) can be used to estimate body iron stores.[185-188] When iron excretion following the injection of DF at a dose of 10 mg/kg is compared to the total nonheme iron concentration of liver biopsies obtained from the same subjects, a positive linear correlation is found (Figure 3; r = 0.83).[179] Studies in which the amount of stainable iron in RE and parenchymal cells is correlated to urinary excretion of chelated iron, or animal studies employing selective radioiron labels of RE and parenchymal cells indicate that iron chelated by DF is mainly obtained from parenchymatous tissues.[190,191] DF-induced iron excretion is enhanced by ascorbic acid and inhibited by vitamin E.[192,193] In patients with cirrhosis, DF-induced excretion is much higher than in control subjects with similar liver iron concentrations.[189] These complicating factors may limit the diagnostic value of DF-induced urinary iron excretion in the assessment

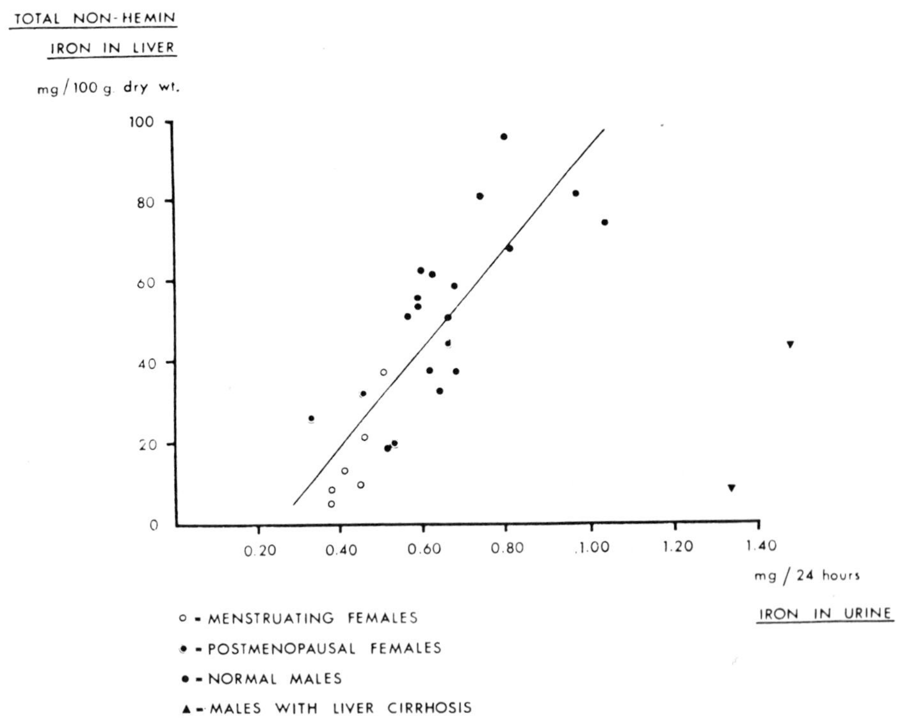

FIGURE 3. Relationship between desferrioxamine-induced urinary iron excretion and total nonheme iron concentration determined in liver biopsy specimens of the same individuals. The two subjects with liver cirrhosis are not included in the correlation study. r = 0.83; $p < 0.001$. (From Hallberg, L., Hedenberg, L., and Weinfeld, A., *Scand. J. Haematol.*, 3, 85, 1966. With permission.)

of body iron stores. In addition, the need for drug injection and subsequent urine collection require a high degree of cooperation on the part of the subjects studied.

Serial phlebotomies of about 400 mℓ at weekly intervals are probably the most accurate method for measuring iron stores, since no assumptions have to be made as to the quantitative relation between the amount of iron removed by phlebotomy and the amount mobilized from stores. Phlebotomy is continued until hemoglobin is reduced to less than 11 g/dℓ and transferrin saturation is below 15%, indicating depletion of iron stores. The total amount of iron removed is calculated by measuring the volume and hemoglobin content of each venesection. The difference between the total amount of iron removed by phlebotomy and the amount of iron lost in reducing the hemoglobin level of the subject represents the total amount of mobilizable storage iron.[194] Minor corrections are also made for the amount of iron absorbed during the study, which is about 2 to 3 mg per day. Published values of total mobilizable iron estimations obtained by quantitative phlebotomy in healthy adult males, females, and blood donors were summarized by Walters et al.[195] and are given in Table 4. At present, serial phlebotomies are still the most accurate method for the assessment of total mobilizable iron stores. However, the method is lengthy and inconvenient and is not suitable for routine clinical use.

Chemical Determination of Hepatic Iron

In specimens obtained by biopsy or at necropsy, clinical determination of hepatic iron may be useful in assessing the iron nutrition of a population, although it does not yield a direct estimate of total body iron stores. Charlton et al. have analyzed the iron content of 3983 liver specimens obtained by necropsy in 18 different countries.[196] They found no difference between individuals dying of cardiovascular disease and those killed by acute trauma. On the other hand, figures were higher in patients dying from neoplastic disease, presumably due to the trapping of iron in reticuloendothelial cells. Age had no effect on liver iron content, except for reduced iron stores in young women because of the increased iron demands of the reproductive period and a progressive increase in liver iron in the Bantu caused by an extremely high dietary intake. After excluding conditions that might have distorted hepatic iron stores by disease or excessive demand, a comparison was made between different countries (Table 5). The lowest iron concentrations were found in subjects from India and New Guinea, and the highest were found in the South African Bantu. There were significant differences between the iron stores of groups from different Western countries.

Serum ferritin measurements were introduced in 1972 by Addison et al.,[197] and several other methods for immunoradiometric assay have been subsequently

Table 4
PUBLISHED VALUES OF STORAGE IRON DETERMINATIONS BY QUANTITATIVE PHLEBOTOMY

Author	(n)	Males	(n)	Females	(n)	Blood donors	Ref.
Olsson (1972)	(11)	750	—	—	(14)	110	219
Balcerzak (1968)	(11)	687	—	—	—	—	175
Pritchard (1964)	(3)	819	(10)	254	—	—	220
Haskins (1952)	(2)	844	—	—	(2)	93	184
Walters (1973)	(7)	900	(10)	210	(5)	400	185
Mean of all series	(34)	767	(20)	232	—	—	—

Modified from Walters, G. O., Miller, F. M., and Worwood, M., *J. Clin. Pathol.*, 26, 770, 1973. With permission.

Table 5
MEDIAN HEPATIC STORAGE IRON CONCENTRATIONS (μg/g)[a]

Location	Race	Lower quartile		Median		Upper quartile	
		Males	Females	Males	Females	Males	Females
Great Britain							
London							
St. George's Hospital	—	65	67	113	119	188	189
Middlesex Hospital	—	107	142	166	177	199	270
West Middlesex Hospital	—	98	103	143	156	243	258
St. Margaret's Hospital	—	132	—	152	285	199	—
Sweden							
Malmö	—	81	73	126	120	207	183
Czechoslovakia							
Prague	—	118	84	230	170	329	243
U.S.							
Seattle	—	103	86	186	133	266	178
Boston	—	114	73	174	115	353	187
Wisconsin	—	161	127	242	205	390	238
South Africa							
Johannesburg	White	121	46	258	128	423	253
	Bantu	373	—	946	128	2068	—
Durban	Bantu	341	203	776	496	1753	1822
	Indian	113	103	183	173	301	290
Rhodesia	Bantu	268	—	633	321	2120	—
Nigeria	Bantu	113	—	133	126	291	—
India							
Unspecified	—	76	—	83	79	185	—
New Delhi	—	48	—	93	116	166	—
Bombay	—	46	—	131	202	238	—
New Guinea							
Rabaul	—	73	—	109	—	167	—
Venezuela							
Caracas	Mestizos	90	108	165	179	270	253
	White	164	—	255	303	267	—
	Negro	56	—	128	66	210	—
Brazil							
Sao Paulo	—	85	—	173	140	259	—
Rio de Janeiro	—	185	—	268	—	350	—
Mexico							
Mexico City	Mestizos	101	—	196	159	274	—
	White	43	—	258	—	310	—
Colombia	—	74	—	117	—	198	—
Taiwan							
Taipeh	—	136	131	181	233	364	393
Japan							
Tokyo	—	52	—	126	226	158	—
Israel							
Jerusalem	—	145	146	204	165	244	239
Mozambique	—	221	—	376	565	1025	—
Costa Rica	—	226	—	243	28	326	—

[a] Excluding patients dying from neoplastic, miscellaneous, and unknown causes, and females under 50 years of age.

Modified from Charlton, R. W., Hawkins, D. M., Mavor, W. O., and Bothwell, T. H., *Am. J. Clin. Nutr.*, 23, 358, 1970.

described.[198,199] Serum ferritin estimation was found to be a quantitative and reproducible method for assessing body iron stores, requiring only a small sample of blood. The normal mean concentration is 123 ng/mℓ in men and 56 ng/mℓ in women, with a 95% confidence range of 12 to 300 ng/mℓ.[200,201] When serum ferritin measurements are compared to storage iron measurements obtained by quantitative phlebotomy, a high degree of correlation is found (Figure 4); ($r = 0.83$, $p < 0.001$), and each ng of ferritin per milliliter represents 8 mg of storage iron.[195] The range of ferritin determinations in iron deficiency, inflammation, liver disease, and iron overload is given in Figure 5. Ferritin determinations are useful in the diagnosis of iron deficiency and the assessment of iron stores after completion of iron therapy,[102] in monitoring the iron status of patients with chronic renal failure on regular dialysis,[203] or evaluating the effects of venesection in idiopathic hemochromatosis or chelation therapy in thalassemia.[204] Reduced serum levels of ferritin are strong evidence of iron depletion, but increased levels do not necessarily mean iron overload. Inflammation, liver disease, and ineffective erythropoiesis are associated with ferritin levels that are disproportionately increased in relation to bone marrow hemosiderin.[201] Disproportionately low serum ferritin levels are found in some patients with precirrhotic hemochromatosis, even in the presence of 5 to 10 g of excess storage iron.[205-207] In hemochromatosis, most of the surplus iron is stored in parenchymal cells, and the relatively low serum ferritin may be explained by the paucity of storage iron in RE cells, which are believed to be the cells responsible for the production of circulating ferritin. Despite these limitations of serum ferritin, it is a very useful laboratory tool for the evaluation of iron stores in most clinical situations and is particularly suitable for surveys involving large numbers of individuals.

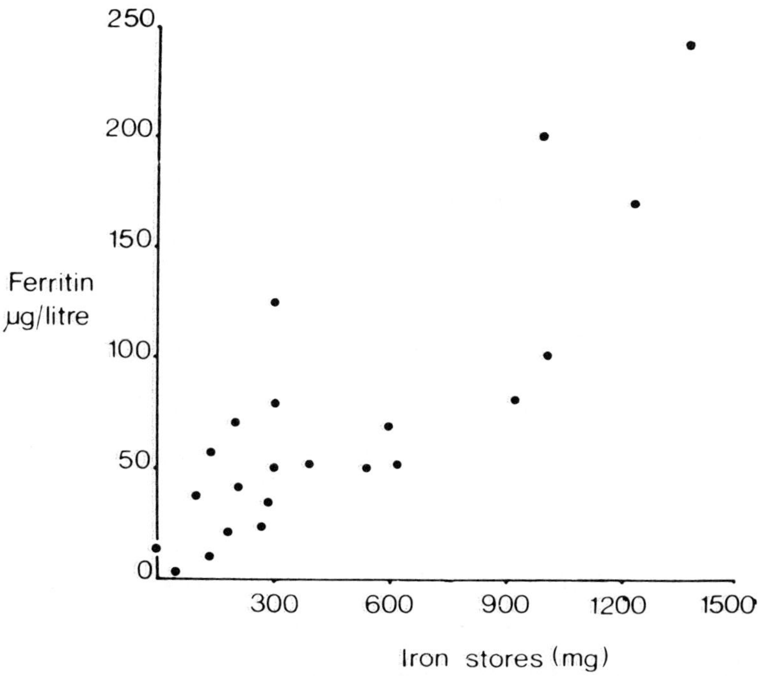

FIGURE 4. Relationship between serum ferritin concentration and mobilizable iron stores determined by serial phlebotomies. $r = 0.83$; $p<0.001$. (From Walters, G. O., Miller, F. M., and Worwood, M., *J. Clin. Pathol.*, 26, 770, 1973. With permission.)

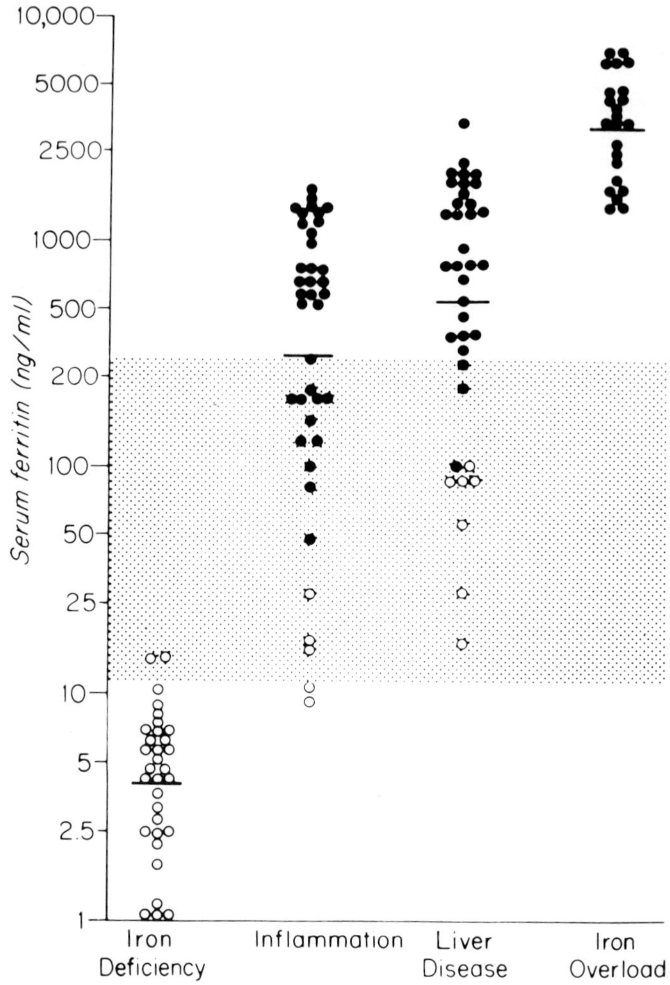

FIGURE 5. Measurements of serum ferritin in uncomplicated iron deficiency, inflammation, liver disease, and iron overload. The shaded area represents the normal range. Patients with iron deficiency defined by a low transferrin saturation or absent marrow iron are represented by open circles. (Reprinted, by permission. From Lipschitz, D. A., Cook, J. D., and Finch, C. A., *The New England Journal of Medicine,* Vol. 290; p. 1213, 1974.

Use of Isotopes in the Study of Iron Turnover

Radioisotopes were first applied to the study of the physiology of iron in the circulation by Hahn et al.[208] in 1939. Within the next 10 years both ^{59}Fe and ^{55}Fe became established as useful radioiron tracers in the study of iron kinetics. It was shown that iron is not taken up directly by circulating erythrocytes[209] and that it is incorporated into hemoglobin by the erythroid precursor cells of the bone marrow. It was also recognized that the rate of radioiron uptake by the marrow was related to the number of erythroid precursors in that tissue.[210,211] The fundamentals of present-day ferrokinetic techniques were laid by Huff et al.[212,213] who first used transferrin-bound radioiron to study the rate of red cell production. Red cell production rates were measured by calculating the rate of clearance from the plasma (T½ ^{59}Fe), the fraction of radioiron incorporated into circulating erythrocytes at days 10 to 14, the plasma iron concentration, and the plasma volume.[214]

Plasma iron turnover (PIT) is calculated as follows:

$$\text{PIT} = \frac{\text{plasma iron (mg/d}\ell\text{)} \times 0.693 \times 1440}{T^{1/2}\ \text{(min)}} = \text{mg/d}\ell\ \text{plasma / day}$$

The above formula can be simplified to:

$$\frac{\text{plasma iron } (\mu g\ \%)}{T^{1/2}\ \text{min}}$$

or converted into mg/dℓ whole blood as a product of:

$$\frac{(100\text{-Hct})}{100}$$

or converted into mg/kg/day as a product of:

$$\frac{\text{plasma volume (m}\ell\text{)}}{\text{weight (kg)} \times 100}$$

Red blood cell utilization (RBCU) expressed as activity of circulating RBC (percent of injected radioiron) is calculated by the formula:

$$\frac{\text{14 day activity / m}\ell\text{ whole blood} \times 100}{\text{0 time activity / m}\ell\text{ whole blood}}$$

Erythrocyte iron turnover (EIT) is the product of PIT × RBCU.

The standard expression of mg/dℓ whole blood per day for PIT and EIT is preferred, since it does not require plasma volume measurement and permits comparison between different individuals. Ferrokinetic data published up to 1970 for various clinical conditions have been reviewed by Finch et al.[214] and are summarized in Table 6. The average normal PIT is 0.70 mg/dℓ whole blood per day and the EIT is 0.56. The standard deviation of the normal mean is ± 24%.[215]

In terms of ferrokinetic measurements, anemias can be divided into three categories: (1) disorders of proliferation, (2) disorders of maturation, and (3) disorders of the mature erythrocyte.

Disorders of proliferation are seen in conditions with impaired erythropoietin production caused by a reduction in tissue metabolism, such as hypofunction of the thyroid, pituitary, or adrenal glands or testes, or in severe renal disease. These conditions are characterized by normal or increased serum iron and T½ ^{59}Fe and reduced or normal PIT and EIT. In renal insufficiency red cell life span is reduced,[216] and a normal EIT in some of the patients reflects a relative insufficiency of erythropoietin response. In iron deficiency serum iron and T½ ^{59}Fe are very low, and PIT and EIT are within the normal range. Iron-deficient erythropoiesis is ineffective[3,217] and the survival of RBC is impaired.[218] Thus, in spite of an apparently normal rate of EIT, the circulating red cell mass cannot be sustained at normal levels in iron deficiency.

Inflammation caused by infection, connective tissue disorders, or malignancy is manifested in low-serum iron, a short T½ ^{59}Fe, and normal PIT and EIT, in a fashion similar to that of iron deficiency. Iron supply is limited because of a block in iron release from tissues.[171] Red cell survival in inflammation is about half normal, and the normal rates of EIT are not sufficient to prevent a reduction in red cell mass. This relative bone marrow failure is caused by the limited supply of transferrin iron and an inadequate erythropoietin response to anemia.[219] Marrow damage ranging from leukemic infiltration of the marrow to complete aplasia is the most simple and straight-

Table 6
FERROKINETIC DATA IN VARIOUS CLINICAL CONDITIONS[a]

Condition	PCV (%)	SI (μg/dl)	T½ (min)	PIT (mg/dl/d)	Utilization (%)	EIT (mg/dl/d)
Normal	45	105	86	0.70	80	0.56
Anemia						
Disorders of proliferation						
Decreased erythropoietin						
Hypothyroidism	31	62	84	0.51	79	0.41
Renal failure						
I Transfused	24	220	221	0.84	34	0.29
II Nontransfused	27	76	79	0.81	81	0.66
Iron deficiency	26	21	20	0.80	94	0.75
Inflammation						
Infection	36	60	47	0.81	86	0.70
Rheum arthritis	37	68	48	0.89	78	0.70
Hodgkin's disease	31	55	42	0.90	76	0.68
Marrow damage						
Aplasia	21	182	351	0.45	0	0
Primary hypoplasia	25	199	310	0.48	26	0.12
Multiple myeloma	30	54	105	0.36	71	0.26
Acute leukemia	23	175	187	0.75	47	0.35
Disorders of maturation						
Nuclear abnormalities						
Pernicious anemia	19	153	51	2.43	28	0.68
Sprue	22	114	62	1.62	46	0.75
Impaired Hb synthesis						
Thalassemia major	24	169	24	5.36	18	0.96
Thalassemia trait	37	151	66	1.44	59	0.85
Refractory anemia with hypercellular marrow	23	152	55	2.13	31	0.66
Myelofibrosis	27	111	62	1.31	44	0.57
Hemolytic anemias						
Hereditary spherocytosis	35	118	27	2.84	61	1.73
Autoimmune hemolytic anemia	29	116	39	2.11	73	1.54
Sickle cell anemia	25	117	29	3.03	63	1.91
PNH	30	136	45	2.10	72	1.51
Polycythemia						
Polycythemia vera	60	86	34	1.01	86	0.87
Secondary polycythemia	57	113	64	0.76	85	0.64
Hemochromatosis	44	213	121	0.98	74	0.73

[a] Average values of data. PCV = packed cell volume; SI = serum iron; PIT = plasma iron turnover; EIT = erythrocyte iron turnover.

From Finch, C. A., Deubelbeiss, K., Cook, J. D., Eschbach, L. A., Harker, L. A., Funk, D. D., Marsaglia, G., Hillman, R. S., Slichter, S., Adamson, J. W., Ganzoni, A., and Giblett, E. R., *Medicine,* 49, 17, 1970. With permission of the Williams & Wilkins Co., Baltimore.

forward manifestation of "disorders of proliferation". EIT is moderately or drastically reduced in this case; serum iron and T½ ^{59}Fe are very high, and PIT reflects mostly nonerythroid iron turnover.

Disorders of maturation are conditions characterized by excessive death of nucleated red cells, or ineffective erythropoiesis. The mechanism responsible for this premature destruction of erythroid cells may be nuclear abnormality, an impairment of hemoglobin synthesis, a heterogenous group of anemias commonly referred to as refractory anemia with hypercellular marrow, and myelofibrosis.

Nuclear abnormality is responsible for ineffective erythropoiesis in the megaloblastic anemia of B12 and folate deficiency. PIT is twice to fourfold normal, but most of the iron turnover is wasted on early death of erythroid precursors, and EIT is only a small fraction of PIT. Following treatment, plasma iron becomes the limiting factor and PIT is often reduced to the range usually found in iron deficiency.[220]

Impaired hemoglobin synthesis is responsible for the extremely severe, ineffective erythropoiesis typical of thalassemia major. Expansion of the erythropoietic tissue throughout the medullary cavities is reflected in a nearly tenfold increase in PIT, with extensive breakdown of developing cells which, in turn, are rapidly catabolized with efficient recircuiting of hemoglobin iron. Because of the premature destruction of erythrocytes, EIT is reduced to about 20% of the PIT.[221] A similar, but less pronounced, discrepancy between PIT and EIT can be found in thalassemia minor and the sideroblastic anemias.[222]

In refractory anemia with hyperplastic marrow and in myelofibrosis ineffective erythropoiesis is the final common expression of a wide range of disorders characterized by abnormal erythroid maturation. The ferrokinetic pattern of these conditions is indistinguishable from that of the megaloblastic anemias or thalassemia.

Hemolytic anemias are characterized by increased serum iron, a very short T½ ^{59}Fe, and increased PIT and EIT. Although EIT is about 30% less than PIT, this discrepancy does not necessarily represent ineffective erythropoiesis, but rather a dilution of the radioiron tracer in the labile iron pool, and, in addition, destruction of young erythrocytes within the 2-week observation period. Premature destruction of erythrocytes is also reflected in the accumulation of radioactivity in organs involved in red cell sequestration and destruction, such as the spleen.

Ferrokinetic studies are useful in defining differences between primary and secondary polycythemia. In both conditions a moderate increase in PIT and EIT may be found, but in polycythemia vera EIT is relatively higher than the rate required to maintain a constant level of circulating red cells, indicating a progressive expansion of the red cell mass. The T½ ^{59}Fe in polycythemia vera is often shorter than in secondary polycythemia, but this difference may be attributed to a coexistent iron deficiency, which is quite common in polycythemia vera.

Ferrokinetics are of limited value in the diagnosis and evaluation of idiopathic hemochromatosis. Although serum iron is usually very high, PIT and EIT are near normal, and nonerythroid iron turnover is not strikingly increased.

The above data, based on simple calculations of PIT and EIT, provide useful information for the clinical assessment of various pathologic conditions. However, the rate of radioiron disappearance from the plasma is a complex function and cannot be accurately expressed as a simple exponential curve. Normally, the slope of the radioiron disappearance curve changes from about 40% per hour initially to less than 1% on the second day because of a reflux of iron into the plasma from more peripheral compartments. Attempts have been made to formulate a reflux model by multicompartmental analysis of plasma radioactivity, but these models have not been validated by correlation with normal and pathologic states.[223-225]

An alternative approach has been the analysis of the radioiron disappearance curve in terms of a probability theory.[226] The distribution of sojourn times for returning particles was calculated from an integrodifferential equation by fitting the plasma iron disappearance curve with a linear combination of exponential functions. This method has been further extended to estimate total reflux based on the area underlying the disappearance curve.[3] Total reflux in turn, was further subdivided into early and late components (Table 7). Total reflux amounts to about ⅓ of total PIT in normal subjects, in iron overload, erythroid hypoplasia, and uremic patients without transfusion requirement. Reflux is over 50% in hemolytic anemia, iron deficiency, and ineffective erythropoiesis. Early reflux has a reentry time of 7 to 10 hr. It is similar in all disease groups, amounting to 0.14 mg iron/dℓ/day with an SD of +0.08. It is not affected by differences in erythropoietic activity, but is positively correlated to the level of plasma iron and plasmatocrit (r = 0.711, $p < 0.001$). Both the reentry time and the amount of iron involved in early exchange are consistent with a lymphatic shunt of transferrin iron. Late reflux is usually larger than early reflux. It is not affected by the size of body iron stores or plasma iron levels, but is very sensitive to erythropoietic activity. Late reflux is very low in aplastic anemia and is greatly increased in hemolytic anemia. The T½ of late reflux is 5 to 15 days as compared to T½ of 7 to 10 hr in early reflux. The close correlation with erythropoietic activity and the time of return identify late reflux with wastage iron of erythropoiesis or iron taken up by the marrow but released without permanent incorporation into circulating erythrocytes.

Having defined the early and late reflux pathways, it is possible to construct a comprehensive model of iron exchange in the body (Figure 6). Fixed tissue turnover represents the amount of iron cleared from the plasma and not returned during the subsequent 2 weeks. It consists of fixed erythrocyte turnover, which indicates effective erythropoiesis, and fixed parenchymal turnover, represented by the hepatic parenchyma as the most important organ. In analogy with early reflux, fixed parenchymal turnover is closely related to the concentration of transferrin iron (r = 0.085, $p <$ 0.001). Total plasma iron turnover is the sum of fixed tissue turnover and total reflux. Since both components of nonerythron turnover, namely early reflux and fixed parenchymal turnover, are proportional to plasma iron supply, they can be derived from the formula:

$$\text{Nonerythron turnover} = \text{S I } (\mu g / d\ell) \times \text{plasmatocrit} \times 0.0035$$

Erythron turnover can be obtained by subtracting nonerythron turnover from PIT. The relation between total erythron turnover and fixed erythrocyte turnover is determined by the efficiency of erythropoiesis.

The handling of iron by RE cells can be studied directly by the use of heat-denatured ^{59}Fe-labeled erythrocytes (^{59}Fe DRBC).[172,173,227] Following a short lag phase required for red cell phagocytosis and heme catabolism, ^{59}Fe derived from hemoglobin enters a labile pool from which it is either promptly returned to circulating transferrin (early release) or is retained (late release) in a more slowly exchanging iron pool (Table 8). The half-life of early and late release in normal man is 33 min and 5.6 days, respectively. Through a wide spectrum of clinical conditions, the half-life of early release was found to be constant, but the proportion of early release ranged from 100% in iron deficiency to as little as 10% in iron overload. The half-life of late release ranged from less than 1 day in iron deficiency or treated hemochromatosis to no measurable release in advanced untreated hemochromatosis. The cumulative release of radioiron within 2 weeks was 100% in patients with iron deficiency and treated hemochromatosis, 93% in normals, and less than 70% in patients with inflammation and untreated hemochromatosis.

Another approach to the study of iron exchange in the body is the in vivo measurement of transferrin ^{59}Fe uptake by the different tissues using surface counting (Figure 7). The distribution of ^{59}Fe radioactivity is measured within 12 days of injection and is expressed in relation to the radioactivity measured over the same organ immediately after injection of labeled transferrin. In normal subjects, ^{59}Fe is rapidly cleared from

Table 7
IRON TURNOVER COMPARTMENTS

	Fixed (mg/dℓ whole blood/day)			Reflux (mg/dℓ whole blood/day)			
	Total	RBC	Parenchymal	Total	Early	Late	Total erythron
Normal subjects	0.50 ± 0.03[a]	0.41 ± 0.02	0.09 ± 0.01	0.25 ± 0.01	0.06 ± 0.01	0.19 ± 0.01	0.60 ± 0.02
Iron overload	0.85 ± 0.05	0.66 ± 0.05	0.18 ± 0.03	0.34 ± 0.03	0.12 ± 0.02	0.23 ± 0.02	0.89 ± 0.07
Iron deficiency	0.32 ± 0.10	0.32 ± 0.09	0.01 ± 0.01	0.37 ± 0.06	0.10 ± 0.03	0.27 ± 0.06	0.59 ± 0.15
Erythroid hypoplasia	0.31 ± 0.04	0.01 ± 0.01	0.30 ± 0.03	0.18 ± 0.02	0.16 ± 0.03	0.02 ± 0.002	0.03 ± 0.01
Renal patients							
I Transfused	0.60 ± 0.09	0.15 ± 0.04	0.45 ± 0.05	0.38 ± 0.03	0.27 ± 0.02	0.11 ± 0.02	0.26 ± 0.06
II Nontransfused	0.56 ± 0.08	0.45 ± 0.06	0.11 ± 0.02	0.36 ± 0.05	0.11 ± 0.02	0.24 ± 0.04	0.69 ± 0.10
Hemolytic anemia	1.56 ± 0.20	1.43[b] ± 0.12	0.13[b] ± 0.07	1.65 ± 0.27	0.15 ± 0.05	1.49 ± 0.25	2.92 ± 0.32
Ineffective erythropoiesis	1.07 ± 0.11	—	—	2.08 ± 0.32	—	—	2.67 ± 0.49

[a] Standard error of the mean.
[b] Values calculated indirectly by estimating the nonerythron iron turnover from plasma iron and plasmatocrit.

From Cook, J. D., Marsaglia, G., Eschbach, J. W., Funk, D. D., and Finch, C. A., *J. Clin. Invest.*, 49, 197, 1970. With permission.

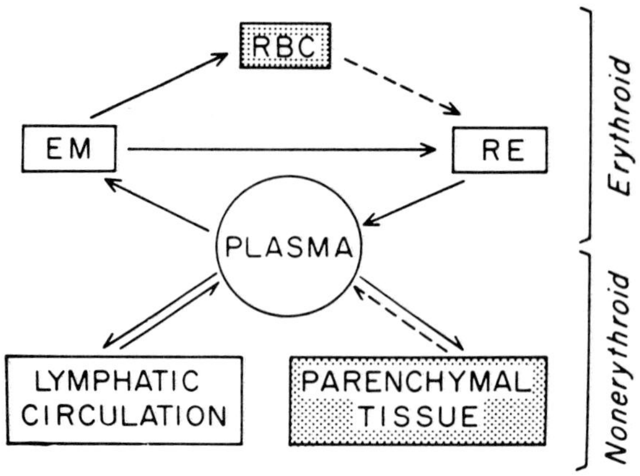

FIGURE 6. A biological model for plasma iron turnover. PIT is divided into iron which remains localized in tissue (shaded areas) and iron which will be returned to the plasma within 2 weeks. Total reflux consists of lymphatic circulation and the sojourn of nonviable erythrocyte precursors via the reticuloendothelial system. The intracellularly fixed tissue turnover is partitioned into an erythrocyte and parenchymal fraction. During a 2-week period of observation, there is no evidence for a return of iron from these sites (interrupted lines). Total erythron iron turnover, including both effective and ineffective erythropoiesis, is represented by the sum of the fixed erythrocyte and late reflux values. (From Cook, J. D., Marsaglia, G., Eschbach, J. W., Funk, D. D., and Finch, C. A., *J. Clin. Invest.*, 49, 197, 1970. With permission.)

Table 8
RETICULOENDOTHELIAL HANDLING OF ^{59}Fe-LABELED ERYTHROCYTES

	Condition				
	Early release		Late release		^{59}Fe/^{55}Fe[a]
	%	T½ (min)	%	T½ (min)	at 15 days
Normal	64	33	36	5.6	92.5
Inflammation	44	42	56	12.0	64.0
Hemochromatosis					
Untreated	57	39	43	∞	69.5
Treated	92	29	8	<0.5	100
Iron deficiency	100	31	0	—	100

[a] Ratio of transferrin ^{55}Fe and DRBC ^{59}Fe in newly formed erythrocytes; used as an index of cumulative ^{59}Fe release from RE cells.

From Fillet, G., These du grade d'Agrege de l'Enseignement Superieur, Universite de Liege, 1977. With permission.

blood with a reciprocal increase in marrow radioactivity. Radioiron is subsequently released from the marrow in newly formed erythrocytes, with a corresponding increase in blood radioactivity. Because of its high vascularity, the spleen reflects blood radioactivity, and there is little change in hepatic radioactivity within the 12-day study period. In hemolytic anemia with a predominantly splenic destruction of erythrocytes, radioactivity accumulates over the spleen, with a reduced proportion of radioactivity

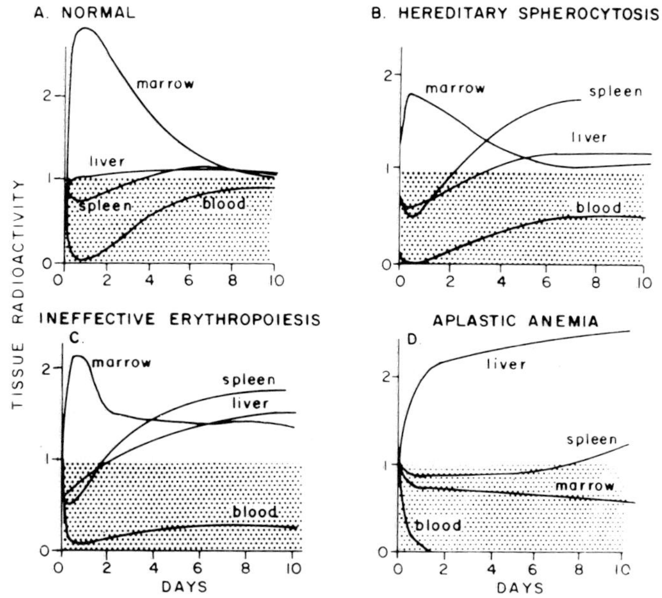

FIGURE 7. Blood and tissue ferrokinetic profiles. All measurements start at 1, representing radioactivity immediately after the injection of radioiron. In hereditary spherocytosis (B), the marrow produces cells which are trapped and subsequently destroyed in the spleen, indicated by the accumulation of radioactivity in the spleen and the reduced proportion of activity appearing in circulating erythrocytes. In ineffective erythropoiesis (C), the marrow is active as shown by its initial uptake of radioiron, but radioactivity subsequently accumulates in the liver, spleen, and marrow, indicating that a large portion of the erythroid activity is wasted on the production of nonviable erythrocytes which are removed by the reticuloendothelial cells of these organs. In aplastic anemia (D), there is no marrow uptake of radioiron and none appears in circulating red cells. Instead, there is pathologic deposition of iron in the parenchymal cells of the liver. (From Finch, C. A., Deubelbeiss, K., Cook, J. D., Eschbach, L. A., Harker, L. A., Funk, D. D., Marsaglia, G., Hillman, R. S., Slichter, S., Adamson, J. W., Ganzoni, A., and Giblett, E. R., *Medicine,* 49, 17, 1970. With permission of the Williams & Wilkins Co., Baltimore.)

in circulating erythrocytes. In ineffective erythropoiesis, radioactivity accumulates over the liver and marrow as well as over the spleen, indicating the production of nonviable erythrocytes which are removed by reticuloendothelial cells of those organs. Finally, in aplastic anemia, there is no marrow uptake of radioactivity and no production of labeled erythrocytes. Iron is accumulated mainly over the liver, reflecting the parenchymal uptake of transferrin ^{59}Fe.[228]

ACKNOWLEDGMENT

This work was supported in part by Grant No. 750 of the United States - Israel Binational Science Foundation.

REFERENCES

1. **Harrison, P. M., Hoare, R. J., Hoy, T. Y., and Macara, I. G.,** Ferritin and haemosiderin: structure and function, in *Iron in Biochemistry and Medicine,* Jacobs, A. and Worwood, M., Eds., Academic Press, London, 1974, 73.
2. **Crichton, R. R., Huebers, H., and Huebers, E.,** Comparative studies on ferritin, in *Proteins of Iron Storage and Transport in Biochemistry and Medicine,* Crichton, R. R., Eds., North-Holland, Amsterdam, 1975, 193.
3. **Cook, J. D., Marsaglia, G., Eschbach, J. W., Funk, D. D., and Finch, C. A.,** Ferrokinetics: a biologic model for plasma iron exchange in man, *J. Clin. Invest.,* 49, 197, 1970.
4. **Callender, S. T., Mallett, B. J., and Smith, M. D.,** Absorption of haemoglobin iron, *Br. J. Haematol.,* 3, 186, 1957.
5. **Turnbull, A., Cleton, F., and Finch, C. A.,** Iron absorption. IV. The absorption of hemoglobin iron, *J. Clin. Invest.,* 41, 1897, 1962.
6. **Hwang, Y. F. and Brown, E. B.,** Effect of desferrioxamine in iron absorption, *Lancet,* 1, 135, 1965.
7. **Conrad, M. E., Weintraub, L. R., Sears, D. A., and Crosby, W. H.,** Absorption of hemoglobin iron, *Am. J. Physiol.,* 211, 1123, 1966.
8. **Hallberg, L. and Solvell, L.,** Absorption of hemoglobin iron in man, *Acta Med. Scand.,* 181, 335, 1967.
9. **Wheby, M. S., Suttle, G. E., and Ford, K. T.,** Intestinal absorption of hemoglobin iron, *Gastroenterology,* 58, 647, 1970.
10. **Callender, S. T., Marney, S. R., and Werner, G. T.,** Absorption of labelled iron from food, *Br. J. Radiol.,* 43, 284, 1970.
11. **Layrisse, M., Martinez-Torres, C., Cook, J. D., Walker, R., and Finch, C. A.,** Iron fortification of food: its measurement by the extrinsic tag method, *Blood,* 41, 333, 1973.
12. **Hallberg, L. and Solvell, L.,** Absorption of a single dose of iron in man, *Acta Med. Scand. Suppl.,* 358(168), 19, 1960.
13. **Brown, E. B.,** The absorption of iron, *Am. J. Clin. Nutr.,* 12, 205, 1963.
14. **Wheby, M. S. and Crosby, W. H.,** The gastrointestinal tract and iron absorption, *Blood,* 22, 416, 1963.
15. **Dowdle, E. B., Schachter, D., and Schenker, H.,** Active transport of ^{59}Fe by everted segments of rat duodenum, *Am. J. Physiol.,* 198, 609, 1960.
16. **Jacobs, P., Bothwell, T. H., and Charlton, R. W.,** Intestinal iron transport: studies using a loop of gut with artificial circulation, *Am. J. Physiol.,* 210, 694, 1966.
17. **Greenberger, N. Y., Balcerzak, S. P., and Ackerman, G. A.,** Iron uptake by isolated intestinal brush borders: changes induced by alterations in iron stores, *J. Lab. Clin. Med.,* 73, 711, 1969.
18. **Hübers, H., Hübers, E., Forth, W., Leopold, G., and Rummel, W.,** Binding of iron to non-ferritin protein in the mucosal cells of normal and iron deficient rats during absorption, *Acta Pharmacol. Toxicol.,* 29(Suppl. 4), 22, 1971.
19. **Richmond, V. S., Worwood, M., and Jacobs, A.,** The iron content of intestinal epithelial cells and its subcellular distribution: studies on normal, iron loaded and iron deficient rats, *Br. J. Haematol.,* 23, 605, 1972.
20. **Conrad, M. E. and Crosby, W. H.,** Intestinal mucosal mechanisms controlling iron absorption, *Blood,* 22, 406, 1963.
21. **Worwood, M. and Jacobs, A.,** The subcellular distribution of ^{59}Fe in small intestinal mucosa: studies with normal, iron deficient and iron loaded rats, *Br. J. Haematol.,* 22, 265, 1972.
22. **Brown, E. B. and Rother, M. L.,** Studies of the mechanism of iron absorption. II. Influence of iron deficiency and other conditions on iron uptake by rats, *J. Lab. Clin. Med.,* 62, 804, 1963.
23. **Worwood, M. and Jacobs, A.,** The subcellular distribution of ^{59}Fe during iron absorption in the rat, *Br. J. Haematol.,* 20, 587, 1971.
24. **Hübers, H., Hübers, E., Simon, J., and Forth, W.,** A method for preparing stable density gradients and their application for fractionation of intestinal mucosal cells, *Life Sci.,* 10, 377, 1971.
25. **Charlton, R. W., Jacobs, P., Torrance, J. D., and Bothwell, T. H.,** Regulation of the intestinal absorption of iron by the rate of erythropoiesis, *Br. J. Haematol.,* 2, 432, 1965.
26. **Sheehan, R. G. and Frenkel, E. P.,** The control of iron absorption in the gastrointestinal mucosal cell, *J. Clin. Invest.,* 51, 224, 1972.
27. **Blanc, B. and Isliker, H.,** Repartition du par dans diverses fraction tissulaires de la mugeuse intestinale au cours de l'absorption, *Helv. Physiol. Pharmacol. Acta,* 23, 145, 1965.
28. **Worwood, M. and Jacobs, A.,** Absorption of ^{59}Fe in the rat: iron binding substances in the soluble fraction of intestinal mucosa, *Life Sci.,* 10, 1363, 1971.
29. **Jacobs, A. and Worwood, M.,** Correlation between iron content and ferritin in hemochromatosis, *Br. J. Haematol.,* 27, 359, 1974.
30. **Pollack, S., Camparro, T., and Arcario, A.,** A search for mucosal iron carrier. Identification of mucosal fractions with rapid turnover of ^{59}Fe, *J. Lab. Clin. Med.,* 80, 322, 1972.

31. **Hübers, H., Hübers, E., Simon, J., and Forth, W.,** Binding of iron to a non-ferritin protein in the mucosal cells of normal and iron deficient rats during absorption, *Life Sci.,* 10, 1141, 1971.
32. **Granick, S.,** Protein apoferritin and ferritin in iron feeding and absorption, *Science,* 103, 107, 1946.
33. **Boender, C. A., Mulder, E., Plaem, J. E., Wael, J., and Verloop, M. C.,** Iron absorption and retention in man, *Nature (London),* 213, 1236, 1967.
34. **Boender, C. A. and Verloop, M. C.,** Iron absorption, iron loss and iron retention in man: studies after oral iron administration of a tracer dose of $^{59}FeSO_4$ and $^{131-}BaSO_4$, *Br. J. Haematol.,* 17, 45, 1969.
35. **Powell, L. W., Campbell, C. B., and Wilson, E.,** Intestinal mucosal uptake of iron and iron retention in idiopathic hemochromatosis as evidence for a mucosal abnormality, *Gut,* 11, 727, 1970.
36. **Brittin, G. M. and Raval, D.,** Duodenal ferritin synthesis during iron absorption in the iron-deficient rat, *J. Lab. Clin. Med.,* 75, 811, 1970.
37. **Brittin, G. M. and Ravel, D.,** Duodenal ferritin synthesis during iron absorption in the iron-deficient rat, *J. Lab. Clin. Med.,* 77, 54, 1971.
38. **Schade, S. G., Felsher, B. F., Bernier, G. M., and Conrad, M. E.,** Effect of cobalt upon iron absorption, *J. Lab. Clin. Med.,* 75, 435, 1970.
39. **Bielig, H. J. and Bayer, E.,** Eisenkomplexe mit 3 ungepaarten Elektronen, *Naturwissenschaften,* 16, 466, 1955.
40. **Conrad, M. E., Benjamin, B. I., Williams, H. L., and Foy, A. L.,** Human absorption of hemoglobin iron, *Gastroenterology,* 53, 5, 1967.
41. **Brown, E. B., Hwang, Y. F., Nicol, S., and Turnberg, J.,** Absorption of radiation-labeled hemoglobin by days, *J. Lab. Clin. Med.,* 72, 58, 1968.
42. **Weintraub, L. R., Weinstein, M. B., Huser, H., and Rafal, S.,** Absorption of hemoglobin iron: the role of heme-splitting substance in the intestinal mucosa, *J. Clin. Invest.,* 47, 531, 1968.
43. **Dawson, R. B., Rafal, S., and Weintraub, L. R.,** Absorption of hemoglobin iron: the role of xantine oxidase in the intestinal heme-splitting reaction, *Blood,* 35, 94, 1970.
44. **Wynter, C. V. A. and Williams, R.,** Iron binding properties of gastric juice in idiopathic haemochromatosis, *Lancet,* 2, 534, 1968.
45. **Forth, W., Rummel, W., and Adres, H.,** Zur Frage der Regulation der Eisenresorption durch Gastroferrin, ein eisenbinden des Protein des Magensafts, *Klin. Wochenschr.,* 46, 1003, 1968.
46. **Jacobs, A.,** Availability and absorption of dietary iron, in *Progress in Gastroenterology,* Vol. 2, Glass, B. J., Ed., Grune & Stratton, New York, 1970, 221.
47. **Kavin, H., Charlton, R. W., Jacobs, P., Green, R., Torrance, J. D., and Bothwell, T. H.,** Effect of the exocrine pancreatic secretions on iron absorption, *Gut,* 8, 556, 1967.
48. **Murray, M. J. and Stein, N.,** Does pancreas influence iron absorption? *Br. J. Haematol.,* 15, 87, 1968.
49. **Jacobs, A., Rhodes, J., and Eakins, J. D.,** Gastric factors influencing iron absorption in anaemic patients, *Scand. J. Haematol.,* 4, 105, 1967.
50. **Jacobs, A.,** Effect of gastric juice and pH in inorganic iron in solution, *Nature (London),* 216, 707, 1967.
51. **Smith, P. M., Studley, F., and Williams, R.,** Iron absorption in idiopathic haemochromatosis and its measurement using a whole body counter, *Clin. Sci.,* 37, 519, 1969.
52. **Crosby, W. H.,** The control of iron balance by the intestinal mucosa, *Blood,* 22, 441, 1963.
53. **Conrad, M. E., Weintraub, L. R., and Crosby, W. H.,** Role of intestine in iron kinetics, *J. Clin. Invest.,* 43, 963, 1964.
54. **Weintraub, L. R., Conrad, M. E., and Crosby, W. H.,** Regulation of the intestinal absorption of iron by the rate of erythropoiesis, *Br. J. Haematol.,* 11, 432, 1965.
55. **Pirzio-Biroli, G., Bothwell, T. H., and Finch, B. A.,** Iron absorption. II. The absorption of radioiron administered with a standard meal in man, *J. Lab. Clin. Med.,* 51, 37, 1958.
56. **Weintraub, L. R., Conrad, M. E., and Crosby, W. H.,** The significance of iron turnover in the control of iron absorption, *Blood,* 24, 19, 1964.
57. **Chirashiri, L. and Izak, G.,** The effect of acute hemorrhages and acute hemolysis on the intestinal iron absorption in the rat, *Br. J. Haematol.,* 12, 611, 1966.
58. **Pearson, W. N., Reich, M., Frank, H., and Salamat, L.,** Effects of dietary iron level on gut iron levels and iron absorption in the rat, *J. Nutr.,* 92, 53, 1967.
59. **Kaufman, R. M., Pollack, S., and Crosby, W. H.,** Iron-deficient diet: effects in rats and humans, *Blood,* 28, 726, 1966.
60. **Balcerzak, S. P. and Greenberger, N. J.,** Iron content of isolated intestinal epithelial cells in relation to iron absorption, *Nature (London),* 20, 270, 1968.
61. **Pollack, S. and Campana, T.,** The relationship between mucosal iron and iron absorption in the guinea pig, *Scand. J. Haematol.,* 7, 208, 1970.
62. **Cook, J. D., Larysse, M., Martinez-Torres, C., Walker, R., Monsen, E., and Finch, C. A.,** Food iron absorption measured by an extrinsic tag, *J. Clin. Invest.,* 51, 805, 1972.

63. **Richmond, V. S., Worwood, M., and Jacobs, M.**, The iron content of intestinal epithelial cells and its subcellular distribution. Studies on normal, iron deficient and iron-overloaded animals, *Br. J. Haematol.*, 23, 605, 1972.
64. **Howard, J. and Jacobs, A.**, Iron transport by rat small intestine in vitro: effect of body iron status, *Br. J. Haematol.*, 23, 595, 1972.
65. **Worwood, M. and Jacobs, A.**, The subcellular distribution of ^{59}Fe in small intestinal mucosa, *Br. J. Haematol.*, 22, 265, 1972.
66. **Taylor, M. R. H. and Gatenby, P. B. B.**, Iron absorption in relation to transferrin saturation and other factors, *Br. J. Haematol.*, 16, 443, 1966.
67. **Pirzio-Biroli, G., and Finch, C. A.**, Iron absorption. III. The influence of iron stores on iron absorption in the normal subject, *J. Lab. Clin. Med.*, 55, 216, 1960.
68. **Heinrich, H. C.**, Iron deficiency without anaemia, *Lancet*, 2, 460, 1968.
69. **Hoglund, S. and Reizenstein, P.**, Studies on iron absorption. V. Effect of gastrointestinal factors on iron absorption, *Blood*, 34, 496, 1969.
70. **Hausmann, K., Kuse, R., Meinecke, K. H., Bartels, H., and Heinrich, H. C.**, Diagnostische Kriterien des prälatenten, latenten und manifesten Eisenmangels, *Klin. Wochenschr.*, 49, 1164, 1971.
71. **Totze, C., Schmerlinska, E., and Heinrich, H. C.**, Cytochemie des Nichthämoglobineisens in Knochenmarkzellen und intestinale Eisenresorption bei verschiedenen Anamien des Kindersalters, *Monatsschr. Kinderheilkd.*, 119, 13, 1971.
72. **Bannerman, R. M., Callender, S. T., Hardisty, R. M., and Smith, R. S.**, Iron absorption in thalassemia, *Br. J. Haematol.*, 10, 490, 1964.
73. **Shahid, M. J. and Haydar, N. A.**, Absorption of inorganic iron in thalassemia, *Br. J. Haematol.*, 13, 713, 1967.
74. **Erlandson, M. E., Walden, B., Stern, G., Hilgartner, M. W., Wehman, J., and Smith, C. H.**, Studies on congenital hemolytic syndromes. IV. Gastrointestinal absorption of iron, *Blood*, 19, 359, 1962.
75. **Brain, M. C. and Herdan, A.**, Tissue iron stores in sideroblastic anaemia, *Br. J. Haematol.*, 11, 107, 1965.
76. **Fletcher, J. and Huens, E. R.**, Significance of the binding of iron by transferrin, *Nature (London)*, 218, 1211, 1968.
77. **Lavie, R. S. and Finch, C. A.**, The in vivo plasma clearance of iron from transferrins of low and high iron saturation, *Clin. Sci.*, 38, 783, 1970.
78. **Krantz, S., Goldwasser, E., and Jacobson, L. O.**, Studies on erythropoiesis. XIV. The relationship of humoral stimulation to iron absorption, *Blood*, 14, 654, 1959.
79. **Beutler, E. and Buttenweiser, E.**, The regulation of iron absorption. A search for humoral factors, *J. Lab. Clin. Med.*, 55, 274, 1960.
80. **Mendel, G. A.**, Studies on iron absorption. I. The relationships between the rate of erythropoiesis, hypoxia, and iron absorption, *Blood*, 18, 727, 1961.
81. **Hathorn, M. K. S.**, The influence of hypoxia on iron absorption in the rat, *Gastroenterology*, 60, 76, 1971.
82. **Apte, S. V. and Brown, E. B.**, Effect of plasma from pregnant women on iron absorption by the rat, *J. Nutr.*, 101, 927, 1969.
83. **Larysse, M. and Martinez-Torres, C.**, Model for measuring the dietary absorption from heme iron. Measurement of the total iron absorption from a complete meal, *Am. J. Clin. Nutr.*, 25, 401, 1972.
84. **Larysse, M., Martinez-Torres, C., Cook, J. D., Walker, R., and Finch, C. A.**, Iron fortification of food: its measurement by the extrinsic tag method, *Blood*, 4, 333, 1973.
85. **Green, R., Charlton, R., Seftel, H., Bothwell, T., Mayet, F., Adams, B., and Finch, C. A.**, Body iron excretion in man, *Am. J. Med.*, 45, 336, 1968.
86. **Hallberg, L., Hagdahl, A. M., Nilsson, L., and Rylo, G.**, Menstrual blood loss in iron deficiency, *Acta Med. Scand.*, 180, 639, 1966.
87. **Kuhn, I. N., Mansen, E. R., Cook, J. D., and Finch, C. A.**, Iron absorption in man, *J. Lab. Clin. Med.*, 71, 715, 1968.
88. **Committee on Iron Deficiency of the AMA Council on Foods and Nutrition.** Iron deficiency in the United States, *JAMA*, 203, 407, 1968.
89. **Wheby, M. S. and Jones, L. G.**, Studies on iron absorption. Role of transferrin in iron absorption, *J. Clin. Invest.*, 42, 1007, 1963.
90. **Wheby, M. S. and Crosby, W. H.**, Studies on iron absorption. The gastrointestinal tract and iron absorption, *Blood*, 22, 416, 1963.
91. **Wheby, M. S.**, Studies on iron absorption, *N. Engl. J. Med.*, 271, 1391, 1964.
92. **Moore, C. V.**, The importance of nutritional factors in the pathogenesis of iron deficiency anemia, *Ser. Haematol.*, 6, 1, 1965.
93. **Peterson, R. E., and Manu, J. D.**, Transport of radioactive iron in the intestinal lymph, *Am. J. Physiol.*, 169, 763, 1952.
94. **Reizenstein, P. G., Cronkite, E. P., Meyer, L. M., and Usenik, A.**, Lymphatics in intestinal absorption of vitamin B_{12} and iron, *Proc. Soc. Exp. Biol. Med.*, 105, 233, 1960.

95. **Hyde, A. S.**, Absorption of radioiron perfused through the duodenuum of the rat, *Am. J. Physiol.*, 191, 265, 1957.
96. **Solvell, L.**, Absorption of radioiron perfused through the duodenuum of the rat, *Acta Med. Scand. Suppl.*, 358(168), 71, 1960.
97. **Charley, P. J., Sarkar, B., Stitt, C., and Saltman, P.**, Chelation of iron by sugars, *Biochim. Biophys. Acta*, 69, 313, 1963.
98. **Laurell, C. B. and Ingelman, B.**, The iron binding protein of swine serum, *Acta Chem. Scand.*, 1, 770, 1947.
99. **Aisen, P. and Brown, E. B.**, The iron-binding function of transferrin in iron metabolism, *Semin. Hematol.*, 14, 31, 1977.
100. **Roberts, R. C., Makey, D. G., and Seal, U. S.**, Human transferrin: molecular weight and sedimentation properties, *J. Biol. Chem.*, 84, 1907, 1966.
101. **Mann, K. G., Fish, W. W., Cox, A. C., and Tanford, C.**, Single chain nature of human serum transferrin, *Biochemistry*, 9, 1348, 1970.
102. **Leibman, A., and Aisen, P.**, Preparation of single crystals of transferrin, *Arch. Biochem. Biophys.*, 171, 717, 1967.
103. **Eriksson, S. and Sjognist, Y.**, Quantitative determination of N-terminal amino acids in some serum proteins, *Biochem. Biophys. Acta*, 45, 290, 1960.
104. **Ferney, R. E. and Komatsu, S. K.**, The role of tyrosyl groups in metal binding properties of transferrins, *Biochemistry*, 6, 1136, 1967.
105. **Jamieson, G. A., Jett, M., and de Barbados, S. L.**, The carbohydrate sequence of glycopeptide chains of human transferrin, *J. Biol. Chem.*, 246, 3686, 1971.
106. **Charlwood, P. A.**, Ultracentrifugal characteristics of human, monkey and rat transferrins, *Biochem. J.*, 88, 394, 1963.
107. **Roop, W. E. and Putnam, F. W.**, Purification and properties of human transferrin C and a slow moving genetic variant, *J. Biol. Chem.*, 242, 2507, 1967.
108. **Surgenor, D. M., Koechlin, B., and Strong, L. E.**, Chemical, clinical and immunological studies on products of human plasma fractionation, metal-combining globulin of human plasma, *J. Clin. Invest.*, 28, 73, 1949.
109. **Morgan, E. H.**, Transferrin and transferrin iron, in *Iron in Biochemistry and Medicine*, Jacobs, A. and Worwood, M., Eds., Academic Press, London, 1974, 29.
110. **MacGillivray, R. T. A. and Brew, K.**, Transferrin: internal homology in the amino acid sequence, *Science*, 190, 236, 1975.
111. **Warner, R. G. and Weber, I.**, Metal combining properties of conalbumin; cupric and ferric citrate complexes, *J. Am. Chem. Soc.*, 75, 5094, 1953.
112. **Lane, R. S.**, DEAE-cellulose chromatography of human transferrin: the effect of increasing iron saturation and copper (II) binding, *Biochim. Biophys. Acta*, 243, 193, 1971.
113. **Lane, R. S.**, Transferrin-reticulocyte binding: evidence for the functional importance of transferrin conformation, *Br. J. Haematol.*, 22, 309, 1972.
114. **Bezkorovainy, A., Rafelson, M. E., Likhite, V.**, Isolation and partial characterization of transferrin from normal human plasma, *Arch. Biochem.*, 103, 371, 1963.
115. **Rosserieau-Motreff, M. Y., Soletewey, F., Lamote, R., and Peeters, H.**, Size and shape determination of apotransferrin and transferrin monomers, *Biopolymers*, 10, 1039, 1971.
116. **Azari, P. R. and Feeney, R. E.**, Resistance of metal complexes of conalbumin and transferrin to proteolysis and thermal denaturation, *J. Biol. Chem.*, 232, 293, 1958.
117. **Glazer, A. N. and McKenzie, H. A.**, The denaturation of proteins. IV. Conalbumin and iron. III. Conalbumin in urea solution, *Biochim. Biophys. Acta*, 71, 109, 1963.
118. **Clark, J. R., Osuga, D. T., and Feeney, R. E.**, A genetically varying minor protein constituent of chicken egg white, *J. Biol. Chem.*, 238, 3621, 1963.
119. **Bezkovainy, A.**, A comparative study of metal-free, iron-saturated and scialic acid-free transferrins, *Biochim. Biophys. Acta*, 127, 535, 1966.
120. **Bron, C., Blanc, C., and Isliker, H.**, Etude electrophoretique de la denaturation de transferrin humaine par l'uree, *Biochem. Biophys. Acta*, 154, 67, 1968.
121. **Faust, C. H. and Tengerdy, R. P.**, The role of antigenic conformation in antigen-antibody complex formation, *Immunochemistry*, 8, 211, 1971.
122. **Scuro, L. A., Dobrilla, G., Lo Carcio, V., Bosello, O., D'Andrea, F., and Innecco, A.**, Transferrin iron-binding capacity and total iron binding capacity. Discrepancy as an index of extra-transferrin iron transport, *Acta Hepato Gastroenterol.*, 19, 90, 1972.
123. **Ezekiel, E.**, The iron binding proteins in milk and the secretion of iron by the mammary gland in the rat, *Biochim. Biophys. Acta*, 107, 511, 1965.
124. **Jordan, S. M. and Morgan, E. H.**, Plasma protein synthesis by tissue slices from pregnant and lactating rats, *Biochim. Biophys. Acta*, 174, 373, 1969.
125. **Baker, E., Shaw, D. C., and Morgan, E. H.**, Isolation and characterization of rabbit serum and milk transferrins: evidence for difference in scialic acid content only, *Biochemistry*, 7, 1371, 1968.

126. **Jordan, S. M., Kaldor, I., and Morgan, E. H.,** Milk and serum iron-binding capacity in the rabbit, *Nature (London),* 215, 76, 1967.
127. **Jordan, S. M. and Morgan, E. H.,** Plasma protein metabolism during lactation in the rabbit, *Am. J. Physiol.,* 219, 1549, 1970.
128. **Morgan, E. H.,** Plasma protein turnover and transmission to the milk in the rat, *Biochim. Biophys. Acta,* 154, 478, 1968.
129. **Soltys, H. D. and Brody, J. I.,** Synthesis of transferrin by human peripheral blood lymphocytes, *J. Lab. Clin. Med.,* 75, 250, 1970.
130. **Gittin, D. and Pericelli, A.,** Synthesis of serum albumin, prealbumin, alpha-foetoprotein, alpha-1-antitrypsin and transferrin by the human yolk sac, *Nature (London),* 228, 995, 1970.
131. **Gitlin, D. and Boseman, M.,** Sites of serum alpha-fetoprotein synthesis in the human and in the rat, *J. Clin. Invest.,* 46, 1010, 1967.
132. **Masters, C. L., Bingold, L. P., and Morgan, E. H.,** Plasma protein metabolism and transfer to the fetus during pregnancy in the rat, *Am. J. Physiol.,* 216, 876, 1969.
133. **Morgan, E. H.,** A study of iron transfer from rabbit transferrin to reticulocytes using synthetic chelating agents, *Biochim. Biophys. Acta,* 244, 103, 1971.
134. **Morgan, E. H. and Peters, T.,** The biosynthesis of rat serum albumin. V. Effect of protein depletion and refeeding on albumin and transferrin synthesis, *J. Biol. Chem.,* 246, 3500, 1971.
135. **Antia, A. V., McFarlane, H., and Soothill, J. F.,** Serum siderophilin in kwashiorkor, *Arch. Dis. Child.,* 43, 459, 1967.
136. **McFarlane, H., Reddy, S., Adcock, K. J., Adeshina, H., Cooke, A. R., and Akere, J.,** Immunoglobulins, transferrin caeruloplasmin and heterophile antibodies in kwashiorkor, *Trop. Geogr. Med.,* 22, 61, 1970.
137. **Githri, D., Landing, B. H., Whipple, A.,** Localization of homologous plasma proteins in tissues of young human beings as demonstrated with fluorescent antibodies, *J. Exp. Med.,* 97, 163, 1953.
138. **Von Ehrenstein, G.,** Iron transport through the lymph stream, *Acta Chem. Scand.,* 10, 703, 1956.
139. **Bogdanikowa, B. and Grabowski, R.,** Serum proteins present in edema fluid, *Clin. Chim. Acta,* 36, 351, 1972.
140. **Parker, W. C. and Bearn, A. G.,** Studies on the transferrins of adult serum, cord serum and cerebrospinal fluid. The effect of neuraminidase, *J. Exp. Med.,* 115, 83, 1962.
141. **Frick, E.,** Quantitative determination of transferrin in normal and pathological cerebrospinal fluid, *Klin. Wochenschr.,* 41, 75, 1963.
142. **Poortmens, J. and Jeanloz, R. W.,** Quantitative immunological determination of 12 plasma proteins excreted in human urine before and after exercise, *J. Clin. Invest.,* 47, 386, 1968.
143. **Morgan, E. H.,** Transferrin and albumin distribution and turnover in the rat, *Am. J. Physiol.,* 211, 1486, 1966.
144. **Morgan, E. H. and Peters, T.,** Intracellular aspects of transferrin synthesis and secretion in the rat, *J. Biol. Chem.,* 246, 3508, 1971.
145. **Morgan, E. H.,** Plasma iron binding capacity and iron stores in altered erythroid metabolism in the rat, *Q. J. Exp. Physiol.,* 48, 176, 1963.
146. **Wasserman, L. R., Sharney, L., Gevirtz, N. B., Schwartz, L., Weintraub, L. R., Tendler, D., Dumont, A. E., Dreiling, D., and Witte, M.,** Studies in iron kinetics. Interpretation of ferrokinetic data in man, *Proc. Soc. Exp. Biol. Med.,* 115, 817, 1964.
147. **Hampton, J. C.,** An electronmicroscope study of the source and distribution of ferritin in hepatic parenchymal cells of the newborn rabbit, *Blood,* 15, 480, 1960.
148. **Cheney, B. A., Lothe, K., Morgan, E. H., Sood, S. K., and Finch, C. A.,** Internal iron exchange in the rat, *Am. J. Physiol.,* 212, 376, 1967.
149. **Hoffenberg, R., Gordon, A. H., Black, E. G., and Louis, L. N.,** Plasma protein catabolism in the perfused rat liver. The effect of alteration of albumin concentration and dietary protein depletion, *Biochem. J.,* 118, 401, 1970.
150. **Waldmann, T. A., Wochner, R. D., and Strober, W.,** The role of the gastrointestinal tract in plasma protein metabolism, *Am. J. Med.,* 46, 275, 1969.
151. **Gardiner, M. E., Finlay-Jones, J. M., and Morgan, E. H.,** Catabolism and urinary excretion of albumin and transferrin before and after intravenous injection of albumin in the rat: with observations in the urinary excretion of IgG globulin, *Biochem. Med.,* 8, 287, 1973.
152. **Jarman, S. and Lassen, N. A.,** Albumin and transferrin metabolism in infectious and toxic diseases, *Scand. J. Clin. Lab. Invest.,* 13, 357, 1961.
153. **Awai, M. and Brown, E. B.,** Studies on the metabolism of I^{131} labeled human transferrin, *J. Lab. Clin. Med.,* 61, 363, 1963.
154. **Cromwell, S. M.,** The metabolism of transferrin, in *Protides of the Biological Fluids,* Peeters, H., Ed., Elsevier, Amsterdam, 1963, 484.
155. **Freeman, T. and Gordon, A. H.,** Albumin catabolism in hypoproteinemic states, studies with ^{131}I-albumin, *Bibl. Haematol.,* 23, 1108, 1966.

156. International Committee for Standardization in Hematology, Proposed recommendation for measurement of serum iron in human blood, *Br. J. Haematol.*, 20, 451, 1971.
157. International Committee for Standardization in Hematology, Studies on standardization of serum iron and iron binding capacity assays, in *Modern Concepts in Hematology*, Izak, G. and Lewis, S. M., Eds., Academic Press, New York, 197, 69.
158. International Committee for Standardization in Hematology, The measurement of total and unsaturated iron binding capacity in serum, *Br. J. Haematol.*, in print, 1978.
159. **Dlott, D., Siegel, M. M., and Bersohn, R.**, A proposed flurometric determination of unsaturated iron-binding capacity, *Am. J. Clin. Pathol.*, 64, 217, 1975.
160. **Mazur, A., Green, S., Saha, A., and Carlton, A.**, Mechanism of release of ferritin iron in vivo by xanthine oxidase, *J. Clin. Invest.*, 37, 1809, 1958.
161. **Grace, N. D., Greenwald, M. A., and Greenberg, M. S.**, Effect of allopurinol on iron mobilization, *Gastroenterology*, 59, 103, 1970.
162. **Kozma, C., Salvador, R. A., and Elion, G. B.**, Allopurinol and iron storage, *Lancet*, 2, 1040, 1967.
163. **Freeden, E. and Osaki, S.**, Ferroxidases and ferrireductases; their role in iron metabolism, *Adv. Exp. Med. Biol.*, 48, 235, 1974.
164. **Bryce, C. F. A. and Crichton, R. R.**, The catalytic activity of horse spleen apoferritin. Preliminary kinetic studies and the effect of chemical modification, *Biochem. J.*, 133, 301, 1973.
165. **Drysdale, J. W. and Munro, H. N.**, Regulation of synthesis and turnover of ferritin in rat liver, *J. Biol. Chem.*, 241, 3630, 1966.
166. **Drysdale, J. W. and Shafritz, D. A.**, In vitro stimulation of apoferritin synthesis by iron, *Biochim. Biophys. Acta*, 383, 97, 1975.
167. **Zahringer, J., Baliga, B. S., and Munro, H. N.**, Novel mechanism for translational control in regulation of ferritin synthesis by iron, *Proc. Natl. Acad. Sci. U.S.A.*, 73, 857, 1976.
168. **Osaki, S., Johnson, D. A., and Frieden, E.**, The mobilization of iron from the perfused mammalian liver by a serum copper enzyme, ferroxidase. I, *J. Biol. Chem.*, 246, 3018, 1971.
169. **Lipschitz, D. A., Bothwell, T. H., Seftel, H. C., Wapnick, A. A., and Charlton, R. W.**, The role of ascorbic acid in the metabolism of storage iron, *Br. J. Haematol.*, 20, 155, 1971.
170. **Wapnick, A. A., Bothwell, T. H., and Seftel, H.**, The relationship between serum iron levels and ascorbic acid stores in siderotic Bantu, *Br. J. Haematol.*, 19, 271, 1970.
171. **Hershko, C., Cook, J. D., and Finch, C. A.**, Storage iron kinetics. VI. The effect of inflammation on iron exchange in the rat, *Br. J. Haematol.*, 28, 67, 1974.
172. **Fillet, G., Cook, J. D., and Finch, C. A.**, Storage iron kinetics. VII. A biologic model for reticuloendothelial iron transport, *J. Clin. Invest.*, 53, 1527, 1974.
173. **Noyes, W. D., Bothwell, T. H., and Finch, C. A.**, The role of the reticuloendothelial cell in iron metabolism, *Br. J. Haematol.*, 6, 43, 1960.
174. **Unger, A. and Hershko, C.**, Hepatocellular uptake of ferritin in the rat, *Br. J. Haematol.*, 28, 169, 1974.
175. **Schade, S. G. and Fried, W.**, The utilization of senescent red cell and hemolysate iron for erythropoiesis, *Proc. Soc. Exp. Biol. Med.*, 151, 78, 1976.
176. **Cook, J. D., Hershko, C., and Finch, C. A.**, Storage iron kinetics. IV. Cellular distribution of ferritin iron stores in rat liver, *Proc. Soc. Exp. Biol. Med.*, 145, 1378, 1974.
177. **Van Wyk, C. P., Linder-Horowitz, M., and Munro, H. N.**, Effect of iron loading on non heme iron compounds in different liver cell populations, *J. Biol. Chem.*, 246, 1025, 1971.
178. **Hershko, C., Cook, J. D., Finch, C. A.**, Storage iron kinetics. II. The uptake of hemoglobin iron by hepatic parenchymal cells, *J. Lab. Clin. Med.*, 80, 624, 1972.
179. **Hershko, C.**, The fate of circulating haemoglobin, *Br. J. Haematol.*, 29, 199, 1975.
180. **Muller-Eberhard, U., Bosman, C., and Liem, H. H.**, Tissue localization of the heme-hemopexin complex in the rabbit and the rat as studied by light microscopy with the use of radioisotopes, *J. Lab. Clin. Med.*, 76, 426, 1970.
181. **Bissell, D. M., Hammaker, L., and Schmid, R.**, Hemoglobin and erythrocyte catabolism in rat liver. The separate roles of parenchymal and sinusoidal cells, *Blood*, 40, 812, 1972.
182. **Bothwell, T. H. and Finch, C. A.**, Iron metabolism, Little, Brown, Boston, 1962, 286.
183. **Douglas, A. S. and Dacie, J. V.**, The incidence and significance of iron-containing granules in human erythrocytes and their precursors, *J. Clin. Pathol.*, 6, 307, 1953.
184. **Henderson, P. A. and Hillman, R. S.**, Characteristics of iron dextran utilization in man, *Blood*, 34, 357, 1969.
185. **Balcerzak, S. P., Westerman, M. P., Heinle, E. W., and Taylor, R. H.**, Measurement of iron stores using deferoxamine, *Ann. Intern. Med.*, 68, 518, 1968.
186. **Ploem, J. E., de Wael, J., Verloop, M. C., and Punt, H.**, Sideruria following a single dose of desferrioxamine-B as a diagnostic test in iron overload, *Br. J. Haematol.*, 12, 396, 1966.
187. **Barry, M., Cartei, G., and Sherlock, S.**, Quantitative measurement of iron stores with diethylenetriamine penta-acetic acid, *Gut*, 11, 291, 1970.

188. **Waxman, H. S. and Brown, E. B.**, Clinical usefulness of iron chelating agents, *Prog. Hematol.*, 6, 338, 1969.
189. **Hallberg, L., Hedenberg, L., and Weinfeld, A.**, Liver iron and desferrioxamine-induced urinary iron excretion, *Scand. J. Haematol.*, 3, 85, 1966.
190. **Harker, L. A., Funk, D. D., and Finch, C. A.**, Evaluation of storage iron by chelates, *Am. J. Med.*, 45, 105, 1968.
191. **Hershko, C., Cook, J. D., and Finch, C. A.**, Storage iron kinetics. III. Study of desferrioxamine action by selective radioiron labels of R.E. and parenchymal cells, *J. Lab. Clin. Med.*, 81, 876, 1973.
192. **Wapnick, A. A., Lynch, S. R., Charlton, R. W., Seftel, H. C., and Bothwell, T. H.**, The effect of ascorbic acid deficiency on desferrioxamine-induced urinary iron excretion, *Br. J. Haematol.*, 17, 563, 1969.
193. **Hershko, C. and Rachmilewitz, E. A.**, The inhibitory effect of vitamin E on desferrioxamine-induced iron excretion in rats, *Proc. Soc. Exp. Biol. Med.*, 152, 249, 1976.
194. **Haskins, D., Stevens, A. R., Finch, S., and Finch, C. A.**, Iron metabolism. Iron stores in man as measured by phlebotomy, *J. Clin. Invest.*, 31, 543, 1952.
195. **Walters, G. O., Miller, F. M., and Worwood, M.**, Serum ferritin concentration and iron stores in normal subjects, *J. Clin. Pathol.*, 26, 770, 1973.
196. Charlton, R. W., Hawkins, D. M., Mavor, W. O., and Bothwell, T. H., Hepatic storage iron concentrations in different population groups, *Am. J. Clin. Nutr.*, 23, 358, 1970.
197. **Addison, G. M., Beamish, M. R., Hales, C. N., Hodgkins, M., Jacobs, A., and Llewellin, P.**, An immunoradiometric assay for ferritin in the serum of normal subjects and patients with iron deficiency and iron overload, *J. Clin. Pathol.*, 25, 326, 1972.
198. **Miles, L. E. M., Lipschitz, D. A., Bieber, C. P., and Cook, J. D.**, Measurement of serum ferritin by a 2-site immunoradiometric assay, *Anal. Biochem.*, 61, 209, 1974.
199. **Halliday, J. W., Gera, K. L., and Powell, L. W.**, Solid phase radioimmunoassay for serum ferritin, *Clin. Chim. Acta*, 58, 207, 1975.
200. **Jacobs, A. and Worwood, M.**, Ferritin in serum. Clinical and biochemical implications, *N. Engl. J. Med.*, 292, 951, 1975.
201. **Lipschitz, D. A., Cook, J. D., and Finch, C. A.**, A clinical evaluation of serum ferritin as an index of iron stores, *N. Engl. J. Med.*, 290, 1213, 1974.
202. **Bentley, D. P. and Jacobs, A.**, Accumulation of storage iron in patients treated for iron deficiency anaemia, *Br. Med. J.*, 2, 64, 1975.
203. **Hussein, S., Prieto, J., O'Shea, M., Hoffbrand, A. V., Baillod, R. A., and Moorhead, J. F.**, Serum ferritin assay and iron status in chronic renal failure and haemodialysis, *Br. Med. J.*, 1, 546, 1975.
204. **Letsky, E. A., Miller, F., Worwood, M., and Flynn, D. M.**, Serum ferritin in children with thalassemia regularly transfused, *J. Clin. Pathol.*, 27, 652, 1974.
205. **Wands, J. R., Rowe, J. A., Mezey, S. E.**, Normal serum ferritin concentrations in precirrhotic hemochromatosis, *N. Engl. J. Med.*, 294, 302, 1976.
206. **Powell, L. W. and Halliday, J. W.**, Serum ferritin in hemochromatosis, *N. Engl. J. Med.*, 294, 1185, 1976.
207. **Crosby, W.-H.**, Normal serum ferritin in precirrhotic hemochromatosis, *N. Engl. J. Med.*, 296, 1116, 1977.
208. **Hahn, P. F., Bale, W. F., Laurence, E. O., and Whipple, G. H.**, Radioactive iron and its metabolism in anemia. Its absorption, transportation and utilization, *J. Exp. Med.*, 69, 739, 1939.
209. **Hahn, P. F., Bale, W. F., Ross, J. F., Hettig, R. A., and Whipple, G. H.**, Radioiron in plasma does not exchange with hemoglobin iron in red cells, *Science*, 92, 131, 1940.
210. **Huff, R. L. and Judd, O. J.**, Kinetics of iron metabolism, in *Advances in Biology and Medical Physics*, Vol. 4, Lawrence, J. H. and Tobias, C. A., Eds., Academic Press, New York, 1956, 223.
211. **Finch, C. A., Gibson, J. G., Peacock, W. C., and Fluharty, R. G.**, Iron metabolism. Utilization of intravenous radioactive iron, *Blood*, 4, 905, 1949.
212. **Huff, R. L., Hennessy, T. G., Austin, R. E., Garcia, J. F., Roberts, B. M., and Lawrence, J. H.**, Plasma and red cell iron turnover in normal subjects and in patients having various hematopoietic disorders, *J. Clin. Invest.*, 29, 1041, 1950.
213. **Huff, R. L., Elmlinger, P. J., Garcia, J. F., Oda, J. M., Cockrell, M. C., and Lawrence, J. H.**, Ferrokinetics in normal persons and in patients having various erythropoietic disorders, *J. Clin. Invest.*, 30, 1512, 1951.
214. **Finch, C. A., Deubelbeiss, K., Cook, J. D., Eschbach, L. A., Harker, L. A., Funk, D. D., Marsaglia, G., Hillman, R. S., Slichter, S., Adamson, J. W., Ganzoni, A., and Giblett, E. R.**, Ferrokinetics in man, *Medicine*, 49, 17, 1970.
215. **Funk, D. D.**, Plasma iron turnover in normal subjects, *J. Nucl. Med.*, 11, 107, 1970.
216. **Adamson, J. W., Eschbach, J., and Finch, C. A.**, The kidney and erythropoiesis, *Am. J. Med.*, 44, 725, 1968.
217. **Pollycove, M.**, Iron metabolism and kinetics, *Semin. Hematol.*, 3, 235, 1966.

218. **Layrisse, M., Linares, J., and Roche, M.,** Excess hemolysis in subjects with severe iron deficiency anemia associated and nonassociated with hookworm infection, *Blood,* 25, 73, 1965.
219. **Cartwright, G. E. and Lee, G. R.,** The anemia of chronic disorders, *Br. J. Haematol.,* 21, 147, 1971.
220. **Finch, C. A., Coleman, D. H., Motulsky, A. G., Donohue, D. M., and Reiff, R. H.,** Erythrokinetics in pernicious anemia, *Blood,* 11, 807, 1956.
221. **Sturgeon, P. and Finch, C. A.,** Erythrokinetics in Cooley's anemia, *Blood,* 12, 64, 1957.
222. **Roath, S., Bourne, M. S., and Israels, M. C. G.,** Ferrokinetics in pyridoxine-responsive anemia, *Acta Haematol.,* 32, 1, 1964.
223. **Pollycove, M. and Mortimer, R.,** A quantitative determination of iron kinetics and hemoglobin synthesis in human subjects, *J. Clin. Invest.,* 40, 753, 1961.
224. **Garby, L., Schneider, W., Sundquist, O., and Vuille, J. C.,** A ferro-erythrokinetic model and its properties, *Acta Physiol. Scand.,* 59 (216), 1, 1963.
225. **Cavill, I. and Ricketts, C.,** The kinetics of iron metabolism, in *Iron in Biochemistry and Medicine,* Jacobs, A. and Worwood, M., Eds., Academic Press, London, 1974, 614.
226. **Hosain, F., Marsaglia, G., and Finch, C. A.,** Blood ferrokinetics in normal man, *J. Clin. Invest.,* 46, 1, 1967.
227. **Fillet, G.,** Etude radioisotopique de la reutilisation du fer chez l'animal et chez l'homme, These du grade d'Agrege de l'Enseignement Superieur, Universite de Liege, 1977.
228. **Hillman, R. S. and Finch, C. A.,** Erythropoiesis; normal and abnormal, *Semin. Hematol.,* 4, 327, 1967.
229. **Olsson, K. S.,** Iron stores in normal men and male blood donors, *Acta Med. Scand.,* 192, 401, 1972.
230. **Pritchard, J. and Mason, R. A.,** Iron stores of normal adults and replenishment with oral iron therapy, *JAMA,* 190, 897, 1964.

Platelets

PLATELET PRODUCTION

Bruce Lee Evatt

Thrombopoietin

Platelet production is most likely mediated by a humoral factor, "thrombopoietin". A substantial amount of experimental evidence favoring a humoral control mechanism has been compiled.[1,2] Thrombocytopenia produced by exchange transfusions or platelet antiserum is followed by transient thrombocytosis, and thrombocytosis secondary to platelet hypertransfusion is followed by transient thrombocytopenia.[3-10] In addition, thrombocytopenia in some members of two families was attributed to a deficiency of a plasma component with thrombopoietic stimulating factor.[11,12]

Initial assays of thrombopoietic-stimulating material in the plasma of thrombocytopenic donors involved measuring changes in platelet counts produced in recipient animals.[1,13,18] However, injection of plasma from thrombocytopenic animals does not regularly cause measurable elevations in the platelet counts of normal recipients, and results of such assays vary greatly;[10] in addition, platelet counts of rodents (the animals most used in experimental studies) fluctuate considerably. Therefore, misinterpretation of apparent variation in circulating platelet counts must be carefully avoided.[19]

The first consistently reproducible measurements of thrombopoietin were obtained when either ^{75}Se-selenomethionine or ^{35}S-sodium sulfate was incorporated in the assay.[10,20] Both ^{75}Se-selenomethionine and ^{35}S-sodium sulfate have been used successfully to measure thrombopoiesis-stimulating factors in the plasma or fractions of plasma proteins obtained from both normal and thrombocytopenic donors (Figures 1—5). These isotopes are incorporated into the cytoplasm of megakaryocytes, and labeled platelets subsequently appear in the circulation after being released from labeled megakaryocytes. Both radionuclides produce similar patterns of incorporation in the platelets, and a relationship has been demonstrated between the level of megakaryocytopoiesis and incorporation of these isotopes into platelets.[10,11,28] However, the most widely used thrombopoietin assays are not quantitative enough for routine clinical use and remain a research tool, and other types of assays are in the developmental stage. These include procedures based upon tissue culture and hemagglutination inhibition,[29-32] which promise to be more quantitative in nature.

The chemical nature of thrombopoietin is unknown at this point. Early investigators described it as being a labile nondialyzable protein moving with the beta globulins on immunoelectrophoresis;[33-34] however, the material they were using was very crude, and the nature of even the most highly purified form of thrombopoietin has not yet been ascertained.[35] Its activity has been separated from erythropoietic activity, but its site of production remains unclear.[35] Some investigators have suggested the kidney as one possible site. Krizsa, using assays for thrombopoietin based upon platelet counts, reported that thrombopoietin activity induced by acute hemorrhage did not appear in the serum of nephrectomized animals; however, nephrectomy did not alter the thrombopoietin response to acute thrombocytopenia.[36] Furthermore, anephretic humans do not become thrombocytopenic.[37] Similarly, Jackson et al. observed that under appropriate conditions, bilateral nephrectomy prevented alterations in megakaryocytopoiesis and proposed that a substance that accelerated platelet production was produced by the kidney in response to severe anemia.[38] McDonald demonstrated thrombopoietin activity in cultures of embryonic kidney cells and suggested that the kidney was one site of thrombopoietin production.[39,40] On the other hand, De Gabriele concluded that the kidney was not the site of thrombopoietin production because normal recovery of platelet levels occurred after thrombocytopenia was induced by platelet antiserum in nephrectomized rats.[17]

Table 1
ASSAYS OF THROMBOPOIETIN

Method of measuring platelet production	Animal used	Advantages	Disadvantages	Ref.
Platelet counts	Mice, rats	—	Imprecise, nonreproducible, lack of sensitivity	15,16,33,34,43
Isotopic methods				
Normal animals as assay animals				
^{75}Se-selenomethionine	Rabbits, mice	Relatively sensitive; Reproducible	Nonquantitative	10,31,35,55
^{35}S-sodium sulfate	Rats, mice			20,27,29,56
Animals with rebound thrombocytosis as assay animals				
^{75}Se-selenomethionine	Mice	Relatively sensitive; Reproducible	Nonquantitative	23,57
^{35}S-sodium sulfate	Mice			58
Animals hypertransfused with platelets as assay animals				
^{75}Se-selenomethionine	Rabbits	Very sensitive, reproducible; Quantitative	Technically extremely difficult	10,28
^{35}S-sodium sulfate	Rats, mice			25,56
Miscellaneous				
Platelet sizing	Guinea pigs, rabbits, mice	Ease of performance	Lack of sensitivity	59,60,61
Measurement of megakaryocytopoiesis	Rats	—	Relatively insensitive, technically difficult	21,48,62,63
Tissue culture	—	—	Presently developmental	30,33
Immunoassay				
Hemagglutinin inhibitor assay	—	Quantitative, rapid, inexpensive	Presently developmental, difficulty obtaining pure thrombopoietin for making antibody	29

The precise mechanism of action of thrombopoietin upon megakaryocytopoiesis is likewise unclear. When platelet production rates were decreased in subjects with thrombocytopenia, the number of megakaryocytes, mitotic index, age composition of megakaryocytes population, and DNA synthesis in the megakaryocyte population were all altered.[27,41-47] After injection of potential thrombopoietic materials, the number of megakaryocytes increased within 2 to 3 days.[21,48] In addition, mitotic indices of megakaryocytes have been reported to be increased in mice 32 hr after injection of thrombopoietic substances.[49] It is possible that thrombopoietin recruits precursor cells of megakaryocytes into identifiable population of megakaryocytes and increases the rate of progression of these cells through the developing megakaryocyte compartments by changing the rate of cytoplasmic development and the number of mitotic divisions.[5,25,27,41,50]

Measurement of Platelet Production in Man

^{75}Se-selenomethionine has been used by several investigators for measuring thrombopoiesis in man.[51,53] The method consists of injecting 100—250 μCi of ^{75}Se-seleno-

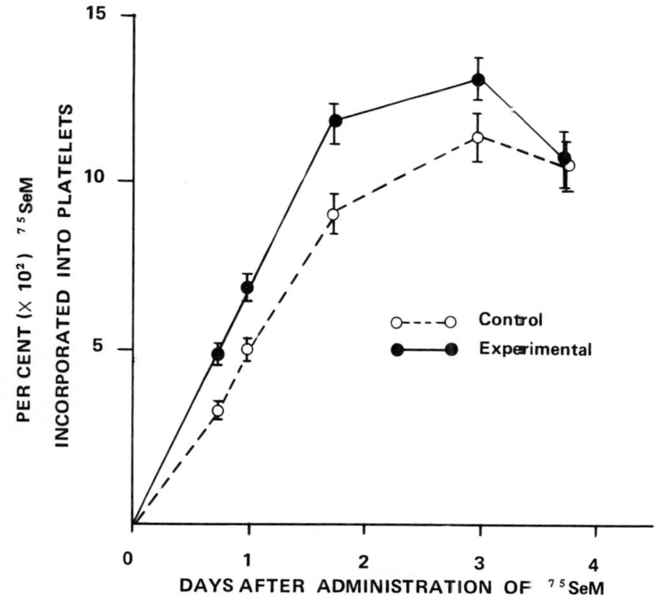

FIGURE 1. Effect of plasma from thrombocytopenic and normal donors upon incorporation of ^{75}SeM into platelets. Platelet-free plasma (75—225 mℓ) from either normal or thrombocytopenic donors was injected into normal recipients in three equally divided doses during the 32-hr period preceding the administration of ^{75}SeM. There were 18 animals in each group. The mean ± 1 SE is shown. Percent of isotope incorporation into platelets was significantly higher in animals that received plasma from thrombocytopenic donors ($P < 0.005$ at 18, 24, and 42 hr). Control animals that received normal plasma did not differ from animals that received 0.9% NaCl (not shown). (From Evatt, B. L. and Levin, J., *J. Clin. Invest.*, 48, 1615, 1969. With permission.)

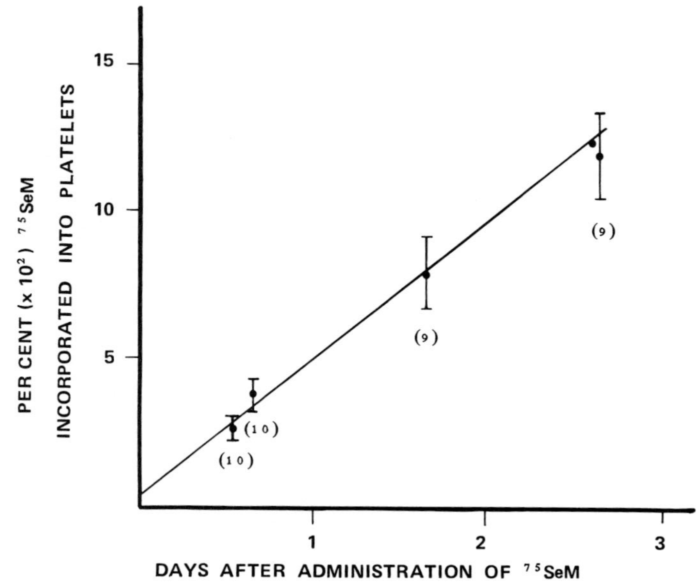

FIGURE 2. Percent of incorporation of ^{75}SeM into circulating platelets in normal mice. Each mouse received 1 μCi of ^{75}SeM intravenously, and blood samples were obtained from successive groups of mice. The mean ± 1 SE is shown, and the numbers in parentheses indicate the number of animals studied. The incorporation of ^{75}SeM into platelets during the 3-day period following administration of isotope was approximately linear; a linear regression analysis of these data indicated a correlation coefficient of 0.998. Maximum ^{75}SeM in circulating platelets occurred 4 days after administration of isotope. (From Levin, J., Evatt, B. L., and Shreiner, D. P. L., *Platelets: Production Function, Transfusion, and Storage,* Baldini, M. G. and Ebbe, S., Eds., Grune & Stratton, New York, 1974, 6. With permission.)

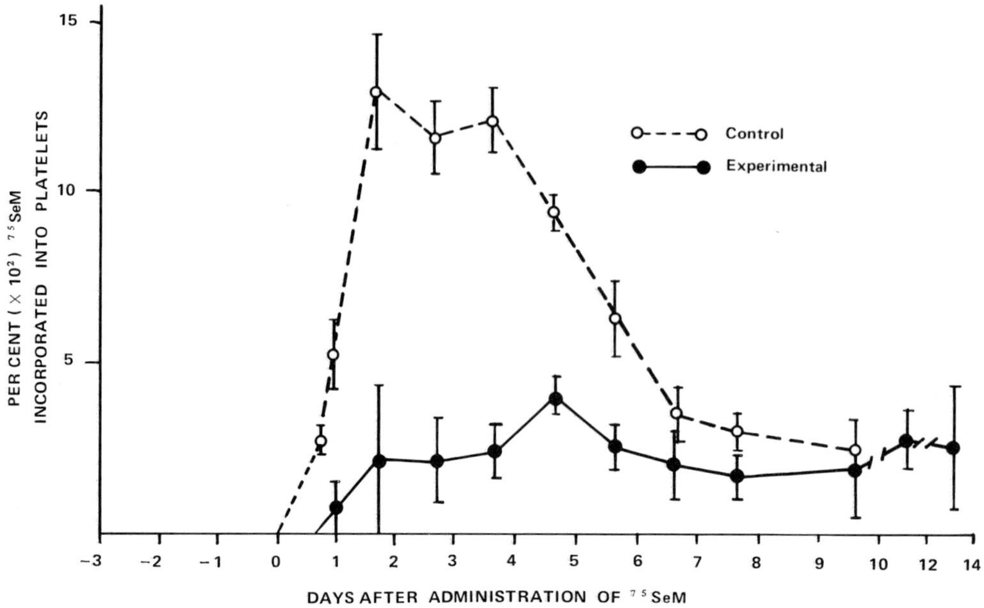

FIGURE 3. Effect of hypertransfusion of platelets upon incorporation of ^{75}SeM into platelets. Two animals were hypertransfused with platelets, starting 3 days before administration of ^{75}SeM. Four control animals received equal volumes of fresh, platelet-free plasma. Thrombocytosis was maintained by daily platelet transfusions for a total period of 6 days. The mean ± 1 SE is shown. Hypertransfusion of platelets produced a marked decrease of incorporation of ^{75}SeM into platelets. (From Evatt, B. L. and Levin, J., *J. Clin. Invest.*, 48, 1615, 1969. With permission.)

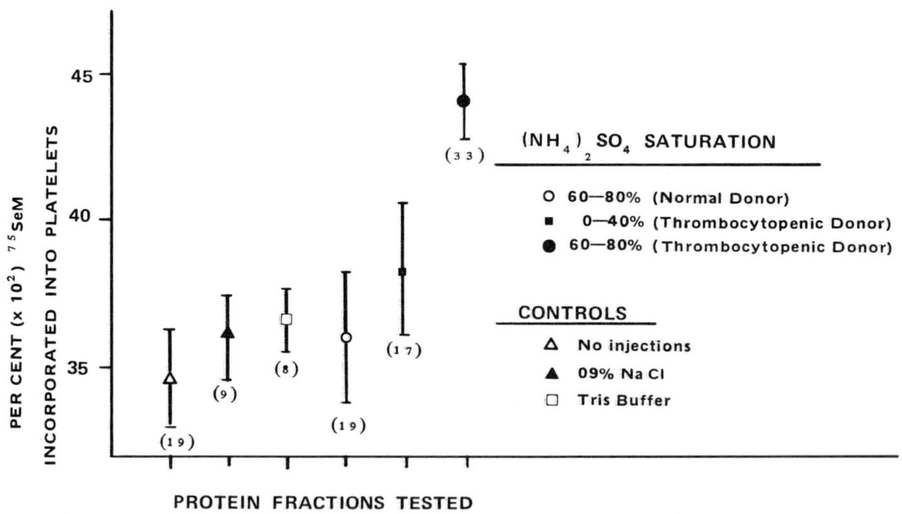

FIGURE 4. Effect of fractions of plasma from normal or thrombocytopenic rabbits upon incorporation of ^{75}SeM into mouse platelets. Each mouse received 1 μCi of ^{75}SeM intravenously after the last of four equally divided doses of proteins and percent dose uptake was measured at 16 hr. The mean ± 1 SE is shown, and the numbers in parentheses indicate the number of animals studied. There was a significant increase ($P < 0.005$) in the level of ^{75}SeM only in the platelets of mice that received fractions precipitated at an $(NH_4)_2SO_4$ saturation of 60 to 80% from plasma of thrombocytopenic rabbits. (From Evatt, B. L., Shreiner, D. P., and Levin, J., *J. Lab. Clin. Med.*, 83, 364, 1974. With permission.)

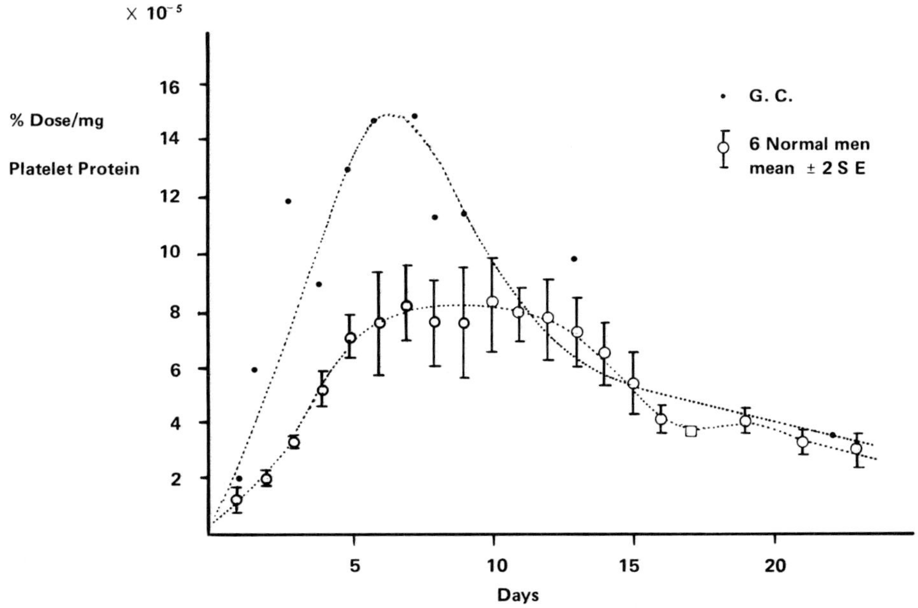

FIGURE 5. Comparison of rate of incorporation and rate of disappearance of ^{75}Se-methionine into platelets of six normal men and platelets of one patient (G.C.) with a myeloproliferative syndrome. (From McIntyre, P. A., Evatt, B., Hodkinson, B. A., and Scheffel, V., *J. Lab. Clin. Med.*, 75, 472, 1970. With permission.)

methionine intravenously and measuring the amount of isotope incorporated into the patients platelets over the next 10 days.[52,53] The method has been demonstrated to be useful in determining platelet production in several clinical entities, but it does have some problems. First of all, the isotope is reused after the catabolism of labeled proteins. Therefore, some "tailing" of the platelet production curve occurs and platelet life span cannot be accurately determined by this method; however, it is feasible to measure relative changes of platelet span. On the other hand, the initial portion of the production curve accurately reflects platelet production, and production rates can be determined. In certain disease states, i. e., those associated with hypersplenism, the ratio of "circulating" to "pooled" platelets may be such that the apparent incorporation of the isotope in the circulating cells is decreased and platelet production could be underestimated.[54] In addition, in clinical conditions in which platelet destruction is excessive, platelets may be destroyed before sufficient quantities are released into the circulation to demonstrate an increased rate of production. Other technical difficulties, such as very low platelet counts, may create problems in isolating enough platelets to make determination of the rate of production reasonably accurate.

REFERENCES

1. **Abildgaard, C. F. and Simone, J. V.**, Thrombopoiesis, *Semin. Hematol.*, 4, 424, 1967.
2. **Cooper, G. W.**, The regulation of thrombopoiesis, in *Regulation of Hematopoiesis*, Vol. 2, Gordon, A. S., Ed., Appleton-Century-Crofts, New York, 1970, 1611.
3. **Craddock, C. G., Adams, W. S., Perry, S., and Lawrence, J. S.**, The dynamics of platelet production as studied by a depletion technique in normal and irradiated dogs, *J. Lab. Clin. Med.*, 45, 906, 1955.
4. **Matter, M., Hartmann, J. R., Kautz, J., DeMarsh, Q. B., and Finch, C. A.**, A study of thrombopoiesis in induced acute thrombocytopenia, *Blood*, 15, 174, 1960.

5. **O'Dell, T. T., Jr., McDonald, T. P., and Asano, M.**, Response of rat megakaryocytes and platelets to bleeding, *Acta Haematol.*, 27, 171, 1962.
6. **Ebbe, S. and Stohlman, F., Jr.**, Megakaryocytopoiesis in the rat, *Blood*, 26, 20, 1965.
7. **Cronkite, E. P., Bond, V. P., Fliedner, T. M., Paglia, D. A., and Adamik, E. R.**, Studies on the origin, production, and destruction of platelets, in *Blood Platelets*, Johnson, S. A., Monto, R. W., Rebuck, J. W., and Hoin, R. C., Eds., Little, Brown, Boston, 1961, 595.
8. **O'Dell, T. T., Jr., Jackson, C. W., and Reiter, R. S.**, Depression of the megakaryocyte-platelet system in rats by transfusion of platelets, *Acta Haematol.*, 38, 34, 1967.
9. **DeGabriele, G. and Penington, D. G.**, Physiology of the regulation of platelet production, *Br. J. Haematol.*, 13, 202, 1967.
10. **Evatt, B. L. and Levin, J.**, Measurement of thrombopoiesis in rabbits using ^{75}Selenomethionine, *J. Clin. Invest.*, 48, 1615, 1969.
11. **Schulman, I., Pierce, M., Lukens, A., and Currimbhoy, Z.**, Studies on thrombopoiesis. I. A factor in normal human plasma required for platelet production; chronic thrombocytopenia due to its deficiency, *Blood*, 16, 943, 1960.
12. **Abildgaard, C. F. and Simone, J. V.**, Thrombopoiesis, *Semin. Hematol.*, 4, 424, 1967.
13. **Steinberg, B., Cheng, F. H. F., Martin, R. A., Dietz, A. A.**, Thrombocytic and thrombopenic factors in normal human serum, *Acta Haematol.*, 33, 341, 1965.
14. **Linman, J. W. and Pierre, R. V.**, Thrombocytosis-promoting activity of normal plasma, *Proc. Soc. Exp. Biol. Med.*, 110, 463, 1962.
15. **Spector, B.**, In vivo transfer of a thrombopoietic factor, *Proc. Soc. Exp. Biol. Med.*, 108, 146, 1961.
16. **O'Dell, T. T., Jr., McDonald, T. P., and Detwiler, T. C.**, Stimulation of platelet production by serum of platelet-depleted rats, *Proc. Soc. Exp. Biol. Med.*, 108, 428, 1961.
17. **DeGabriele, G. and Penington, D. G.**, Regulation of platelet production: 'thrombopoietin', *Br. J. Haematol.*, 13, 210, 1967.
18. **Schulman, I., Abildgaard, C. F., Cornet, J., Simone, J. A., and Currimbhon, Z.**, Studies on thrombopoiesis. II. Assay of human plasma thrombopoietic activity, *J. Lab. Clin. Med.*, 66, 604, 1965.
19. **O'Dell, T. T., Jr., McDonald, T. P., and Howsden, F. L.**, Native and foreign stimulators of platelet production, *J. Lab. Clin. Med.*, 64, 418, 1964.
20. **Cooper, G. W., Cooper, B., and Chang, C-Y.**, Demonstration of a circulating factor regulating blood platelet production using ^{35}S-sulfate in rats and mice, *Proc. Soc. Exp. Biol. Med.*, 134, 1123, 1970.
21. **O'Dell, T. T., Jr. and McDonald, T. P.**, Two mechanisms of sulfate-S^{35} uptake by blood platelets of rats, *Am. J. Physiol.*, 206, 580, 1964.
22. **Cohen, P., Cooley, M. H., Gardner, F. H.**, The use of selenomethionine (Se^{75}) as a label for canine and human platelets, *J. Clin. Invest.*, 44 (Abstr.), 1036, 1965.
23. **Penington, D. G.**, Assessment of platelet production with ^{75}Se-selenomethionine, *Br. Med. J.*, 4, 782, 1969.
24. **McIntyre, P. A., Evatt, B., Hodkinson, B. A., and Scheffel, U.**, Selenium-75 selenomethionine as a label for erythrocytes, leukocytes, and platelets in man, *J. Lab. Clin. Med.*, 75, 472, 1970.
25. **Harker, L. A.**, Regulation of thrombopoiesis, *Am. J. Physiol.*, 218, 1376, 1970.
26. **O'Dell, T. T., Jr., Jackson, C. W., and Reiter, R. S.**, Depression of the megakaryocyte-platelet system in rats by transfusion of platelets, *Acta Haematol.*, 38, 34, 1967.
27. **Harker, L. A.**, Kinetics of thrombopoiesis, *J. Clin. Invest.*, 47, 458, 1968.
28. **Shreiner, D. P. and Levin, J.**, Detection of thrombopoietic activity in plasma by stimulation of suppressed thrombopoiesis, *J. Clin. Invest.*, 49, 1709, 1970.
29. **McDonald, T. P.**, The hemagglutination-inhibition assay for thrombopoietin, *Blood*, 41, 219, 1973.
30. **Metcalf, D., MacDonald, H. R., Odartchenko, N., and Sordat, B.**, Growth of mouse megakaryocyte colonies in vitro, *Proc. Natl. Acad. Sci. U.S.A.*, 72, 1744, 1975.
31. **Nakeff, A. and Roozendaal, K. J.**, Thrombopoietin activity in mice following immune-induced thrombocytopenia, *Acta Haematol.*, 54, 340, 1975.
32. **Nakeff, A. and Daniels-McQueen, S.**, In vitro colony assay for a new class of megakaryocyte precursor: colony-forming unit megakaryocyte (CFU-M), *Proc. Soc. Exp. Biol. Med.*, 151, 587, 1976.
33. **LeXuan, C. and Ebbe, S.**, Assay of plasma thrombopoietic activity in rats, *Med. Exp.*, 7, 317, 1962.
34. **Linman, J. W. and Pierre, R. V.**, Studies on thrombopoiesis. III. Thrombocytosis-promoting effects of "thrombocythemic" and "polycythemic" plasmas, *J. Lab. Clin. Med.*, 62, 374, 1963.
35. **Evatt, B. L., Spivak, J. L., and Levin, J.**, Relationships between thrombopoiesis and erythropoiesis: with studies of the effects of preparations of thrombopoietin and erythropoietin, *Blood*, 48, 547, 1976.
36. **Krizsa, F.**, Study on the development of posthaemorrhagic thrombocytosis in rats, *Acta Haematol.*, 46, 228, 1971.
37. **Evatt, B. L. and Sapier, D.**, unpublished observations.

38. **Jackson, C. W., Simone, J. V., and Edwards, C. C.**, The relationship of anemia and thrombocytosis, *J. Lab. Clin. Med.*, 84, 357, 1974.
39. **McDonald, T. P., Clift, R., Lange, R. O., Nolan, C., Tribby, I. I. E., and Barlow, G. H.**, Thrombopoietin production by human embryonic kidney cells in culture, *J. Lab. Clin. Med.*, 85, 59, 1975.
40. **McDonald, T. P.**, Role of the kidneys in thrombopoietin production, *Exp. Hematol.*, 4, 27, 1976.
41. **Ebbe, S. and Stohlman, F., Jr.**, Megakaryocytopoiesis in the rat, *Blood*, 26, 30, 1965.
42. **O'Dell, T. T., Jr., Jackson, C. W., Friday, T. J., and Du, K. P.**, Assay of megakaryocytopoiesis in thrombocytopenic rats, *Br. J. Haematol.*, 21, 233, 1971.
43. **O'Dell, T. T., Jr.**, Humoral regulation of thrombocytopoiesis, in *Humoral Control of Growth and Differentiation*, Vol. 1, Gordon, A. S., Ed., Academic Press, New York, 1973.
44. **O'Dell, T. T., Jr.**, Megakaryocytopoiesis and its response to stimulation and suppression, in *Platelets: Production, Function, Transfusion, and Storage*, Baldini, M. G. and Ebbe, S., Eds., Grune & Stratton, New York, 1974, 11.
45. **O'Dell, T. T., Jr., Jackson, C. W., and Gosslee, D. G.**, Maturation of rat megakaryocytes studied by microspectrophotometric measurement of DNA, *Proc. Soc. Exp. Biol. Med.*, 119, 1194, 1965.
46. **Paulus, J. M.**, DNA metabolism and development of organelles in guinea pig megakaryocytes: a combined ultrastructural, autoradiographic and cytophotometric study, *Blood*, 35, 298, 1970.
47. **Paulus, J. M.**, Cytophotometric measurements of DNA in thrombopoietic megakaryocytes, *Exp. Cell Res.*, 53, 310, 1968.
48. **Krizsa, F., Gergely, G., and Rák, K.**, Megakaryocyte response in posthaemorrhagic thrombocytosis of mice, *Acta Haematol.*, 39, 112, 1968.
49. **McDonald, T. P.**, Assays for thrombopoietin, *Scand. J. Haematol.*, 18, 5, 1977.
50. **Penington, D. G. and Olson, J. E.**, Megakaryocytes in states of altered platelet production: cell numbers, size, and DNA content, *Br. J. Haematol.*, 18, 447, 1970.
51. **Brodsky, I., Siegel, N. H., Kahn, S. B., Ross, E. M., and Petkov, G.**, Simultaneous fibrinogen and platelet survival with (^{75}Se) Selenomethionine in man, *Br. J. Haematol.*, 18, 341, 1970.
52. **McIntyre, P. A., Evatt, B., Hodkinson, B. A., and Scheffel, U.**, Selenium ^{75}Selenomethionine as a label for erythrocytes, leukocytes and platelets in man, *J. Lab. Clin. Med.*, 75, 472, 1970.
53. **Najean, Y. and Ardaillou, N.**, The use of ^{75}Selenomethionine for the in vivo study of platelet kinetics, *Scand. J. Haematol.*, 6, 395, 1969.
54. **Aster, R. H.**, Pooling of platelets in the spleen: role in the pathogenesis of "hypersplenic" thrombocytopenia, *J. Clin. Invest.*, 45, 645, 1966.
55. **Evatt, B. L., Shreiner, D. P., and Levin, J.**, Thrombopoietic activity of fractions of rabbit plasma: studies in rabbits and mice, *J. Lab. Clin. Med.*, 83, 364, 1974.
56. **Cooper, G. W., Cooper, B., Ossias, A. L., and Zanjani, E. D.**, A hypertranfused mouse assay for thrombopoietic factors, *Blood*, 42, 423, 1973.
57. **Penington, D. G.**, Isotope bioassay for 'thrombopoietin', *Br. Med. J.*, 1, 606, 1970.
58. **McDonald, T. P.**, Bioassay for thrombopoietin utilizing mice in rebound thrombocytosis, *Proc. Soc. Exp. Biol. Med.*, 144, 1006, 1973.
59. **Weiner, M. and Karpatkin, S.**, Use of the megathrombocyte to demonstrate thrombopoietin, *Thromb. Diath. Haemorrh.*, 28, 24, 1972.
60. **Weintraub, A. H. and Karpatkin, S.**, Heterogeneity of rabbit platelets. II. Use of the megathrombocyte to demonstrate a thrombopoietic stimulus, *J. Lab. Clin. Med.*, 83, 896, 1974.
61. **McDonald, T. P.**, A comparison of platelet size, platelet count and platelet ^{35}S incorporation as assays for thrombopoietin, *Br. J. Haematol.*, 34, 257, 1976.
62. **O'Dell, T. T., Jr., Jackson, C. W., Friday, T. J., and Charsha, D. E.**, Effects of thrombocytopenia on megakaryocytopoiesis, *Br. J. Haematol.*, 17, 91, 1969.
63. **O'Dell, T. T., Jr., Murphy, J. R., and Jackson, C. W.**, Stimulation of megakaryocytopoiesis by acute thrombocytopenia in rats, *Blood*, 48, 765, 1976.
64. **Levin, J., Evatt, B. L., and Shreiner, D. P. L.**, Measurement of plasma thrombopoiesis stimulating activity using selenomethionine-^{75}Se: studies in rabbits and mice, in *Platelets: Production Function, Transfusion, and Storage*, Baldini, M. G. and Ebbe, S., Eds., Grune & Stratton, New York, 1974, 66.

KINETICS OF ISOTOPICALLY LABELED PLATELETS

Bruce Lee Evatt

Many investigators have studied the life spans of platelets in the circulation in order to characterize thrombocytopenic disorders and to determine the function or fate of platelets under normal and pathologic conditions. In early attempts to measure platelet life spans in patients with such disorders, the rate of platelet clearance after a platelet transfusion was approximated by direct counting of platelets. Although such an approximation was reasonable under certain conditions, direct counting methods were unsuitable for normal subjects. The development of methods of labeling platelets with isotopic markers permitted investigators to more accurately assess the behavior of circulating platelets under numerous conditions. The type of isotope used and the manner in which it is presented to the subject are determined by whether production of platelets or survival of platelets is to be studied. Each isotope has advantages and disadvantages that must be considered when choosing an isotope for a study.

The ideal isotopic marker is one that requires little or no manipulation of platelets, is nontoxic to the platelet or the subjects, is not metabolized, does not elute or transfer from one platelet to another, and is not reutilized by the megakaryocyte for new platelet production after the labeled platelets have been cleared from the bloodstream.[1] No compound now available for the study of platelet kinetics satisfies all these criteria.

The general types of isotopes used in the study of platelet kinetics are shown in Table 1. Isotopes used for labeling platelets may be classified into two broad categories: those that are incorporated into the cytoplasm of megakaryocytes and subsequently released into the circulation within newly formed platelets and those that attach directly to the platelets. Isotopes in the first category produce a cohort label of a population of platelets that have an approximately uniform age, whereas isotopes in the second category directly label an entire population of platelets with respect to age.

Table 1
FORMS OF ISOTOPES USED FOR STUDIES OF PLATELET KINETICS

	Used for megakaryocyte labels	Ref.
	^{32}P-sodium phosphate	31—34
	^{35}S-methionine	35
	^{35}S-sodium sulfate	36—38
	^{75}Se-selenomethionine	39,40,45
	Used for platelet labels	
In vitro label	^{51}Cr-sodium chromate	5,9,10,16,20,41
	^{14}C-serotonin	42,43
	^{111}Indium	29,30
	^{32}P-diisopropylflurophosphate (DFP)	23
In vivo label	^{3}H-diisopropylflurophosphate (DFP)	44
	^{32}P-diissopropylflurophosphate (DFP)	20,26,44
	^{14}C-Serotonin	42,43

Optimal conditions for platelet labeling in platelet survival studies are given in Table 2. Primary considerations are temperature, type of anticoagulant, amount of manipulation, manner of resuspension, and type of container used for harvesting the platelets. If these conditions are not well-controlled and are less than optimal, the appearance of the platelet survival curves may change dramatically.

Effect of Temperature

When harvested at 0 to 10°C, platelets lose their normal disc-like configuration and become spherical.[2] When examined under the electron microscope, they are frequently shown to have lost the peripheral microtubules.[3-4] Such platelets, when labeled, show a reduced viability.[5,6] Similarly, platelets maintained at 37°C have high metabolic demands and show decreased viability after being stored for short periods.[7] Temperatures of 20°C have been shown to produce platelets with the greatest recovery of injected cells.[8]

Effect of Anticoagulant

The choice of anticoagulant has a profound effect upon platelet survivals. In the original studies, ethylenediamine tetracetic acid (EDTA) was used as an anticoagulant in collecting blood for platelet survivals because of the ease with which platelets could be resuspended.[9] After infusion, however, platelets thus prepared quickly disappeared from the circulation and were sequestered predominantly in the liver.[10-11] EDTA damages membrane transport and is thought to be directly responsible for the decrease in survival time of such platelets. Sodium citrate, on the other hand, is harmless to platelets but permits them to clump irreversibly because of the small amounts of adenosine diphosphate (ADP) released by the platelets when they are centrifuged during the preparation procedure. This clumping may be reduced by lowering the pH of the media to 6.5, thereby diminishing the sensitivity of the platelet ADP.[12-13] The ACD anticoagulant is usually acidified by adding additional citrate acid.

Effect of Preparation Methods

During the isolation procedure, manipulation must be kept to a minimum if platelet survival is to be optimal. During repeated centrifugation, platelets become temporarily spherical and partially release some of their constituents,[14] with a resultant loss of some of their ability to aggregate.[15] In addition, for optimal platelet survival, resuspension should be carried out with gentle rocking procedures.

Plasma appears to be the most suitable media for storage and manipulation of pla-

Table 2
OPTIMAL CONDITIONS FOR PLATELET LABELING USE IN SURVIVAL STUDIES

Type of platelets	Autologous platelets (if unavailable: HB, antigen neg and ABO-rh compatibility)
Isotope used for random in vitro labeling	^{51}Cr-sodium chromate (preservative free)
Type of anticoagulant	ACD[a] or CPD[b] Added 0.15 M citric acid to lower pH to 0.5
Temperature	20 to 25°C
Type of container	Pyrogen-free sterile plastic transfusion bags
Method of resuspension	Gentle rocking

[a] ACD, NIH solution A: 2.2 g trisodium citrate (dihydrate); 0.8 g citric acid (monohydrate); 2.5 g dextrose; water to 100 mℓ.

[b] CPD, 63 mℓ/one unit pack contains 0.206 g citric acid (monohydrate); 1.66 g trisodium citrate (dihydrate); 0.140 g sodium dihydrogen phosphate (monohydrate); and 1.61 g dextrose.

telets in vitro. Platelets incorporate greater amounts of chromium 51, however, when suspended in isotonic sodium chloride than in plasma.[16-17] Platelets lose potassium rapidly from prolonged incubation in saline, however, and may demonstrate decreased viability.[18]

Plastic containers seem to be best because they are easy to handle. Results of recent studies suggest that the type of plastic used is of some importance.[7] Other studies suggest, however, that the viability of platelets stored in ACD is the same whether glass or plastic containers are used.[19]

Labeling Procedure Recommended by ICSH[20]

The panel on the Diagnostic Application of Radioisotopes in Hematology of the International Committee for Standardization of Hematology (ICSH) has recommended the following technique for platelet isolation and for labeling with ^{51}Cr.

Platelet Isolation and Labeling

All operations should be carried out with sterile techniques. The patient is weighed, and the platelet count is performed. After the analyst has considered the patient's age, weight, clinical condition, and platelet count, an appropriate volume of blood is decided upon. This will be 200—500 mℓ. For every 100 volumes of blood to be taken, 15 volumes of ACD are measured into the sterile transfusion bag (with two dry satellite bags attached). The blood is then taken into the bag. Donor blood collected not more than 2 hr previously and maintained at a temperature between 20 and 25°C may be used.

The entire bag is then centrifuged at 300 g (as calculated at the bottom of the container) for 15 min, including acceleration but not deceleration. The supernatant platelet-rich plasma (PRP) is transferred with the help of the "plasma extractor" into the first satellite bag. Approximately 5 mℓ of ACD or 1 mℓ of 0.15 M citric acid per 100 mℓ of PRP is added. This brings the pH of the PRP to 6.5 ± 0.2. The platelets are sedimented into a pellet by centrifugation at 1500 g for 15 min.

All but 5 mℓ of the supernatant platelet-poor plasma (PPP) is transferred into the second satellite bag, without disturbing the pellet. The platelets in the pellet are resuspended by repeated gentle inversion of the bag. One to two μCi of ^{51}Cr per kg body weight as sodium chromate (^{51}Cr) is added to the platelet suspension. The upper limit of activity should be used when autologous platelets are used in thrombocytopenic patients, and the lower limit should be used in studies of children. The mixture is incubated without shaking for 30 min at a temperature between 20 and 25°C.

All but 40 mℓ of the PPP in the second satellite bag is returned to the incubated mixture. Two hundred mℓ of filtered air is introduced into the bag before centrifugation to produce a good air-plasma interface; this facilitates the complete removal of the supernatant. The bag is centrifuged at 1500 g for 15 min to form a second platelet pellet. The radioactive PPP is then carefully removed without disturbing the platelet pellet. Approximately 20 mℓ of nonradioactive PPP is gently layered over the platelet pellet in such a way that the pellet is not disturbed; the PPP is then carefully decanted and discarded. (The object is to remove as much unbound ^{51}Cr from the bag as possible.)

The labeled platelets in the pellet are gently resuspended in 10 to 20 mℓ of nonradioactive PPP. It is desirable, especially if whole blood radioactivity measurement is to be used, to remove the contaminating ^{51}Cr-labeled red cells before injecting the labeled platelet suspension. The red cells are sedimented by centrifuging the suspension in tubes at 200 g for 5 min. The labeled supernatant platelet suspension is collected by aspiration. Although the adequacy of red cell removal can frequently be judged visually, it should be assessed more objectively by preparing standards in both saline and ammonium oxalate.

Standards are prepared in duplicate by adding 0.1 mℓ of the labeled platelet suspension to each of four counting tubes, two containing 2 mℓ of ammonium oxalate solution 10 g/ℓ and two containing saline. The four tubes are centrifuged at 200 g for 30 min. The supernatants are removed without disturbing the platelet pellet and discarded. The four tubes are then capped and saved for counting. A known amount of labeled platelet suspension, usually 10 to 20 mℓ containing 5 to 15 μCi (ℓ), is injected intravenously and the time is noted. Samples should be obtained at 30 min, 2 hr, and daily for 10 days after injection (Table 3).

Model of Platelet Kinetics for Determination of Platelet Life Span in Humans

Platelet kinetics performed in the normal state have led to a controversy on the true nature of platelet survival. Much of this controversy has been introduced because platelet studies performed with the different isotopes produce survival curves that are correlated with the different types of platelet utilization. For instance, if the platelet destruction was absolutely random, presumably in support of hemostasis, platelets would be cleared before they reach senility and would produce an exponential type of decay curve. On the other hand, if the platelets were cleared at the time they became effete, clearance of the isotopically labeled platelets would be linear with time. If both of these conditions were present, the survival curves would be intermediate between the two.[1,21-22] In general, survival curves obtained with platelets labeled with ^{14}C-serotonin and ^{32}P-orthophosphate are exponential, whereas curves obtained with platelets labeled with ^{51}chromium have been found to be both linear[5,10,23,24] or intermediate between linear and exponential.[16,25] Survival curves with P-diisopropyl flurophosphate (DFP) ^{32} have been described as linear.[23,26]

The different types of survival curves that have been established clearly indicate that mathematical models have not been generally agreed upon for approximating platelet survival curves. This disagreement becomes important when certain clinical studies are performed. For example, a 20% change in platelet survival time may be crucial in clinical interpretation, as for example, in assessing the effect of drugs upon platelet utilization. The model chosen should not be left to the investigator's personal preference.

Recently, Murphy et al. developed a model in which platelets could receive a variable number of insults before being destroyed.[27] If, for example, platelet utilization was entirely independent of platelet age, a large number of "hits" would be removed, and the disappearance of the isotopic label would be expected to be linear with time. On the other hand, a totally random destruction due to a low order of "hits" would be expected to give an isotope clearance that would closely approximate the exponential.[21,28] With a mathematical curve-fitting technique based upon this model, the closest approximation of the data to curves could be induced without observer bias. Although this model does not correct for the differences observed with the use of different isotopes, it is promising as a useful tool in objectively computing platelet survival times. The reader is referred to the ICSH recommendations for a discussion of the types of methods used in computing platelet half-life.[20]

Obviously, the ideal label for platelets has not been established. Recent work using Indium^{111} as a platelet label[29,30] has been very promising. It is apparent that this high energy gamma emitter gives a survival curve similar to that of chromium and that is also useful as an imaging isotope (Figure 1). Its usefulness as a human platelet label is now under investigation in several laboratories.

Nonradioisotope Technique for Platelet Kinetics

As an alternative to determining platelet survival in the circulation by using radioisotope-labeled platelets, a simple nonradioisotopic method has been described.[57] This method is easy to perform and produces platelet curves that closely correlate with those

Table 3
CHARACTERISTICS OF DIRECT PLATELET LABELS[a]

Isotope	Binding characteristics	Toxicity	Elution, reutilization fate
^{3}H or ^{32}P — DFP	Binds irreversibly to enzymes that contain serine group and serine hydroxyls of other proteins,[46] labels RBC, granulocytes, platelets; not lymphocytes	Highly toxic, anticholinesterase in amounts > 4 mg, normal amount (> 0.03 mg/kg), produce no ill effects	Little or no elution or reutilization,[23,49] some ^{32}P may be incorporated into newly formed platelets
^{14}C-serotonin	Transported across platelet membrane, stored in dense granules[47,48]	Physiological effects of serotonin in amounts greater than 2 mg, (Normal label < 0.5 mg)	Measured life span may be shorter because serotonin exchanges with body components,[43] 80—90% excreted in urine within 15 days,[42] 5% via GI tract[43]
^{51}Cr-sodium chromate	20% bound to platelet stroma; 80% to low molecular weight, dialyzable compounds, and nucleotides,[50,51] 10% released in coagulation	Usual dose of 5 μg nontoxic, exposure of >10 μg/mℓ for longer than 30 min produces decreased platelet aggregation to connective tissue[52]	Less than 15% elution,[5,10,53] ultimately deposited in liver and spleen from effete platelets released at 3% per day into urine[10]
^{111}In-8-hydroxy-quinoline	Unknown binding in platelets, known to bind to intracellular components and soluble fractions of leukocytes,[54-56] up to 70% of label bound to platelets[30]	None in amounts used for labeling	Less than 4% eluted from platelets,[30] after 6 days 43% in liver, 13.3% in spleen, subsequent excretion in urine

[a] For megakaryocyte labels, see chapter on "Platelet Production" in this volume.

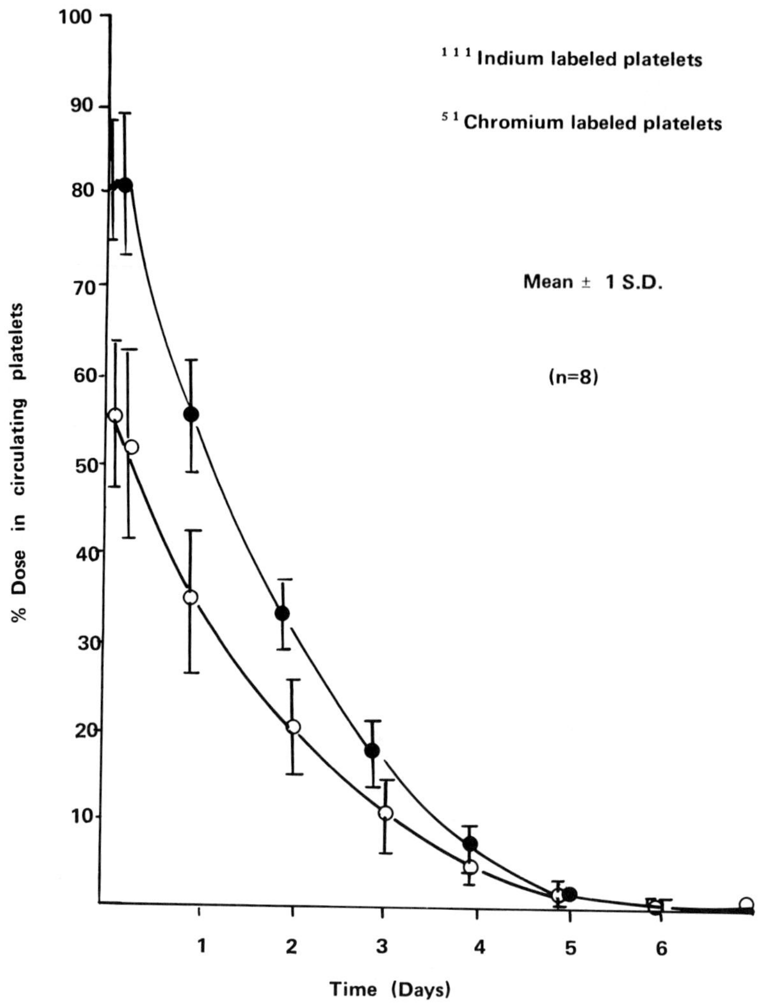

FIGURE 1. The percent dose of ^{111}In and ^{51}Cr radioactivity bound to circulating platelets is plotted against time in days. Each experimental group was composed of eight rabbits. The values plotted are the mean ±1 standard deviation. (From Scheffel, U., McIntyre, P. A., Evatt, B., et al., *Johns Hopkins Med. J.*, 140, 285, 1977. With permission.)

obtained by using the ^{51}Cr-sodium chromate radiosotopic method. It is based upon the observation that acetylsalicylic acid (aspirin) inhibits the peroxidation of platelet lipids, which are produced by a variety of agents, such as epinephrine, thrombin, and the sulfhydryl-blocking agent N — ethylmaleimide.[58] The aspirin effect persists throughout the life span of the platelet; therefore, if base-line lipid peroxidation is obtained, serial determinations of lipid peroxidation after aspirin ingestion reflect the disappearance of aspirin-treated platelets as they are replaced with normal platelets. The method is described below,[57] and Figure 2 shows a comparison of survival curves obtained by using chromium 51 and by aspirin-inhibited peroxidation.

Principal

Lipid peroxidation is measured as the malonaldehyde after its reaction from 2-thiobarbituric acid.

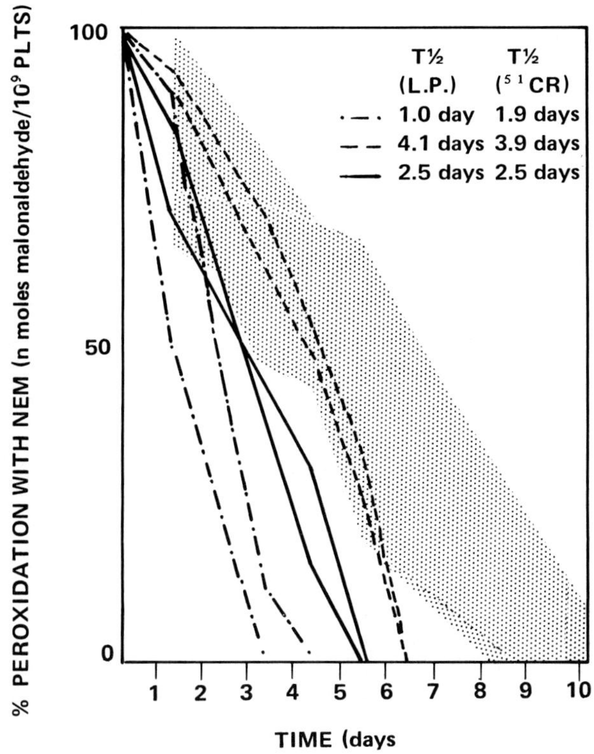

FIGURE 2. Comparison of ^{51}Cr and lipid peroxide (L.P.) platelet survivals. Two curves are presented for each of the three patients, showing the similarity in results. (From Stuart, M. J., Murphy, S., and Oski, F. A., *N. Engl. J. Med.*, 292, 1310, 1975. With permission.)

Materials

Prepare a 0.53% solution of 2-thiobarbituric acid in 2.3% perchloric acid and store at 4°. (800 mg 2-thiobarbituric acid + 10 mℓ concentrated NaOH + 50 mℓ distilled water). Adjust pH to 7.4 by adding concentrated perchloric acid and adjust volume to 100 mℓ with distilled water. To this 100 mℓ solution, add 50 mℓ of 7% perchloric acid.

Collection and Preparation of Sample

Collect venous blood in 2.3% sodium citrate, 9 to 1 ratio. Centrifuge whole blood at 22° for 15 min at 150 × g. Remove the platelet-rich plasma and determine the platelet count. Divide this material into aliquots and spin at 600 × g for 15 min. Invert the tubes for 2 min to allow any residual plasma to drain off.

Method

Incubate platelet buttons for 60 min at 37° with thrombin, 0.5 U/mℓ final concentration; resuspend in 0.15 M phosphate buffered saline, pH 7.4. Terminate the reaction by adding 2 mℓ of 2.3% perchloric acid containing 0.53% of 2-thiobarbituric acid.

Agitate the platelets with a Vortex® mixer and heat for 15 min in a boiling water bath and cool to 22°C. Read the supernatant color at 532 nanometers and express the results in nanomoles of malonaldehyde per 10^9 platelets. The molar absorption of malonaldehyde is 1.37×10^{-5}. Reproducibility is ± 7%. Platelets in normal individuals should have a mean half-life of about 4 days. Results are best expressed as percent initial peroxidation vs. a fraction of time after the aspirin ingestion. The test can only be employed for patients who have not taken aspirin before the test; it is contraindicated in patients who cannot take a single dose of aspirin.

The method has not yet become widely accepted, primarily because of the problems in the amount of variation observed in the platelet lipid peroxidation. It has been suggested that the 10-mℓ blood sample obtained for the test is insufficient for accurate results and that larger samples should be used.* In any event, the test should not be performed for normal individuals having a platelet count of less than 120,000. Neither should it be used for patients with platelet counts of less than 65,000 who have disorders such as idiopathic (immune) thrombocytopenic purpura (ITP) in which the platelets are larger than normal. The simplicity of the test makes it an attractive potential alternative to isotopic techniques, and further investigation is warranted.

REFERENCES

1. **Aster, Richard, H.**, Factors affecting the kinetics of isotopically labeled platelets in platelet kinetics, in *Platelet Kinetics*, Paulus, J. M., Ed., North-Holland, Amsterdam, 1971.
2. **Zucker, M. B. and Borrelli, J.**, Reversible alterations in platelet morphology produced by anticoagulants and by cold, *Blood*, 9, 602, 1954.
3. **White, J. G. and Krivit, W.**, An ultrastructural basis for the shape changes induced in platelets by chilling, *Blood*, 30, 625, 1967.
4. **Behnke, O. M.**, Some possible practical implications of liability of blood platelet microtubules, *Vox Sang.*, 13, 502, 1967.
5. **Baldini, M., Costea, N., and Dameshek, W.**, The viability of stored human platelets, *Blood*, 16, 1669, 1960.
6. **Levin, R. H. and Freireich, E. J.**, Effect of storage up to 48 hr on response to transfusions of platelet-rich plasma, *Transfusion*, 4, 251, 1964.
7. **Murphy, S. and Gardner, F. H.**, Platelet preservation. Effect of storage temperature on maintenance of platelet viability. Deleterious effect of refrigerated storage, *N. Engl. J. Med.*, 280, 1094, 1969.
8. **Aster, R. H.**, Platelet transfusion therapy, *The Platelet*, Brinkhous, K., Ed., Williams & Wilkins, Baltimore, 1970.
9. **Aas, K. and Gardner, F.**, Survival of blood platelets labeled with chromium, *J. Clin. Invest.*, 37, 1257, 1958.
10. **Aster, R. H. and Jandl, J. H.**, Platelet sequestration in man. I. Methods, *J. Clin. Invest.*, 43, 843, 1964.
11. **Davey, M. G. and Lander, H.**, The behavior of infused human platelets during the first 24 hr after infusion, *Br. J. Haematol.*, 10, 94, 1964.
12. **Aster, R. H.**, The anticoagulants of choice for platelet transfusion, *Transfusion*, 6, 32, 1966.
13. **Flatow, F. A. and Freireich, E. J.**, The increased effectiveness of platelet concentrates prepared in acidified plasma, *Blood*, 27, 449, 1966.
14. **Mourad, N.**, Studies on release of certain enzymes from human platelets, *Transfusion*, 8, 363b, 1968.
15. **Sivertsen, U.**, Changes in Platelet Aggregation During Storage, Proc. XIII Int. Congr. Haematol., Munich, 1970, 43.
16. **Davey, M. G.**, The survival and destruction of human platelets, *Bibl. Haematol.*, 22, 1, 1966.
17. **Abrahamsen, A. F.**, Platelet survival studies in man — with special reference to thrombosis and atheroschlerosis, *Scand. J. Haematol.*, Suppl. 3, 1, 1968.
18. **Cooley, M. H. and Cohen, P.**, Potassium transport in human blood platelets, *J. Lab. Clin. Med.*, 70, 69, 1967.
19. **Rolivic, Z. and Baldini, M.**, Comparative studies of the viability of human platelets stored at 4°C in plastic and glass containers, *Transfusion*, 7, 204, 1967.

* Working Party on Platelets, International Committee on Thrombosis and Hemostasis, Discussion, VIth Congress of the International Society on Thrombosis and Hemostasis, June 26, 1977, Philadelphia, Pa.

20. **Belcher, E. H., et al.**, Recommended methods for radioisotope platelet survival studies. A report by the panel on Diagnostic Application of Radioisotopes in Haematology of the International Committee for Standardization in Hematology, *Blood,* 50, 1137, 1977.
21. **Mustard, J. F., Rowsell, J. C., and Murphy, E. A.**, Platelet economy (platelet survival and turnover), *Br. J. Haematol.*, 12, 1, 1966.
22. **Murphy, E. A., Robinson, G. A., Rowsell, A. C., and Mustard, J. F.**, The pattern of platelet disappearance, *Blood,* 30, 26, 1967.
23. **Bithell, T. C., Athens, J. W., Cartwright, G. E., and Wintrobe, M. M.**, Radioactive diisopropylfluorophosphate as a platelet label: an evaluation of in vitro and in vivo techniques, *Blood,* 29, 354, 1967.
24. **Seidl, S.**, *Die Thrombozytentransfusion Untersuchurgen mit Radioaktiv markierten thrombozyten,* Gurton Fisher, Stuttgart, 1968.
25. **Kotilainen, M.**, Platelet kinetics in normal subjects and haematological disorders with special reference to thrombocytopenia and to the role of the spleen, *Scand. J. Haematol.*, Suppl. 5, 5—97, 1969.
26. **Zucker, M. D., Ley, A. B., and Mayer, K.**, Studies on platelet life-span and platelet depots by use of DFP^{32}, *J. Lab. Clin. Med.*, 58, 405, 1961.
27. **Murphy, E. A. and Francis, M. E.**, The estimation of blood platelet survival. II. The multiple Int model, *Thromb. Diath. Haemorrh.*, 25, 53, 1971.
28. **Murphy, E. A. and Francis, M. E.**, The estimation of blood platelet survival. I. General principles of the study of cell survival, *Thromb. Diath. Haemorrh.*, 22, 281, 1969.
29. **Thakur, M. L., Welch, M. J., Joist, J., Heinrich, J., and Coleman, R. E.**, $Indium^{111}$ labeled platelets. Studies on preparation and evaluation of in vitro and in vivo function, *Thromb. Res.*, 9, 345, 1976.
30. Scheffel, U., McIntyre, P. A., Evatt, B., Dvornicky, J. A., Jr., Natarajan, T. K., Bolling, D. R., and Murphy, E. A., Evaluation of $Indium^{111}$ as a new high photon yield gamma-emitting "physiological" platelet label, *Johns Hopkins Med. J.*, 140, 285—293, 1977.
31. **Firkin, B. G. and Williams, W. J.**, Incorporation of radioactive phosphorous into phospholipids of human leukemic leukocytes and platelets, *J. Clin. Invest.*, 40, 423, 1961.
32. **Adelson, E., Kaufman, R. M., Leaf, A. A., Kirby, J. C., and Rheingold, J. J.**, Physiology of platelet destruction as revealed by tagging of cohorts. I. Studies in dogs, *J. Lab. Clin. Med.*, 62, 385, 1963.
33. **Ebbe, S., Baldini, M., and Donovan, J.**, Comparative studies of platelet survival by different methods in the rabbit, *Blood,* 25, 584, 1965.
34. **Adelson, E., Rheingold, J. J., and Crosby, W. H.**, Studies of platelet survival by tagging in vivo with P^{32}, *J. Lab. Clin. Med.*, 50, 570, 1957.
35. **O'Dell, T. T., Jr., Tausche, F. G., and Furth, J.**, Platelet life-span as measured by transfusion of isotopically labeled platelets in rats, *Acta Haematol.*, 13, 45, 1955.
36. **Cronkite, E. P.**, Regulation of platelet production, Brookhaven Symposia, *Biology,* 10, 96, 1958.
37. **O'Dell, T. T., Jr., Tausche, F. G., and Gude, W. D.**, Uptake of radioactive sulfate by elements of the blood and the bone marrow of rats, *Am. J. Physiol.*, 180, 491, 1955.
38. **Vodopick, H. A. and Kniseley, R. M.**, Sulfur-35 studies in man: platelet survival and plasma and urinary radioactivity assayed by beta liquid scintillation spectrometry, *J. Lab. Clin. Med.*, 62, 109, 1963.
39. **Cohen, P., Cooley, M. H., and Gardner, F. H.**, The use of selenomethionine (Se^{75}) as a label for canine and human platelets, *J. Clin. Invest.*, 44, 1036, 1965.
40. **Evatt, B. L. and Levin, J.**, Measurement of thrombopoiesis in rabbits using ^{75}Selenomethionine, *J. Clin. Invest.*, 48, 1615, 1969.
41. **Najean, Y., Ardaillou, N., and Dresch, C.**, Platelet life-span, *Ann. Rev. Med.*, 20, 47, 1969.
42. **Heyssel, R. M.**, Determination of human platelet survival utilizing C^{14} labeled serotonin, *J. Clin. Invest.*, 40, 2134, 1961.
43. **Zucker, M. B., Hellman, L., and Zumoff, B.**, Rapid disappearance of ^{14}C-labeled serotonin from platelets in platelets with carcinoid syndrome, *J. Lab. Clin. Med.*, 63, 137, 1964.
44. **Adelson, E., Kaufman, R. M., Berdequez, C., Lear, A. A., and Rheingold, J. J.**, Platelet tagging with tritium-labeled diisopropylfluorophosphate, *Blood,* 26, 744, 1965.
45. **McIntyre, P. A., Evatt, B., Hodkinson, B. A., and Scheffel, U.**, Selenium ^{75}Selenomethionine as a label for erythrocytes, leukocytes and platelets in man, *J. Lab. Clin. Med.*, 75, 472, 1970.
46. **Athens, J. W., Mauer, A. M., Ashenbrucker, G. E., Cartwright, G. E., and Wintrobe, M. M.**, Leukokinetic studies. I. A method for labeling leukocytes with diisopropylfluorophosphate (DFP^{32}), *Blood,* 14, 303, 1959.
47. **Zucker, M. B.**, Serotonin: hematologic aspects, *Prog. Hematol.*, 2, 206, 1962.
48. **White, J. G.**, Dense bodies of human platelets — origin of serotonin storage particles from platelet granules, *Am. J. Pathol.*, 53, 791, 1968.
49. **Cooney, D. P., Smith, B. A., and Fawley, D. E.**, The use of ^{32}diisoprophyflurophosphate (^{32}DFP) as a platelet label: evidence for reutilization of the isotope in man, *Blood,* 31, 791, 1968.

50. **Aster, R. H. and Enright, S. E.**, A platelet and granulocyte membrane defect in paroxysmal nocturnal hemoglobinuria, *J. Clin. Invest.*, 48, 1199, 1969.
51. **Steiner, M. and Baldini, M.**, Subcellular distribution of ^{51}Cr and characterization of its binding sites in human platelets, *Blood*, 35, 727, 1970.
52. **Kattlove, H. E. and Spaet, T. H.**, The effect of chromium on platelet function in vitro, *Blood*, 25, 659, 1970.
53. **Harker, L. A. and Finch, C. A.**, Thrombokinetics in man, *J. Clin. Invest.*, 48, 963, 1969.
54. **Thakur, M. L., Coleman, R. E., and Welch, M. H.**, In-111 labeled leukocytes for the localization of abscesses, *J. Nucl. Med.*, 17, 560, 1976.
55. **Thakur, M. L., Coleman, R. E., and Welch, M. J.**, Indium-111 labeled leukocytes for the localization of abscesses. Preparation, analysis, tissue distribution and comparison with gallium-67 citrate in dogs, *J. Lab. Clin. Med.*, 89, 217, 1977.
56. **Segal, A. W.**, Indium-111-labeled leukocytes for localization of abscesses, *Lancet II*, 1056, 1976.
57. **Stuart, M., Murphy, S., and Oski, F.**, A simple nonradioisotope method for the determination of platelet life-span, *N. Engl. J. Med.*, 292, 1310, 1975.

PLATELET BIOCHEMISTRY

H. Holmsen, J. B. Smith, J. L. Daniel, S. Holme, and T. K. Bills

Several aspects of platelet biochemistry are relatively well elucidated and will be briefly reviewed here. Only human platelets are considered. Because great changes in metabolism occur when platelets are activated, it is convenient to consider the biochemistry of a resting and a stimulated platelet separately. We have chosen to discuss energy metabolism, adenine nucleotide compartmentalization, lipid composition and metabolism, contractile and microtubule proteins, glycoproteins, secretable proteins, and serotonin in the resting platelet. We will describe the biochemical characteristics of a stimulated platelet: energy and adenine nucleotide metabolism, arachidonate oxidation, functional effects of some prostaglandins, participation of contractile and microtubule proteins in function, and intracellular regulation of platelet responses by Ca^{2+}, cAMP, and cGMP.

Platelets have no nucleus and lack DNA. Only traces of RNA are present, and protein synthesis is small and probably insignificant. Our knowledge about amino acid metabolism in platelets is scanty, but it should be pointed out that taurine is present in exceptionally large amounts, although nothing is known about the function of this amino acid. These areas of platelet biochemistry are not dealt with here.

The Resting Platelet

In circulating blood, the resting platelet has a discoid shape and a volume of 7 μ^3. Human platelets are, however, extremely excitable and respond to exposure to anticoagulants, foreign surfaces, physical stress (e.g., centrifugation, gel filtration), pH changes, etc., by losing their discoid shape and becoming spheres with long pseudopods. Their excitability makes it difficult for the biochemist to establish the true basic rates of reactions and pathways, since these are altered when platelets are stimulated. As a result, the rates of certain metabolic conversions, levels of certain substances, the conformation of certain proteins, etc., for "resting" platelets may be somewhat different from the resting platelets in circulation.

Energy Metabolism and Compartmentalization of Adenine Nucleotides (H. Holmsen)

Figure 1 shows schematically the major pathways of energy and adenine nucleotide metabolism in platelets (Table 1). In the figure, ATP, ADP, and AMP represent adenine nucleotides in the metabolic pool, whereas °ATP and °ADP designate the nonmetabolic or storage pool of adenine nucleotides. Although the different pathways are not interconnected in Figure 1, ATP, ADP, and AMP are in equilibrium. The metabolic adenine nucleotides are not synthesized *de novo* in vitro, but can be synthesized from preformed purines (adenine, hypoxanthine) or from adenosine.[1,8] For the sake of clarity the reduction and oxidation sites for NADH-NAD in extramitrochondrial reactions are not shown.

Lipid Metabolism (T. K. Bills)

Lipid performs a major structural role in platelets by constituting the plasma membrane, which separates the cytoplasm of the platelet from its plasma environment,[80] and the membranes of the intracellular organelles, including mitochondria, α-granules, and dense granules. Lipid comprises 15 to 17% of platelet dry weight.[81] Of this, 67% is phospholipid, 25% neutral lipid, and 8% glycosphingolipid. The phospholipids include phosphatidylcholine (40%), phosphatidylethanolamine (28%) — of which half is in the plasmalogen form, sphingomyelin (18%), phosphatidylserine (9%), and phos-

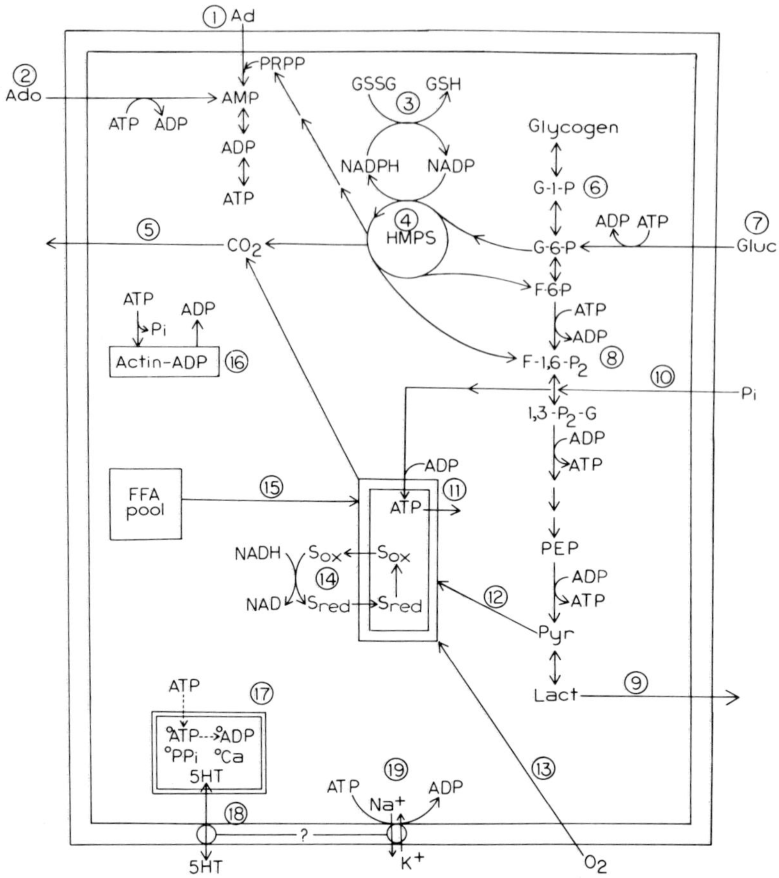

FIGURE 1. Energy and adenine nucleotide metabolism in the resting platelet. The processes marked by encircled numbers are explained in Table 1.

phoinositides (4%) — of which 60% is monophosphoinositide, 30% diphosphoinositide, and 10% triphosphoinositide.[81] It has been estimated that 63% of platelet phospholipid is located in the plasma membrane, and it has been shown that there is an asymmetric distribution of phospholipids between the outer and inner surfaces of this membrane.[82] Extensive analyses of the fatty acid composition of phospholipids have been done.[81,83,84]

Cholesterol is the major neutral lipid in platelets (95%). Small amounts of triglyceride (2.4%), free fatty acids (2.4%), and cholesterol esters (0.2%) are present. Hematosides are the major glycosphinlogipid in platelets.[85] Resting platelets are capable of synthesizing a number of lipids including triglycerides[86] and free fatty acids.[87] The synthesis of phospholipids in platelets is depicted in Figure 2, Table 2. The synthesis of prostaglandins and thromboxanes occurs in stimulated platelets and is depicted in Figure 4, Table 7.

Contractile Proteins (J. L. Daniel)

The known properties of contractile, regulatory, and microtubule proteins isolated from platelets are shown in Table 3. Information about the absolute content of the various proteins in platelets is either missing or at great variance in the literature, and has been omitted in Table 3.[102,104] Platelets appear to contain the capability to synthesize platelet actomyosin protein.[121] Subcellular localization of platelet actin and myosin is not completely clear. Early attempts to demonstrate actomyosin in the external pla-

Table 1
ENERGY AND ADENINE NUCLEOTIDE METABOLISM IN RESTING PLATELET

Index key	Name of process/pathway	Rate μmoles/min×10^{11} cells	Description	Comments	Ref.
1	Adenine uptake and conversion	0.01	Specific uptake; km = 1.6×10^{-7} M; adenine not free intracellularly; converted to AMP by adenine phosphoribosyl transferase (km = 5×10^{-6} M, both substrates); radioactive adenine labels metabolic adenine nucleotide pool	Uptake rate probably dependent on [PRPP]; PRPP synthetase present; [guanine/hypoxanthine phosphoribosyl transferase present; uptake of guanine and hypoxanthine slow, probably important in vivo]	1—5
2	Adenosine uptake and conversions	Low km = 0.08; High km = 10	Two uptake systems; low km (9.8×10^{-6} M), high km (9.4×10^{-3}M); intracellularly low [adenosine] phosphorylated (adenosine kinase, Km = 2×10^{-6} (adenosine), 9×10^{-4} M (ATP), high [adenosine] deaminated (adenosine deaminase, km = 1×10^{-4} M; radioactive adenosine labels metabolic adenine nucleotide pool	Inhibition: low km system: papaverine; high km system: adenine, both systems: metabolic inhibitors; uptake unrelated to inhibition of platelet function; unclassified inhibitors: dipyridamole, quasidine, pyrimidine derivatives	6—12
3	Glutathione metabolism	—	[GSH] = 2 μmol/10^{11} cells; kept constant by GSH reductase	[Protein-bound SH] high in platelets; glutathione peroxidase present	13, 14
4	Hexose monophosphate shunt (HMPS)	0.02—0.03	As in generalized cell; measured as $^{14}CO_2$ production from [1−^{14}C] glucose; 0.5—2% enters HMPS	Produces NADPH for GSH homeostasis (# 3) and fatty acid synthesis; hydroperoxides, stimulate HMPS and adenine uptake; suggests PRPP synthesis from R-5-P	5, 15—20
5	CO_2 production	0.09	From glucose; 40% in HMPS and 60% in tricarboxylic acid cycle	CO_2 from fatty acid (see # 15)	15, 21—22.
6	Glycogenolysis	0.9	Maximal rate, AMP-dependent and -independent phosphorylase; Ca^{2+} required for activation; amylo - 1.6 - glucosidase hydrolyses limit dextrin	cAMP no effect; [Glycogen] = < 60 μmol (glucose)/10^{11} cells, present in granules; 1—4 bonds split much faster than 1 - 6 bonds; regulation of glycogenolysis unclear; isolation of platelet stimulates	23—28
	Glycogen synthesis	0.5—1.2	Maximal rate; G-6-P-dependent and -independent glycogen synthase	Little incorporation of glucose in vitro; regulation of glycogen synthesis unclear	25, 29—33
7	Glucose uptake	0.3—2.3 (glucose) 4 (2-deoxy-glucose)	At saturating permeant concentration (> 1 mM)	Glucose, 2-deoxyglucose, mannose, fructose transported by same mechanism; Regulation obscure; markedly affected by + and − 0_2	15, 16, 34, 35

Table 1 (continued)
ENERGY AND ADENINE NUCLEOTIDE METABOLISM IN RESTING PLATELET

Index key	Name of process/pathway	Rate μmoles/ min×10^{11} cells	Description	Comments	Ref.
8	Glycolysis	See # 9	As in generalized cell, 10 enzymatic reactions, with activities 10—160 times glycolytic flux; Pasteur and Crabtree effects; not reversible[b]	Phosphofructokinase[a] and glucose uptake major regulatory steps. Glycolysis inhibited by 2-deoxyglucose, MIA, F^-; flux dependent on glucose supply (both exogenous and from glycogen) and state of platelet; major site of ATP production	36—49
9	Lactate production	1.5—2.5 (aerobic) 3—8 (anaerobic)	End product of glycolysis, accumulates extracellularly	See # 8	
10	P_i uptake and conversions	0.9	At [Pi] = 1.2 mM; Pi incorporated into nucleotide di- and triphosphates (not monophosphate) and derivatives, glycolytic intermediates, certain phospholipids	$^{32}P_i$ - labels metabolic adenylate pool; [Pi] = 3—5 μ mol/10^{11} cells platelets; control of uptake and possible compartmentalization unknown; incorporation into phospholipid dependent on mitochondrial respiration; in vitro different from in vivo pattern	50—56
11	Oxidative phosphorylation	2.1	Measured as the initial rate of lowering of [ATP] when ox. phos. is abruptly inhibited	May account for 40—50% of total ATP production; in rat platelets 55% in presence of glucose, 90% in its absence	57, 58
12	Oxidation of pyruvate	0.003—0.023	1% of glucose metabolized enters tricarboxylic acid cycle	—	15
13	Oxygen consumption	0.25—0.6	85% mitochondrial, i.e., antimycin-sensitive	15% antimycin-insensitive; due to lipid peroxidation and microsomal oxidation	41, 46
14	Oxidation of cytosolic NADH	?	NADH not permeable to mitochondria; "shuttles" required	α-Glycerophosphate-dihydroxyacetone phosphate substrate shuttle possible	61
15	Fatty acid oxidation	0.008	Measured for palmitate, equivalent to 0.95 μmol ATP produced/min/10^{11} cells	Classical β-oxidation; carnitine cycle present; oxidation rate dependent on presence/ absence of glucose	62—64
16	ADP turnover in actin-ADP	1.0	10—40% metabolic ADP bound to actin; the ADP-actin bond breaks in acid, not in ethanol; difference used to study turnover of ADP in intact platelets	Thought to represent ATP consumption (40% of total) related to maintenance of a certain G-F actin equilibrium	65, 66

Table 1 (continued)
ENERGY AND ADENINE NUCLEOTIDE METABOLISM IN RESTING PLATELET

Index key	Name of process/pathway	Rate μmoles/ min×10^{11} cells	Description	Comments	Ref.
17	Storage pool of adenine nucleotides, Ca^{2+}, pyrophosphate and serotonin (5HT)	—	Substances in dense granules; 5HT readily exchangeable; Ca^{2+} and PPi not exchangeable; very slow exchange between granular and cytoplasmic ATP	60% of platelet ATP and ADP present in storage pool, ATP/ADP = 0.7 [platelet content: 5—7 μmol ATP, 2.5—4 μmol ADP/10^{11} cells]; ^{31}P-nuclear magnetic resonance not observed from stored nucleotides and PPi. Dense granule content markedly reduced in Storage Pool Deficiency	67—75
18	Serotonin uptake	0.378	Multistep process, see Table 5	—	76
19	Na^+-K^+ transport	—	Ouabain-sensitive Na^+/K^+ pump present	Connection with serotonin uptake suggested	77—79

[a] Activators: F-6-P, Mg ADP^-, Mg^{2+}, cAMP, OH^-, SO_4^{2-}, Pi. Inhibitors: Mg ATP^{2-}, ATP^{4-}, citrate, H^+.

[b] No gluconeogenesis; P-enolpyruvate carboxykinase, pyruvate carboxykinase and F - 1.6 - P_2ase not present.

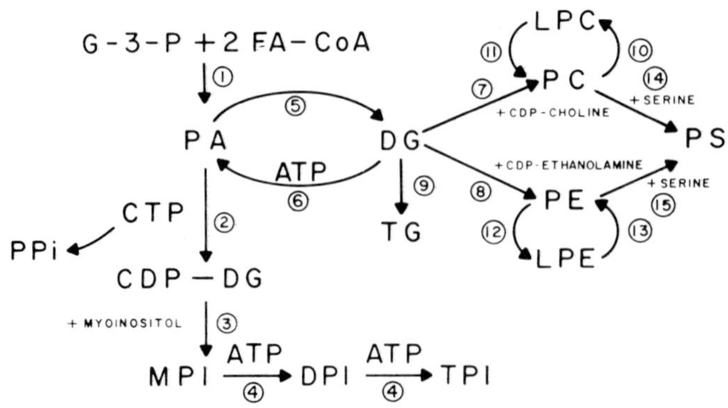

FIGURE 2. Phospholipid synthesis. The processes marked by encircled numbers are described in Table 2.

telet surface[122] have not been confirmed when more recent technology has been applied.[123,124] However, actin may become exposed during activation.[124] Crawford and co-workers have shown that actin is associated with isolated platelet membranes and also with granules.[125,126] However, it is not certain that this association occurs as an artifact during preparation in light of the "sticky" nature of actin.[127] Myosin is apparently found mainly in the cytoplasm.[128]

Tubulin, the major protein of microtubules, is morphologically seen as a microtubule circumferential band.[129] Whether a nonpolymerized pool of tubulin exists in resting platelets is not known.

Glycoproteins and Secreted Proteins (S. Holme)

It is well established that the exterior of cell membranes[132,133] is rich in glycoproteins. They have been shown to span the membrane, with an intracellular terminating part of the polypeptide chain associated with proteins located at the internal surface of the membrane and with the carbohydrate containing moiety in a prominent position of the external surface. Presently, platelet glycoproteins are studied intensively in many laboratories. Their structure, location, and orientation on the platelet membrane are thought to be of importance in platelet contact interactions.[134-137] However, much confusion exists regarding the number and molecular weights of the membrane glycoproteins, probably because different and inadequate techniques for isolation and identification are used. Two main approaches have been utilized:

1. Labeling of membrane proteins with ^{125}I, using lactoperoxidase catalyzed iodination of washed human platelets. Originally, three glycoprotein fractions termed GPI, GPII, and GPIII were defined on periodic acid-Schiff (PAS)-staining and counting of slices of sodium dodecyl sulfate polyacrylamide gels (SDS-PAGE) after electrophoresis of reduced samples of solubilized whole platelets.[138] Recently, six surface glycoproteins have been isolated by using a nonreduced-reduced two dimensional gel electrophoresis system based on alteration of the molecular weights of the glycoproteins by reducing the disulfides[139] (Table 4A).
2. Separation and identification on SDS-PAGE with PAS-staining of reduced samples of isolated platelet membranes. Three glycoprotein bands have been described (Table 4B). A prominent glycoprotein which migrates at the same rate as membrane-bound glycoprotein I is often found located in the cytosol fraction following platelet lysis.[134] Probably this protein is identical with the one described by Lombart[145] and named glycocalicin due to its presumed origin from the platelet glycocalyx.[147] It has been suggested that this protein is involved in ristocetin or bovine factor VIII-induced aggregation.[140,148] The field of platelet glycoproteins is pres-

Table 2
PHOSPHOLIPID SYNTHESIS

Figure key	Activity	Substrate	Product	Properties	Ref.
1	Acyl-CoA: sn-glycero-3-phosphate O-acyltransferase	sn-glycerol-3-phosphate (G-3-P) + fatty acyl-Co A (FA-Co A)	Phosphatidic acid (PA)	May be specific enzyme for each species of FA-Co A; some catalyze acylation of saturated FA-Co A at the 1-position, others unsaturated FA-Co A at the 2-position	88
2	CTP: diacyl glycerophosphate-cytidyl transferase	Phosphatidic acid (PA) + cytidine triphosphate (CTP)	Cytidine diphosphate diglyceride (CDP - DG) + pyrophosphate (PPi)	Requires Mg^{2+}; enzyme may be specific for 1-stearoyl-2-arachidonyl-phosphatidic acid	89
3	Cytidine diphosphate diglyceride: myoinositol, phosphatidyltransferase	Cytidine diphosphate diglyceride (CDP-DG) + myoinositol	Monophosphoinositide (MPI) + cytidine monophosphate (CMP)	Requires Mn^{2+}; substrate specificity has not been determined	90
4	Phosphoinositide kinase	Monophosphoinositide (MPI) or diphosphoinositide (DPI) + adenosine triphosphate (ATP)	Diphosphoinositide (DPI) or triphosphoinositide (TPI) + adenosine diphosphate (ADP)	Occurs in the resting state but formation of DPI and TPI is increased during aggregation	83
5	Phosphatidate phosphatase	Phosphatidic acid (PA)	Diglyceride (DG) + inorganic phosphate	Requires Mg^{2+}; enzyme attacks all PA species	91
6	Diglyceride kinase	Diglyceride (DG) + adenosine triphosphate (ATP)	Phosphatidic acid (PA) + adenosine diphosphate (ADP)	Requires Mg^{2+}; substrate specificity has not been determined	92
7	Cholinephosphotransferase	Diglyceride (DC) + cytidine-diphosphate choline (CDP-choline)	Phosphatidylcholine (PC) + cytidine monophosphate (CMP)	This reaction proceeds at a much greater rate than either step 8 or 9; this enzyme utilizes all DG species	93
8	Ethanolamine-phosphotransferase	Diglyceride (DG) + cytidine-diphosphate ethanolamine (CDP-ethanolamine)	Phosphatidylethanolamine (PE) + cytidine monophosphate (CMP)	Requires Mn^{2+}; can utilize either DG or 1-alkyl-2-acyl-glycerol the plasmalogen precursor; this enzyme may selectively utilize DG containing arachidonic acid at the 2-position	94
9	Acyl-CoA: diglyceride O-acyltransferase	Diglyceride (DG) + fatty acyl-Co A (FA-Co A)	Triglyceride (TG)	—	86

Table 2 (continued)
PHOSPHOLIPID SYNTHESIS

Figure key	Activity	Substrate	Product	Properties	Ref.
10	Phospholipase A_2	Phosphatidylcholine	Lyso-phosphatidyl-choline (LPC) + free fatty acid (FFA)	Stimulated by thrombin; utilizes only PC containing arachidonic acid at the 2-position	95, 96
11	Acyl-CoA: phospholipid acyltransferase	Lyso-phosphatidylcholine (LPC) + fatty acyl-Co A (FA-Co A)	Phosphatidylcholine (PC)	May be specific enzyme for specific FA-Co A species	97
12	Phospholipase A_2	Diacyl-phosphatidyl-ethanol-amine	Lyso-phosphatidyl-eth-anolamine (LPE) + free fatty acid (FFA)	Requires Ca^{2+}; shows no specificity with respect to PE species	98
13	Acyl-CoA: phospholipid acyltransferase	Lyso-phosphatydylethanol-amine (LPE) + fatty acyl-Co A (FA-Co A)	Phosphatidylethanol-amine (PE)	—	97
14	Choline: serine transferase	Phosphatidyl-choline (PC) + serine	Phosphatidylserine (PS) + choline	Has not been demonstrated in human platelets	—
15	Ethanolamine: serine transferase	Phosphatidylethanolamine (PE) + serine	Phosphatidylserine (PS) + ethanolamine	This enzyme does not show specificity with respect to PE species	89

Table 3
PLATELET CONTRACTILE AND MICROTUBULE PROTEINS

Protein	Molecular weight (daltons)	Subunits	Polymers	Sedimention coefficient	Interactions	Comments	Ref.
Actin	42,000—45,000	—	6 nM double helical filaments with 39 nm repeat	2.75; 3.15	Binds 1 mol ADP/mol in polymer form; activates myosin Mg ATPase	Similar to muscle actin but contains some sequence differences; maybe two forms	99—106
Filamin (actin-binding protein)	? (dimer in chicken gizzard)	270,000	—	8.85 (chicken gizzard)		—	104, 107, 108

α-Actinin	95,000 (skeletal muscle)	95,000?			Both probably cause actin gelation and alignment of actin filaments	—	107
Profilin	16,000	16,000	—	—	Binds to G-actin	Causes actin to remain depolymerized; proposed to regulate polymerization state of actin	131
Myosin	460,000; 540,000	Heavy chain 200,000; light chain 20,000; 16,000	Forms bipolar filament, 320 nm long, 10 nm wide	6.85, 5.55, 6.25	Displays K-EDTA ATPase and Ca ATPase; interacts with actin to give Mg ATPase	—	109—113
Myosin light chain kinase	80,000, Ca^{2+}-insensitive	80,000	—	?	Phosphorylates the 20,000 dalton subunit of platelet myosin, elevating actomyosin ATPase	Phosphorylation of platelet myosin increases during platelet stimulation; 80,000 dalton kinase likely to be Ca-insensitive proteolytic fragment of 100,000 dalton kinase	114—116, 130
	~ 117,000 Ca^{2+}-sensitive	100,000, 17,000					
Tropomyosin	dimer? (60,000)	30,000	Forms paracrystals with 34.5 nm axial repeat	?	Binds to platelet actin	Smaller than skeletal muscle tropomyosin	117
Troponin	?	?	?	?	—	Existence open to question; troponin C-like protein shown to be modulator of phosphodiesterase	118, 119
Tubulin	110,000 (dimer)	$\alpha = 55,000$ $\beta = 52,000$	Form 25 nm microtubules	6.05	Binds cochicine and GDP; phosphorylated by endogenous kinase	Amino acid composition very similar to brain tubulin	120
Microtubule; associated	> 200,000	May be several	—	—	Associated with tubulin, may include an ATPase	Not as well characterized as other microtubule associated proteins	101

Table 4A
SURFACE LABELED GLYCOPROTEINS

Original terminology	Nomenclature synonyms (1977)[139]	Nomenclature synonyms	Apparent molecular weight (nonreduced—reduced)	Relative staining properties: Coomassie Blue	Relative staining properties: PAS	Comments
I	Ia		153,000—167,000	+	+	I weakly labeled with ^{125}I by lactoperoxidase or by diazotized (^{125}I)-dicodosulfanililic acid; Ia contains interchain disulfides
	Ib		170,000—143,000	+	+ + + +	Ib disulfide linked to small polypeptides
II	IIa		138,000—158,000	+	+	Contains interchain disulfides; decreased iodination in Bernard Soulier platelets[134]
	IIb	IIa[140]	142,000—132,000	+ +	+ + +	Disulfide linked to small polypeptides; decreased iodination in Glanzmann's thrombasthenia[133]
III	III	IIb[141]	99,000—110,000	+ + + +	+ + +	Contains interchain disulfides; decreased iodination in Bernard Soulier and Glanzmann's thrombasthenia[135,136]
	IV		97,000	+	+ +	—

[a] Major glycoprotein.[142]

Table 4B
ISOLATED MEMBRANE GLYCOPROTEINS

Major band	Apparent molecular weight: Phillips[135]	Apparent molecular weight: Nurden[144]	Properties[140,143]	Comments
I	150,000	155,000	High content of sialic acid; stains predominantly with PAS, but poorly with Coomassie blue	Gives rise to a large molecular weight trypsin resistant acidic macroglycopeptide on proteolytic digestion;[144,145] (Molecular weight 120,000; 60% carbohydrate; 22% sialic acid)[146] GP I much reduced in Bernard-Soulier platelets;[143] reduction of bovine factor VIII and ristocetin-induced aggregation in parallel with hydrolysis of GP I[136]
II	124,000	135,000	Less sialic acid than GP I; stains predominantly with PAS and Coomassie blue	No staining in Glanzmann's Thrombasthenia[144]
III	106,000	103,000	Contains little or no sialic acid; stains predominantly with PAS and Coomassie blue	Reduced in Glanzmann's Thrombasthenia[144]

ently under rapid development, and newer techniques have already shown subdivision of the glycoprotein fractions described here. The complexity of these subfractions makes it difficult at present to make a clear classification of the subfractions and their origin.

Proteins secreted by the platelets can tentatively be divided into three categories: (1) proteins identical or similar to plasma proteins, (2) cationic proteins, and (3) platelet specific proteins. The most described proteins in each category are presented in Table 4C. The physiological significance of the secreted proteins in Category 1 and 2 regarding hemostasis, inflammation, and cell growth is evident. On the other hand, the biological role of the platelet specific proteins is still unclear.

Serotonin (H. Holmsen)

There are several aspects to the interaction between platelets and serotonin. The amine causes shape change and aggregation of the cells, it is taken up and stored in the dense granules, it is metabolized in the cells under various circumstances, and it is liberated from the cells by a wide variety of agents. There is much literature about serotonin-platelet interactions, because the platelet has been used as a model to study general pharmacological principles for amine uptake, storage, and liberation. The evidence that is presented in Table 5 has been chosen selectively to illuminate some apparent main features of the interaction between platelets and serotonin.

In short, Table 5 serves to illustrate that:

1. The platelet surface has two distinctly different "receptors" for serotonin. One receptor receives a signal for platelet responses, i.e., shape change and aggregation. Another receptor, or transport system, facilitates the transport of serotonin. The action of various inhibitors clearly distinguishes between the two receptors.

2. There is strong evidence that the transfer of serotonin across the plasma membrane is driven by a downhill Na^+ gradient from the outside to the inside of this membrane. Chloride ions appear to be necessary for the transport and may be cotransported with serotonin.

3. A quite different transport system is present at the membrane surrounding the dense granules, which undirectionally transports serotonin into the matrix of these granules.

4. Once inside the dense granule, serotonin is bound to some (hitherto undefined) structures.

5. Liberation of serotonin can occur by at least four distinguishable mechanisms: (A) the contents of the storage granules are rapidly extruded, secretion, (B) inhibition of the granule membrane transport system causes slow liberation, (C) serotonin can be displaced from its storage sites by other amines, and (D) specific aminophores can transport serotonin through the granule and plasma membrane, apparently independent of the different transport systems. When serotonin is liberated slowly, a considerable part is oxidized by monoamine oxidase, and the products accumulate in the medium.

It appears as if the storage mechanism makes the uptake of serotonin by intact cells an irreversible process. In platelets from patients with storage pool deficiency, or thrombin-treated platelets, the storage mechanism is destroyed. Such platelets take up

Table 4C
SECRETED PROTEINS

Category	Localization	Comments
1. Similar to plasma		
Fibrinogen	α-Granules;[149] secreted by thrombin[150,151] or collagen[149]	Approximately 9% of total platelet protein;[149] resembles plasma fibrinogen in immunological properties, electrophoretic behavior, sedimentation coefficient, light absorption spectra, total amino acid composition, and N-terminal amino acids;[153,154] differs in intrinsic velocity, increased amount of sialic acid, hexose and hexosamine, behavior on agar gel immunoelectrophoresis, plasmin degradation, and degradation products[153,155,156]
2. Cationic		
Vascular permeability factor	α-Granules; serum, prepared from PRP 2+	Heat stable, molecular weight 30,000; causes increased vascular permeability (Evans Blue) in mouse and rabbit skin[157]
Growth factor	Released by various aggregating agents from granules[157a,158]	Approximately 50 ng/mℓ PRP of purified growth factor, PGF; molecular weight 13,700, isoelectric point at pH 9.7;[161-163] indication of immunological identity of PGF with pituitary growth factor[160]
3. Platelet specific		
Platelet factor 4, (high affinity-PE_4)	Released by various aggregating agents from α-granules[164-166] different from acid hydrolases;[152] liberated during storage[167]	Composed of a single protein chain containing 70 amino acids; molecular weight 7,800;[168] antiheparin activity;[165] may be liberated from platelets by mechanism other than platelet release with thrombin and collagen[167]
β-thromboglobulin	Released by thrombin;[169] liberated during storage and centrifugation[170]	Molecular weight 36,000; 6 subunits; migration as α-globulin;[171] increased level in PFP from patients with thromboembolism and deep venous thrombosis[172]

Table 5
INTERACTION BETWEEN PLATELETS AND SEROTONIN

(AGGREGATION, UPTAKE, STORAGE, LIBERATION)

No.	Process	Inhibitors	Cofactors	Comments	Ref.
1	Induction of shape change and aggregation	Methysergide, bromo-LSD, chlorpromazine, cinanserin (rat), flupenthixol, chlorprothixene	Ca^{2+}, fibrinogen stirring (aggregation)	$K_a = 2.3 \times 10^{-8}$ M (rat) chlorpromazine different in vivo and in vitro; 5, 6-dihydroxytryptamine similar to serotonin; inhibitors little effect on uptake	173-181
2	Uptake by intact cells	Imipramine, amitriptyline, choline cardic glycosides, Lilly -110140, reserpine	Na^+, Cl^-, Li^+ (enchances), membrane sialic acid, metabolizing cells, active Na^+ - K^+ pump; intact storage mechanism	Normal level; 0.3 μmole/10^{11} cells; capacity; 1.6 μmole/10^{11} cells; rate: 0.4 μmole/min/10^{11} cells; $K = 2.3 \times 10^{-7}$ M; uptake dependent on downhill Na^+ gradient from outside to inside; inhibitors little effect on aggregation; Cl^- cotransport I and II; extracellular and intracellular serotonin exchangeable where storage capacity exceeded	182-195
3	Transport across plasma membrane (I)	Imipramine, amitryptaline gramicidin, nigericin; not inhibited by reserpine, cinanserin	Na^+, Cl^-	$K_a = 5 \times 10^{-7}$ M; transport along downhill Na^+ gradient	196
4	Intracellular, extragranular metabolism	Aerobiosis, N_2, monoamines, monoamine oxidase inhibitors	O_2, Monoamine oxidase in mitochondria, aldehyde dehydrogenase	Serotonin oxidized to 5-hydroxytryptophol, 5-0H indole acetaldehyde, 5-0H indole acetic acid	197-201
5	Transport across dense granule membrane (II)	Reserpine, prenylamine, cardiac glycosides, metabolic inhibitors have no effect	—	Reserpine binds to dense granule; imipramine was little effect	202-206
6	Storage in dense granules	Other amines; impaired in platelets from patients with Storage Pool Deficiency	ATP, divalent cation? Glycoprotein?	Serotonin bound to ATP-Me^{2+} micelles? Serotonin bound to glycoprotein? After emptying (by reserpine) osmiophility lost, sp. gravity unchanged (rabbit)	207-212

Table 5 (continued)
INTERACTION BETWEEN PLATELETS AND SEROTONIN

(AGGREGATION, UPTAKE, STORAGE, LIBERATION)

No.	Liberation	Inducer	Comments	Ref.
7	Secretion	See Table 6	Rapid extrusion of serotonin together with other dense granule constituents (ATP, ADP, Ca, PPi); inhibited by elevated [cAMP],cyclo-oxygenase inhibitors, metabolic inhibitors; no oxidation of serotonin	See Tables 7 and 8
	Inhibition of transport I		Liberation by imipramine, amitryptaline, cardiac glycosides not reported	182-195
	Inhibition of transport II	Reserpine	Slow process; serotonin oxidized	220
	Exchange	Tyramine, DL-amphetamine, quinidine, methylene blue?	Relatively rapid; little serotonin oxidation; inducer stored in granule	220-223
	Aminophore	X - 537 A	—	224, 225

serotonin for a short while (initial rates are the same as in normal platelets), then the uptake levels off, and serotonin oxidation products begin to appear.

The Stimulated Platelet

A great number of agents stimulate platelets to change shape from a disc form to a spheric one,[226] to aggregate,[227] to produce prostaglandins and thromboxanes,[228] and to secrete the constituents from the various storage granules.[229] Typical inducers of these platelet responses that may be operative in vivo are low molecular substances such as ADP, epinephrine, prostaglandins G_2 and H_2, and vasopressin; proteolytic enzymes such as thrombin and trypsin; and fibrous proteins such as collagen. These inducers require metabolically intact platelets for adequate responses. During this sequence of responses, substances are made available by the platelets themselves that are potent inducers of platelet responses, and a positive feedback of the overall reaction is created.[230] Some agents cause platelet clumping, which is independent of cellular metabolism and is referred to as agglutination. Nonphysiological agglutinating agents that are used for diagnostic purposes are bovine factor VIII-related protein[231] and the antibiotic ristocetin.[232] Physiologically important agents such as antiplatelet antibodies and platelet-unrelated antigen-antibody complexes may cause platelet clumping by the agglutination pathway, but the secretion often observed[233,234] may be by the metabolism-dependent pathway, as caused by close platelet contact.[235,236]

Energy and Adenine Nucleotide Metabolism (H. Holmsen)

The sequence of the response shape change, aggregation, prostaglandin-thromboxane formation, and secretion is dependent on a continuous supply of ATP,[237,238] and a number of metabolic changes are known to occur concomitantly with the response sequence. However, many of the metabolic changes last long after the functional responses have been terminated. This makes it difficult to discern the cause-effect relationship between metabolic and functional responses, i.e., whether the metabolic change is involved in reactions necessary for the functional response to occur, or whether the metabolic response is a result of alterations caused by the functional response.

The metabolic changes that are known to be initiated during the sequence of functional responses are illustrated in Figure 3 and described in more detail in Table 6. No attempts have been made to give priority to the metabolic changes according to their possible relative importance as integrated parts of the mechanism(s) underlying the functional responses. Figure 3 and Table 6 also describe briefly the functional responses of platelets.

Arachidonate Oxygenation (J. B. Smith)

It is assumed that the liberation of arachidonic acid from phospholipids by phospholipase A_2 is the rate limiting step for its oxygenation. However, it is possible that inhibition of the acylation of lysophospholipid would increase the oxygenation of arachidonic acid.

The fact that prostaglandin cyclooxygenase is inhibited by aspirin has been useful in elucidating the role of prostaglandins in platelet response. Aspirin abolishes shape change, aggregation, and secretion induced by arachidonic acid, showing that the effects of arachidonic acid depend entirely on the formation of prostaglandin endoperoxides. In contrast, aspirin has little or no effect on shape change, aggregation, and secretion induced by thrombin, indicating that its effects are largely independent of prostaglandin formation. Partial inhibition of aggregation and secretion has been noted with collagen, indicating a partial dependence on prostaglandin formation.

Steps 1 through 5 in Figure 4 occur in stimulated platelets, whereas steps 6 and 7

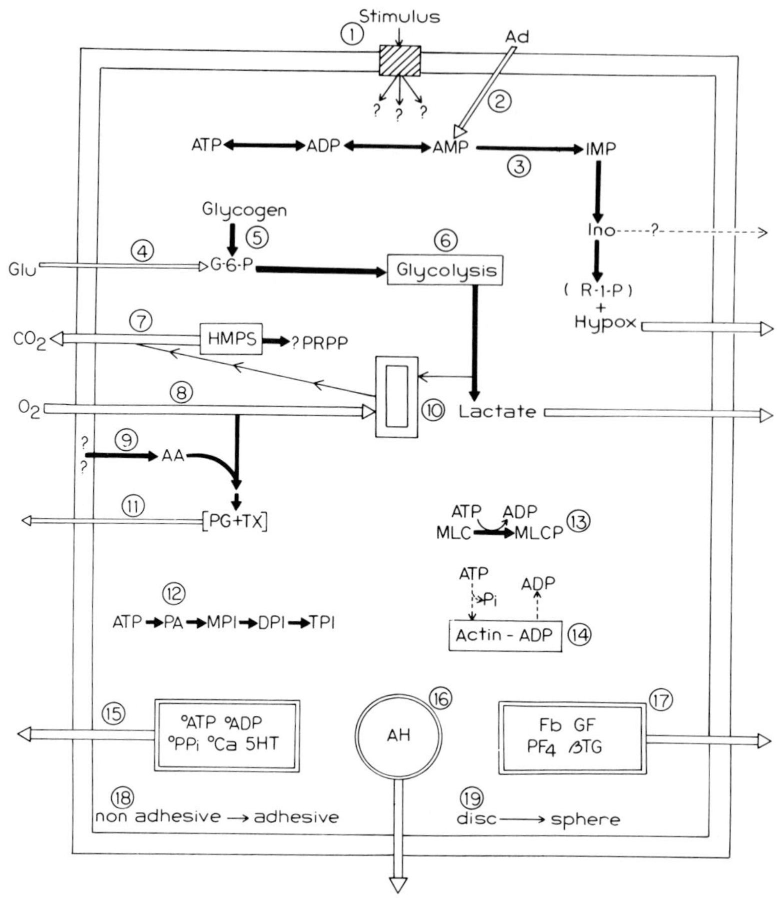

FIGURE 3. Energy and adenine nucleotide metabolism in a stimulated platelet. Description of various responses. The processes marked with encircled numbers are described in Table 6. The wide - lined arrows indicate that rate of process is increased relative to rate in resting platelet. The open - lined arrows indicate transfer across membrane. Broken-lined arrows indicate slower rate than in resting platelet.

occur in other tissues. These steps are described in detail in Table 7. Many of the products formed from arachidonic acid have potent biological activities (Table 8). A major consideration is that prostaglandin endoperoxides are converted by platelets into thromboxane A_2, a potent vasoconstrictor that induces aggregation. They are converted by blood vessel walls into prostacyclin, a vasodilator that is a potent inhibitor of platelet aggregation.

Contractile and Microtubule Proteins (J. L. Daniel)

The exact role of these proteins in platelet function is not yet defined. However, many investigators have assumed a role for platelet actomyosin in either shape change, aggregation, secretion, or clot retraction. White,[331] using morphological data, has suggested that platelet stimulation initiates a "contractile wave" mediated by actomyosin and resulting in the disassembly and reassembly of platelet microtubules. Other morphological evidence shows the appearance of microfilaments[332] in pseudopods during shape change. Microfilaments have been identified as actin filaments using heavy meromyosin labeling.[333] Actin filaments in pseudopods are oriented as if the membrane were functioning as a skeletal muscle Z-line.[348] Pseudopod formation can be reversed and platelets can resume discoid shape.[331] Involvement of actomyosin in clot retraction

Table 6
ENERGY AND ADENINE NUCLEOTIDE METABOLISM IN STIMULATED PLATELETS

DESCRIPTION OF VARIOUS RESPONSES

Index key	Process	Typical inducers	Description	Comments	Ref.
1	Stimulation or induction	ADP, epinephrine, thrombin, collagen, serotonin, vasopressin	Interaction between inducer and membrane receptor	Specific receptor for each inducer; inducer does not penetrate membrane; a "second messenger" is liberated to cytoplasm and activates cellular responses	239-245
2	Adenine uptake	ADP, thrombin	Uptake increased after stimulation; V_{max} and K_m increase	Uptake maximally increased by shape change (# 19), may reflect increased [PRPP]	235, 246
3	Decrease in metabolic adenylate pool	ADP, epinephrine, thrombin, collagen, bovine factor VIII	Balanced by accumulation of extracellular hypoxanthine	Occurs only during secretion; maximally 40% decrease; irreversible, may reflect noncompensated usage	247-251
	Decrease in adenylate energy charge	ADP, serotonin	Decrease from 0.93 to 0.91 in less than 3 sec	Occurs during shape change; may reflect sudden noncompensated usage of ATP	238, 252, 253
4	Glucose uptake	ADP, collagen	Up to eightfold increase	Transient	254-256
5	Glycogenolysis	Thrombin	Activation of phosphorylase by Ca^{2+}; liberation (?) of amylo - 1, 6 - glucosidase (pig)	First metabolic response in rat platelets; lasts after function	257-259
6	Glycolysis	Thrombin, collagen, ADP, epinephrine	Threefold increase in lactate production; regulation at phosphofructokinase step (by AEC?)	Unclear whether increase results from changes caused by function or function requires increased ATP production; increase transient	256, 257, 260-266
7	CO_2 production	Thrombin, collagen	Increase in HMPS and mitochondrial oxidation	Mitochondrial (glucose) oxidation starts after function is terminated	255, 256, 267
8	O_2 uptake	Thrombin, collagen, arachidonic acid, ADP, epinephrine, A 23187	Rapid O_2 consumption by arachidonate oxidation (see Figure 4, Table 8) and by mitochondria	The greater part inhibited by ETYA,[a] but not CN^- or antimycin; this "burst in O_2 uptake" short lasting	268-271

Table 6 (continued)
ENERGY AND ADENINE NUCLEOTIDE METABOLISM IN STIMULATED PLATELETS

DESCRIPTION OF VARIOUS RESPONSES

Index key	Process	Typical inducers	Description	Comments	Ref.
9	Arachidonate liberation	ADP, epinephrine, thrombin, collagen	From platelet phospholipids; see Figure 4, Table 8	Mechanism unclear, phospholipase A_2 suggested	
10	Mitochondrial processes	Thrombin, ADP, latex particles, epinephrine	See # 7 and 8	Increase in fatty acid oxidation and citric acid cycle	254, 256, 271-273
11	Prostaglandin-thromboxane formation	See # 9	See Figure 4, Table 8	—	
12	Phosphoinositide synthesis	ADP, thrombin, collagen	Increased ^{32}P incorporation into phosphatidic acid, mono-, di-, and triphosphoinositide	Major changes during shape change	274-276
13	Myosin light chain phosphorylation	Thrombin, collagen	See Table 3	See section on "Intracellular Regulation"	
14	Turnover of ADP in actin-ADP	Thrombin + Ca	Decrease in ADP turnover in ethanol insoluble protein fraction	Demonstrable when filaments (F-actin) are clearly seen	277
15	Dense granule secretion	Thrombin, collagen, ADP, epinephrine, arachidonic acid	Discharge of dense granule contents (See Table 1) to extracellular medium	Secretion rapid (< 20 sec with thrombin)	251, 278-281
16	Acid hydrolase secretion	Thrombin, collagen, A 23187	Discharge of acid hydrolase containing granules (lysosomes)	Slower than dense granule secretion, not induced by ADP, epinephrine, arachidonate; secreted hydrolases: β-N-acetyglucosaminidase, β-galactosidase, β-glucosaminidase, elastinase, collagenase; not secreted: acid p-nitrophenylphosphate	251, 282-285
17	α-Granule secretion	See # 15	Discharge of contents in α-granules: platelet factor 4, β-thromboglobulin, growth factor	See Table 4B	

18	Aggregation	All inducers	Membrane transformed from nonadhesive to adhesive and platelets aggregate when brought in close contact	Requires extracellular fibrinogen, Ca^{2+}, may be other plasma-proteins; biochemical difference nonadhesive/adhesive membrane not known; glycoprotein II (Table 4A) appears necessary	288-291
19	Shape change	All inducers, not epinephrine	Shape changes from disc to sphere with pseudopods	Very fast (< 3 sec); independent of extracellular Ca^{2+}; precedes aggregation and secretion; function unknown	292-294

[a] Eicosa 5, 8, 11, 14 tetraynoic acid.

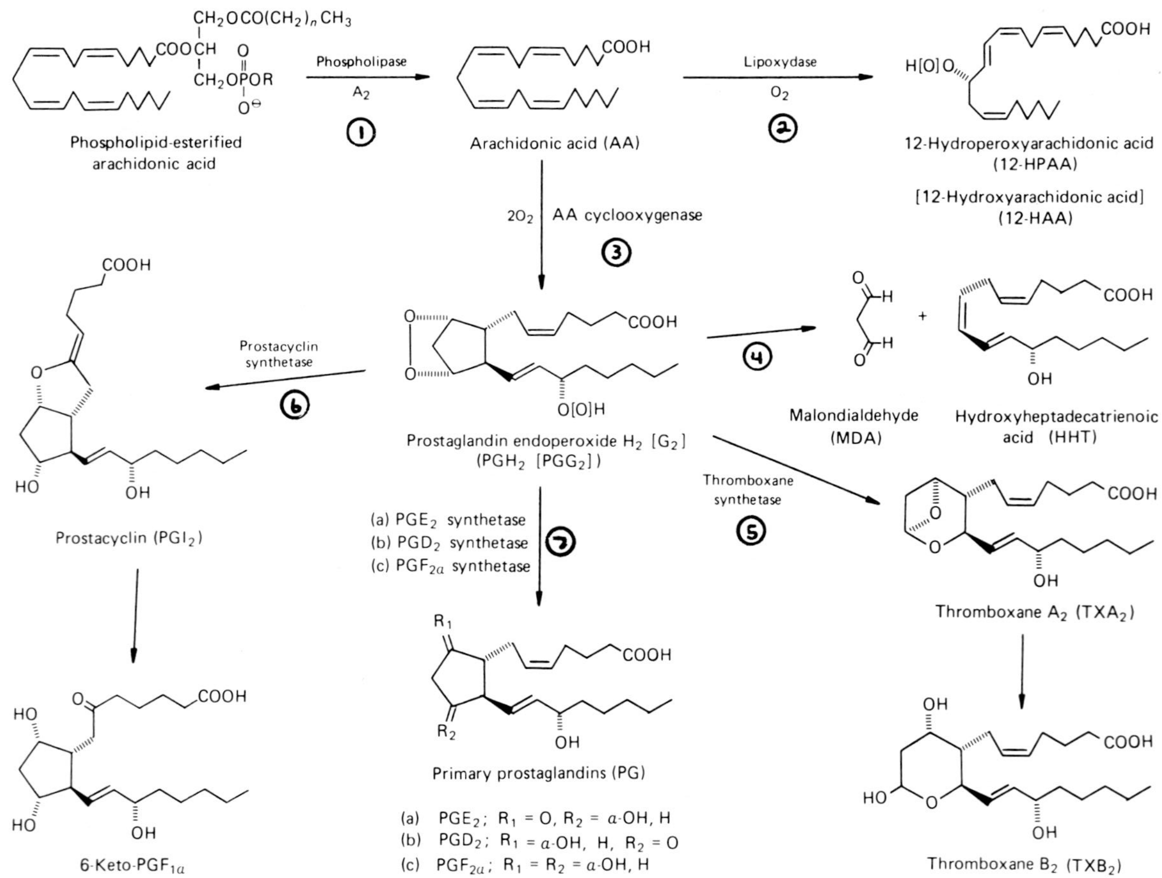

FIGURE 4. Pathways of arachidonate oxygenation. The processes as marked by numbers are described in Table 7. (The figure was kindly provided by Dr. K. C. Nicelaou, University of Pennsylvania, Philadelphia.)

Table 7
PATHWAYS OF ARACHIDONATE OXYGENATION

Key to diagram	Name of activity	Occurrence	Properties	Ref.
1	Phospholipase A_2	Platelets-subcellular distribution not known	Attacks 2-position of phosphatidylcholine and phosphatidylinositol; activated when platelets are incubated with thrombin, collagen, or calcium ionophore (A23187)	295-298
2	Arachidonate lipoxygenase (lipoxydase)	Platelets-soluble and membrane bound	Introduces molecular O_2 at C-12 (ω 9) of arachidonic acid; differs from plant lipoxygenase (ω 6) specificity; inhibited by ETYA (5, 8, 11, 14-eicosatetraynoic acid) but not aspirin or indomethacin	299-302
3	Cyclooxygenase	Platelet microsomes; also sheep seminal vesicle microsomes (SSVM)	Introduces two molecules of O_2 in a concerted cyclisation of arachidonic acid; most studied in SSVM; purified enzyme requires haemin for activity; reductive breakdown of PGG_2 deactivates cyclooxygenase; enzyme inhibited by ETYA and indomethacin; is acetylated by aspirin with associated inhibition	299, 303-311
3a	Peroxidase	Not studied in platelets; occurs in SSVM	Reduces 15-hydroperoxy group of PGG_2; requires suitable reducing substance as proton donor (hydroquinone, tryptophan, serotonin, phenol); pure prostaglandin synthetase of SSVM contains both cyclooxygenase and peroxidase; peroxidase protects cyclooxygenase from inactivation by PGG_2 and is not inhibited by aspirin or indomethacin	304, 305
4	Spontaneous	Aqueous medium	Formation of HHT and MDA is promoted at acid pH	304
5	Thromboxane synthetase	Platelet microsomes	Catalyzes rearrangement of PGG_2 or PGH_2 into TxA_2; the enzyme is not inhibited by aspirin or indomethacin; TxA_2 is unstable ($t\frac{1}{2}$ at 37° = 32 sec) and incorporates one molecule of water to form the stable TxB_2	299, 308, 314, 315
6	Prostacyclin synthetase	Blood vessel walls-microsomal fraction	Catalyzes rearrangement of PGG_2 or PGH_2 into PGI_2; the enzyme is not inhibited by aspirin or indomethacin; PGI_2 is unstable at neutral pH ($t\frac{1}{2}$ = 300 sec) and incorporates one molecule of water to form stable 6-keto-$PGF_{1}\alpha$	316-317
7	Prostaglandin isomerases and reductases	SSVM	Probably of minor importance in platelet function; prostaglandin endoperoxides are unstable ($t\frac{1}{2}$ = 300 sec) and rearrange into PGE_2 and PGD_2 (ratio 3:1). Formation of PGD_2 is promoted by serum albumins of certain species	303, 304, 312, 313

Table 8
PROSTAGLANDINS AND THROMBOXANES THAT INFLUENCE PLATELET AGGREGATION AND, WITH THE EXCEPTION OF PGE_1, ARE PRODUCED FROM ARACHIDONIC ACID

Prostaglandin	Effect on platelets	Comments	Ref.
PGD_2	Inhibits aggregation	Causes good inhibition in human platelet-rich plasma (PRP) at 20 nM; less effective on animal platelets; increases platelet cyclic AMP	318-320
PGE_1	Inhibits aggregation	Causes good inhibition in PRP from most species at 20 nM; increases platelet cyclic AMP; formed from 8, 11, 14-eicosatrienoic acid	321-324
PGG_2	Induces aggregation	Causes aggregation in human PRP at 1 μM	303, 325
PGH_2	Induces aggregation	Causes aggregation in human PRP at 3 μM	303, 325
PGI_2	Inhibits aggregation	Causes good inhibition in PRP from most species at 1 nM; potent vasodilator; increases platelet cyclic AMP	317, 327-329
TxA_2	Induces aggregation	Not yet isolated; appears to be more active than PGG_2 as an aggregating agent; potent vasoconstrictor	314, 330

was assumed since antibodies against partially purified actomyosin inhibited clot retraction; however, recent studies using more specific antibodies have failed to confirm this observation.[334-336] Clot retraction does, however, show many features similar to muscle contraction.[337] Cytochalasin B has been used to study the role of platelet contractile proteins, but these studies are ambiguous due to lack of precise knowledge about the mode of action of this drug.[338-340] Studies of phosphorylation of platelet proteins have provided useful information about the functional role of contractile proteins. Adelstein and co-workers[341,342] have shown that purified platelet myosin is phosphorylated by a kinase in vitro and that this phosphorylation enhances actomyosin ATPase activity.[343] Phosphorylation of platelet myosin has been shown in intact platelets in response to stimuli.[344,345] The time course of phosphorylation of myosin is similar to that of platelet secretion. Other studies indicate that this phosphorylation is linked to the secretory process and not aggregation.[346] Colchicine appears to bind specifically to tubulin and to prevent microtubule assembly. Studies with this drug show it does not block aggregation or clot retraction.[338,347] However, microtubules appear necessary for maintenance of normal discoid shape.

Intracellular Regulation of Platelet Responses: Proposed Ca^{2+} Translocations and the Cyclic AMP/Cyclic GMP Systems (H. Holmsen)

Human platelets contain 20 to 28 μ moles Ca/10^{11} platelets or 90 to 140 n-moles/mg protein.[349-351] More than 65% of platelet Ca is secretable,[352-354] and the Ca content in platelets from patients with Storage Pool Deficiency[355] and Chediak Higashi's Syndrome[356] is less than 35% of that in normal platelets. Microprobe analysis[357] and subcellular fractionation[358] have shown that the dense granules are rich in Ca. These facts show that the majority of platelet Ca is located in the dense granules and is thereby inaccessible for intracellular processes.

There is no evidence as to where the remaining platelet Ca is localized. If the remaining Ca^{2+} was present solely in cytoplasm, its concentration would be in the range of 8 to 10 mM, which is inconceivable for many obvious reasons. It has been demonstrated that platelet microsomes can accumulate Ca in a process that requires ATP and Mg^{2+} [359-361] and that the accumulation is promoted by cAMP.[362] This suggests that Ca is

Table 9
INTRACELLULAR REGULATION OF PLATELET RESPONSES

PROPOSED Ca^{2+} TRANSLOCATIONS AND THE CYCLIC AMP/CYCLIC GMP SYSTEMS

Index key #	Name of process or compartment	Description	Comments	Ref.
1	Induction	Agonist-receptor interaction; Ca^{2+} liberated from plasma membrane pool?	See Table 6, Index key # 1	380
2	Plasma membrane Ca pool	—	Plasma membrane not separated from intracellular membranes with current fraction techniques	359-362
3	Cytoplasmic Ca pool	—	Should not exceed 10^{-7} M in resting cells (analogy with skeletal muscle)	381
4	Ca reservoir	In intracellular membrane structures	Dense tubular system suggested; morphologically similar to sarcoplasmic reticulum	382
5	Adenyl cyclase	ATP → cAMP + PPi[a] increase in [cAMP] powerfully inhibits platelet responses	Membrane enzyme with catalytic site on inside, regulatory site on outside	383-392
6	Cyclic nucleotide phosphodiesterase	cAMP → AMP + Pi[b] cGMP → GMP + Pi[c]	Both soluble and particulate forms	389, 393-397
7	Activation of Ca pump	cAMP activates ATP-dependent Ca accumulation in vesicles	Removal of cytoplasmic Ca^{2+} may be cause of inhibition of response	362
8	Ca^{2+} enhanced Ca^{2+} liberation from intracellular Ca-reservoir	—	—	
9	TXA_2-enhanced Ca^{2+} liberation from intracellular Ca-reservoir	Ionophoric action of TXA_2	If correct, TXA_2 does not require membrane receptor	398
10	Shape change	Increase in [Ca_{cyt}] induces process	Chlortetracycline inhibits; ADP inducer	399, 400
11	Aggregation	Increase in [Ca_{cyt}] induces process	Chlortetracycline as probe, ADP and epinephrine as inducers	399

Table 9 (continued)
INTRACELLULAR REGULATION OF PLATELET RESPONSES

PROPOSED Ca^{2+} TRANSLOCATIONS AND THE CYCLIC AMP/CYCLIC GMP SYSTEMS

Index key #	Name of process or compartment	Description	Comments	Ref.
12	Secretion	Increase in $[Ca_{cyt}]$ induces process	TMB-8 (Ca antagonist) inhibits secretion	370
13	Phospholipase A_2 activation	Increase in $[Ca_{cyt}]$ induces process	cAMP inhibits (calf platelets) - indirect evidence	401
14	Activation of contractile processes	Increase in $[Ca_{cyt}]$ induces process	Platelet actomyosin ATPase regulated Ca^{2+}? Regulation of myosin light chain kinase by Ca^{2+} not shown	402-404
15	Breakdown of microtubules	Increase in $[Ca_{cyt}]$ induces process	Microtubule depolymerizes with Ca^{2+}	405
16	c-GMP system	cGMP synthesized from GTP by guamyl cyclase, and hydrolyzed by cyclic phosphodiesterase	Cyclase soluble; stimulated by fatty acids and serotonin; cGMP level increased during aggregation; not if platelets are stimulated but not aggregated; role of cGMP obscure	406-411

[a] Activators: Prostaglandins D_2, E_1, and I_2 (see Table 8). Inhibitor: 3′, 5′-deoxyadenosine.

[b] Inhibitors: Papaverine, dipyridamole, methylxanthines.

[c] Three kinetically different PDE_1 with different K_m for cAMP and cGMP. Inhibitors equally effective for both substrates.

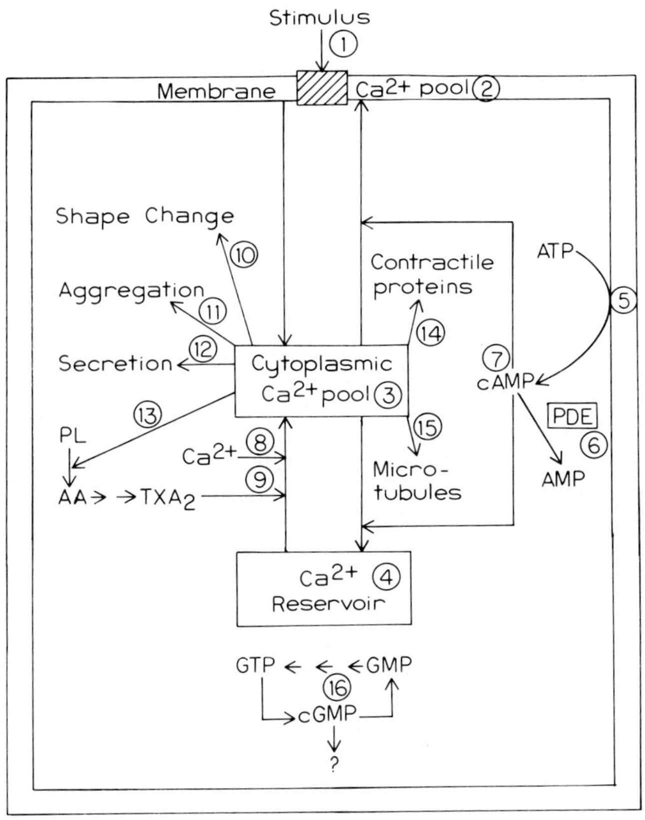

FIGURE 5. Intracellular regulation of platelet responses: proposed Ca^{2+} translocations and the cyclic AMP/cyclic GMP systems. The processes marked with encircled numbers are described in Table 7.

present in membranous structures in platelets (analogous to sarcoplasmic reticulum in skeletal muscle) and that cAMP may act to stimulate transfer of Ca from cytoplasm to the membrane stores.

No changes in the distribution of Ca between cytoplasm and membrane after stimulation have been reported. However, the divalent ionophore A 23187 induces the entire shape change-aggregation-secretion sequence without uptake of Ca from the medium,[363-369] and the calcium antagonist TMA-8 inhibits secretion.[370] This is to date the only obtainable evidence that Ca may be a "second messenger" in the mechanisms underlying platelet responses. A rapid influx of exogenous Ca takes place after the platelet responses are manifested,[352,364,371,372] but is unrelated to the actual mechanisms underlying the various responses.

It follows from the above that we know nothing about the extragranular, nonsecretable fraction of platelet Ca. Despite this, Ca^{2+} has been implied by numerous workers as the "second messenger", the link between the agonist-receptor interaction and those reactions directly connected with the execution of the functional responses. The proposed mechanisms for Ca-involvement are schematically illustrated in Figure 5 and described in Table 9.

Aspects of regulation of platelet responsiveness through the cyclic AMP and GMP systems are also reviewed in Figure 5 and Table 9. Protein kinases that are activated by cAMP have been demonstrated,[373-377] but their function is not known. Some distinct protein fractions are phosphorylated in intact platelets during stimulation.[378,379]

REFERENCES

1. **Holmsen, H. and Rozenberg, M. C.**, Adenine nucleotide metabolism of blood platelets. III. Adenine phosphoribosyl transferase and nucleotide formation from exogenous adenine, *Biochim. Biophys. Acta,* 157, 266, 1968.
2. **Sixma, J. J., Trieshnigg, A. M., and Holmsen, H.**, Adenine nucleotide metabolism of blood platelets. VIII. Mechanism of adenine uptake by intact cells, *Biochim. Biophys. Acta,* 298, 3, 1973.
3. **Jershushalmy, Z., Sperling, O., Pinkhas, J., Krynska, M., and DeVries, A.**, Phosphoribosylpyrophosphate synthetase and purine phosphoribosyltransferases in human and rabbit blood platelets, *Haemostasis,* 1, 279, 1972/73.
4. **Rivard, G. E., McLaren, J. D., and Brunst, R. F.**, Incorporation of hypoxanthine into adenine and guanine nucleotides by human platelets, *Biochim. Biophys. Acta,* 381, 144, 1975.
5. **Boer, P., Lipstein, B., DeVries, A., and Sperling, O.**, The effect of ribose 5-phosphoribosyl-1-pyrophosphate availability on de novo synthesis of purine nucleotides in rat liver slices, *Biochim. Biophys. Acta,* 432, 10, 1976.
6. **Sixma, J. J., Lips, J. P. M., Trieschnigg, A. M. C., and Holmsen, H.**, Transport and metabolism of adenosine in human blood platelets, *Biochim. Biophys. Acta,* 443, 33, 1976.
7. **Holmsen, H., Day, H. J., and Storm, E.**, Adenine nucleotide metabolism of blood platelets. VI. Subcellular localization of nucleotide pools with different functions in the platelet release reaction, *Biochim. Biophys. Acta,* 186, 254, 1969.
8. **Holmsen, H. and Rozenberg, M. C.**, Adenine nucleotide metabolism of blood platelets. I. Adenosine kinase and nucleotide formation from exogenous adenosine and AMP, *Biochim. Biophys. Acta,* 155, 326, 1968.
9. **Haslam, R. J.**, Interactions of the pharmacological receptors of blood platelets with adenylate cyclase, *Ser. Haematol.,* 6, 333, 1976.
10. **Born, G. V. R. and Mills, D. C. B.**, Potentiation of the inhibitory effect of adenosine on platelet aggregation by drugs that prevent its uptake, *J. Physiol.,* 202, 41, 1969.
11. **Markwardt, F. and Hoffman, A.**, Effects of papaverine on cyclic AMP phosphodiesterase of human platelets, *Biochem. Pharmacol.,* 19, 2519, 1970.
12. **Rozenberg, M. C., Ledwidge, C. M., Wilcken, D. E. L., and McKeon, M.**, The inhibition of adenosine phosphorylation in platelets by dipyridamole, *J. Lab. Clin. Med.,* 77, 88, 1971.
13. **Karpatkin, S. and Weiss, H. J.**, Deficiency of gluthathione peroxidase associated with high levels of reduced gluthione in Glanzmann's thrombasthenia, *N. Engl. J. Med.,* 287, 1062, 1972.
14. **Fantl, P.**, Thiol groups of blood platelets in relation to clot retraction, *Nature (London),* 198, 95, 1963.
15. **Chaudry, A. A., Sagone, A. L., Jr., Metz, E. N., and Balcerzak, S. P.**, Relationship of glucose oxidation to aggregation of human platelets, *Blood,* 41, 249, 1973.
16. **Cowan, D.**, Platelet metabolism in acute leukemia, *J. Lab. Clin. Med.,* 82, 54, 1973.
17. **Deykin, D. and Desser, R. K.**, The incorporation of acetate and palmitate into lipids by human platelets, *J. Clin. Invest.,* 47, 1590, 1968.
18. **Majerus, P. W., Smith, M. B., and Clamon, G. H.**, Lipid metabolism of human platelets. I. Evidence for a complete fatty acid synthesizing system, *J. Clin. Invest.,* 48, 156, 1969.
19. **Holmsen, H. and Robkin, L.**, Hydroperoxides stimulate HMPS, unpublished observations.
20. **Kosow, D. P.**, Glucose 6-phosphate dehydrogenase of human platelets. Kinetics and regulatory properties, *Arch. Biochem. Biophys.,* 162, 186, 1974.
21. **Doery, J. C. G., Hirsh, J., and Cooper, J.**, Energy metabolism in human platelets: interrelationships between glycolysis and oxidative metabolism, *Blood,* 36, 159, 1970.
22. **Waller, H. D., Lohr, G. W., Grignani, F., and Gross, R., Uber den Energiestoffwechsel normaler menschlicher thrombozyten,** *Thromb. Diath. Haemorrh.,* 3, 520, 1959.
23. **Chaiken, R., Pagano, D., and Detwiler, T. C.**, Regulation of platelet phosphorylase, *Biochim. Biophys. Acta,* 403, 315, 1975.
24. **Karpatkin, S., Braun, J., and Charmatz, A.**, Requirement of divalent cation for human platelet phosphorylase activity, *Biochim. Biophys. Acta,* 220, 22, 1970.
25. **Aguilar, J. and Rosell-Perez, M.**, Studies on glycogen metabolism in human platelets. II. Metabolite levels and enzymes of the glycogen cycle, *Rev. Esp. Fisiol.,* 31, 163, 1975.
26. **Gear, A. R. L. and Schneider, W.**, Control of platelet glycogenolysis activation of phosphorylase by calcium, *Biochim. Biophys. Acta,* 392, 111, 1975.
27. **Sixma, J. J., Akkerman, J. W. N., Lips, J., and Holmsen, H.**, Excerpta Medica, Amsterdam, 522, 1978.
28. **Scott, R. B. and Still, W. J. S.**, Glycogen in human blood platelets. Isolation by ultracentrifugation and characteristics of the isolated particles, *Blood,* 35, 517, 1970.
29. **Aguilar, J. and Rosell-Perez, M.**, Studies on glycogen metabolism in the human platelet. I. Characteristics and regulation of the glycogen synthetase, *Rev. Esp. Fisiol.,* 31, 151, 1975.

30. **Karpatkin, S. and Charmatz, A.**, Heterogeneity of human platelets. III. Glycogen metabolism in platelets of different sizes, *Br. J. Haematol.*, 19, 135, 1970.
31. **Vainer, H., Besson, P., Jeanneau, C., and Caen, J.**, La glycogene-synthetase dans les plaquettes et les populations plaquettaires anormales de syndrome myeloproliferatifs, *Nouv. Rev. Fr. Hematol.*, 9, 514, 1969.
32. **Scott, R. B.**, Activation of glycogen phosphorylase in blood platelets, *Blood*, 30, 321, 1967.
33. **Steiner, M. and Kuramoto, A.**, Energy metabolism of aggregating platelets, *Ser. Haematol.*, 4, 98, 1971.
34. **Doery, J. C. G., Hirsh, J., and de Gruchy, G. C.**, Platelet metabolism and function, *Haematologia*, 4, 405, 1970.
35. **Solomon, H. M. and Gaut, Z. N.**, Accumulation and metabolism of 2-deoxy-D-glucose-1-^{14}C in the human platelet, *Biochem. Pharmacol.*, 19, 2631, 1970.
36. **Kerby, G. P. and Taylor, S. M.**, The influence of buffers on human platelet aggregation and energy metabolism, *Proc. Soc. Exp. Biol. Med.*, 136, 452, 1971.
37. **Doery, J. C. G., Hirsh, J., and Mustard, J. F.**, Energy metabolism in washed human platelets responsive to ADP: comparison with platelets in plasma, *Br. J. Haematol.*, 25, 657, 1973.
38. **Akkerman, J. W. N., Gorter, G., Wester, J., and Sixma, J. J.**, Preparation of concentrated platelet suspensions by dehydration against polyethyleneglycol 20,000, *Scand. J. Haematol.*, 17, 71, 1976.
39. **Doery, J. C. G., Hirsh, J., and de Gruchy, G. C.**, Platelet glycolytic enzymes: effect of cellular disruption procedures on activity, *Br. J. Haematol.*, 19, 145, 1970.
40. **Detwiler, T. C.**, Levels of intermediates and cofactors of the glycolytic pathway and the citric acid cycle in rat platelets, *Biochim. Biophys. Acta*, 177, 161, 1969.
41. **Akkerman, J. W. N., Gorter, G., Sixma, J. J., and Staal, G. E. J.**, Variations in levels of gycolytic intermediates in human platelets during platelet-collagen interaction, *Biochim. Biophys. Acta*, 421, 296, 1976.
42. **Akkerman, J. W. N., Gorter, G., Sixma, J. J., and Staal, G. E. J.**, Human platelet 6-phosphofructokinase. Purification, kinetic parameters and the influence of sulphate ions on enzyme activity, *Biochim. Biophys. Acta*, 370, 102, 1974.
43. **Akkerman, J. W. N., Gorter, G., Sixma, J. J., and Staal, G. E. J.**, Influence of Mg^{2+}, ITP^{4-} on human platelet phosphofructokinase, *Biochim. Biophys. Acta*, 370, 113, 1974.
44. **Akkerman, J. W. N., Gorter, G., Sixma, J. J., and Staal, G. E. J.**, Influence of sulphate on effects on ADP, 3′,5′-cyclic AMP and citrate on human platelet phosphofructokinase activity, *Int. J. Biochem.*, 5, 853, 1974.
45. **Akkerman, J. W. N., Gorter, G., Over, J., Sixma, J. J., and Staal, G. E. J.**, Human platelet 6-phosphofructokinase. Relation between inhibition by Mg ATP^{2-} and cooperativity towards fructose 6-phosphate and investigations on the formation of a ternary complex, *Biochim. Biophys. Acta*, 397, 395, 1975.
46. **Nishimura, J. and Minakami, S.**, Effect of hydrogen ion concentration on energy metabolism in pig platelets, *Biochim. Biophys. Acta*, 396, 1, 1975.
47. **Czapek, E. E., Deykin, D., and Salzman, E. W.**, Platelet dysfunction in glycogen storage disease type 1, *Blood*, 41, 235, 1973.
48. **Soyama, K., Shimada, N., Kusunoki, T., and Nakamura, T.**, The diagnostic value of thrombocytic glucose 6-phosphatease in patients with von Gierke's disease and its heterozygotes, *Clin. Chim. Acta*, 44, 327, 1973.
49. **Schrijver, J., Koster, J. F., and Hulsmann, W. C.**, Insignificance of gluconeogensis in human blood platelets, *Eur. J. Clin. Invest.*, 5, 7, 1975.
50. **Holmsen, H.**, Incorporation in vitro ^{32}P into blood platelet acid-soluble organophosphates and their chromatographic identification, *Scand. J. Clin. Lab. Invest.*, 17, 230, 1965.
51. **Wu, R., Sessa, G., and Hamerman, D.**, Pi transport and clycolysis in leucocytes and platelets, *Biochim. Biophys. Acta*, 93, 614, 1964.
52. **Firkin, B. G. and Williams, W. J.**,The incorporation of radioactive phosphorus into the phospholipids of human leukemic leukocytes and platelets, *J. Clin. Invest.*, 40, 423, 1961.
53. **Cohen, P., Broekman, M. J., Verkley, A., Lisman, J. W. W., and Derksen, A.**, Quantification of human platelet inositides and the influence of ionic environment on their incorporation of orthophosphate-^{32}P, *J. Clin. Invest.*, 50, 762, 1971.
54. **Paysant, M., Bursztein, C., Maupin, B., and Polonovski, J.**, Metabolisme phospholopidque du sang. IV. Incorporation in vitro du ^{32}P dans les phospholipides plaquettaires du sang humain, *Bull. Soc. Chim. Biol.*, 44, 477, 1962.
55. **Grossman, C. M. and Bartos, F.**, Succinate dependence of in vitro incorporation of ^{32}P-orthophosphate into human platelet phosphatide, *Arch. Biochem. Biophys.*, 128, 231, 1968.
56. **Karpatkin, S. and Langer, R. M.**, Biochemical energetics of stimulated platelet plug formation. Effect of thrombin, adenosine diphosphate, and epinephrine on intra- and extracellular adenine nucleotide kinetics, *J. Clin. Invest.*, 47, 2158, 1968.

57. **Holmsen, H.,** unpublished observations.
58. **Detwiler, T. C.,** Effects of deoxyglucose on platelet metabolism, *Biochim. Biophys. Acta,* 244, 303, 1971.
59. **Murer, E. H.,** Clot retraction and energy metabolism of platelets. Effects and mechanism of inhibitors, *Biochim. Biophys. Acta,* 172, 266, 1969.
60. **Kirkland, S. J. and Baum, H.,** Mitochondrial respiration and the thrombin-induced release reaction of platelets, *Biochem. Pharmacol.,* 23, 1859, 1974.
61. **Fukami, M. H. and Salganicoff, L.,** personal communication.
62. **Cohen, P. and Wittels, B.,** Energy substrate metabolism in fresh and stored human platelets, *J. Clin. Invest.,* 49, 119, 1970.
63. **Sander, J. and Farstad, M.,** Carnitine palmityltransferase and its relation to Palmityl-CoA synthetase in blood platelets from fasting, healthy subjects, *Scand. J. Lab. Clin. Invest.,* 32, 183, 1973.
64. **Donabedian, R. and Nemerson, Y.,** Fatty acid oxidation by human platelets and its stimulation by thrombin, *Am. J. Physiol.,* 221, 1283, 1971.
65. **Holmsen, H.,** Ethanol-insoluble adenine nucleotides in platelets and their possible role in platelet function, *Ann. N.Y. Acad. Sci.,* 201, 109, 1972.
66. **Daniel, J. L. and Holmsen, H.,** unpublished observations.
67. **Holmsen, H.,** Collagen-induced release of adenosine diphosphate from blood platelets incubated with radioactive phosphate in vitro, *Scand. J. Clin. Invest.,* 17, 239, 1965.
68. **Holmsen, H., Day, H. J., and Storm, E.,** Adenine nucleotide metabolism of blood platelets. VI. Subcellular localization of nucleotide pools with different functions in the platelet release reaction, *Biochim. Biophys. Acta,* 186, 254, 1969.
69. **Holmsen, H., Østvold, A. C., and Day, H. J.,** Behavior of endogenous and newly absorbed serotonin on the platelet release reaction, *Biochem. Pharmacol.,* 22, 2599, 1973.
70. **Mürer, E. H. and Holme, R.,** A study of the release of calcium from human blood platelets and its inhibition by metabolic inhibitors, N-ethylmaleimide and aspirin, *Biochim. Biophys. Acta,* 222, 197, 1970.
71. **Fukami, M. H., Holmsen, H., Dangelmaier, C. A., and Bauer, J.,** Pyrophosphate in human platelets: secretion, subcellular localization and metabolic status, *Fed. Proc.,* 37, 1756, 1978.
72. **Reimers, H. J., Mustard, J. F., and Packham, M. A.,** Transfer of adenine nucleotides between the releasable and nonreleasable compartments of rabbit blood platelets, *J. Cell Biol.,* 67, 61, 1975.
73. **Ugurbil, K., Shulman, R., Holmsen, H., and Costa, J.,** High resolution ^{31}P-NMR of human platelets, *Biophys. J.,* 21, 147a, 1978.
74. **Holmsen, H. and Weiss, H. J.,** Further evidence for a deficient storage pool of adenine nucleotides in platelets from some patients with thrombocytopathia — "Storage Pool Disease", *Blood,* 39, 197, 1972.
75. **Lages, B., Scrutton, M. C., Holmsen, H., Day, H. J., and Weiss, H. J.,** Metal ion contents of gel-filtered platelets from patients with Storage Pool Disease, *Blood,* 46, 119, 1975.
76. **Drummond, A. H. and Gordon, J. L.,** Uptake of 5-hydroxytryptamine by rat blood platelets and its inhibition by adenosine 5′-diphosphate, *Br. J. Pharmacol.,* 56, 417, 1976.
77. **Baadenhuijsen, H. and Haanen, C.,** Platelet membrane function studies on platelets from patients with hereditary thrombopathic thrombocytopenia, *Haemostasis,* 3, 98, 1974.
78. **Sneddon, J. M.,** Relationship between internal Na^+/K^+ and the accumulation of ^{14}C-5-hydroxytryptamine by rat platelets, *Br. J. Pharmacol.,* 43, 834, 1971.
79. **Barthel, W., Haustein, K. O., and Markwardt, F.,** On the relations between serotonin uptake and function of the transport-ATPase system of blood platelets, *Acta Biol. Med. Germ.,* 31, 713, 1973.
80. **Barber, A. J. and Jamieson, G. A.,** Isolation and characterization of plasma membranes from human blood platelets, *J. Biol. Chem.,* 245, 6357, 1970.
81. **Douste-Blazy, L., Chap, H., and Gautheron, P.,** Platelet lipid composition, *Haemostasis,* 2, 85, 1974.
82. **Chap, H. J., Zwaal, R. F. A., and Van Deenen, L. L. M.,** Action of highly purified phospholipases on blood platelets. Evidence for an asymmetric distribution of phospholipids in the surface membrane, *Biochim. Biophys. Acta,* 467, 146, 1977.
83. **Cohen, P., Broekman, M. J., Verkley, A., Lismann, J. W. W., and Derksen, A.,** Quantification of human platelet inositides and the influence of ionic environment on their incorporation of orthophosphate - 32P, *J. Clin. Invest.,* 50, 762, 1971.
84. **Iacono, J. M., Fellner, D. C., Paoletti, R., Ishikawa, I., Frigeni, V., and Fumagelli, R.,** Comparison of blood platelets and erythrocyte lipids in man in three age groups from three regions: Milan, Cincinnati and Sicily, *Haemostasis,* 2, 141, 1973.
85. **Marcus, A. J., Ullman, H. L., and Safier, L. B.,** Studies on human platelet gangliosides, *J. Clin. Invest.,* 51, 2602, 1972.
86. **Deykin, D. and Desser, R. K.,** The incorporation of acetate and palmitate into lipids by human platelets, *J. Clin. Invest.,* 47, 1590, 1968.

87. **Majerus, P. S., Smith, M. B., and Clamon, G. H.**, Lipid metabolism in human platelets. I. Evidence for a complete fatty acid synthesizing system, *J. Clin. Invest.*, 48, 156, 1969.
88. **Okuma, M., Yamashita, S., and Numa, S.**, Enzymic studies on phosphatidic acid synthesis in human platelets, *Blood,* 41, 379, 1973.
89. **Call, F. L. and Williams, W. J.**, Biosynthesis of cytidine diphosphate diglyceride by human platelets, *J. Clin. Invest.*, 49, 392, 1970.
90. **Lucas, C. T., Call, F. L., and Williams, W. I.**, The biosynthesis of phosphatidylinositol in human platelets, *J. Clin. Invest.*, 49, 1949, 1970.
91. **Call, F. L. and Williams, W. J.**, Phosphatidate phosphatase in human platelets, *J. Lab. Clin. Med.*, 82, 663, 1973.
92. **Call, F. L. and Rubert, M.**, Diglyceride kinase in human platelets, *J. Lipid Res.*, 14, 466, 1973.
93. **Elsbach, P., Pettis, P., and Marcus, A.**, Lysolecithin metabolism by human platelets, *Blood,* 37, 675, 1971.
94. **Call, F. L. and Rubert, M.**, Synthesis of ethanolamine phosphoglycerides by human platelets, *J. Lipid Res.*, 16, 352, 1975.
95. **Bills, T. K., Smith, J. B., and Silver, M. J.**, Metabolism of 14-C arachidonic acid by human platelets, *Biochim. Biophys. Acta,* 424, 303, 1976.
96. **Bills, T. K., Smith, J. B., and Silver, M. J.**, Selective release of arachidonic acid from the phospholipids of human platelets in response to thrombin, *J. Clin. Invest.*, 60, 1, 1977.
97. **Cohen, P., Derksen, A., and van den Bosch, H.**, Pathways of fatty acid metabolism in human platelets, *J. Clin. Invest.*, 49, 128, 1970.
98. **Jesse, R. L. and Cohen, P.**, Arachidonic acid release from diacyl phosphatidylethanolamine by human platelet membranes, *Biochem. J.*, 158, 283, 1976.
99. **Probst, E. and Lüscher, E. F.**, Studies on thrombosthenin A, the actin-like moiety of the contractile protein from blood platelets. I. Isolation, characterization and evidence for two forms of thrombosthenin A, *Biochim. Biophys. Acta,* 278, 577, 1972.
100. **Booyse, F. M., Hoveke, T. P., and Rafelson, M. E., Jr.**, Human platelet actin: isolation and properties, *J. Biol. Chem.*, 284, 4083, 1973.
101. **Crawford, N.**, Platelet microfilaments and microtubules, in *Platelets in Biology and Pathology,* Gordon, J. L., Ed., Elsevier/North-Holland, Amsterdam, 1976, 121.
102. **Pollard, T. D.**, Functional implications of the biochemical and structural cytoplasmic contractile protein, in *Molecules and Cell Movement,* Inoué, S. and Stephens, R.E., Eds., Raven Press, New York, 1975, 259.
103. **Bettex-Galland, M. and Lüscher, E. F.**, Thrombosthenin: a contractile protein from thrombocytes. Its extraction from human blood platelets and some of its properties, *Biochim. Biophys. Acta,* 49, 536, 1961.
104. **Lucas, R., Detwiler, T. C., and Stracher, A.**, The identification and isolation of a high molecular weight (270,000 dalton) actin binding protein from human platelets, *J. Cell Biol.*, 70, 259a, 1976.
105. **Elzinga, M., Maron, B. J., and Adelstein, R. S.**, Human heart and platelet actins are products of different genes, *Science,* 191, 94, 1976.
106. **Abramowitch, J. W. A., Stracher, A., and Detwiler, T. C.**, A second form of actin: platelet microfilaments depolymerized by ATP and covalent cations, *Arch. Biochem. Biophys.*, 167, 230, 1975.
107. **Schollmeyer, J. E., Rao, G. H. R., and White, J. G.**, A platelet actin binding protein, *Circulation,* 54 (2), 2, 1976.
108. **Shizuta, Y., Gallo, M., Davies, P., Pastan, I., and Lewis, M. S.**, Purification and properties of filamin an actin binding protein from chicken gizzard, *J. Biol. Chem.*, 251, 6562, 1976.
109. **Pollard, T. D., Thomas, S. M., and Niederman, R.**, Human platelet myosin. I. Purification by a rapid method applicable to other nonmuscle cells, *Anal. Biochem.*, 60, 258, 1974.
110. **Booyse, F. M., Hoveke, T. P., Zschocke, D., and Rafelson, M. E., Jr.**, Human platelet myosin: isolation and properties, *J. Biol. Chem.*, 246, 4291, 1971.
111. **Adelstein, R. S. and Conti, M. A.**, The characterization of contractile proteins from platelet and fibroblasts, *Cold Spring Harbor Symp. Quant. Biol.*, 37, 599, 1972.
112. **Niederman, R. and Pollard, T. D.**, Human platelet myosin. II. In vitro assembly and structure of myosin filaments, *J. Cell Biol.*, 67, 72, 1975.
113. **Cove, D. H. and Crawford, N.**, Platelet contractile proteins: separation and characterization of the actin and myosin-like components, *J. Mechanochem. Cell Motil.*, 3, 123, 1975.
114. **Daniel, J. L. and Adelstein, R. S.**, Isolation and properties of platelet myosin light chain kinase, *Biochemistry,* 15, 2370, 1976.
115. **Adelstein, R. S. and Conti, M. A.**, Phosphorylation of platelet myosin increases actin-activated myosin ATPase activity, *Nature (London),* 265, 597, 1975.
116. **Daniel, J. L., Holmsen, H., and Adelstein, R. S.**, Thrombin-stimulated myosin phosphorylation in intact platelets and its possible involvement in secretion, *Thromb. Haemostasis,* 38, 984, 1977.
117. **Cohen, I. and Cohen, C.**, A tropomyosin-like protein from human platelets, *J. Mol. Biol.*, 68, 383, 1972.

118. **Cohen, I., Kaminski, E., and De Vries, A.**, Actin-linked regulation of the human platelet contractile system, *FEBS Lett.*, 34, 315, 1973.
119. **Muszbek, L., Kuznicki, J., and Drabikowski, W.**, Troponin C like protein of blood platelets, *FEBS Lett.*, 80, 308, 1977.
120. **Castle, A. G. and Crawford, N.**, Phosphorylation of platelet microtubule proteins by an endogenous protein kinase, *Biochim. Soc. Trans.*, 4, 691, 1976.
121. **Booyse, F. M. and Rafelson, M. E., Jr.**, Studies on human platelet. I. Synthesis of platelet protein in a cell-free system, *Biochim. Biophys. Acta*, 166, 689, 1968.
122. **Nachman, R. L., Marcus, A. J., and Safier, L. B.**, Platelet thrombosthenin: subcellular localization and function, *J. Clin. Invest.*, 46, 1380, 1967.
123. **Pollard, T. D., Fuijuwara, K., Handin, R., and Weiss, G.**, Contractile proteins in platelet activation and contraction, *Ann. N. Y. Acad. Sci.*, 283, 218, 1977.
124. **Bouvier, C. A., Gabbiani, G., Ryan, G. B., Badonnel, M. C., Majno, G., and Lüscher, E. F.**, Binding of anti-actin autoantibodies to platelets, *Thromb. Haemostasis*, 37, 321, 1977.
125. **Taylor, D. G., Mapp, R. J., and Crawford, N.**, The identification of actin associated with pig platelet membranes and granules, *Biochem. Soc. Trans.*, 3, 161, 1975.
126. **Taylor, D. G., Williams, V. M., and Crawford, N.**, Platelet membrane actin. Solubility and binding studies with ^{125}I-actin, *Biochem. Soc. Trans.*, 4, 156, 1976.
127. **Bray, D.**, Sticky actin, *Nature (London)*, 256, 616, 1975.
128. **Harris, G. L. A. and Crawford, N.**, The identification and subcellular localization of thrombosthenin "M", the myosin-like component of pig platelets, *J. Mechanochem. Cell Motil.*, 3, 135, 1975.
129. **Behnke, O.**, Further studies on microtubules. A marginal bundle in human and rat thrombocytes, *J. Ultrastruct. Res.*, 13, 469, 1965.
130. **Dabrowska, R., Sherry, J. M. F., and Hartshorne, D. J.**, *Motility in Cell Function*, Pepe, F., Ed., Academic Press, New York, 1978, in press.
131. **Markey, F., Lindberg, U., and Eriksson, L.**, Human platelets contain profilin, a potential regulator of actin polymerizability, *FEBS Lett.*, 88, 75, 1978.
132. **Parsons, D. F. and Subjeck, J. R.**, Morphology of the polysaccharide coat of mammalian cells, *Biochim. Biophys. Acta*, 352, 218, 1972.
133. **Hughes, R. C.**, Glycoproteins as components of cellular membranes, *Prog. Biophys. Mol. Biol.*, 26, 189, 1973.
134. **Nurden, A. T. and Caen, J. P.**, Role of surface glycoproteins in human platelet function, *Thromb. Haemostasis*, 35, 139, 1976.
135. **Phillips, D. R., Jenkins, C. S. P., Lüscher, E. F., and Larrieu, M. J.**, Molecular differences of exposed surface proteins on thrombasthenic platelet plasma membrane, *Nature (London)*, 257, 599, 1975.
136. **Jenkins, C. S. P., Phillips, D. R., Clemetson, K. J., Meyer, D., Larrieu, M.-J., and Lüscher, E. F.**, Platelet membrane glycoproteins implicated in ristocetin-induced aggregation: studies of the proteins on platelets from patients with Bernard-Soulier syndrome and von Willebrand's disease, *J. Clin. Invest.*, 57, 112, 1976.
137. **Okumura, T. and Jamieson, G. A.**, Platelet glycocalicin: a single receptor for platelet aggregation induced by thrombin or ristocetin, *Thromb. Res.*, 8, 701, 1972.
138. **Phillips, D. R.**, Effect of trypsin on the exposed polypeptides and glycoproteins in the human platelet membrane, *Biochemistry*, 11, 4582, 1972.
139. **Phillips, D. R. and Agin, P. P.**, Platelet plasma membrane glycoproteins. Evidence for the presence of nonequivalent disulfide bonds using nonreduced-reduced two-dimensional gel electrophoresis, *J. Biol. Chem.*, 252, 2121, 1977.
140. **George, J. N., Potterf, R. D., Lewis, P. C., and Sears, D. A.**, Studies on platelet plasma membranes. I. Characterization of surface proteins of human platelets labeled with diazotized (^{125}I)-diiodosulfanilic acid, *J. Lab. Clin. Med.*, 88, 232, 1976.
141. **Tanner, M. J. A., Boxer, C. H., Cumming, J., and Verrier-Jones, J.**, A set of surface proteins common to the circulating human platelet and lymphocyte, *Biochem. J.*, 141, 909, 1974.
142. **Nachman, R. L., Hubbard, A., and Ferris, B.**, Iodination of the human platelet membrane, *J. Biol. Chem.*, 248, 2928, 1973.
143. **Nurden, A. T. and Gaen, J. P.**, Specific rates for platelet surface glycoproteins in platelet function, *Nature (London)*, 255, 720, 1975.
144. **Nurden, A. T. and Gaen, J. P.**, An abnormal platelet glycoprotein pattern in three cases of Glanzmann's thrombasthenia, *Br. J. Haematol.*, 28, 253, 1974.
145. **Lombart, C., Okumura, T., and Jamieson, G. A.**, Isolation of a surface glycoprotein of human platelets, *FEBS Lett.*, 41, 30, 1974.
146. **Pepper, D. S. and Jamieson, G. A.**, Isolation of a macroglycopeptide from human platelets, *Biochemistry*, 9, 3706, 1970.

147. Okumura, T. and Jamieson, G. A., Platelet glycocalicin. I. Orientation of glycoproteins on the human platelet surface, *J. Biol. Chem.*, 251, 5944, 1976.
148. Solum, N. O., Hagen, I., and Peterka, M., Human platelet glycoproteins. Further evidence that the "GPI band" from whole platelets contains three different polypeptides one of which may be involved in the interaction between platelets and factor VIII, *Thromb. Res.*, 10, 71, 1977.
149. Lopaciuk, S., Lovette, K. M., McDonagh, J., Chuang, H. Y. K., and McDonagh, R. P., Subcellular distribution of fibrinogen and factor XIII in human blood platelets, *Thromb. Res.*, 8, 453, 1976.
150. Davey, M. G. S. and Lüscher, E. F., Release reactions of human platelets induced by thrombin and other agents, *Biochim. Biophys. Acta*, 165, 490, 1968.
151. Keenan, J. P. and Solum, N. O., Quantitative studies on the release of platelet fibrinogen by thrombin, *Br. J. Haematol.*, 23, 461, 1972.
152. Broekman, J. J., Handin, R. I., and Cohen, P., Distribution of fibrinogen and platelet factors 4 and XIII in subcellular fractions of human platelets, *Br. J. Haematol.*, 31, 51, 1975.
153. Solum, N. O. and Lopaciuk, S., Bovine platelet proteins. III. Some properties of platelet fibrinogen, *Thromb. Diath. Haemorrh.*, 21, 428, 1969.
154. Doolittle, R. F., Takagi, T., and Cottrell, B. A., Platelet and plasma fibrinogens are identical gene products, *Science*, 185, 368, 1974.
155. Ganguly, P., Isolation of some properties of fibrinogen from human blood platelets, *J. Biol. Chem.*, 247, 1809, 1972.
156. James, H. L., Bradford, H. R., and Ganguly, P., Platelet fibrinogen. Identity and initial observations on the mode of its degradation by plasmin, *Biochim. Biophys. Acta*, 386, 209, 1975.
157. Nachman, R. L., Wersler, B., and Ferris, B., Increased vascular permeability by human platelet granule cationic extract, *J. Clin. Invest.*, 49, 274, 1970.
157a. Busch, C., Wasteson, Å., and Westermark, B., Release of a cell growth promoting factor from human platelets, *Thromb. Res.*, 8, 493, 1976.
158. Ihnatowycz, I. O., Moore, S., and Mustard, T. F., Platelet growth factor (PFG) stimulation of DNA synthesis in smooth muscle cells in vitro, *Fed. Proc.*, 36 (Abstr.), 430, 1977.
159. Antoniades, H. N., Stathakos, D., and Scher, C. D., Isolation of a cationic polypeptide from human serum that stimulates proliferation of 3T3 cells, *Proc. Natl. Acad. Sci. U.S.A.*, 72, 2635, 1975.
160. Antoniades, H. N. and Scher, C. D., Radioimmunoassay of a human serum growth factor for Balb tc-3T3 cells: derivation from platelets, *Proc. Natl. Acad. Sci. U.S.A.*, 74, 1973, 1977.
161. Ross, R., Glomset, J., Kariya, B., and Harker, L., A platelet-dependent serum factor that stimulates the proliferation of arterial smooth muscle cells in vitro, *Proc. Natl. Acad. Sci. U.S.A.*, 71, 1207, 1974.
162. Ross, R. and Glomset, J., The pathogenesis of atherosclerosis, *N. Engl. J. Med.*, 295, 369, 1976.
163. Westermark, B. and Wasteson, A., Å platelet factor stimulating human normal glial cells, *Exp. Cell Res.*, 98, 170, 1976.
164. Niewiarowski, S., Poplawski, A., Lipinski, B., and Farbiszewski, R., The release of platelet clotting factors during aggregation and viscous metamorphosis, *Exp. Biol. Med.*, 3, 121, 1968.
165. Walsh, P. N. and Gagnatelli, G., Platelet antiheparin activity: storage site and release mechanism, *Blood*, 44, 157, 1974.
166. Da Prada, M., Jakabova, R., Lüscher, E. F., Pletscher, A., and Richards, J. G., Subcellular localization of the heparin neutralizing factor in blood platelets, *J. Physiol.*, 257, 495, 1976.
167. Niewiarowski, S., Rucinski, B., Millman, M., and Hawiger, J., Immunoassay of human platelet factor 4 (antiheparin factor) and its significance for evaluation of the platelet function. Platelet function testing, Proc. Workshop on Platelets in Philadelphia, October 1976, Day, H. J., Holmsen, H., and Zucker, D., Eds., U. S. Government Printing Office, in press.
168. Morgan, F. J., Chesterman, C. N., McGready, J. R., and Begg, G. S., Studies on the chemistry of human platelet factor 4, *Haemostasis*, 6, 53, 1977.
169. Moore, S., Pepper, D. S., and Cash, J. D., The isolation and characterization of a platelet specific β-globulin (β-thromboglobulin) and the detection of anti-urokinase and anti-plasmin released from thrombin-aggregated washed platelets, *Biochim. Biophys. Acta*, 379, 360, 1975.
170. Ludlam, C. A. and Cash, J. D., Studies on the liberation of β-thromboglobulin from human platelets in vitro, *Br. J. Haematol.*, 33, 239, 1976.
171. Moore, S., Pepper, D., and Cash, J., Platelet antiheparin activity: the isolation and characterization of platelet factor 4 released from thrombin-aggregated washed human platelets and its dissociation into subunits and the isolation of membrane-bound antiheparin activity, *Biochim. Biophys. Acta*, 379, 370, 1975.
172. Ludlam, C. A. and Anderton, J. L., Platelet β-thromboglobulin. Platelet function tests, Proc. Workshop on Platelets in Philadelphia, October 1976, Day, H. J., Holmsen, H., Zucker, D., Eds., U. S. Government Printing Office, in press.
173. Mitchell, J. R. A. and Sharp, A. A., Platelet clumping in vitro, *Br. J. Haematol.*, 10, 78, 1964.
174. Michal, F. and Penglis, F., Inhibition of serotonin-induced platelet aggregation in relation to thrombus production, *J. Pharmacol. Exp. Ther.*, 166, 276, 1969.

175. Boullin, D. J., Woods, H. F., Grimes, R. P. J., Grahame-Smith, D. G., Wiles, D., Gelder, M. G., and Kolakowska, T., Increased platelet aggregation responses to 5-hydroxytryptamine in patients taking chlorpromazine, *Br. J. Clin. Pharmacol.*, 2, 29, 1975.
176. Boullin, D. J., Grahame-Smith, D. G., Grimes, R. P. J., and Woods, H. F., Inhibition of 5-hydroxytryptamine-induced human blood platelet aggregation by chlorpromazine and its metabolites, *Br. J. Pharmacol.*, 53, 121, 1975.
177. Drummond, A. H. and Gordon, J. L., Specific binding sites for 5-hydroxytryptamine on rat blood platelets, *Biochem. J.*, 150, 129, 1975.
178. Boullin, D. J., Grimes, R. P. J., and Orr, M. W., The actions of flupenthixol upon 5-hydroxytryptamine-induced aggregation and the uptake of 5-hydroxytryptamine and dopamine by human blood platelets, *Br. J. Pharmacol.*, 55, 555, 1975.
179. Barzaghi, F., Baumgartner, H. R., Carruba, M., Mantegazza, P., and Pletscher, A., The 5-hydroxytryptamine-like actions of 5, 6-dihydroxytryptamine, *Br. J. Pharmacol.*, 48, 245, 1973.
180. Born, G. V. R., Juengjaroen, K., and Michal, F., Relative activities on and uptake by human blood platelets of 5-hydroxytryptamine and several analogues, *Br. J. Pharmacol.*, 44, 117, 1972.
181. Drummond, A. H., Whigham, K. A. E., and Prentice, C. R. M., Effects of chlorprothixene isomers on platelet 5-hydroxytryptamine receptors: evidence for different 5-hydroxytryptamine conformations at uptake and stimulatory sites, *Eur. J. Pharmacol.*, 37, 385, 1976.
182. Yates, C. M., Todrick, A., and Tait, A. C., Effect of imipramine and some analogues on the uptake of 5-hydroxytryptamine by human blood platelets in vitro, *J. Pharm. Pharmacol.*, 16, 460, 1964.
183. Lingjaerde, O., Jr., Uptake of serotonin in blood platelets: dependence on sodium and chloride, and inhibition by choline, *FEBS Lett.*, 3, 103, 1969.
184. Lingjaerde, O., Jr., Uptake of serotonin in blood platelets in vitro. I. The effects of chloride, *Acta Physiol. Scand.*, 81, 75, 1971.
185. Todrick, A. and Tait, A. C., The inhibition of human platelet 5-hydroxytryptamine uptake by tricyclic antidepressive drugs. The relation between structure and potency, *J. Pharm. Pharmacol.*, 21, 751, 1969.
186. Barthel, W. and Markwardt, F., Untersuchungen über den einfluss von herzglykosiden auf die 5-HT-aufnahme der blutplättchen, *Biochem. Pharmacol.*, 20, 2597, 1971.
187. Genefke, I. K., The active uptake of 5-hydroxytryptamine in rat and human blood platelets under the influence of lithium in vivo and in vitro, *Acta Psychol. Scand.*, 48, 394, 1972.
188. Sneddon, J. M., Sodium-dependent accumulation of 5-hydroxytryptamine by rat blood platelets, *Br. J. Pharmacol.*, 37, 680, 1969.
189. Zucker, M. B. and Borrelli, J., Absorption of serotonin (5-hydroxytryptamine) by canine and human platelets, *Am. J. Physiol.*, 186, 105, 1956.
190. Szabados, L., Mester, L., Michal, F., and Born, G. V. R., Accelerated uptake of 5-hydroxytryptamine by human blood platelets enriched in a sialic acid, *Biochem. J.*, 148, 335, 1975.
191. Horng, J. S. and Wong, D. T., Effects of serotonin uptake inhibitor. Lilly 110140 on transport of serotonin in rat and human blood platelets, *Biochem. Pharmacol.*, 25, 865, 1976.
192. Kibby, M. R., Kinetics of 5-hydroxytryptamine exchange in rabbit blood platelets and its analysis by digital computer, *Biochemistry*, 119, 39, 1970.
193. Murphy, D. L., Colburn, R. W., Davis, J. M., and Bunney, W. E., Jr., Stimulation by lithium of monoamine uptake in human platelets, *Life Sci.*, 8, 1187, 1969.
194. Sneddon, J. M., Relationship between internal Na^+/K^+ and the accumulation of ^{14}C-5-hydroxytryptamine by rat platelets, *Br. J. Pharmacol.*, 43, 834, 1971.
195. Barthel, W., Haustein, K.-O., and Markwardt, F., On the relations between serotonin uptake and function of the transport-ATPase system of blood platelets, *Acta Biol. Med. Germ.*, 31, 713, 1973.
196. Rudnick, G., Active transport of 5-hydroxytryptamine by plasma membrane vesicles isolated from human blood platelets, *J. Biol. Chem.*, 252, 2170, 1977.
197. Bartholini, G., Pletscher, A., and Bruderer, H., Formation of 5-hydroxytryptophol from endogenous 5-hydroxytryptamine by isolated blood platelets, *Nature (London)*, 203, 1281, 1964.
198. Da Prada, M., Bartholini, G., and Pletscher, A., Formation of 5-hydroxytryptophol by blood platelets after thrombin and reserpine, *Experientia*, 21, 135, 1965.
199. Bartholini, G. and Pletscher, A., Two types of 5-hydroxytryptamine release from isolated blood platelets, *Experientia*, 20, 376, 1964.
200. Broekman, M. J., Westmoreland, N. P., and Cohen, P., An improved method for isolating alpha granules and mitochondria from human platelets, *J. Cell Biol.*, 60, 507, 1974.
201. Paasonen, M. D., Release of 5-hydroxytryptamine from blood platelets, *J. Pharm. Pharmacol.*, 17, 681, 1965.
202. Da Prada, M. and Pletscher, A., Isolated 5-hydroxytryptamine organelles of rabbit blood platelets: physiological properties and drug-induced changes, *Br. J. Pharmacol.*, 34, 591, 1968.
203. Hughes, F. B., Shore, P. A., and Brodie, B. B., Serotonin storage mechanism and its interaction with reserpine, *Experientia*, 14, 178, 1958.

204. Minter, B. and Crawford, N., Subcellular localization of reserpine and 5-hydroxytryptamine in blood platelets after reserpine-induced release, *Biochem. J.*, 109, 42, 1968.
205. Da Prada, M. and Pletscher, A., Storage of exogenous monoamines and reserpine in 5-hydroxytryptamine organelles of blood platelets, *Eur. J. Pharmacol.*, 7, 45, 1969.
206. Da Prada, M. and Pletscher, A., Differential uptake of biogenic amines by isolated 5-hydroxytryptamine organelles of blood platelets, *Life Sci.*, 8, 65, 1969.
207. Pletscher, A., Da Prada, M., Berneis, K. H., and Tranzer, J. P., New aspects on the storage of 5-hydroxytryptamine in blood platelets, *Experientia*, 27, 993, 1971.
208. Pignatti, P. F. and Cavalli-Sforza, L. L., Serotonin binding proteins from human blood platelets: an experimental model system for studies on properties of synaptic vesicles, *Neurobiology*, 5, 65, 1975.
209. Davis, R. B. and White, J. G., Localization of 5-hydroxytryptamine in blood platelets: an autoradiographic and ultrastructural study, *Br. J. Haematol.*, 15, 93, 1968.
210. Da Prada, M., Pletscher, A., Tranzer, J. P., and Knuchel, H., Action of reserpine on subcellular 5-hydroxytryptamine organelles of blood platelets, *Life Sci.*, 7, 477, 1968.
211. Pareti, F. I., Day, H. J., and Mills, D. C. B., Nucleotide and serotonin metabolism in platelets with defective secondary aggregation, *Blood*, 44, 789, 1974.
212. Weiss, H. J., Tschopp, T. B., Rogers, J., and Brand, H., Studies of platelet 5-hydroxytryptamine (serotonin) in storage pool disease and albinism, *J. Clin. Invest.*, 54, 421, 1974.
213. Valdorf--Hansen, J. F. and Zucker, M. B., Effect of temperature and inhibitors on serotonin-^{14}C release from human platelets, *Am. J. Physiol.*, 220, 105, 1971.
214. Harada, K. and Zucker, M. B., Simultaneous development of platelet factor 4 activity and release of ^{14}C-serotonin, *Thromb. Diath. Haemorrh.*, 25, 41, 1971.
215. Frohlich, M. M. and Balazs, V., Pathological serum protein (cryoglobulin) as nucleic acid-protein complex, *Naturwissenschaften*, 24, 639, 1964.
216. Takagi, H., Kuruma, I., and Nomura, Y., Mechanism of 5-hydroxytryptamine release induced by bacterial lipopolysaccharide from blood platelets. I. A possible participation of proteolytic enzyme in plasma, *Jpn. J. Pharmacol.*, 18, 59, 1968.
217. Humphrey, J. H. and Jaques, R., The release of histamine and 5-hydroxytryptamine (serotonin) from platelets by antigen-antibody reactions (in vitro), *J. Physiol.*, 128, 9, 1955.
218. Markwardt, F. and Barthel, W., Untersuchungen über die freisetzung von serotonin aus blutplättchen durch thrombin, *Arch. Exp. Pathol.*, 249, 176, 1964.
219. Buckingham, S. and Maynert, E. W., The release of 5-hydroxytryptamine, potassium and amino acids from platelets, *J. Pharmacol. Exp. Ther.*, 143, 332, 1964.
220. Da Prada, M., Bartholini, G., and Pletscher, A., Effect of monoamine liberators on the metabolism of 5-hydroxytryptamine in blood platelets, *Biochem. Pharmacol.*, 14, 1721, 1965.
221. Davis, J. W. and Wilson, S. J., The effect of quinidine on the uptake and release of serotonin by platelets in vitro, *Exp. Biol. Med.*, 131, 1107, 1969.
222. Bridges, J. M. and Baldini, M., Effect of quinidine and related compounds on uptake and release of serotonin by blood platelets, *Nature (London)*, 210, 1364, 1966.
223. Schick, P. K. and Yu, B. P., Methylene blue-induced serotonin release in human platelets, *J. Lab. Clin. Med.*, 82, 546, 1973.
224. Worner, P. and Brossmer, R., Selective release of serotonin from platelets by diffusion facilitated by the ionophore X-537A, *Thromb. Res.*, 7, 567, 1975.
225. Murer, E. H., Davenport, K., and Day, H. J., Metabolic aspects of the secretion of stored compounds from blood platelets. IV. Effects of ionophore X537A on washed platelets, *Biochim. Biophys. Acta*, 428, 369, 1976.
226. Born, G. V. R., Observations on the change in shape of blood platelets brought about by adenosine diphosphate, *J. Physiol.*, 209, 487, 1970.
227. Born, G. V. R. and Cross, M. J., The aggregation of blood platelets, *J. Physiol.*, 168, 1963.
228. Samuelsson, B., The role of prostaglandin endoperoxides and thromboxanes in human platelets, in *Prostaglandins in Haematology*, Silver, M. J., Smith, J. B., and Kocsis, J. J., Eds., Spectrum, New York, 1977, 1.
229. Holmsen, H., Biochemistry of the platelet release reaction, in *Ciba Found. Symp.*, Biochemistry and Pharmacology of Blood Platelets, 35, 175, 1975.
230. Holmsen, H., Prostaglandin endoperoxide-thromboxane synthesis and dense granules secretion as positive feedback loops in the propagation of platelet responses during the basic platelet reaction, *Thromb. Haemostasis*, 38, 1042, 1977.
231. Forbes, C. D. and Prentice, C. R. M., Aggregation of human platelets by purified porcine and bovine antihemophilic factor, *Nature (London)*, 241, 149, 1973.
232. Howard, M. A., Sawers, R. J., and Firkin, B. G., Ristocetin: a means of differentiating von Willebrand's Disease into two groups, *Blood*, 41, 687, 1973.

233. **Mueller-Eckhardt, C. H. and Lüscher, E. F.**, Immune reactions of human blood platelets. II. The effect of latex particles coated with gamma-globulin in relation to complement activation, *Thromb. Diath. Haemorrh.*, 20, 168, 1968.
234. **Pfueller, S. L., Weher, S., and Lüscher, E. F.**, Studies of mechanism of human platelet release reaction induced by immunologic stimuli. III. Relationship between binding of soluble IGG aggregates to FC receptor and cell response in presence and absence of plasma, *J. Immunol.*, 118, 514, 1977.
235. **Massini, P. and Lüscher, E. F.**, The induction of the release reaction in human blood platelets by close cell contact, *Thromb. Diath. Haemorrh.*, 25, 13, 1971.
236. **O'Brien, J. R. and Woodhouse, M. A.**, Platelets: their size, shape and stickiness in vitro: degranulation and proprinquity, in *Experimental Biology and Medicine*, Haanen, C. and Jurgens, J., Eds., S. Karger, Basel, New York, 1968, 90.
237. **Murer, E. H., Hellem, A. J., and Rozenberg, M. C.**, Energy metabolism and platelet function, *Scand. J. Clin. Lab. Invest.*, 19, 280, 1967.
238. **Holmsen, H., Setkowsky, C. A., and Day, H. J.**, Effects of antimycin and 2-deoxyglucose on adenine nucleotides in human platelets. The role of metabolic ATP levels in primary aggregation, secondary aggregation and shape change of human platelets, *Biochem. J.*, 144, 385, 1974.
239. **Macfarlane, D. E. and Mills, D. C. B.**, The effects of ATP on platelets: evidence against the central role of released ADP in primary aggregation, *Blood*, 46, 309, 1975.
240. **Mills, D. C. B. and Macfarlane, D. E.**, Platelet receptors, in *Platelets in Biology and Pathology*, Gordon, J. L., Ed., Elsevier/North-Holland, Amsterdam, 1976, 159.
241. **Michal, F. and Penglis, F.**, Inhibition of serotonin-induced platelet aggregation in relation to thrombus production, *J. Pharmacol. Exp. Ther.*, 166, 276, 1969.
242. **Barthell, W. and Markwardt, F.**, Aggregation of blood platelets by adrenaline and its uptake, *Biochem. Pharmacol.*, 24, 1903, 1975.
243. **Tollefsen, D. M., Feagler, J. R., and Majerus, P. W.**, The binding of thrombin to the surface of human platelets, *J. Biol. Chem.*, 249, 2646, 1974.
244. **Haslam, R. J. and Rosson, G. M.**, Aggregation of human blood platelets by vasopressin, *Am. J. Physiol.*, 223, 958, 1972.
245. **Chiang, T. M., Beachey, E. H., and Kang, A. H.**, Binding of collagen alpha chains to human platelets, *J. Clin. Invest.*, 59, 405, 1977.
246. **Sixma, J. J., Trieshnigg, A. M., and Holmsen, H.**, Adenine nucleotide metabolism of blood platelets. VIII. Mechanism of adenine uptake by intact cells, *Biochim. Biophys. Acta*, 298, 3, 1973.
247. **Ireland, D. M.**, Effect of thrombin on the radioactive nucleotides of human washed platelets, *Biochem. J.*, 105, 857, 1967.
248. **Holmsen, H., Day, H. J., and Storm, E.**, Adenine nucleotide metabolism of blood platelets. VI. Subcellular localization of nucleotide pools with different functions in the platelet release reaction, *Biochim. Biophys. Acta*, 186, 254, 1969.
249. **Holmsen, H., Day, H. J., and Setkowsky, C. A.**, Secretory mechanisms: behavior of adenine nucleotides during platelet release reaction induced by adenosine diphosphate and adrenaline, *Biochem. J.*, 129, 67, 1972.
250. **Østvold, A. C., Lindberg, M. E., Solum, N. O., and Holmsen, H.**, Release of nonmetabolic adenine nucleotides during the interaction between bovine fibrinogen/factor VIII and human platelets, *Haemostasis*, 4, 3, 1975.
251. **Holmsen, H.**, Biochemistry of the platelet release reaction, biochemistry and pharmacology of blood platelets, *Ciba Found. Symp.*, 35, 175, 1975.
252. **Mills, D. C. B.**, Changes in the adenylate energy charge in human blood platelets induced by adenosine diphosphate, *Nature (London)*, 243, 220, 1973.
253. **Kattlove, H. E.**, Platelet ATP in ADP-induced aggregation, *Am. J. Physiol.*, 226, 325, 1974.
254. **Stjernholm, R. L., Bryce Larke, R. P., and Wheelock, J. E. F.**, Carbohydrate metabolism in the human platelet, *J. Reticuloendo. Soc.*, 10, 309, 1971.
255. **Cowan, D.**, Platelet metabolism in acute leukemia, *J. Lab. Clin. Med.*, 82, 54, 1973.
256. **Chaudry, A. A., Sagone, A. L., Jr., Metz, E. N., and Balcerzak, S. P.**, Relationship of glucose oxidation to aggregation of human platelets, *Blood*, 41, 249, 1973.
257. **Detwiler, T. C.**, Control of energy metabolism in platelets. The effects of thrombin and cyanide on glycolysis, *Biochim. Biophys. Acta*, 256, 163, 1972.
258. **Fukami, M. H., Salganicoff, L., and Bauer, J.**, Pig Platelet Amylo-1.6-Glucosidase-Subcellular Localization and Possible Activation by Thrombin. Vth Congress International Society on Thrombosis and Haemostasis Paris, Abstr. 438, 1975.
259. **Karpatkin, S.**, Studies on human platelet glycolysis. Effect of glucose, cyanide insulin, citrate, and agglutination and contraction on platelet glycolysis, *J. Clin. Invest.*, 46, 409, 1967.
260. **De Vreker, G. G. and De Vreker, R. A.**, Aspects of platelet metabolism during aggregation, *Rev. Belge Pathol.*, 31, 79, 1965.

261. Warshaw, A. L., Laster, L., and Shulman, N. R., The stimulation by thrombin of glucose oxidation in human platelets, *J. Clin. Invest.*, 45, 1923, 1966.
262. Kuramoto, A., Steiner, M., and Baldini, M. G., Metabolic basis of platelet phagocytosis, *Biochim. Biophys. Acta*, 201, 471, 1970.
263. Gross, R. and Schneider, W., Energy metabolism, in *The Circulating Platelet*, Johnson, S. A., Ed., Academic Press, New York, 1971, 123.
264. Corn, M., Effect of thrombin on glycolysis of fresh and stored platelets, *J. Appl. Physiol.*, 21, 62, 1966.
265. Akkerman, J. W. N., Gorter, G., Sixma, J. J., and Staal, G. E. J., Variations in levels of gycolytic intermediates in human platelets during platelet-collagen interaction, *Biochim. Biophys. Acta*, 421, 296, 1976.
266. Fukami, M. H., Holmsen, H., and Salganicoff, L., Adenine nucleotide metabolism of blood platelets. IX. Time course of secretion and changes in energy metabolism in thrombin-treated platelets, *Biochim. Biophys. Acta*, 44, 633, 1976.
267. McElroy, F. A., Kinlough-Rathbone, R. L., Ardlie, N. G., Packham, M. A., and Mustard, J. F., The effect of aggregating agents on oxidative metabolism of rabbit platelets, *Biochim. Biophys. Acta*, 253, 64, 1971.
268. Murer, E. H., Release reaction and energy metabolism in blood platelets with special reference to the burst in oxygen uptake, *Biochim. Biophys. Acta*, 162, 320, 1968.
269. Muenzer, J., Weinbach, E. C., and Wolfe, S. M., Oxygen consumption of human blood platelets. I. Effect of thrombin, *Biochim. Biophys. Acta*, 376, 237, 1975.
270. Fukami, M. H., Holmsen, H., and Bauer, J., Thrombin-induced consumption malondialdehyde formation and serotonin secretion in human platelets, *Biochim. Biophys. Acta*, 428, 253, 1976.
271. Holmsen, H., CN-insensitive O_2 uptake in platelet treated with ADP, epinephrine and A23187, unpublished observation.
272. Okuma, M., Steiner, M., and Baldini, M., Studies on lipid peroxides in platelets. I. Methods for assay and effect of storage, *J. Lab. Clin. Med.*, 75, 283, 1970.
273. Donabedian, R. and Nemerson, Y., Fatty acids oxidation by human platelets and its stimulation by thrombin, *Am. J. Physiol.*, 221, 1283, 1971.
274. Lloyd, J. V. and Mustard, J. F., Changes in ^{32}P-content of phosphatidic acid and the phosphoinositides of rabbit platelets during aggregation induced by collagen or thrombin, *Br. J. Haematol.*, 26, 243, 1974.
275. Lloyd, J. V., Nishizawa, E. E., Haldar, J., and Mustard, J. F., Changes in ^{32}P-labeling of platelet phospholipids in response to ADP, *Br. J. Haematol.*, 23, 571, 1972.
276. Lloyd, J. V., Nishizawa, E. E., Joist, J. H., and Mustard, J. F., Effect of ADP-induced aggregation on $^{32}PO_4$ incorporation into phosphatidic acid and the phosphoinoistides of rabbit platelets, *Br. J. Haematol.*, 24, 589, 1973.
277. Daniel, J. L., Robkin, L., Salganicoff, L., and Holmsen, H., Measurement of the nucleotide exchange rate as a possible determination of the cellular state of actin, in *Motility in Cell Function*, Pepe, F. A., Ed., Academic Press, New York, in press, 1979.
278. Holmsen, H., Prostaglandin endoperoxide — thromboxane synthesis and dense granule secretion as positive feedback loops in the propagation of platelet responses during the basic platelet reaction, *Thromb. Haemostasis*, 1977.
279. Silver, M. J., Smith, J. B., Ingerman, C., and Kocsis, J. J., Arachidonic acid-induced human platelet aggregation and prostaglandin formation, *Prostaglandins*, 4, 863, 1973.
280. Lages, B., Scrutton, M. C., and Holmsen, H., Secretion by gel filtered platelets: response of platelet Ca^{2+}, Mg^{2+}, and K^{+} to secretory agents, *J. Lab. Clin. Med.*, in press, 1977.
281. Wiley, J. S., Kuchibhotla, J., Shaller, C. C., and Colman, R. W., Potassium uptake and release by human blood platelets, *Blood*, 48, 185, 1976.
282. Holmsen, H., Day, H. J., and Stormorken, H., The platelet release reaction, *Scand. J. Haematol.*, 8, 1, 1969.
283. Holmsen, H. and Day, H. J., The selectivity of the thrombin induced platelet release reaction: subcellular localization of released and retained constituents, *J. Lab. Clin. Med.*, 75, 840, 1970.
284. MacIntyre, D. E., McMillan, R. M., and Gordon, J. L., Secretion of lysosomal enzymes by platelets, *Biochem. Soc. Trans.*, 5, 1177, 1977.
285. Mills, D. C. B., Robb, I. A., and Roberts, G. C. K., The release of nucleotides, 5-hydroxytryptamine and enzymes from human blood platelets during aggregation, *J. Physiol.*, 195, 715, 1968.
286. Robert, B., Szigeti, M., Robert, L., Legrand, Y., Pignaud, G., and Caen, J., Release of elastolytic activity from platelets, *Nature (London)*, 227, 1248, 1970.
287. Chesney, C. McI., Harper, E., and Colman, R. W., Human platelet collagenase, *J. Clin. Invest.*, 53, 1647, 1974.
288. Mustard, J. F. and Packham, M. A., Factors influencing platelet function: adhesion, release, and aggregation, *Pharmacol. Rev.*, 22, 97, 1970.

289. **Smith, J. B. and Macfarlane, D. E.**, Platelets, in *The Prostaglandins,* Vol. 2, Ramwell, P. W., Ed., Plenum Press, 1974, 293.
290. **Holmsen, H.**, The platelet: its membrane, physiology and biochemistry, in *Clinics in Haematology,* O'Brien, J. R., Saunders, London, 1972, 235.
291. **Sixma, J. J.**, Methods for platelet aggregation, in *Platelet Function and Thrombosis — A Review of Methods,* Manucci, P. M. and Gorini, S., Eds., Plenum Press, New York, 79.
292. **Born, G. V. R.**, Observations on the change in shape of blood platelets brought about by adenosine diphosphate, *J. Physiol.,* 209, 487, 1970.
293. **Feinberg, H., Michel, H., and Born, G. V. R.**, Determination of the fluid volume of platelets by their separation through silicone oil, *J. Lab. Clin. Med.,* 84, 926, 1974.
294. **White, J. G.**, Shape change, *Thromb. Diath. Haemorrh.,* Suppl. 60, 159, 1973.
295. **Bills, T. K., Smith, J. B., and Silver, M. J.**, Metabolism of [^{14}C] arachidonic acid by human platelets, *Biochim. Biophys. Acta,* 424, 303, 1976.
296. **Bills, T. K., Smith, J. B., and Silver, M. J.**, Platelet uptake, release and oxidation of [^{14}C] arachidonic acid, in *Prostaglandins in Hematology,* Silver, M. J., Smith, J. B., and Kocsis, J. J., Eds., Spectrum Publications, New York, 1977, 27-55.
297. **Pickett, W. C., Jesse, R. L., and Cohen, P.**, Initiation of phospholipase A_2 activity in human platelets by the calcium ionophore A23187, *Biochim. Biophys. Acta,* 486, 209, 1977.
298. **Russell, F. A. and Deykin, D.**, The effect of thrombin on the uptake and transformation of arachidonic acid by human platelets, *Am. J. Hematol.,* 1, 59, 1976.
299. **Hamberg, M. and Samuelsson, B.**, Prostaglandin endoperoxides. Novel transformations of arachidonic acid in human platelets, *Proc. Natl. Acad. Sci. U.S.A.,* 71, 3400, 1974.
300. **Nugteren, D. H.**, Arachidonate lipoxygenase in blood platelets, *Biochim. Biophys. Acta,* 380, 299, 1975.
301. **Ho, P. P. K., Walters, C. P., and Sullivan, H. R.**, A particulate arachidonate lipoxygenase in human blood platelets, *Biochem. Biophys. Res. Comm.,* 76, 398, 1977.
302. **Turner, S. R., Tainer, J. A., and Lynn, W. S.**, Biogenesis of chemotactic molecules by the arachidonate lipoxygenase of platelets, *Nature (London),* 257, 680, 1975.
303. **Hamberg, M., Svensson, J., Wakabayashi, T., and Samuelsson, B.**, Isolation and structure of two prostaglandin endoperoxides that cause platelet aggregation, *Proc. Natl. Acad. Sci. U.S.A.,* 71, 345, 1974.
304. **Nugteren, D. H. and Hazelhof, E.**, Isolation and properties of intermediates in prostaglandin biosynthesis, *Biochim. Biophys. Acta,* 326, 448, 1973.
305. **Miyamoto, T., Yamamoto, S., and Hayaishi, O.**, Prostaglandin synthetase system — resolution into oxygenase and isomerase components, *Proc. Natl. Acad. Sci. U.S.A.,* 71, 3645, 1974.
306. **Egan, R. W., Paxton, J., and Kuehl, F. A., Jr.**, Mechanism for irreversible self-deactivation of prostaglandin synthetase, *J. Biol. Chem.,* 251, 7329, 1976.
307. **Van der Ouderaa, F. J., Buytenhek, M., Nugteren, D. H., and Van Dorp, D. A.**, Purification and characterization of prostaglandin endoperoxide synthetase from sheep vesicular glands, *Biochim. Biophys. Acta,* 487, 315, 1977.
308. **Hamberg, M., Svensson, J., and Samuelsson, B.**, Prostaglandin endoperoxides. A new concept concerning the mode of action and release of prostaglandins, *Proc. Natl. Acad. Sci. U.S.A.,* 71, 3824, 1974.
309. **Roth, G. J. and Majerus, P. W.**, The mechanism of the effect of aspirin on human platelets. I. Acetylation of a particulate fraction protein, *J. Clin. Invest.,* 56, 624, 1975.
310. **Roth, G. J., Stanford, N., and Majerus, P. W.**, Acetylation of prostaglandin synthetase by aspirin, *Proc. Natl. Acad. Sci. U.S.A.,* 72, 3073, 1975.
311. **Smith, J. B. and Willis, A. L.**, Aspirin selectively inhibits prostaglandin formation by human platelets, *Nature New Biol.,* 231, 236, 1971.
312. **Hamberg, M. and Fredholm, B. B.**, Isomerization of prostaglandin H_2 into prostaglandin D_2 in the presence of serum albumin, *Biochim. Biophys. Acta,* 431, 189, 1976.
313. **Christ-Hazelhof, E., Nugteren, D. H., and Van Dorp, D. A.**, Conversions of prostaglandin endoperoxides by glutathione-S-transferases and serum albumins, *Biochim. Biophys. Acta,* 450, 450, 1976.
314. **Hamberg, M., Svensson, J., and Samuelsson, B.**, Thromboxanes: a new group of biologically active compounds derived from prostaglandin endoperoxides, *Proc. Natl. Acad. Sci. U.S.A.,* 72, 2994, 1975.
315. **Sun, F. F.**, Biosynthesis of thromboxanes in human platelets. I. Characterization and assay of thromboxane synthetase, *Biochem. Biophys. Res. Commun.,* 74, 1432, 1977.
316. **Moncada, S., Gryglewski, R., Bunting, S., and Vane, J. R.**, An enzyme isolated from arteries transforms prostaglandin endoperoxides to an unstable substance that inhibits platelet aggregation, *Nature (London),* 263, 663, 1976.
317. **Johnson, R. A., Morton, D. R., Kinner, J. H., Gorman, R. R., McGuire, J. C., and Sun, F. F.**, The chemical structure of prostaglandin X (prostacyclin), *Prostaglandins,* 12, 195, 1976.

318. Smith, J. B., Silver, M. J., Ingerman, C. M., and Kocsis, J. J., Prostaglandin D_2 inhibits the aggregation of human platelets, *Thromb. Res.*, 5, 291, 1974.
319. Nishizawa, E. E., Miller, W. L., Gorman, R. R., Bundy, G. L., Svensson, J., and Hamberg, M., Prostaglandin D_2 as a potential antithrombotic agent, *Prostaglandins*, 9, 109, 1975.
320. Mills, D. C. B. and Macfarlane, D. E., Stimulation of human platelet adenylate cyclase by prostaglandin D_2, *Thromb. Res.*, 5, 401, 1974.
321. Kloeze, J., Influence of prostaglandins on platelet adhesiveness and platelet aggregation, in *Prostaglandins, Proceedings of the II Nobel Symposium*, Bergstrom, S. and Samuelsson, B., Eds., Interscience, London, 1966, 241.
322. Kloeze, J., Relationship between chemical structure and platelet-aggregation activity of prostaglandins, *Biochem. Biophys. Acta*, 187, 285, 1969.
323. Robison, G. A., Arnold, A., and Hartman, R. C., Divergent effects of epinephrine and prostaglandin E_1 on the level of cyclic AMP in human blood platelets, *Pharmacol. Res. Commun.*, 1, 325, 1973.
324. Harwood, J. P., Moskowitz, J., and Krishna, G., Dynamic interactions of prostaglandin and norepinephrine in the formation of adenosine 3′5′ monophosphate in human and rabbit platelets, *Biochim. Biophys. Acta*, 261, 444, 1972.
325. Malmsten, C., Hamberg, M., Svensson, J., and Samuelsson, B., Physiological role of an endoperoxide in human platelets: hemostatic defect due to platelet cyclo-oxygenase deficiency, *Proc. Natl. Acad. Sci. U.S.A.*, 72, 1446, 1975.
326. Willis, A. L., Vane, F. M., Kuhn, D. C., Scott, C. G., and Petrin, M., An endoperoxide aggregator (LASS), formed in platelets in response to thrombotic stimuli-purification, identification and unique biological significance, *Prostaglandins*, 8, 453, 1974.
327. Moncada, S., Gryglewski, R., Bunting, S., and Vane, J. R., An enzyme isolated from arteries transforms prostaglandin endoperoxides to an unstable substance that inhibits platelet aggregation, *Nature (London)*, 263, 663, 1976.
328. Gorman, R. R., Bunting, S., and Miller, O. V., Modulation of human platelet adenylate cyclase by prostacyclin (PGX), *Prostaglandins*, 13, 377, 1977.
329. Tateson, J. E., Moncada, S., and Vane, J. R., Effects of prostacyclin (PGX) on cyclic AMP concentrations in human platelets, *Prostaglandins*, 13, 389, 1977.
330. Needleman, P., Moncada, S., Bunting, S., Vane, J. R., Hamberg, M., and Samuelsson, B., Identification of an enzyme in platelet microsomes which generates thromboxane A_2 from prostaglandins, *Nature (London)*, 261, 558, 1976.
331. White, J. G., Fine structural alterations induced in platelets by adenosine diphosphate, *Blood*, 31, 604, 1968.
332. Zucker-Franklin, D., Nachman, R. L., and Marcus, A. J., Ultrastructure of thrombosthenin, the contractile protein of blood platelets, *Science*, 157, 945, 1967.
333. Behnke, O., Kristensen, B. I., and Nelson, L. E., Electron microscopical observations on actinoid and myosinoid filaments in blood platelets, *J. Ultrastruct. Res.*, 37, 351, 1971.
334. Nachman, R. L., Marcus, A. J., and Safier, L. B., Platelet thrombosthenin: subcellular localization and function, *J. Clin. Invest.*, 46, 1380, 1967.
335. Pollard, T. D., Fuijuwara, K., Handin, R., and Weiss, G., Contractile proteins in platelet activation and contraction, *Ann. N. Y. Acad. Sci.*, 283, 218, 1977.
336. Bouvier, C. A., Gabbiani, G., Ryan, G. B., Badonnel, M. C., Majno, G., and Lüscher, E. F., Binding of anti-actin autoantibodies to platelets, *Thromb. Haemostasis*, 37, 312, 1977.
337. Cohen, I. and DeVries, A., Platelet contractile regulation in an isometric system, *Nature (London)*, 246, 36, 1973.
338. White, J. G., Platelet microtubules and microfilaments: effects of cytochalasin B on structure and function, in *Platelet Aggregation*, Caen, J., Ed., Masson et Cie, Paris, 1971, 15.
339. Spudich, J. A. and Lin, S., Cytochalasin B, its interaction with actin and actomyosin from muscle, *Proc. Natl. Acad. Sci. U.S.A.*, 69, 442, 1972.
340. Haslam, R. J., Davidson, M. M. L., and McClenaghan, M. D., Cytochalasin B, the blood platelet release reaction and cyclic GMP, *Nature (London)*, 253, 455, 1975.
341. Adelstein, R. S. and Conti, M. A., The characterization of contractile proteins from platelet and fibroblasts, *Cold Spring Harbor Symp. Quant. Biol.*, 37, 599, 1972.
342. Daniel, J. L. and Adelstein, R. S., Isolation and properties of platelet myosin light chain kinase, *Biochemistry*, 15, 2370, 1976.
343. Adelstein, R. S. and Conti, M. A., Phosphorylation of platelet myosin increases actin-activated myosin ATPase activity, *Nature (London)*, 256, 597, 1975.
344. Daniel, J. L., Holmsen, H., and Adelstein, R. S., Thrombin-stimulated myosin phosphorylation in intact platelets and its possible involvement in secretion, *Thromb. Haemostasis*, 38, 984, 1977.
345. Lyons, R. M., Stanford, N., and Majerus, P. W., Thrombin-induced protein phosphorylation in human platelets, *J. Clin. Invest.*, 56, 924, 1975.

346. **Haslam, R. J. and Lynham, J. A.**, Increased phosphorylation of specific blood proteins in association with the release reaction, *Biochem. Soc. Trans.*, 4, 694, 1976.
347. **Boyle-Kay, F. M. and Fudenberg, H. H.**, Inhibition and reversal of platelet activation by cytochalasin B or cocemid, *Nature (London)*, 244, 288, 1973.
348. **Nachmias, V. and Asch, A.**, Regulation and polarity: results with myxomycate plasmodium and with human platelets, *Cold Spring Harbor Conf. Cell Proliferation*, 3, 771, 1976.
349. **Aledort, L. M., Hirsch, C., Udkow, M., and Puszkin, E.**, Effect of anticoagulants on calcium and magnesium content of human platelets, *Transfusion*, 9, 212, 1969.
350. **Cousin, C. and Caen, J.**, Dosage du magnesium et du calcium dans les plaquettes sanguines humaines, *Rev. Fr. Etud. Clin. Biol.*, 9, 520, 1964.
351. **Lages, B., Scrutton, M. C., and Holmsen, H.**, Studies on gel filtered human platelets: isolation and characterization in a medium containing no added Ca^{2+}, Mg^{2+}, K^{+}, *J. Lab. Clin. Med.*, 85, 811, 1975.
352. **Murer, E. H. and Holme, R.**, A study of the release of calcium from human blood platelets and its inhibition by metabolic inhibitors, N-ethylmaleimide and aspirin, *Biochim. Biophys. Acta*, 222, 197, 1970.
353. **Detwiler, T. C. and Feinman, R. D.**, Kinetics of the thrombin-induced release of calcium (II) by platelets, *Biochemistry*, 12, 282, 1973.
354. **Lages, B., Scrutton, M. C., and Holmsen, H.**, Secretion by gel filtered human platelets: response of platelet Ca^{2+}, Mg^{2+}, and K^{+} to secretory agents, *J. Lab. Clin. Med.*, in press, 1977.
355. **Lages, B., Scrutton, M. C., Holmsen, H., Day, H. J., and Weiss, H. J.**, Metal ion contents of gel-filtered platelets from patients with storage pool disease, *Blood*, 46, 119, 1975.
356. **Boxer, G. J., Holmsen, H., Robkin, L., Bang, N. U., Boxer, L. A., and Baehner, R. L.**, Abnormal platelet function in Chediak-Higashi syndrome, *Br. J. Haematol.*, 35, 521, 1977.
357. **Skaer, R. J., Peters, P. D., and Emmines, J. P.**, The localization of calcium and phosphorus in human platelets, *J. Cell Sci.*, 15, 679, 1974.
358. **Fukami, M. H. and Bauer, J.**, An improved method for the isolation of serotonin storage granules from human platelets, *Fed. Proc.*, 36 (Abstr.), 4285, 1977.
359. **Grette, K.**, Relaxing factor in extracts of blood platelets and its function in the cells, *Nature (London)*, 198, 188, 1963.
360. **Statland, B. E., Heagan, B. M., and White, J. G.**, Uptake of calcium of platelets relaxing factor, *Nature (London)*, 223, 521, 1969.
361. **Robblee, L. S., Shepro, D., and Belamarich, F. A.**, Calcium uptake and associated adenosine triphosphatase activity of isolated platelet membranes, *J. Gen. Physiol.*, 61, 462, 1976.
362. **Kaser-Ganzmann, R., Jakabova, M., George, J. N., and Lüscher, E. F.**, Stimulation of calcium uptake in platelet membrane vesicles by adenosine 3′,5′-cyclic monophosphate and protein kinase, *Biochim. Biophys. Acta*, 466, 429, 1977.
363. **Feinman, R. D. and Detwiler, T. C.**, Platelet secretion induced by divalent cation ionophores, *Nature (London)*, 249, 172, 1974.
364. **Massini, P. and Lüscher, E. F.**, Some effects of ionophores for divalent cations on blood platelets. Comparison with the effects of thrombin, *Biochim. Biophys. Acta*, 372, 109, 1974.
365. **White, J. G., Rao, G. H. R., and Gerrard, J. M.**, Effects of the ionophore A23187 on blood platelets. I. Influence on aggregation and secretion, *Am. J. Pathol.*, 77, 135, 1974.
366. **Murer, E. H., Stewart, G. J., Rausch, M. A., and Day, H. J.**, Calcium ionophore A23187 (Eli Lilly). Effect on platelet function, structure and metabolism, *Thromb. Diath. Haemorrh.*, 34, 72, 1975.
367. **Kinlough-Rathbone, R. L., Chahil, A., Packham, M. A., Reimers, H. J., and Mustard, J. F.**, Effect of A23187 on thrombin-degranulated washed rabbit platelet, *Thromb. Res.*, 7, 435, 1975.
368. **Feinstein, M. B. and Fraser, C.**, Human platelet secretion and aggregation induced by calcium ionophores. Inhibition by PGE_1 and dibutyryl cyclic AMP, *J. Gen. Physiol.*, 66, 561, 1975.
369. **Holmsen, H. and Setowsky-Dangelmaier, C. A.**, Adenine nucleotide metabolism of blood platelets. X. Formaldehyde stops centrifugation-induced secretion after A23187 stimulation and causes breakdown of metabolic ATP, *Biochim. Biophys. Acta*, 497, 46, 1977.
370. **Charo, I. F., Feinman, R. D., and Detwiler, T. C.**, Inhibition of platelet secretion by an antagonist of intracellular calcium, *Biochem. Biophys. Res. Commun.*, 72, 1462, 1976.
371. **Kinlough-Rathbone, R. L., Chahil, A., and Mustard, J. F.**, Divalent cations and the release reaction of pig platelets, *Am. J. Physiol.*, 226, 235, 1974.
372. **Robblee, L. S., Shepro, D., Belamarich, F. A., and Towle, C.**, Platelet calcium flux and the release reaction, *Ser. Haematol.*, 6, 311, 1973.
373. **Salzman, E. W. and Weisenberger, H.**, Role of cyclic AMP in platelet function. IV. Cardiovascular pharmacology, *Adv. Cyclic Nucleotide Res.*, 1, 231, 1972.
374. **Bishop, G. A. and Rozenberg, M. C.**, The effect of ADP, calcium and some inhibitors of platelet aggregation on protein phosphokinases from human blood platelets, *Biochim. Biophys. Acta*, 384, 112, 1975.

375. Steiner, M., Endogenous phosphorylation of platelet membrane proteins, *Arch. Biochem. Biophys.*, 171, 245, 1975.
376. Booyse, F. M., Marr, J., Yang, D. C., Guiliani, D., and Rafelson, M. E., Jr., Adenosine cyclic 3′,5′ monphosphate-dependent protein kinase from human platelets, *Biochim. Biophys. Acta,* 422, 60, 1976.
377. Assaf, S. A., Human platelet protein kinase phosphorylation reaction with platelet membrane and cytoplasmic enzymes and crystallization of a cyclic AMP-independent protein kinase, *Ann. N. Y. Acad. Sci.*, 283, 159, 1977.
378. Lyons, R. M., Stanford, N., and Majerus, P. W., Thrombin-induced protein phosphorylation in human platelets, *J. Clin. Invest.*, 56, 924, 1975.
379. Haslam, R. J. and Lynham, J. A., Increased phosphorylation of specific blood platelet proteins in association with the release reaction, *Biochem. Soc. Trans.*, 4, 694, 1976.
380. Holmsen, H., Classification and possible mechanisms of action of some drugs that inhibit platelet aggregation, *Ser. Haematol.*, 8, 50, 1976.
381. Huxley, A. F., Muscular contraction, *J. Physiol.*, 243, 1, 1974.
382. White, J. G., Interaction of membrane systems in blood platelets, *Am. J. Pathol.*, 66, 295, 1972.
383. Salzman, E. W. and Levine, L., Cyclic 3′,5′-adenosine monophosphate in human blood platelets. II. Effect of N^6-2′-0-dibutytyl cyclic 3′,5′-adenosine monophosphate on platelet function, *J. Clin. Invest.*, 50, 131, 1971.
384. Brodie, G. N., Baenziger, N. L., Chase, L. R., and Majerus, P. W., The effects of thrombin on adenyl cyclase activity and a membrane protein from human platelets, *J. Clin. Invest.*, 51, 81, 1972.
385. Haslam, R. J., Interactions of the pharmacological receptors of blood platelets with adenylate cyclase, *Ser. Haematol.*, 6, 333, 1973.
386. Krishna, G. and Harwood, J. P., Requirement for guanosine triphosphate in the prostaglandin activation of adenylate cyclase of platelet membranes, *J. Biol. Chem.*, 247, 2253, 1972.
387. McDonald, J. W. D. and Stuart, R. K., Regulation of cyclic AMP levels and aggregation in human platelets by prostaglandin E_1, *J. Lab. Clin. Med.*, 81, 838, 1973.
388. Mills, D. C. B. and Macfarlane, D. E., Stimulation of human platelet adenylate cyclase by prostaglandin D_2, *Thromb. Res.*, 5, 401, 1974.
389. Mills, D. C. B. and Smith, J. B., The influence on platelet aggregation of drugs that affect the accumulation of adenosine 3′,5′-cyclic monophosphate in platelets, *Biochem. J.*, 121, 185, 1971.
390. Robinson, G., Cole, B., Arnold, A., and Hartmann, R., Effects of prostaglandins on function and cyclic AMP levels of human blood platelets, *Ann. N. Y. Acad. Sci.*, 180, 324, 1971.
391. Smith, J. B., Silver, M. J., Ingerman, C. M., and Kocsis, J. J., Prostaglandin D_2 inhibits the aggregation of human platelets, *Thromb. Res.*, 5, 291, 1974.
392. Vigdahl, R. L., Mongin, J., and Marquis, N. R., Platelet aggregation. IV. Platelet phosphodiesterase and its inhibition by vasodilators, *Biochem. Biophys. Res. Commun.*, 42, 1088, 1971.
393. Amer, M. S. and Mayol, R. F., Studies with phosphodiesterase. III. Two forms of the enzyme from blood platelets, *Biochim. Biophys. Acta,* 309, 149, 1973.
394. Song, S. Y. and Cheung, W. Y., Cyclic 3′,5′-nucleotide phosphodiesterase: properties of the enzyme of human blood platelets, *Biochim. Biophys. Acta,* 242, 593, 1971.
395. Hodaka, H. and Asano, T., Human blood platelet 3′,5′-cyclic nucleotide phosphodiesterase: isolation of low-km and high-km phosphodiesterase, *Biochim. Biophys. Acta,* 429, 485, 1976.
396. Markwardt, F. and Hoffman, A., Effects of papaverine on cyclic AMP phosphodiesterase of human platelets, *Biochem. Pharmacol.*, 19, 2519, 1970.
397. Salzman, E W., Rubino, E. B., and Sims, R. V., Cyclic 3′,5′-adenosine monophosphate in human blood platelets. III. The role of cyclic AMP in platelet aggregation, *Ser. Haematol.*, 3, 100, 1970.
398. Gerrard, J. M., Peterson, D., Townsend, D., and White, J. G., Prostaglandins and platelet contraction, *Circulation,* 54 (Abstr.), 767, 1976.
399. Lebreton, G. C., Sandler, W. C., and Feinberg, H., Effect of D_2O and chlortertracycline on ADP-induced platelet shape change and aggregation, *Thromb. Res.*, 8, 477, 1976.
400. LeBreton, G. C., Dinerstein, R. J., Roth, L. J., and Feinberg, H., Direct evidence for intracellular divalent cation redistribution associated with platelet shape change, *Biochem. Biophys. Res. Commun.*, 71, 362, 1976.
401. Lapetina, E. G., Schmitges, C. J., Chandrabose, K., and Cuatrecasas, P., Cyclic adenosine 3′,5′-monophosphate and prostacyclin inhibit membrane phospholipase activity in platelets, *Biochem. Biophys. Res. Commun.*, 76, 828, 1977.
402. Cohen, I., Kaminski, E., and DeVries, A., Actin-linked regulation of the human platelet contractile system, *FEBS Lett.*, 34, 315, 1973.
403. Thorens, S., Schau, M. C., and Lüscher, E. F., A calcium-sensitizing system from human platelets and its activity on muscle and platelet actomyosin, *Experientia,* 29, 349, 1973.
404. Daniel, J. L. and Adelstein, R. S., Isolation and properties of platelet myosin light chain kinase, *Biochemistry,* 15, 2370, 1976.

405. **Crawford, N.**, Platelet microfilaments and microtubules, in *Platelets in Biology and Pathology*, Gordon, J. L., Ed., Elsevier/North-Holland, Amsterdam, 1976, 121.
406. **Haslam, R. J. and McClenaghan, M. D.**, Effects of collagen and of aspirin on the concentration of guanosine 3′,5′-cyclic monophosphate in human blood platelets: measurement by a prelabeling technique, *Biochem. J.*, 138, 317, 1974.
407. **Haslam, R. J.**, Roles of cyclic nucleotides in platelet function, in *Biochemistry and Pharmacology of Platelets, Ciba Found. Symp.*, 35, 121, 1975.
408. **Rodan, G. A. and Feinstein, M. B.**, Interrelationships between Ca^{2+} and adenylate and guanylate cyclases in control of platelet secretion and aggregation, *Proc. Natl. Acad. Sci. U.S.A.*, 73, 1829, 1976.
409. **Chiang, T. M., Dixit, S. N., and Kang, A. H.**, Effect of cyclic 3′,5′-guanosine monophosphate on human platelet function, *J. Lab. Clin. Med.*, 88, 215, 1976.
410. **Glass, D. B., Fry, W., III, Carr, D. W., and Goldberg, N. D.**, Stimulation of human platelet guanylate cyclase by fatty acids, *J. Biol. Chem.*, 252, 1279, 1977.
411. **Agarwal, K. C. and Steiner, M.**, Effect of serotonin on cyclic nucleotides of human platelets, *Biochem. Biophys. Res. Commun.*, 69, 962, 1976.

PLATELET ULTRASTRUCTURE*

Dorothea Zucker-Franklin and George Grusky

Since the properties and functions of blood platelets are discussed in detail elsewhere in this volume, this chapter will be devoted entirely to a description of the ultrastructural features of the cell that are believed to subserve these functions. For the sake of clarity, schematic drawings of platelets in cross and longitudinal thin section (±600 Å) have been included to aid the reader in identifying structures represented in the electron micrographs.

In the circulation, platelets are disc-shaped anuclear cells with a diameter of 1.5 to 3.0 μm. The schematic drawings in Figures 1A and 1B** represent idealized equatorial and longitudinal sections, respectively. The thin sections used for electron microscopy can only be approximations of these planes. Insofar as possible, the discussion will follow the sequence of the structures encountered from the outside to the inside of the cell.

The platelet, like any other mammalian cell, is limited by a trilaminar membrane, i.e., the plasma membrane. Like other membranes, it is rich in phospholipids; however, the phospholipids in the platelet membrane seem to be organized in a manner that is particularly favorable for fulfilling the function of platelet factor 3.[1] It will be recalled that platelet factor 3 is not a real factor, but rather the property of platelet membranes that causes them to interact with plasma-clotting factors in the coagulation cascade.[2] The external surface of the membrane bears a coat that is rich in acid mucopolysaccharides and glycoproteins.[3,4] In Figure 2, this coat material has been delineated with the help of ruthenium red.[5]

Although its biochemical constituents have not been fully analyzed, it seems likely, on the basis of morphological observations, that the platelet coat plays a role in platelet adhesion and aggregation. During platelet aggregation, "bridges" form between adjacent platelets (Figure 3A). These bridges appear to consist of coat material.[6] Moreover, when platelets are aggregated with collagen, such bridges can also be resolved between platelets and the periodic dense bands of the collagen fibril[7] (Figure 3B), which underscores the widely held theory that the multimeric conformation of fibrillar collagen has a crucial effect on platelets.[8-11] The coat material remains associated with the platelet membrane during all phases of adhesion, aggregation, and release.

At the cytoplasmic aspect of the plasma membrane, 7 nm filaments oriented parallel and at right angles to the membrane may be resolved (Figure 4).[12] It is believed that external stimuli are transmitted via the membrane to the submembranous filaments and that the latter mediate the complicated contour changes platelets undergo during aggregation and thrombus formation. The plasma membrane with its surface coat and submembranous filaments invaginates to form the so-called open canalicular system (Figures 5 to 8). Whether or not all components of this system remain in continuity with the extracellular environment has not been fully elucidated. It is clear, however, that any substance or particle that adheres to the membrane will eventually become interiorized in this fashion. Figures 5 to 7 illustrate how a soluble substance (peroxidase), a small particulate substance (ferritin), and a large particle (latex) are taken into this surface-connecting system. This process requires energy. When both oxidative phosphorylation and glycolysis are inhibited, the canalicular system remains distended and apparently in continuity with the exterior (Figure 8).[13] In sections that do not show

* Supported by USPHS Research Grants nos. AM12274 and AM01431.

** All figures for this chapter follow text.

the continuity of the canalicular spaces with the surface, the structures nevertheless remain identifiable by virtue of the submembranous filaments that occupy their cytoplasmic aspect (Figure 9). The membrane system just described is also responsible for the demarcation of individual platelet "fields" within the giant platelets that are often seen in blood specimens of patients with accelerated thrombocytopoiesis (Figure 10). Whether such giant platelets will disintegrate in circulating blood to give rise to individual platelets is not certain.

In the peripheral cytoplasm of the intact, well-fixed platelet, it is difficult to resolve any filaments, but a circumferential band of microtubules is a striking feature (Figures 1, 2, 11, and 12). The microtubules appear to subserve a cytoskeletal function, i.e., they maintain the asymmetric shape of the cell. Microtubules are also occasionally seen in the pseudopods of platelets that have been involved in the clotting process (Figure 13). Like microtubules in other cells, they depolymerize at 4°C and following treatment with colchicine or vincristine. In the process of platelet aggregation, the annular band of microtubules may also disappear and be transiently replaced by a band of microfilaments (Figure 14).[6] Therefore, it is possible that circumferentially oriented filaments consist of tubulin rather than actin, although this has not been proven. During the release reaction induced by aggregating agents or when platelets are subjected to a hypotonic environment, 7 nm filaments become visible throughout the platelet cytoplasm (Figure 9), as well as in pseudopods forming under such conditions (Figure 15). It has been established beyond reasonable doubt that these filaments represent the contractile proteins of platelets which were first extracted and recognized by Bettex-Galland and Lüscher in 1959.[14] The 7 nm filaments can be "decorated" with heavy meromyosin (HMM^{S-1}) *in situ* or when extracted and purified in vitro. All actin filaments examined to date have had the ability to form ATP-dissociable complexes with HMM.[15,16] The characteristic "arrowhead" complexes which form in vitro when HMM is reacted with filaments extracted from platelets are illustrated in Figure 16.[17] Biochemical analysis has confirmed that the thin filaments are similar, though not identical, to muscle actin.[18,19]

As in smooth muscle, the morphologic demonstration of myosin was more difficult. Moreover, the content of myosin in platelets is very low when compared to the concentration of actin.[20] The first observation suggesting that myosin could be demonstrated *in situ* was the appearance of tactoids when platelets were exposed to high concentrations of $MgCl_2$ and ATP (Figure 17A.)[17] Under similar conditions, myosin polymerized in trypsin-treated smooth muscle.[21-23] Myosin was subsequently extracted and characterized morphologically (Figure 17B)[17] as well as biochemically.[24] These contractile proteins are estimated to constitute about 15% of the total protein of the cell. However, their precise function, i.e., how they translate their interaction into mechanoskeletal deformation of the cell is not yet fully understood. The recognition that the submembranous filaments are oriented parallel as well as at right angles to the plasma and canalicular membranes has led us to postulate that they are instrumental in effecting a peristaltic movement throughout this system.[12] In fact, during aggregation when the canalicular system becomes displaced toward the center of the cell, its various components appear to become connected by filaments (Figure 18).

Apart from the open canalicular system, the platelet possesses an organelle referred to as the dense tubular system because it usually contains an amorphous substance that is similar in electron density to the cytoplasm.[3] To date, the function of this membrane system has generated more speculation than information. The only experimental evidence available so far indicates that the system contains a peroxidase or catalase-like enzyme[25,26] that is based on its reactivity with H_2O_2 and 2,3 diaminobenzidine used for demonstrating such enzymes on the ultrastructural level.[27]

Among the most conspicuous organelles of the platelet are the granules, which are easily resolved with the light microscope. Since the granules disappear during the release reaction, much effort has been expended in investigating their functional significance. How fragmentary the relevant data still are is therefore amazing. Morphologically, the granules appear heterogeneous, which to a certain extent has been substantiated by biochemical analysis of the isolated structures. Some of the granules may be classified as lysosomes since they have been shown to contain acid hydrolases.[28] Other granules are extremely electron dense (Figure 19). Since the number of these very dense granules appears to be directly proportional to the serotonin content of the platelet,[29] it is believed that they contain 5-hydroxytryptamine and perhaps also the nonmetabolic pool of adenine nucleotides and catecholamines. However, independent of their morphology or biochemical content, all granules appear to clump in the center of the platelet prior to their dissolution during the release phenomenon (Figure 20).

In addition to the structures already described, the platelet possesses a few mitochondria and a variable number of glycogen particles (Figure 2), which play the same role in energy metabolism as they do in other cells. Ribosomes and rare profiles of rough endoplasmic reticulum are only seen in very young platelets in conditions of accelerated thrombocytopoiesis.

Finally, it should be added that all the structures mentioned in this survey with the exception of the 7 nm filaments have also been identified in replicas obtained from freeze-fractured platelets (Figure 21). The possibility that there are membrane specializations that may account for the unique function of the platelet in coagulation and hemostasis is currently under intense study by this method.

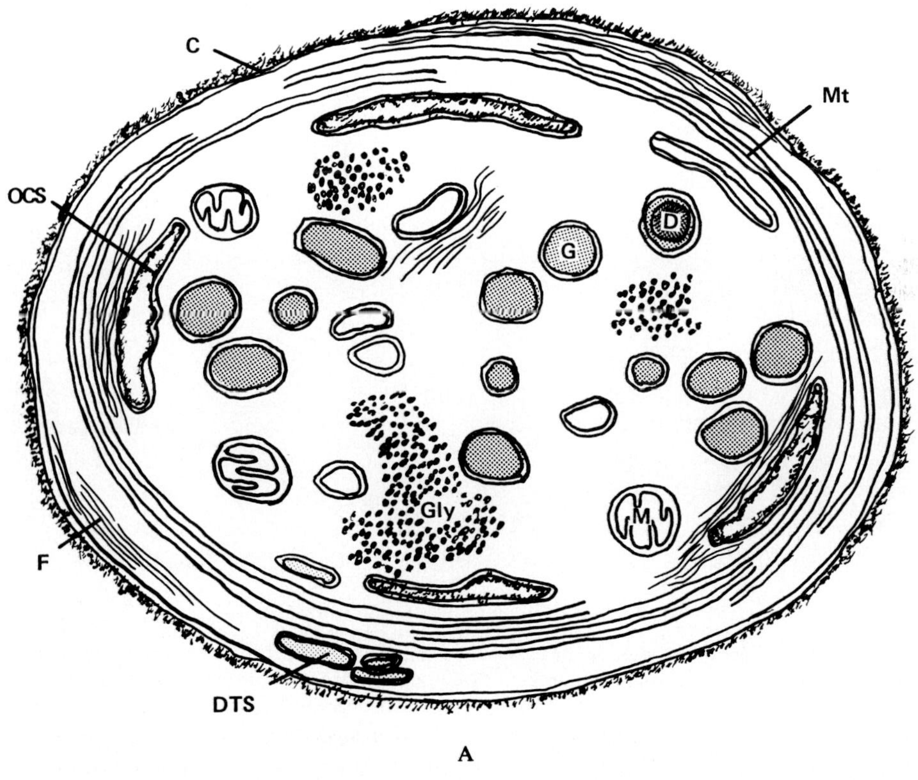

A

FIGURE 1. Schematic drawing of a circulating platelet in equatorial section (A) and in cross section (B) showing a characteristic complement of organelles. Key = C—coat; Mt — microtubules; OCS — open canalicular system; DTS — dense tubular system; M — mitochondria; G — granules; D — dense granules; Gly — glycogen; F — filaments.

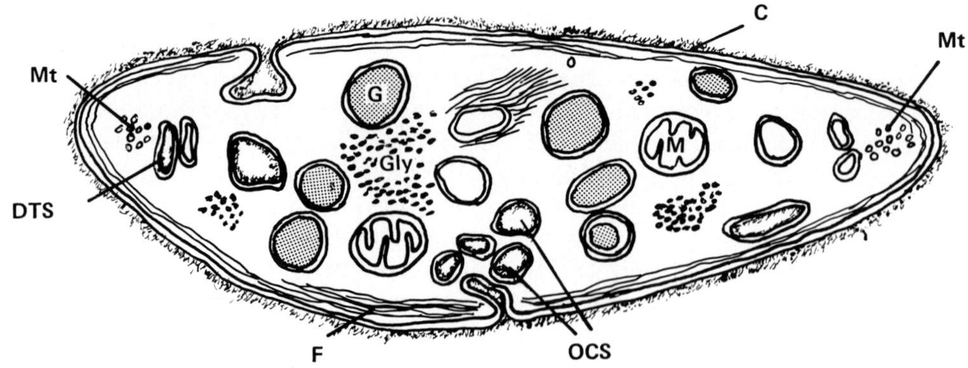

FIGURE 1B

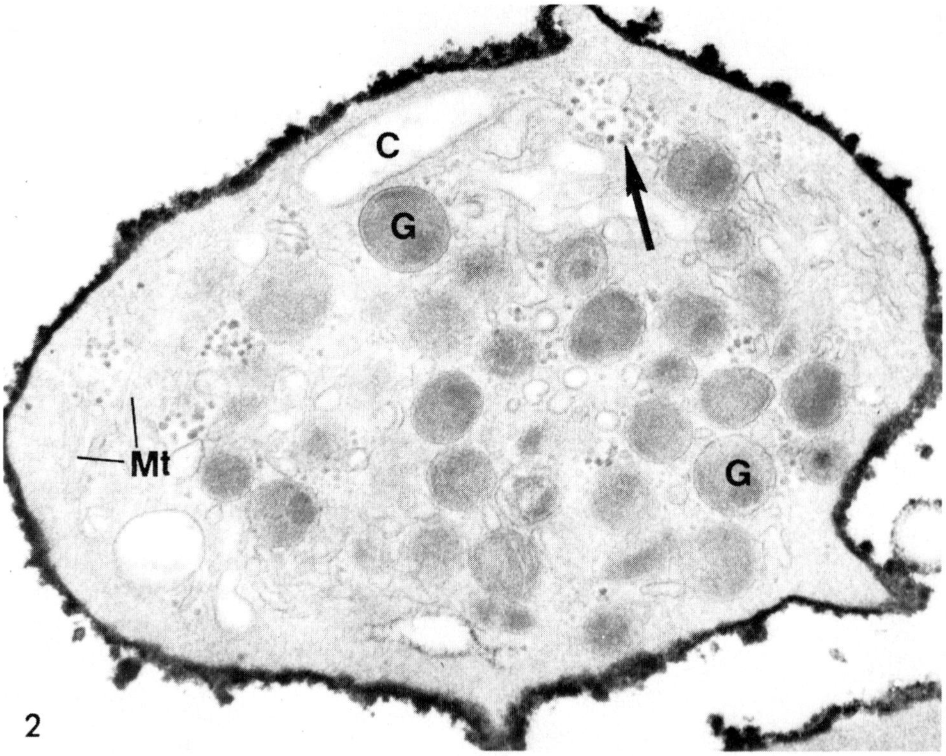

FIGURE 2. Glutaraldehyde fixation in the presence of ruthenium red has enhanced the electron density of the platelet coat. The coat averages 20 nm in thickness and is composed of sulfated acid mucopolysaccharides derived from the megakaryocyte. It is associated with both the surface membranes and those that compose the open canalicular system. G — granule; glycogen (arrow); Mt — microtubules; G — canalicular system. (Magnification × 34,000.)

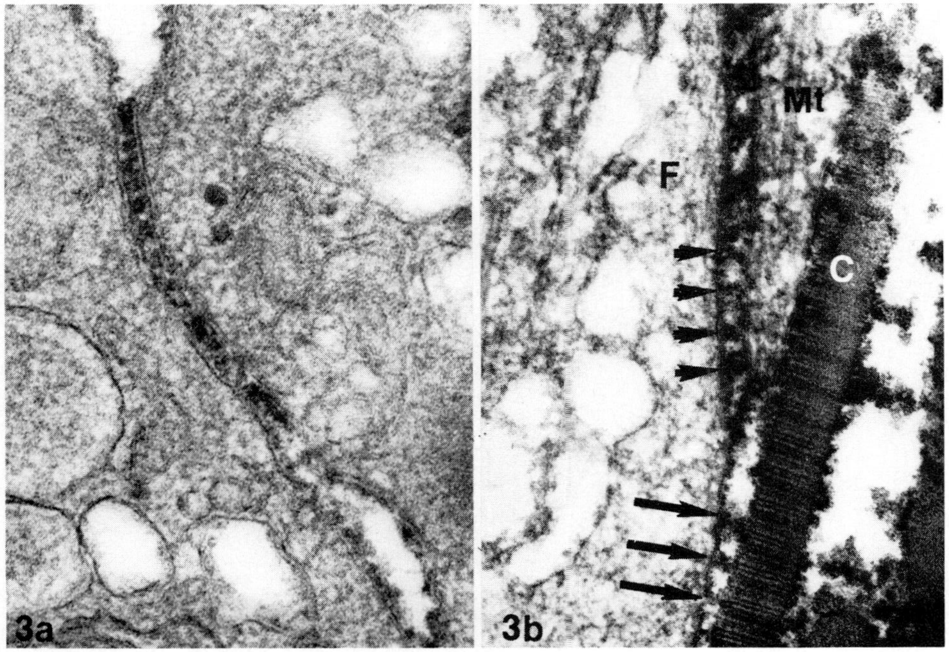

FIGURE 3. (A) Detail of platelets aggregated with 10^{-3} M ADP and fixed in glutaraldehyde containing ruthenium red. Electron dense bridges are located between the membranes of adjacent platelets at regular intervals. The membranes involved appear morphologically unaltered. (Magnification × 125,000.) (B) Detail of platelets aggregated with purified cartilage collagen (C) and fixed in the presence of ruthenium red. "Bridges" between adjacent platelets (short arrows) demonstrate the same spacing as those formed between a platelet and collagen (long arrows). Microtubules (Mt) and microfilaments (F) are visible within the platelet cytoplasm. (Magnification × 78,000.)

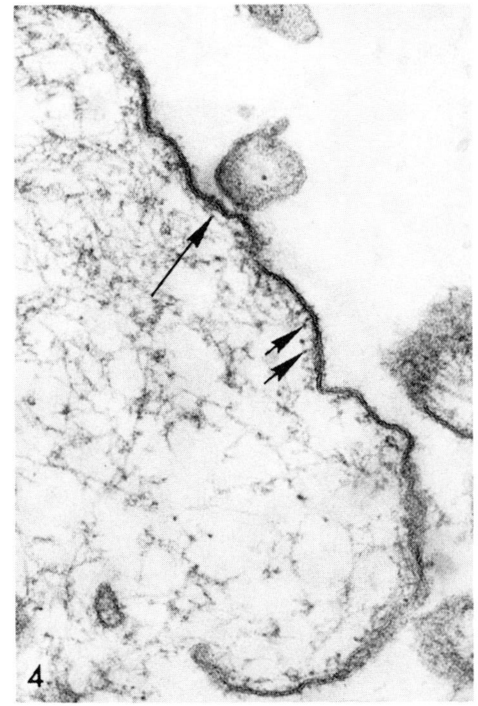

FIGURE 4. Osmotic shock has revealed the presence of filaments in close association with the cytoplasmic surfaces of the platelet membrane systems. Situated at a distance of ±10 nm from the membrane and having a spacing of ±15 nm, the filaments average 7 nm in diameter and may be seen in both longitudinal section (long arrows) and in cross section (short arrows). (Magnification × 81,000.)

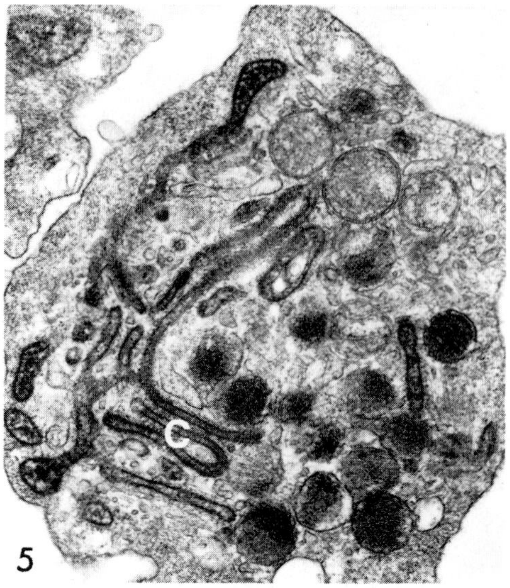

FIGURE 5. Platelet incubated with horseradish peroxidase at 37°C followed by treatment with diaminobenzidine in the presence of hydrogen peroxide prior to post fixation in osmium tetroxide. The open canalicular system (C) is clearly delineated by the deposition of an electron dense precipitate. (Magnification × 17,000.)

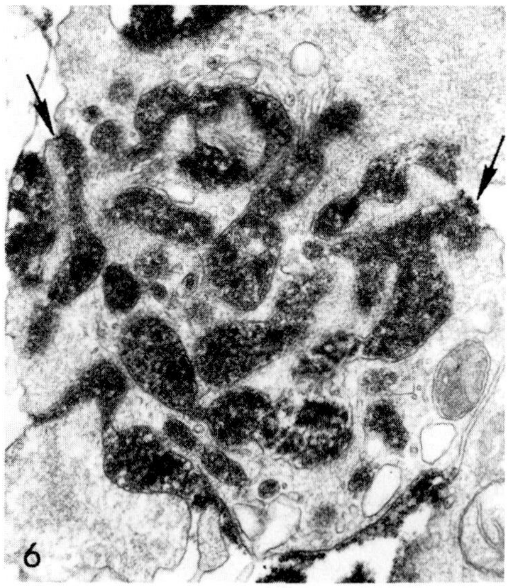

FIGURE 6. Platelet incubated with cationized ferritin shows interiorization and concentration of the electron dense particles within the open canalicular system. Arrows indicate continuity between the OCS and the platelet exterior. (Magnification × 31,000.)

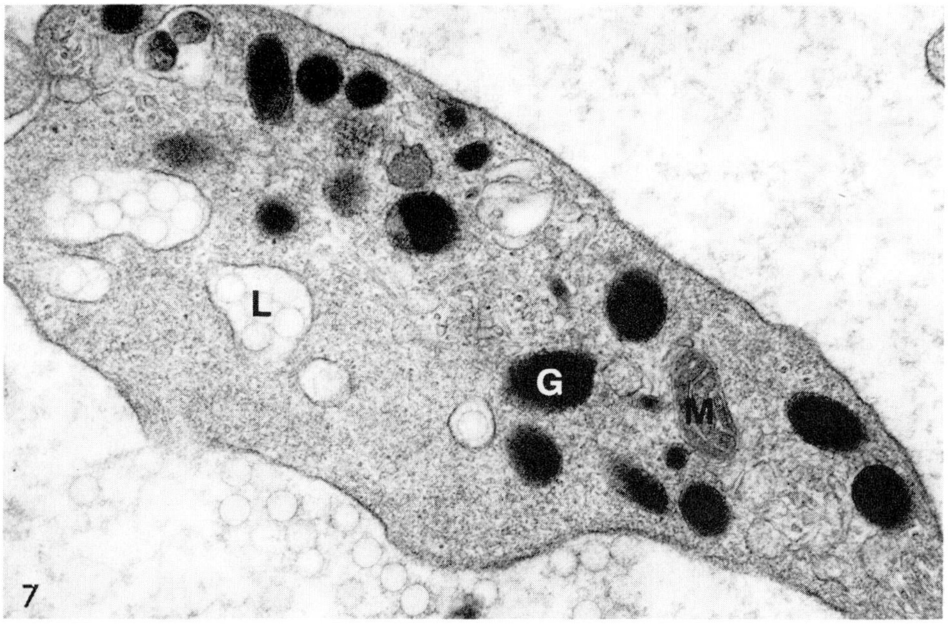

FIGURE 7. Platelet after incubation at 37°C with 0.3 μm latex particles. Although dependent on energy metabolism, the process may not represent true phagocytosis, but rather the pari passu interiorization by membrane flow of particles (L) adherent to the platelet surface. G — granules; M — mitochondrion. (Magnification × 32,000.)

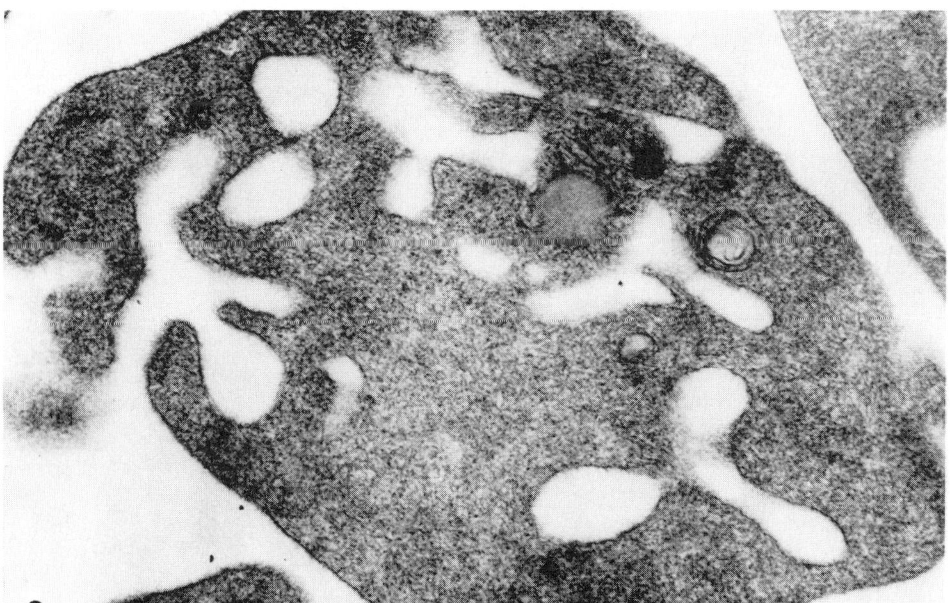

FIGURE 8. Platelet after incubation in a nitrogen atmosphere in the presence of 10^{-4} M sodium iodoacetate. The dilatation of the open canalicular system clearly demonstrates its continuity with the platelet exterior. (Magnification × 43,000.)

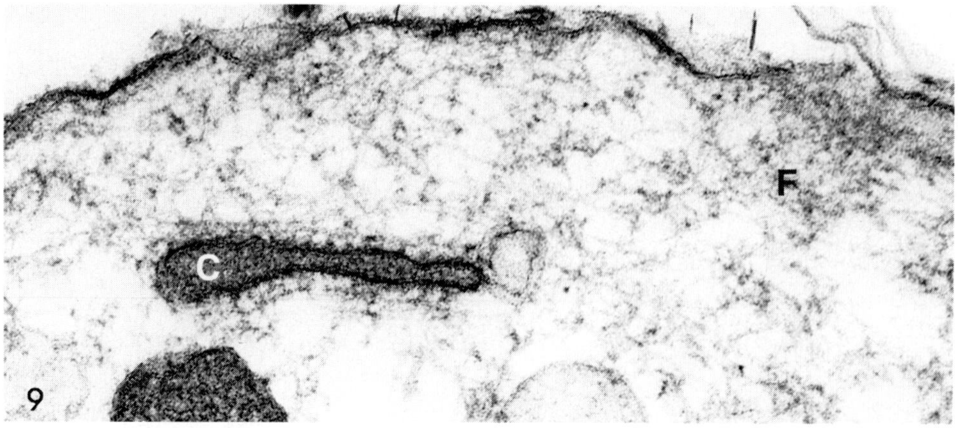

FIGURE 9. Detail of platelet cytoplasm after osmotic shock. Filaments are associated with the canalicular system (C) seen in longitudinal and cross section. In addition cytoplasmic 7 nm filaments (F) are clearly evident throughout the platelet cytoplasm and below the plasma membrane. (Magnification × 101,000.)

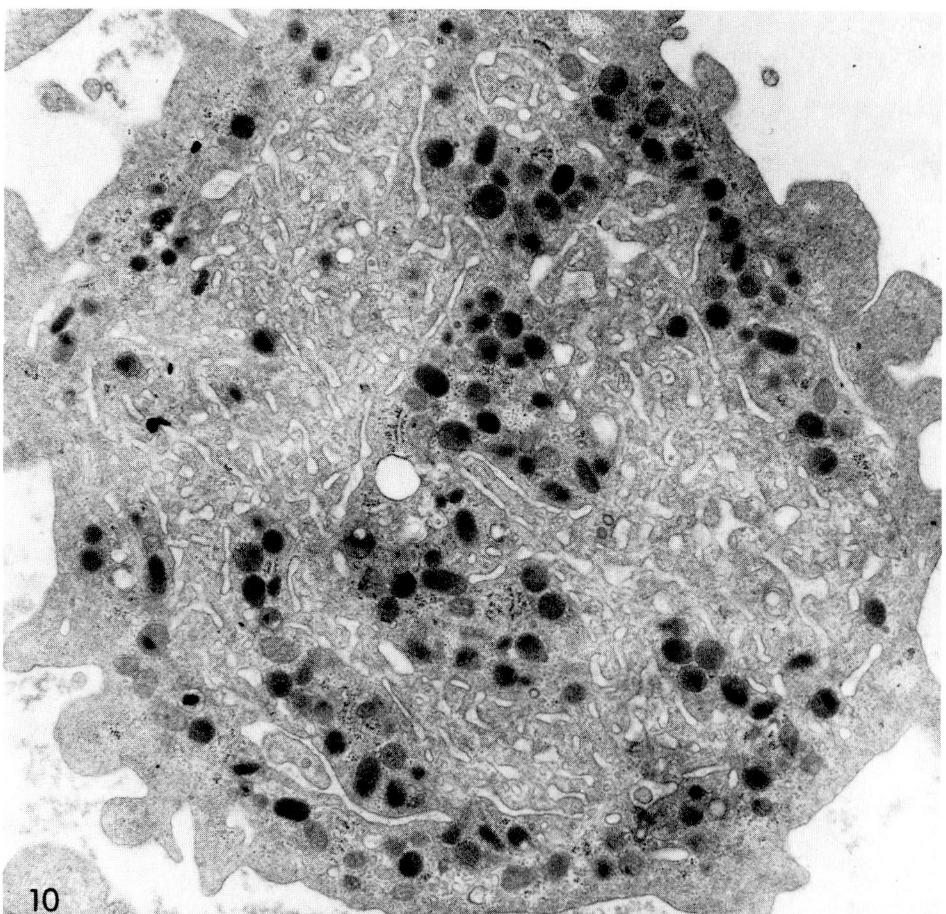

FIGURE 10. Giant platelet containing an extensive membrane system demarcating individual platelet fields. (Magnification × 15,000.)

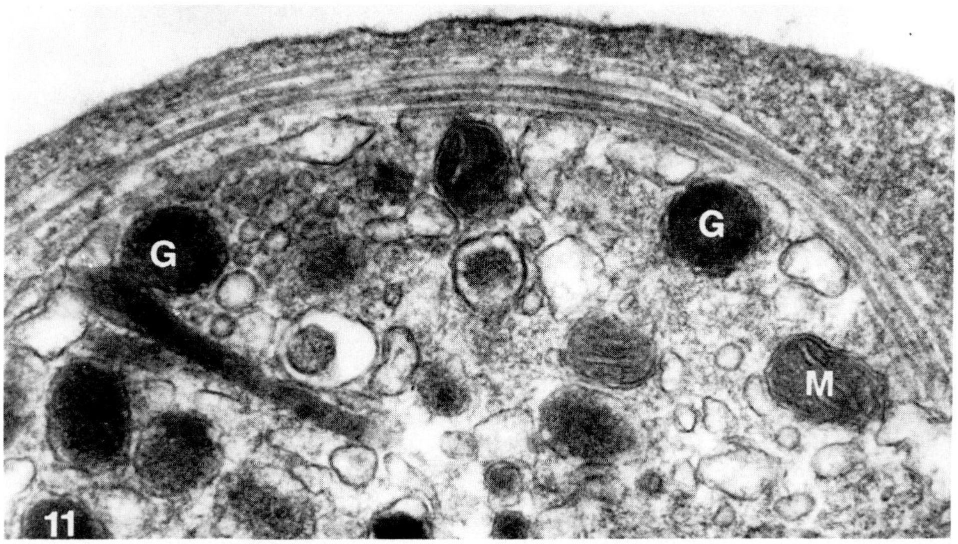

FIGURE 11. The circumferential band of microtubules may be seen in longitudinal aspect of platelets which have been sectioned through the equatorial plane. Their function appears to be cytoskeletal, since the disappearance of the intact tubules is accompanied by the loss of the characteristic discoid shape. G — granules; M — mitochondrion. (Magnification × 50,000.)

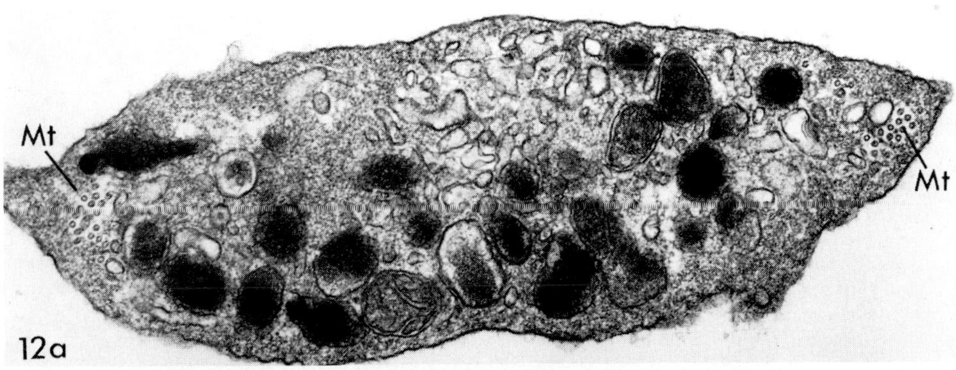

FIGURE 12a. In cross section, 10—20 microtubules (Mt) may be seen at either end of the platelet profile. (Magnification × 36,000.)

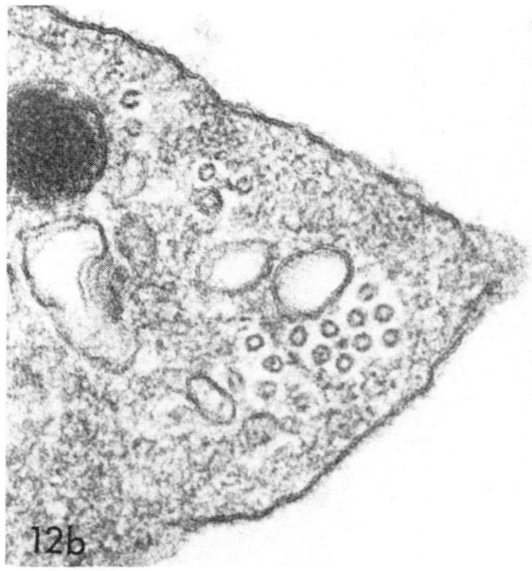

FIGURE 12b. Detail of the platelet illustrated in Figure 12a shows the circumferential band of microtubules at higher magnification. (Magnification × 87,000.)

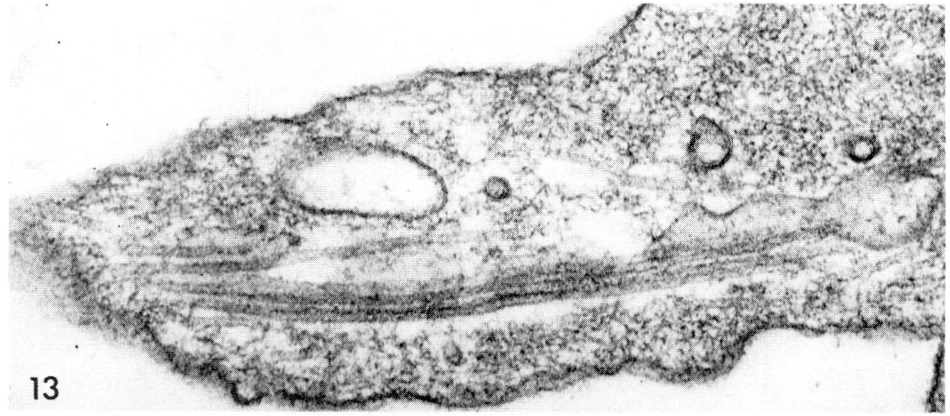

FIGURE 13. Pseudopod of platelet formed during clotting. Microtubules appear to run in parallel with extended process. (Magnification × 9,000.)

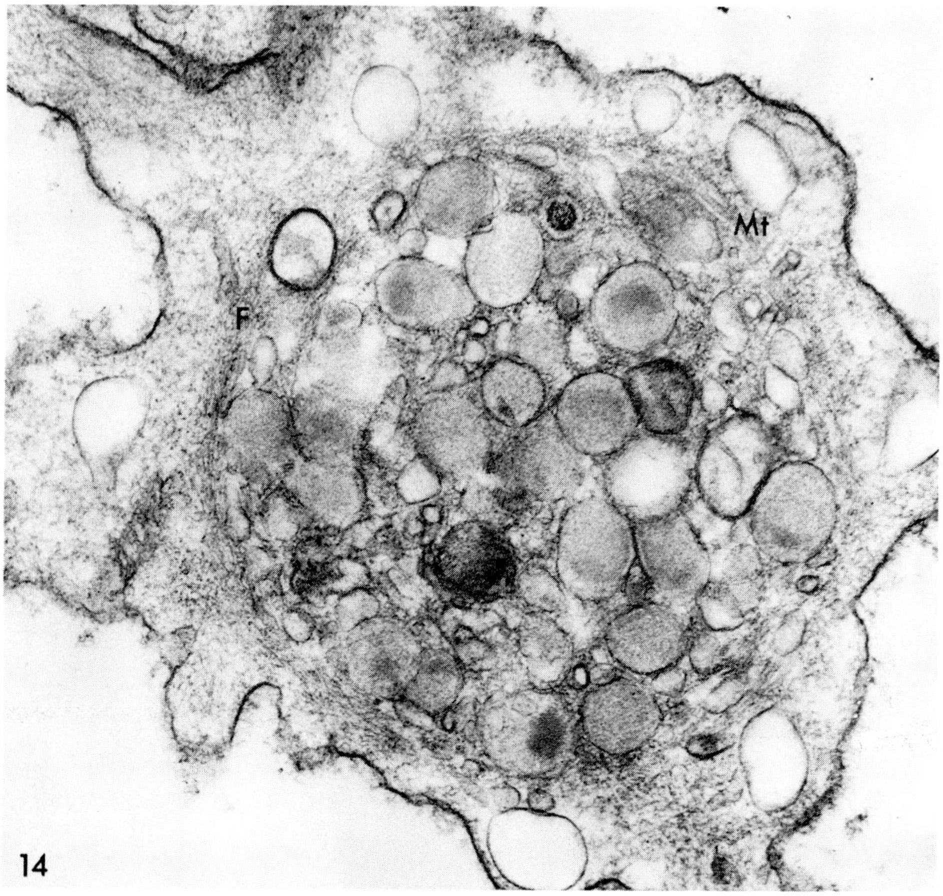

FIGURE 14. Brief treatment of platelets with ADP prior to glutaraldehyde fixation results in the partial dissociation of the band of microtubules (Mt). The area formerly occupied by tubules is now filled with circumferentially arranged filaments (F) and at higher magnification (not shown here) may demonstrate continuity with the ends of the dissociating microtubules. (Magnification × 43,000.)

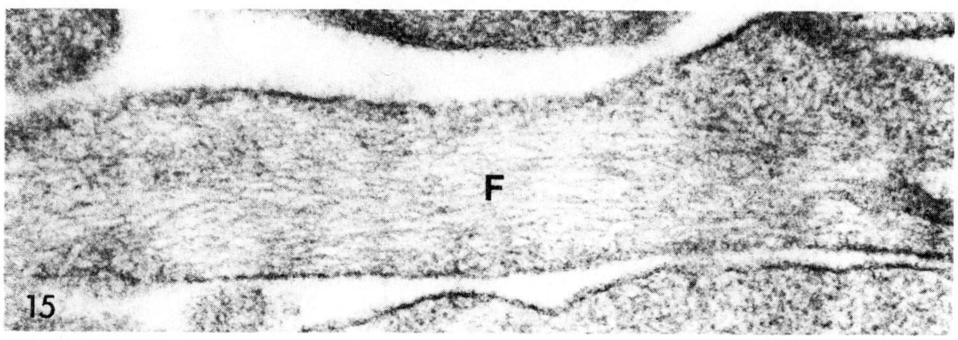

FIGURE 15. Detail of a platelet pseudopod containing microfilaments (F). Longitudinal sections of pseudopods often display masses of 7 nm filaments arranged parallel to the long axis of the cytoplasmic extension. (Magnification × 74,000.)

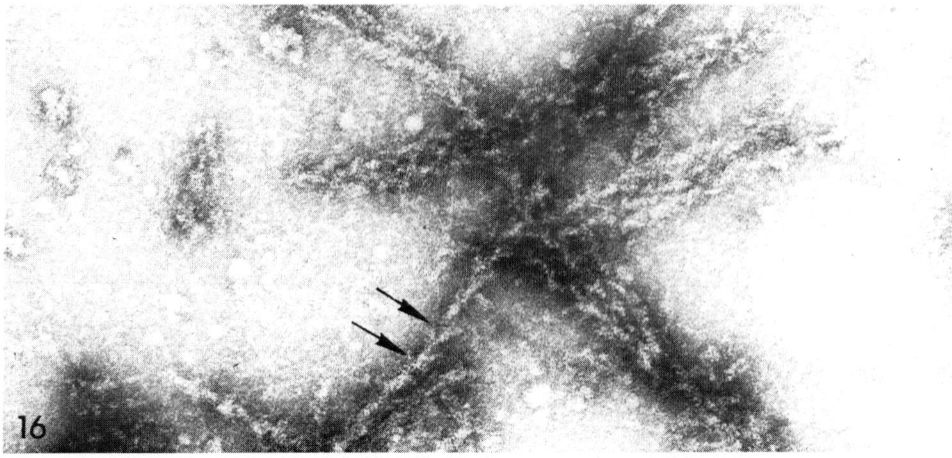

FIGURE 16. After extraction from bovine platelets, 7—8 nm filaments form "arrowhead" complexes (arrows) when reacted with heavy meromyosin with a fixed polarity and an average periodicity of 36 nm. Morphologically, these complexes are indistinguishable from those formed between heavy meromyosin and muscle actin. (Magnification × 120,000.)

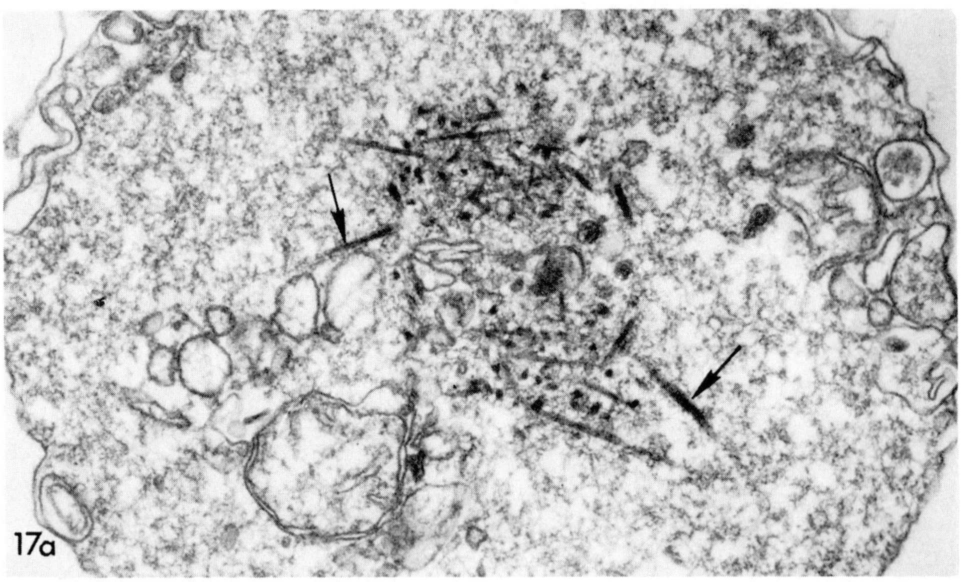

A

FIGURE 17. (A) Platelet after incubation in 2 mM ATP and 50 mM $MgCl_2$ contains aggregates of thick filaments (arrows) which resemble myosin filaments observed in trypsin-treated smooth muscle. These "tactoids" average 25—35 nm in diameter and 0.5 μm in length. (Magnification × 48,000.) (B) A myosin aggregate isolated from bovine platelets. It is 0.3 μm in length and has a smooth central shaft composed of parallel arrays of thinner filaments. The ends of the aggregates are either bulbous or tapered and resemble myosin isolated from smooth and striated muscle. (Magnification × 160,000.)

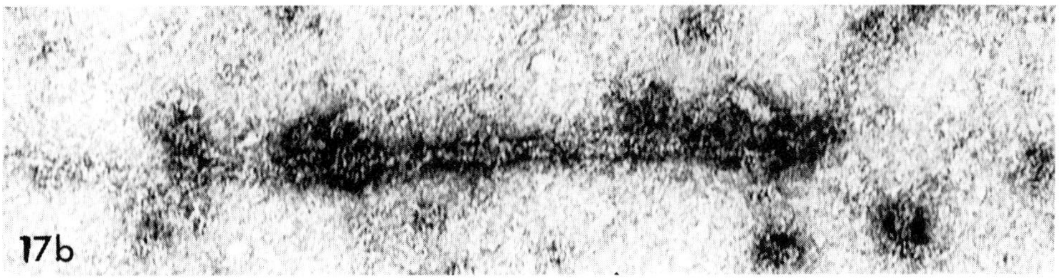

FIGURE 17 B

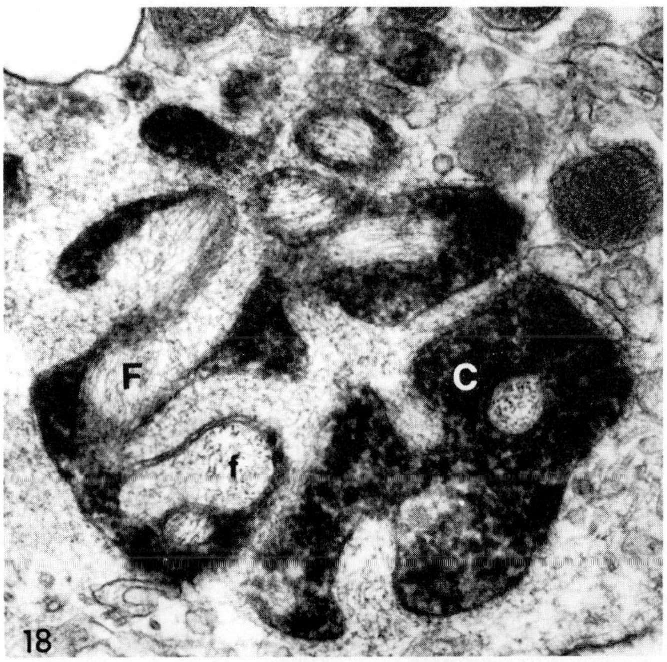

FIGURE 18. Platelet open canalicular system following incubation with peroxidase and treatment with 10^{-5} M ADP. The cytoplasmic aspect of the coalescing OCS is replete with filaments which are seen in longitudinal (F) and in cross section (f) and appear to be closely associated with the canalicular membranes. (Magnification × 52,000.)

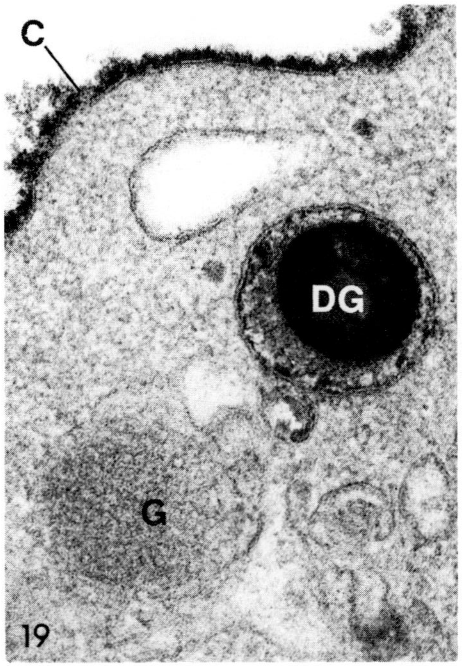

FIGURE 19. Detail of platelet cytoplasm containing a "dense granule" (DG) believed to store serotonin — not to be confused with the other granules which are often referred to as α granules. Some of the granules are lysosomes. C — coat; G — granule. (Magnification × 187,000.)

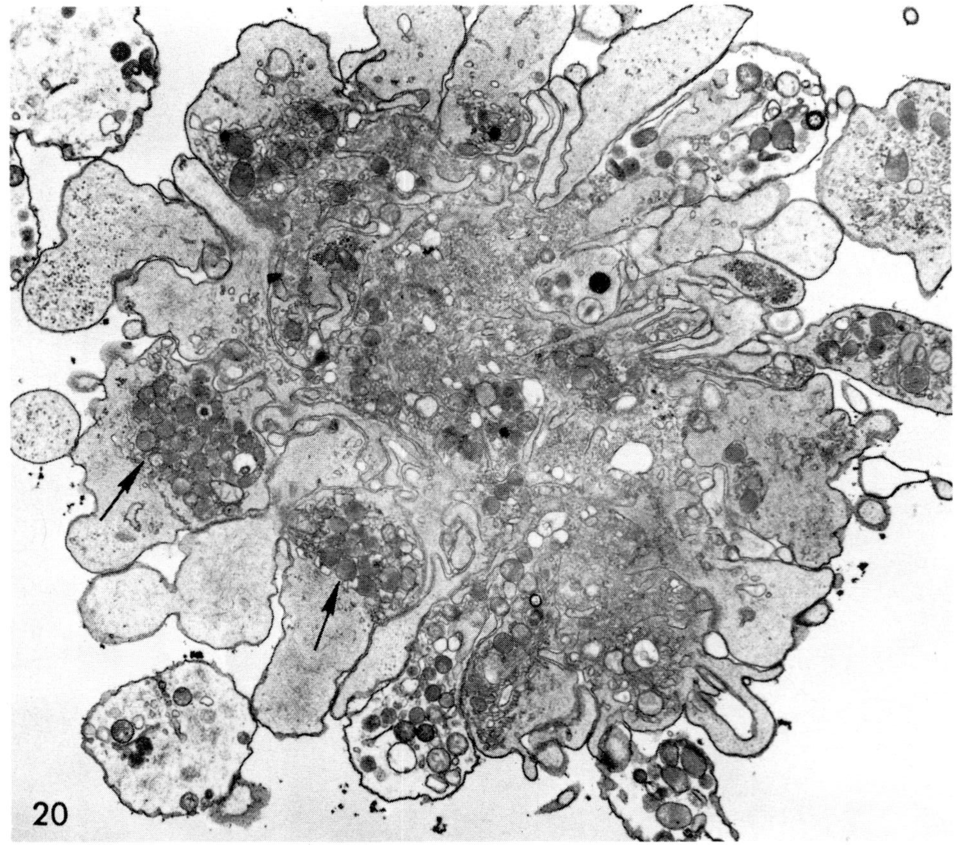

FIGURE 20. Platelets fixed one minute after the addition of thrombin. The platelets at the center of the aggregate have begun to undergo viscous metamorphosis, while those at the periphery retain much of their complement of granules. Note the centralization of the granulomere (arrows) which occurs prior to degranulation. (Magnification × 10,000.)

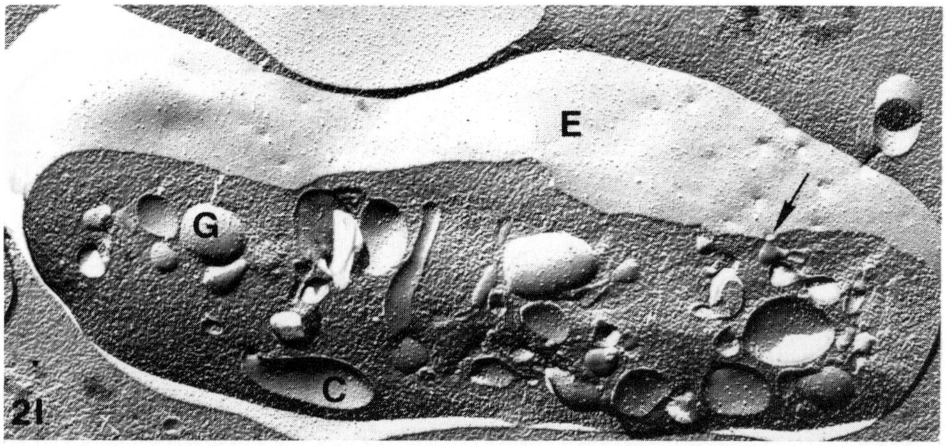

FIGURE 21. Freeze-fractured platelet showing the particles on the outer membrane (E face). A connection to the open canalicular system is clearly evident (arrow). C — canaliculi; G — granule. (Magnification × 30,000.)

REFERENCES

1. **Marcus, A. S., Ullman, H. L., and Safier, L. B.,** Lipid composition of subcellular particles of human blood platelets, *J. Lipid Res.,* 10, 108, 1969.
2. **O'Brien, J. R.,** Some effects on blood coagulation of erythrocytes and other cells, *J. Clin. Pathol.,* 12, 45, 1959.
3. **Behnke, O.,** Electron microscopic observations on the membrane system of rat blood platelets, *Anat. Rec.,* 158, 121, 1967.
4. **Behnke, O.,** Electron microscopical observations on the surface coating of human blood platelets, *J. Ultrastructure Res.,* 24, 51, 1968.
5. **Luft, J. H.,** Ruthenium red and violet. II. Fine structural localization in animal tissues, *Anat. Rec.,* 171, 369, 1971.
6. **Zucker-Franklin, D.,** Microfibrils of blood platelets: their relationship to microtubules and the contractile protein, *J. Clin. Invest.,* 48, 165, 1969.
7. **Zucker-Franklin, D. and Rosenberg, L.,** Platelet interaction with modified articular cartilage. Its possible relevance to joint repair, *J. Clin. Invest.,* 59, 641, 1977.
8. **Muggli, R. and Baumgartner, H. R.,** Collagen induced platelet aggregation: requirement for tropocollagen multimers, *Thromb. Res.,* 3, 715, 1973.
9. **Jaffe, R. and Deykin, D.,** Evidence for a structural requirement for the aggregation of platelets by collagen, *J. Clin. Invest.,* 53, 875, 1974.
10. **Brass, L. F. and Bensusan, H. B.,** The role of collagen quaternary structure in the platelet: collagen interaction, *J. Clin. Invest.,* 54, 1480, 1974.
11. **Simons, E. R., Chesney, C., Colman, R. W., Harper, E., and Samberg, E.,** The effect of the conformation of collagen on its ability to aggregate platelets, *Thromb. Res.,* 7, 123, 1975.
12. **Zucker-Franklin, D.,** The submembranous fibrils of human blood platelets, *J. Cell Biol.,* 47, 293, 1970.
13. **Zucker-Franklin, D.,** The ultrastructure of megakaryocytes and platelets, in *Regulation of Hematopoiesis,* Vol. 2, Gordon, A. S., Ed., Appleton-Century-Crofts, New York, 1970, 1553.
14. **Bettex-Galland, M. and Luscher, E. F.,**Extraction of an actomyosin-like protein from human thrombocytes, *Nature (London),* 184, 276, 1959.
15. **Huxley, H. E.,** Electron microscope studies on the structure of natural and synthetic protein filaments from striated muscle, *J. Mol. Biol,* 7, 281, 1963.

16. **Ishikawa, H., Bischoff, R., and Holtzer, H.,** Formation of arrowhead complexes with heavy meromyosin in a variety of cell types, *J. Cell Biol.,* 43, 312, 1969.
17. **Zucker-Franklin, D. and Grusky, G.,** The actin and myosin filaments of human and bovine blood platelets, *J. Clin. Invest.,* 51, 419, 1972.
18. **Adelstein, R. S. and Conti, M. A.,** The characterization of contractile proteins from platelets and fibroblasts, *Cold Spring Harbor Symp. Quant. Biol.,* 37, 599, 1972.
19. **Booyse, F. M., Hoveke, T. P., and Rafelson, M. E.,** Human platelet actin-isolation and properties, *J. Biol. Chem.,* 248, 4083, 1973.
20. **Pollard, T. D., Thomas, S. M., and Niederman, R.,** Human platelet myosin. I. Purification by a rapid method applicable to other nonmuscle cells, *Anal. Biochem.,* 60, 258, 1974.
21. **Kelly, R. E. and Rice, R. V.,** Ultrastructural studies on the contractile mechanism of smooth muscle, *J. Cell Biol.,* 42, 683, 1969.
22. **Schoenberg, C. F.,** An electron microscope study of the influence of divalent ions on myosin filament formation in chicken gizzard extracts and homogenates, *Tissue Cell,* 1, 83, 1969.
23. **Rosenbluth, J.,** Myosin-like aggregates in trypsin-treated smooth muscle cells, *J. Cell Biol.,* 48, 174, 1971.
24. **Adelstein, R. S., Pollard, T. D., and Kuehl, M.,** Isolation and characterization of myosin and two myosin fragments from human blood platelets, *Proc. Natl. Acad. Sci. U.S.A.,* 68, 2703, 1971.
25. **Breton-Gorius, J. and Guichard, J.,** Ultrastructural localization of peroxidase activity in human platelets and megakaryocytes, *Am. J. Pathol,* 66, 277, 1972.
26. **White, J. G.,** Iteractins of membrane systems in blood platelets, *Am. J. Pathol.,* 66, 295, 1972.
27. **Karnovsky, M. J.,** The ultrastructural basis of capillary permeability studied with peroxidase as a tracer, *J. Cell Biol.,* 35, 213, 1967.
28. **Marcus, A. J., Zucker-Franklin, D., Safier, L. B., and Ullman, H. L.,** Studies on human platelet granules and membranes, *J. Clin. Invest.,* 45, 14, 1966.
29. **Tranzer, J. P., DaPrada, M., and Pletscher, A.,** Ultrastructural localization of 5-hydroxytryptamine in blood platelets, *Nature (London),* 212, 1574, 1966.
30. **Hoak, J. C.,** Freeze-etching studies of human platelets, *Blood,* 40, 514, 1972.

LABORATORY TESTS IN PLATELET FUNCTION

H. James Day

Introduction

The physiological role of platelets in the vascular system appears to be an important component in the initiation of hemostasis. At the same time, platelets can contribute to the thrombotic process through an interreaction with the vessel wall and a stimulation of the latter structure which may lead to the development of atherosclerosis.[1,2]

Platelets ordinarily circulate in the blood as disc-shaped cells which do not adhere to either normal endothelium or to each other. Upon a disturbance of the endothelial lining of the vessel wall, platelets adhere first to submembranous structures such as collagen, connective tissue, microfibrils, etc., followed by other platelets migrating to the site of the injury and undergoing a series of biochemical and physical changes which have been well characterized[1,2,3,4] including synthesis of prostaglandin and a secretory process.

During the secretory process, known as the release reaction, platelets secrete chemical substances such as adenosine diphosphate (ADP), serotonin (5HT), vascular permeability factor, platelet factor 4, calcium, lysosomal enzymes, and a smooth, muscle-stimulating substance. During this secretory phase, platelets make available to the coagulation system, a phospholipid termed platelet factor 3 (PF3). ADP is capable of producing further platelet aggregation after which the original platelet aggregate begins to grow in size until it reaches the stage of a platelet hemostatic plug. This ADP, perhaps in addition to the above previously mentioned calcium and 5HT, causes other platelets to stick to one another or aggregate in response to highly specific stimuli, which are in turn aggregating agents when used in vitro.

The platelets are also capable of activating coagulation factors such as factor XI, factor XII, and factor V; the intrinsic system of coagulation is thereby activated, resulting in the fibrinogen to fibrin reaction.[5] Under these circumstances, platelets formed on the surface of the platelet mass no longer aggregate but adhere to the polymerizing fibrin. This fibrin leads to a stabilization of the hemostatic plug and serves to limit the size of the intraluminal mass. Normally, this mass will break off and will be swept downstream into the small arterial circulation and will not cause any circulatory embarrassment. However, under specific circumstances, such as in patients with homocystinuria or perhaps those in whom an atherosclerotic plaque is already present (in the coronary arteries), the platelet mass grows until it becomes a large thrombus leading to distal circulatory anoxia and, in some circumstances, sudden death. It is therefore obvious that hemostasis and thrombosis are intimately interrelated.

Much of the information gained as to the role of platelets in hemostasis has accrued from the study of platelet function in vitro.

The Platelet Function Tests

A series of platelet function tests has been developed for testing platelets in vitro due to the inherent difficulties in assessing platelet function in vivo. These tests measure the ability of platelets to adhere, aggregate, and release their hemostatic promoting activities. Table 1 is a listing of the commonly used platelet function tests. An encyclopedic discussion of all these platelet function tests is beyond the scope of this review. The interested reader may seek greater details in a recently published symposium.[6]

The most commonly used platelet function tests are bleeding time, platelet aggregation, platelet glass bead retention, platelet factor 3 availability, and clot retraction. Measurement of the bleeding time is the single most important in vivo indicator of

Table 1
TESTS OF PLATELET FUNCTION

Bleeding time	Duke Ivy	Borchgrevink template

Clot retraction
Platelet Factor 3 availability
- Direct
- Clotting assay — serum prothrombin time

Platelet aggregation
- Visual
- Light transmission and light scattering
- Microscopic
- Filtration pressure method
- Detection of aggregates in freshly drawn blood
- Spontaneous aggregation
- Glass bead trapping of platelet aggregates

Platelet adhesion and aggregation (adhesion)

Adhesion

- Glass slides and cover slips
- Rotating glass tube, coated with collagen
- Aggregometry technique for platelet-collagen adhesion

Adhesion-aggregation-retention

- In vivo method of Borchgrevink
- Rotating glass bulb
- Glass wool
- Glass bead column

hemostatic function. While in vitro methods have aided pharmacological and clinical research and have identified patients with hemostatic defects, results of the studies of the tendency toward thrombosis are sometimes confusing. It is important to realize that techniques, such as those based upon platelet adhesion to glass beads (platelet glass bead retention) and measurement of platelet aggregation in platelet-rich plasma, measure phenomena which occur in vitro and do not necessarily reflect in vivo behavior. In addition, tests performed in platelet-rich plasma are by definition devoid of red and white blood cells which obviously have a meaningful role in contributing toward the migration of platelets to the vessel wall and perhaps the generation of the hemostatic plug and thrombotic mass. Thus the screen filtration pressure method and perhaps the Chandler loop technique have greater physiological significance but generally have been superseded by the performance of the far more simple test of platelet aggregation in citrated platelet-rich plasma. Similarly, the development of the platelet aggregation method has almost totally eliminated the necessity of performance of an estimation of clot retraction, and availability of phospholipid (PF3) in the assessment of platelet function for similar information is made available by the platelet aggregation test, as will be discussed below.

The ideal system for testing platelet function would be an in vivo device which is attached to the subject with minimal preparation and trauma. Such a device would allow blood to react at physiological pH, temperature, pressure, and flow conditions. It would need an artificial blood vessel wall or submembranous components with which to interact. It is obvious that platelet function cannot be studied in this way at this time. To date, the test most likely fulfilling this description is the bleeding time method which measures all of the in vivo parameters. The main deficiency of the bleeding time method is that in spite of enormous improvement in standardization, it still is relatively gross; one must be content with recording the flow of blood from a cut surface, the assumption being that once bleeding stops, the hemostatic plug is intact. At this time, the bleeding time test is probably incapable of detecting any abnormal reactions of the platelets to the vessel wall in thrombotic tendencies.

The platelet function tests as outlined below represent those that are currently performed in most laboratories around the world. They do not necessarily represent the best tests of any of the platelet functions, but it is the purpose of this review to detail the methodology and interpretation of the results of those which are currently being used.

The Bleeding Time

In many ways, the bleeding time is the broad spectrum test of platelet function. It measures the entire sequence of events in the formation of the hemostatic plug as may be obtained from interpretation of the data related to the time it takes from infliction of a wound to the cessation of bleeding; therefore, it is a test which takes into account many platelet functions. It is the most commonly employed test of in vivo platelet function. Prolongation of the bleeding time reflects either a qualitative (thrombocytopathia) or quantitative (thrombocytopenia) defect in platelets, abnormalities in plasma factors such as fibrinogen and vWF, or a defective vessel wall as may occur in some inborn errors of metabolism such as Ehlers-Danlos syndrome. When the bleeding time is abnormal, other more specific tests of platelet function are performed which will yield definitive answers as to the exact pathological condition affecting the platelet. As of this writing, only a prolongation of the bleeding time is accepted as evidence of abnormality in the function of platelets resulting in a hemostatic defect, although claim has been made that a specifically performed bleeding time test (stress bleeding time) may yield shortened times in those patients with thrombosis.[7]

The advent of ingenious gadgeting has brought increased acceptance of the carefully performed bleeding time test as one of the better tests of platelet function. Modifications of the original pin prick of the ear lobe technique as described by Duke in 1910[8] were generally unsuccessful and only succeeded in scarifying many ear lobes with multiple incisions. The ear lobe test suffered from lack of reproducibility, a great coefficient of variation, and asymmetry in the ear lobes of tested individuals. It is still done on newborn infants and young children in some institutions, although simpler methods such as incision of the heel or finger may be better for those small subjects.

The next advance in standardization was that of Ivy et al.[9] They chose to make skin punctures on the forearm 2 in. below the anticubital fossa with the venous and capillary pressure standardized at precisely 40 mm Hg by an inflated sphygmomanometer cuff on the upper arm. The skin punctures were hard to standardize, although various devices were made available in an effort to produce a "standard puncture wound." The problem lay in the variability in the depth of the puncture produced by spring-loaded lancets, surgical blades, ice picks, etc. At times, superficial venules were pierced; at other times the skin was never pierced due to the reluctance of a kind-hearted laboratory worker.

A significant modification was to make three very superficial (1 mm deep) linear cuts 12 mm long with a surgical blade. This technique, as introduced by Borchgrevink and Waaler,[10] allowed for greater precision and usefulness with good reproducibility. Bleeding time determinations were remarkably similar between one arm and the other, and the coefficient of variation between individual cuts was lower than with the Ivy technique. Limitations of the technique were found in operator variability, variation in length and depth of incision, etc.

An attempt at even greater reproducibility was the introduction of the "standardized template bleeding time".[11] The venous pressure is maintained at 40 mm Hg by an inflated sphygmomanometer cuff on the upper arm as in the Ivy technique. A template with a linear slit 11 mm long is pressed firmly on the forearm. A scalpel with a guard so arranged that the blade protrudes 1 mm through the template slit is used to make a standard incision which is blotted every 30 sec.

The method is highly reproducible and the data generated from several centers indicate that the method is capable of yielding bleeding time data that for the first time might be comparable when performed in different laboratories. Modifications of the types of devices have been made by several investigators culminating in the introduction of several mechanical devices which inflict a standard incision 5 mm long and 1 mm deep in each of two sites.[12,13]

Evidence obtained with this type of template bleeding time device strongly suggests that aspirin prolongs the bleeding time of normal people,[11,14] although other, older techniques indicated the same tendency. The prolongation of the bleeding time by aspirin indicates that prostaglandin formation by the platelets is important in the normal hemostatic sequence; it has been well demonstrated that aspirin blocks prostaglandin formation by acetylation of the cyclooxygenase.[15]

Harker and Slichter[14] have demonstrated that in thrombocytopenic patients with impaired platelet production, the normal mean bleeding time of 4.9 ± 1.5 min (± 15.0) is prolonged linearly in relation to the decrease in the platelet count from 100,000 per c.mm. Thus, at a platelet count of 125,000, a normal bleeding time might be expected if the platelets are functionally adequate; at 75,000 per c.mm, an 8 min bleeding time, at 50,000 per c.mm, a bleeding time of 10 min, etc., and at a platelet count of less than 10,000 per c.mm, a bleeding time of more than 15 min.

This type of quantitative analysis of the bleeding time allows the clinical investigator to diagnose the not-too-rare definitive condition of thrombocytopenia-thrombocytopathia. In this clinical situation, the bleeding time is prolonged beyond that which might be expected with comparable platelet counts: for example, with a platelet count of 100,000 per c.mm, the bleeding time might be 8 min and with 75,000 per c.mm, 10 min, etc.

Variations in the performance of the template bleeding time do not seem to have any great effect upon the reproducibility of the results. Thus Mielke et al.[11] have failed to note any difference in results obtained if two or three incisions are made in the forearm through the use of a 9-mm incision at 1-mm depth 2 in. below the anticubital fossa. The incisions may be either horizontal or vertical. The horizontal incision may produce a slightly longer bleeding time (1 min prolongation), but these results are probably not significant. From a theoretical viewpoint, horizontal incisions are preferable to vertical incisions, since the latter tend to separate more readily because of the anatomy of the skin and subcutaneous tissue and may result in more scarring. This latter complication may be avoided by using an antiseptic solution to cleanse the wound and application of a butterfly bandage to approximate the wound edges.

Several authors have shown that the template bleeding time test is more sensitive to defects in prostaglandin synthesis than either the Ivy or the Duke technique and is thereby the most sensitive test for detection of platelet function defects either congenital or acquired.

The template bleeding time is prolonged in patients with von Willebrand's disease following aspirin ingestion, release defects due to storage pool deficiency or due to defects in prostaglandin synthesis (aspirin-like release defects), thrombasthenia, Bernard-Soulier syndrome, uremia, etc. It should be noted that a "normal" bleeding time may be detected in patients with mild degrees of hemostatic defects due to abnormal platelet function at any time during the laboratory investigation of these individuals. Under these circumstances, repeated determinations of the bleeding time may have to be performed.

The Glass Bead Column Platelet Retention Test or Platelet "Adhesion" in Vitro

Platelets have the ability to interact with many different surfaces. Wright[16] showed that platelets are removed from anticoagulated blood by adherence when rotated in a flask containing glass-wool fiber. She was able to quantitate this phenomenon. Hellem [17,18] standardized the total exposed glass surface by the adoption of a glass bead column utilizing glass beads of uniform size and shape packed into a plastic tube sealed at both ends by nylon mesh. Hellem passed native or anticoagulated blood propelled either by a hand-held syringe or a constant infusion pump through the plastic columns. Under these circumstances the only cellular elements retained by the glass beads are the platelets; the majority of the white cells and all of the red cells traverse the column without being retained. The number of platelets retained by the glass bead column are obtained by serial counting of the platelets in the effluent emerging at regular intervals from the syringe tip and relating to the basal platelet count of the blood specimens before it passes over the column. The percentage retention represents the difference between the number of platelets in the control sample in the syringe and that of the sample obtained from the average platelet count of the fourth and fifth aliquot of blood or plasma passed over the column.

There are many tests of platelet adhesiveness (see Table 1) which measure both adhesion and adhesion-aggregation. No discussion will be made of any methods except for the glass bead column platelet retention test, since this is the most widely used form of testing in clinical situations. The literature is replete with results of the various tests performed on patients with problems of bleeding or thrombosis, and the reports are often contradictory.

Several modifications have been made in the basic glass bead column technique since the original description by Hellem. Salzman[19] employed a vacuum-containing tube which drew the blood through the glass bead column. It utilized shorter plastic tubes and fewer glass beads, which meant that the platelets were in contact with the glass beads for a minimal time. This fact plus variability in the force of the vacuum led to gradual decline in the use of this test by most investigators, due to nonreproducibility of results in spite of its simpler technique.

Bowie et al.[20] modified the Hellem glass bead column by utilizing heparinized whole blood. This change allows the blood to be drawn, mixed with various agents, incubated, or, in the case of hospitalized patients, allows the sample to be returned from the bedside to the laboratory before the test is run. Various other modifications have been made, but it is apparent that the basic method developed by Hellem and later modified by him[21] and others[19,20,22] continues to have a place in the platelet function laboratory and provides useful information.

As stated previously, all in vitro platelet function studies are an exercise in phenomenology, and platelet glass bead retention is no exception. The mechanisms by which platelets are retained in the glass bead column are not fully understood. Red blood cells influence the viscosity and hence the blood flow through the glass bead filter by their "tumbling" effect, which promotes contact of the platelets with the foreign surface and with each other under conditions in which a constant speed of infusion is achieved through the use of the mechanical pump. In those cases in which a pump is not utilized, conditions are chaotic and the results are nonreproducible.

Plasma proteins are obviously important; the initial adhesion of platelets to glass requires ionized calcium, fibrinogen, and possibly gamma-globulin. The absolute need for the latter is still uncertain. In studies with washed platelet suspensions, gamma-globulin promotes adhesion, but this may represent the effect of aggregates of gamma-globulin rather than the unaggregated protein having an influence upon platelets. However, platelets suspended in serum or in afibrinogenemic plasma depend upon the presence of fibrinogen alone to promote adherence. These studies and others demonstrate the need for fibrinogen in platelet glass bead retention. Weiss and Rogers[23] found afibrinogenemic individuals to have decreased glass bead retention.

Other requirements for the initial *adhesion* of platelets to glass besides those mentioned above are platelets which are responsive to ADP (thus thrombasthenic platelets do not adhere as they are not responsive to any agent) but do not include the necessity of von Willebrand factor. *Retention*, on the other hand, seems to involve formation of platelet aggregates in the column requiring both ADP, which is probably released from the platelets, and plasma vWF. The poor retention found in blood from patients with release defects such as storage pool disease suggests that the necessary ADP is derived from the storage granules. A lack of parallel release of ^{14}C-serotonin and failure of aspirin to inhibit retention indicate that the usual release reaction is not involved. At this writing, the interaction of ADP and vWF is not well understood. Zucker[24] has recently shown that ADP added before blood is passed through the column inhibits retention, and ADP inhibits platelet agglutination caused by ristocetin plus vWF.

Variables Affecting Platelet Glass Bead Retention

Platelet glass bead retention is affected by many variables, all of which need to be standardized so that reproducible results can be obtained in different laboratories. Some of the lack of confidence in this method of platelet function testing which has developed over the years may have arisen because many laboratories have attempted to introduce modifications which may not have been the most helpful in providing consistent results and subsequently led to nonreproducibility by others. In addition, inasmuch as platelet glass bead retention involves platelet aggregation and adherence, retention, the same factors which affect aggregation have a similar effect upon the results derived from this test.

Presence of other blood cells — As mentioned above, red blood cells promote contact of the platelets to the glass beads in the column. Platelet retention increases as the hematocrit rises and falls in the anemic individual. White blood cells degrade ADP, and a high proportion of white cells decreases platelet aggregation and possibly retention.

Glass beads — In his methods, Hellem[17,18] suggested washing the glass beads with a caustic solution to remove impurities. Washing the beads does not seem necessary with the method of Bowie et al.[20] in which retention is very high in normals. Any such artifact which may be introduced by suspended foreign matter on most glass beads currently available seems to be negligible. Platelet retention may change with increasing age of the glass bead column, but this too does not seem to be important in the Bowie test. Zucker et al.[25] recommends storing the column in a desiccator because moisture reduces platelet retention. This may be especially helpful to those inhabitants of climates subject to conditions of variable humidity who may have less than ideal climate control.

Plastic tubing — The type of plastic tube used for the column seems to be important and can have a profound effect upon platelet retention. With the use of polyvinyl tubes, platelet retention is high. The opposite situation (low retention) occurs with tubes of polyethylene and Teflon,® while those tubes made with silastic give intermediate results.[26] There is evidence that contaminating substances are leached from polyvinyl plastic and that this causes an increase in platelet retention. Similar phenomena may be responsible for the changes seen with aging of columns mentioned above.

Anticoagulant — Native blood would appear to have several obvious advantages over blood containing an anticoagulant, yet the time limitations imposed by working with native blood prevent the method from being universally employed and point to the convenience of working with anticoagulated blood. Anticoagulants that chelate calcium usually result in decreased platelet retention,[20] therefore making heparin the anticoagulant of choice if the concentration is standardized. Platelet retention seems to increase when the concentration of heparin is increased over 1 unit/mℓ.

Flow rate and contact time — If the contact time is decreased due to a rapid flow rate, platelet retention decreases.[20] The retention can be adjusted by adjusting the number of beads and the flow rate. This may eventually result in the utilization of this technique — through further modification — to look for decreased retention in patients with bleeding disorders and increased retention in patients with a tendency toward thrombosis.

It should be noted that platelet retention increases as blood passes through the column. This may explain the variation in results obtained from different laboratories since some investigators pool the effluent from the syringe tip while others collect aliquots and do serial counts. The latter method seems to yield the most satisfactory and reproducible results.

Collection and storage of samples — A poor venipuncture and excess shaking of the blood will decrease platelet retention. Studies of this phenomenon by Coller and Zucker[22] have indicated that decreased retention occurs if air bubbles are passed through the pump or if the blood is inverted in the collection tube or syringe, passed from one syringe to another, or slowly centrifuged and remixed (all called disturbance phenomena). If the blood is left 1 to 2 hr at room temperature after disturbance, the retention returns to normal, indicating the reversibility of the process. Hellem[17,18] reported that the most reproducible results were obtained if the undisturbed blood was passed through the glass bead column between 30 to 60 min after venipuncture. Periods of storage greater than 1 hr result in decreased retention with values approaching zero in 24 hr.

The Value of Platelet Glass Bead Retention in Clinical Medicine

Hemostatic Defects

The glass bead column platelet retention test has been used as a tool for diagnosis of many hemostatic disorders, involving both primary and secondary platelet function defects (Table 2). Of the secondary disorders, myeloproliferative syndromes — often associated with thrombocytosis — demonstrate decreased adhesiveness, which possibly reflects a qualitatively abnormal platelet. Similar results have been obtained in uremia where decreased platelet retention is noted, which is reversible after dialysis. Part of this may be due to changes in plasma volume reflected in changes in hematocrit before and after hemodialysis. An abnormality in platelet glass bead interaction has been demonstrated in scurvy, which is reversible in 3 days after vitamin C. In multiple myeloma, paraproteinemia apparently results in decreased platelet retention by coating the glass beads and the platelets, making the adherence and aggregation phases less operative.

Patients with qualitative platelet disorders have decreased glass bead retention of their platetets. These disorders include the primary platelet function defects of Glanzmann's thrombasthenia and release defects due to storage pool deficiency or to defects in prostaglandin synthesis.

It is in von Willebrand's disease that the test has its greatest application. Although reduced platelet retention is not diagnostic of any specific condition, it does indicate a qualitative platelet defect as in von Willebrand's disease. In a patient lacking other secondary causes of platelet function defects such as paraproteinemia or uremia and if aggregometry is normal, decreased platelet glass bead retention probably indicates a variant of von Willebrand's disease and appropriate confirmatory studies should be done. When the test is well standardized, it has the same spectrum as the bleeding time method. In fact, there are some subjects with von Willebrand's disease who may have

Table 2
DISORDERS OF PLATELET FUNCTION

Disorder	Bleeding time	Glass bead retention	Aggregation 1st phase	Aggregation 2nd phase	Aggregation Ristocetin	PF3 availability	Clot retention	Comment
Thrombasthenia	↑	↓	↓	↓	N	↓	↓	Membrane defect
Release defect								
Storage pool disease	↑	↓	N	↓	N	↓	N	Decreased storage granule content
Aspirin or aspirin-like	↑	N or ↓	N	↓	N	↓	N	Normal storage granule content
Bernard-Soulier syndrome	↑	↓	N	N	↓	↓	N	Giant platelets
von Willebrand's disease	↑	↓	N	N	↓	N	N	Lack of vWF in plasma

a normal bleeding time and an abnormal glass bead retention (or vice versa). Weiss[27] suggested that platelet glass bead retention might be considered to be "a very sensitive bleeding time." The increasing availability of factor VIII antigen and von Willebrand cofactor assay may supersede the glass bead retention test in the diagnosis of von Willebrand's disease, although the latter may remain helpful in those patients with this disease who have taken oral contraceptives, are pregnant, or have received recent transfusions. In these situations, patients develop normal factor VIII coagulant activity, factor VIII antigen, and vWF, but the platelet retention test remains abnormal.

The test still plays an important role in the diagnosis of qualitative platelet abnormalities if only as a screening test or a "very sensitive bleeding time". In these clinical situations, when the bleeding time is normal or prolonged, the platelet retention is usually reduced. Usually, when the bleeding time is prolonged, the platelet retention is greatly reduced. At times, they are not strictly in harmony; the bleeding time may show greater prolongation than the glass bead retention reduction in some von Willebrand's variants.

Thrombotic Tendencies

The use of the platelet retention test to predict thrombotic tendencies has been disappointing in general. Several variations of the test have been applied to the diagnosis of conditions associated with thrombosis and emboli. It seems likely that the various modifications or "methods" proclaimed to show positive results in specific disease entities such as acute myocardial infarction or severe atherosclerosis may be influenced by changes in the plasma proteins in these diseases, although the many modifications of these tests from one investigator to another make satisfactory comparisons difficult. All adhesion and aggregation tests which show "hyperfunctioning" platelets in patients with various disease states associated with thrombosis probably do so because of an alteration in the plasmatic environment.

Platelet Aggregation and Agglutination

Aggregation of platelets in platelet-rich plasma (PRP) or in artificial media has proved to be a useful way of assessing congenital, acquired, and drug-induced abnormalities of platelet function. The following is a discussion of this method of testing of platelet function, including an elaboration upon the theory behind the aggregation phenomenon, review of methods of study, discussion of variables affecting the results, and clinical value of this test.

Mechanism of Aggregation

In vivo, it seems probable that platelets are exposed to epinephrine, collagen, thrombin, and serotonin. If platelets see ADP in vivo, it is most likely to arise from stored endogenous ADP released by cell-cell contact. There are probably specific receptors on the platelet surface for all or most of aggregation-inducing agents. It would appear that serotonin and probably ADP, the latter in a medium containing physiological concentrations of calcium, are primary aggregating agents, and other mechanisms are not operative. With certain concentrations of ADP (in a low calcium medium such as citrated PRP) and with epinephrine, primary aggregation is followed by secondary aggregation in association with the formation of arachidonate, prostaglandin endoperoxides, and thromboxane A2 from platelets and the release of the contents of platelet granules.[28,29,30] It would then appear that the second wave of platelet aggregation is caused by intermediates of the arachidonate pathway and released ADP. Sodium arachidonate and its intermediates in the thromboxane pathway are in themselves aggregating and release-inducing agents.

Ristocetin, an antibiotic which was never used extensively clinically due to the development of thrombocytopenia in recipients, agglutinates platelets in the presence of von Willebrand factor.[31,32] This phenomenon serves as a useful tool in diagnosis of the clinically important syndrome, von Willebrand's disease. This agglutination probably involves the formation of electrostatic linkages between the platelets and may be followed by the same type of secondary aggregation seen with high concentrations of ADP in citrated PRP.

Platelets exposed to collagen in PRP adhere, release ADP, and form prostaglandin endoperoxides and thromboxane A2,[33] resulting in the aggregation of other platelets not adherent to the collagen. It would therefore appear that collagen causes aggregation of platelets through two separate mechanisms.

Thrombin produces aggregation through the two mechanisms listed above — ADP release and prostaglandin production and through an as yet poorly defined third mechanism.[34] The divalent calcium ionophores probably act in the same fashion besides causing a change in the internal platelet calcium which leads to aggregation and release of granule contents.

Those aggregation inducers acting by more than one mechanism seem to utilize these mechanisms synergistically to augment the reaction.[34] Thus, if one of the synergistic mechanisms is impaired or completely blocked, the aggregation response may be greatly inhibited, particularly with low concentrations of aggregating agents.[34]

With the exception of epinephrine, platelets change from a disc to a sphere shape in the presence of the aggregating agents. In the presence of fibrinogen and divalent cations in a stirred system, aggregation follows the initial shape change.

Methods of Studying Aggregation: Light Transmission and Light Scattering

In this section, only the method of study of platelet aggregation using light transmission and light scattering will be discussed. A review of other methods such as the screen filtration pressure methods, micro or macroscopic examination for aggregates, Chandler loop, etc., may be found in a recent publication.[35]

The most commonly used method for study of platelet aggregation is the one in which PRP is stirred and the light transmission is recorded.[36] The same technique can be used for studying washed or separated platelets resuspended in an artificial media, a property valuable in studying PRP's with low platelet counts.[37] The method also allows for a study of platelet shape-change phenomenon, a reaction which to date has only research interest.

Following the introduction of an aggregating agent to the medium (plasma or artificial), the platelet undergoes disc-to-sphere transformation and forms pseudopods (a reaction known as shape-change), which is recorded as a decrease in light transmission on the graphic display. This occurs with all aggregating agents except epinephrine. The period between introduction of the aggregating agent and onset of change (shape-change or aggregation) is known as the lag phase, the length of which may be important in diagnosing some disease states if a standard reference collagen reagent is utilized.[38]

Following this decrease in light transmission (shape-change) there is an increase in light transmission reflecting aggregation of the platelets into larger aggregates. It has been estimated that 80% of the platelets must be aggregated into small aggregates before any increase in light transmission is recorded.[39] Although this figure may vary depending upon the sensitivity of the instrument employed, it seems likely that the majority of the platelets are already aggregated with the onset of increase in light transmission.

Depending on the type and concentration of aggregating agent, the increase in light transmission, usually called aggregation, may do one of three things (Figure 1): (a) it may reach a maximum after which there is no further change in light transmission, (b) it may proceed through an aggregation phase, which is followed by a disaggregation phase recorded as a subsequent decrease in light transmission and return to new baseline values, or (c) it may undergo a second wave of aggregation indicated by a further increase in light transmission until a new maximum is obtained (full aggregation) (Figure 2). In PRP, only certain specific concentrations of ADP, epinephrine, thrombin, and ristocetin cause the biphasic response associated with ADP and amine release from the platelet.[40] The cause of the second phase of aggregation is attributed to released ADP and generation of prostaglandins.[34] When high concentrations of ADP (Figure 1) or ristocetin are used, only a single full aggregation response is recorded (maximal light transmission) which reflects fusion of the two separate phases of the reaction on the graphic recording.

With collagen-induced aggregation, a lag phase is apparent which depends upon the polymerization time of the collagen and will vary with the collagen reagent used. Thrombopathic platelets may have a long lag time with a standard collagen reagent, which is due to a delay in their release of ADP. Platelets will then adhere to the collagen fibrils, synthesize prostaglandins, and undergo the release reaction. The ADP re-

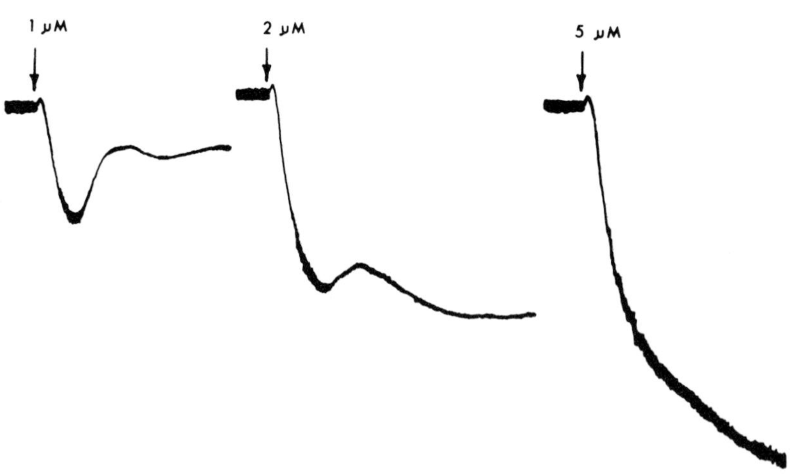

FIGURE 1. Effect of varying concentrations of ADP upon platelet aggregation patterns (see text).

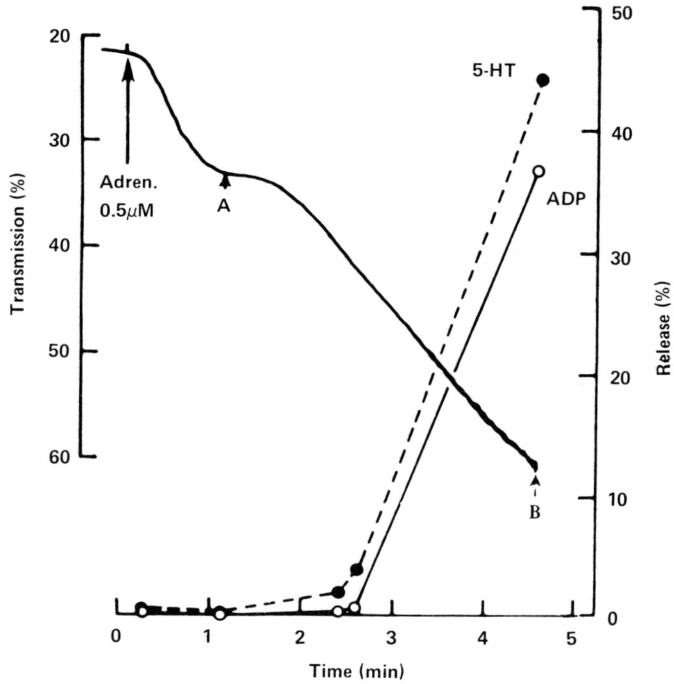

FIGURE 2. Biphasic aggregation pattern induced by adrenaline with superimposed measurement of released 5HT (---) and ADP (——). Note beginning of release with onset of second phase aggregation with minimal release between 2 and 3 min after application of aggregation inducer.

leased from the platelets will allow the aggregates to grow in size until full aggregation is recorded. The fact that aspirin will abate but not abolish this aggregation phenomenon indicates that more than prostaglandin synthesis is involved.

It has been shown that when ADP as an aggregating agent is tested in citrated PRP, the second phase of aggregation with its accompanying release reaction is an artifact caused by a low concentration of calcium.[30] When tested in a solution containing significant concentrations of calcium, ADP causes first phase aggregation alone. It is likely that close platelet contact caused by ADP or epinephrine in the presence of a low concentration of ionized calcium activates the pathway leading to the formation of prostaglandin endoperoxides and thromboxane A2 from platelet arachidonate.

Variables Affecting Platelet Aggregation Testing

Anticoagulants

Citrate is the primary anticoagulant used in platelet-rich plasma-platelet aggregation test procedures. While the preceding section has dealt with the "artifact" of ADP-induced biphasic platelet aggregation, citrate still remains a useful anticoagulant in most coagulation laboratories and seems to be the most suitable for all aspects of platelet function testing with the exception of platelet glass bead retention which utilizes heparin.

Ts'ao et al.[41] and Han and Ardlie[42] point out that small increases in the citrate concentration have an inhibitory effect upon platelet aggregation. The effect is greatest with epinephrine-induced aggregation, least with collagen-induced aggregation, and intermediate with ADP-induced aggregation. The authors note the importance of controlling the citrate: blood ratio of platelet aggregation results when the blood of different donors are to be compared in that the hematocrits of various patients may vary, necessitating an adjustment in the concentration of citrate. Sufficient citrate must be present to prevent generation of traces of thrombin as the proteolytic enzyme per se can potentiate and thereby influence the aggregation responses recorded.[30] The citrate inhibiting effect has been previously noted for platelet adhesiveness.[17,18] EDTA has no role as an anticoagulant in studying platelet aggregation except for a study of shape change, as platelets do not aggregate in the presence of EDTA but they do change shape. At this writing, shape change has minimal clinical relevance as most platelet function abnormalities described to date have the shape change mechanism intact except for lack of shape change with ADP in platelets with the Bernard-Soulier syndrome.

Heparin is a complex anticoagulant when used in the study of platelet aggregation. Heparin is capable of enhancing the primary phase of aggregation to a greater degree than that seen with citrate since citrate reduces the concentration of ionized calcium.[43] Blood drawn in heparin frequently contains aggregates, since heparin is capable of inducing aggregation of platelets in citrated plasma depending upon the type and concentration of heparin used. Heparin is capable of causing a thrombocytopenia when used clinically, which may be due to the platelet aggregation effect. Zucker[43] sums up the role of heparin as an anticoagulant for platelet aggregation by stating that "heparin enhances primary aggregation, induces aggregation by causing the release reaction, and as a result, may reduce the release reaction subsequently, provoked by other stimuli such as epinephrine."

pH

The pH of the plasma or suspending fluid influences the extent and type of aggregation pattern obtained after challenge with various aggregating agents.[44,49] Maximal aggregation occurs at a pH in the range of 7.4 to 8.0; only platelet shape change occurs below 6.4 or above 10.

Han and Ardlie[42] found that second-wave aggregation did not occur if the pH of the plasma rose above pH 8. They could prevent such a loss of reactivity by maintenance of the atmosphere surrounding the platelet-rich plasma with 5% CO_2. Zucker[45] and others[44] have called attention to the harmful effects of a loss of CO_2 from the specimen while the samples are maintained on the laboratory bench. Several methods have been devised to prevent such loss of CO_2, including capping, sealing, and flowing CO_2 over the specimens and using controlled atmosphere chambers.

Effect of Storage of PRP

The time aggregation is performed after drawing of the blood is as important as with the platelet retention test, although this may vary with the agent used to induce aggregation. Rossi and Louis[47] found that as PRP is allowed to stand at room temperature, it becomes progressively more responsive to the aggregating effects of epinephrine and collagen. Thus at 5 min minimal aggregation was seen with these agents, but after 45 min the addition of the same concentration of aggregation inducer caused a full aggregation effect. The effect of time was more pronounced with epinephrine than collagen, but suggested a need for strict adherence to a standard performance time of the test. Reuter et al.[48] postulated that the scope of time dependence may be due to changes in the permeability of the platelet membrane for ADP, resulting in leakage of ADP from the platelet interior and thereby acting in a synergistic fashion to augment the effect of varying concentrations of aggregation inducers. These authors were able to demonstrate an increase in ADP in the supernatant plasma as time passed.

Storage of citrated PRP at room temperature has a distinctly less deleterious effect on the platelet than storage at 4°C.[48] Platelets stored under these latter conditions have an increased tendency to aggregate because the inactivation of the temperature-dependent oxydative phosphorylation system results in a decreased synthesis of ATP and therefore an increased membrane permeability for ADP.[48]

Citrated PRP loses its aggregability after storage at 20°C for varying periods of time. Thus platelet aggregation was shown to be less after 3 hr at 20°C than after 2 hr under the same conditions.

Praga and Pagliani[49] stress the importance of the time that PRP is incubated in the cuvette holder of the aggregometer. When citrated PRP which has been maintained at 20°C is added to a cuvette holder maintained at 37°C and ADP is used as an aggregating agent, slight variations in the activated PRP temperature (not that of the cuvette holder) may result in qualitative changes of aggregation curves such as appearance of a second wave or disaggregation, especially when low concentrations of ADP (<1 μM) are used.

Conditions of Stirring

Coller and Gralnick[50] demonstrated that stir bar size and shape affected aggregation patterns. In general, stir bars that mixed more effectively gave greater aggregation. Small differences in stir bar length resulted in significant differences in aggregation and could make the difference between the presence or absence of the second wave of ADP and epinephrine aggregation. It appeared that Teflon®-coated stir bars produced faster equilibration of the aggregating agent and the platelets in the PRP than noncoated steel bars due to the increased thickness of the Teflon® coating. An unexpected finding was that there was an enhancement of the second wave of epinephrine aggregation by some of the longer steel wire bars compared to the Teflon®-coated bar despite less effectiveness in mixing. O'Brien[51] had previously shown that 1000 rpm was the ideal speed for the stirrer motor; this has been confirmed.[52]

Preparation of PRP

The ideal PRP would contain the maximum harvest of platelets in the maximum volume of plasma with a minimum number of red and white blood cells. Utilizing present techniques, a recovery of 37 to 42% plasma, a platelet count in excess of 3.0×10^5 mm^{-3}, and less than 2 to 4 RBC per high power field (×400) is as nearly ideal as can be achieved. The time of centrifugation must be kept short in order to obtain platelets which are still functional. A reasonable volume of plasma is required for platelet aggregation tests, and it is desirable to have a representative sample of the platelet population. Woods et al.[53] performed a detailed study of the factors influencing preparation of PRP and found that centrifugation of citrated whole blood for just over Gmax-221G (Gav = 193.6) for 10 min gave a satisfactory harvest of PRP. They determined that the G force used was critical; if too high, too many platelets were lost, if too low, too many red cells contaminated the preparation. It is to be stressed that G-av forces are to be used and not RPM, since each centrifuge has different radii. Centrifuge tubes with vertical walls and flat bottoms may be preferable to conical tubes.[53]

Number of Platelets

Platelet counts of the PRP between 200,000 to 400,000 per mm^3 are satisfactory for most studies. Abnormal results may occur in patients with high platelet counts with a resulting platelet count of over 500,000 to 600,000. This seems to be due to an intrinsic defect in the platelets. Satisfactory platelet aggregation curves may be obtained with platelet counts as low as 75,000.[54]

Effects of Drugs

Platelet aggregation may be inhibited by a wide variety of drugs, most of which contain aspirin or other antiinflammatory agents. Since well over 500 compounds that contain aspirin are marketed, most of which are sold without prescription,[55] the subject under study may inadvertently be taking an aspirin-containing drug and not know it. Since aspirin prevents prostaglandin synthesis, the second phase of aggregation is ablated and collagen-induced aggregation is reduced. Other drugs such as phenothiazine, benzodiazepine, tricyclic antidepressants, glyceryl guanacolate, antihistamines, furadantin, and carbenicillin are all said to affect platelet aggregation. It is best to ask the patients to avoid all drugs prior to testing and to repeat all abnormal patient platelet responses before a definitive diagnosis is made.

Interpretation of Aggregation Data

Analysis of aggregation curves via mathematically derived formula by computer analysis has been proposed by several groups of investigators.[56,57] Such sophistication hardly seems warranted at this point, because the aggregometer tracings are recording a gross phenomenon which is occurring in the cuvette and may have little relevance to what occurs in vivo or for that matter early in vitro. The analogy between reading an electrocardiogram and the tracings from a recorder connected to a platelet aggregometer may be correct. The maximal change in light transmission seems to be the most important parameter to be tested; thus percentage of aggregation (referring to the delta optical density change before and after aggregation agent addition) is probably an acceptable unit for assigning a numerical value to platelet aggregation. The initial rate of change and time required to reach maximal aggregation are also useful parameters. A platelet aggregation response is said to be abnormal when significantly less change in optical density (aggregation response or percentage of aggregation) occurs in a platelet-rich plasma preparation from a given subject than that obtained in a population of normal individuals tested under similar conditions and with identical concentrations of aggregating agent.[55] Comparison of aggregation curves produced by thrombin, ionophores such as A23187, arachidonate, and collagen are only possible when low concentrations of these agents are used; when higher concentrations are utilized it is best to use serotonin or nucleotide release as a means of comparison. The antibiotic ristocetin, which causes agglutination and not aggregation of platelets, produces dose-responsive curves in platelet-rich plasma which can be used as an indirect measure of the von Willebrand's factor in plasma.[58,32,35]

Several commercial aggregometers are available in both the Eastern and Western Hemisphere and appear to be reliable in the hands of various investigators. The choice of a single channel aggregometer vs. one with multiple channels seems to rest with the preference of the individual scientist and the use to which the apparatus is to be put; multiple cuvettes appear most useful for pharmacological manipulation, whereas single channel or dual channel appear adequate for patient evaluation. The best advice to anyone who wishes to acquire an aggregometer would be to investigate several of the types available and make the final determination on the basis of the needs of the individual laboratory.

Clinical Value of Platelet Aggregation (Table 2)

Platelet aggregation has become accepted as one of the principal tests for detecting abnormalities of platelet function which may be either congenital or acquired. Recent review articles detail clinical and laboratory descriptions of these conditions.[35,58,45,52,59] The following discussion will be restricted to the changes one might see in aggregation tracings. In the majority of conditions in which platelets do not aggregate normally, some improvement of hemostasis exists with the exception of an isolated lack of second phase aggregation to epinephrine which may be "normal" finding in up to 40% of "normal" blood donors.[7]

Thrombasthenia

In this disorder (Figure 3), neither primary nor secondary aggregation occurs with all known aggregating agents. Agglutination with ristocetin, adherence to collagen, shape change, and release of granular contents is intact. The hemostatic defect is usually severe.

Abnormalities of the Release (Secretion) Reaction

These are of two main types: (1) storage pool deficiency and (2) nonstorage pool deficiency or "aspirin-like" defect. Both defects produce similar aggregation patterns (Figure 4): lack of second-phase aggregation with ADP and epinephrine with only primary aggregation recorded followed by rapid disaggregation. Collagen-induced aggregation is greatly diminished, especially when lower concentrations of collagen are used.

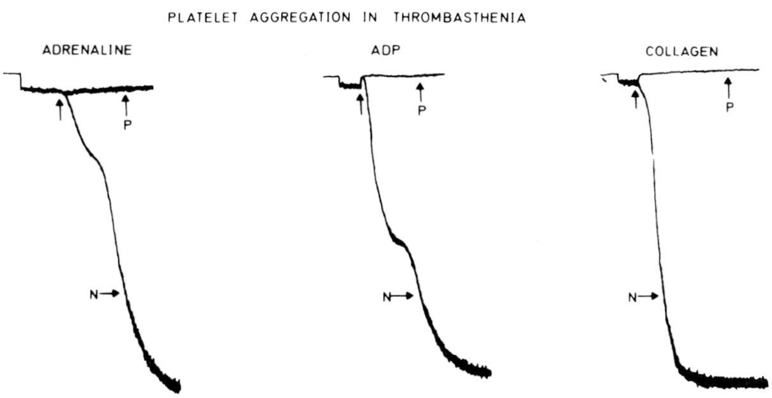

FIGURE 3. Platelet aggregation in thrombasthenia. Note absence of any aggregation pattern with the three reagents and presence of shape change with ADP and collagen. P = patient; N = normal control.

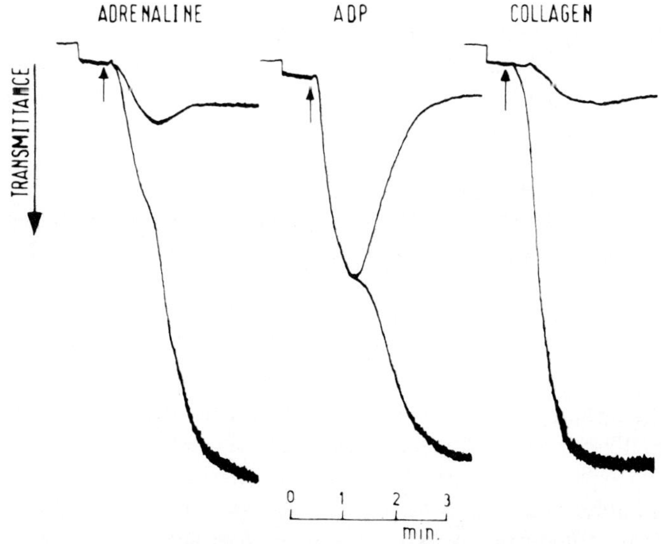

FIGURE 4. Platelet aggregation in a release defect (Storage Pool deficiency). Note only first phase aggregation with adrenaline and ADP followed by rapid disaggregation. Collagen-induced aggregation is deficient in comparison to normal.

The two conditions are separated by measurement of the storage pool ADP, ATP, serotonin, and calcium, all of which are diminished in the first type of release abnormality — storage pool deficiency. Radioactive serotonin uptake and release has proven a useful simple test to identify this group of patients.[59] The second platelet release abnormality "aspirin-like" or "nonstorage pool deficiency" is associated with a normal storage pool, but an aggregometry tracing is recorded resembling that following aspirin ingestion. Defects in prostaglandin synthesis have been reported in this group of patients, and this subclassification of release defects may be better termed prostaglandin defects in the future.

Storage pool defects have been reported in Hermansky-Pudlak syndrome, Albinos, Wiskott-Aldrich syndrome, thrombocytopenia with absent radii, and Chediak-Higashi syndrome.

In all cases, the defect in hemostasis usually is mild.

von Willebrand Disease

In this syndrome, associated with a deficiency or abnormality in a plasma factor (vWF), platelet aggregation with all aggregating agents is normal. Agglutination with ristocetin is defective or absent in some cases. The platelets play a passive role in this latter reaction, because platelets which have been fixed with gluteraldehyde or formalin will agglutinate in PRP provided vWF is present.

Bernard-Soulier Syndrome

In this disorder characterized by giant platelets, all aggregation responses to the standard aggregating agents such as ADP, collagen, thrombin, and epinephrine are normal. Shape change in the presence of ADP may not occur, but the most useful diagnostic test appears to be lack of agglutination to ristocetin or bovine factor VIII.

Others

Platelet aggregation is defective in several thrombocytopenic disorders such as the May-Hegglin anomaly, "Swiss cheese" platelet disorder, Gray platelet syndrome, etc. In the majority of these cases, defective collagen-induced aggregation is most common, and response to ADP is diminished. As a whole, the group has been termed thrombocytopenic-thrombocytopathic.

Defective platelet aggregation has been identified in a group of diseases known as "acquired storage pool deficiencies" which are seen in association with such diseases as lupus, nephritis, autoimmune phenomenon, etc.[60]

Platelet Factor 3 (PF3) Availability

Platelets function in the coagulation sequence by supplying the phospholipid (PF3) necessary for the generation of thrombin. In this way, PF3 availability tests measure in test tubes the clot-promoting effect of platelets.

PF3 shortens the clotting time, and various commercial reagents containing phospholipid obtained from different sources function in a similar manner. Stypven reagent, prepared from the venom of the Russel viper, accelerates coagulation by interacting with coagulation factors V and X and thus increasing the formation of prothrombinase. The prothrombinase then indirectly accelerates thrombin formation and, secondarily, the conversion of fibrinogen into fibrin.

The test for platelet factor 3 availability may be performed by using the Stypven reagent or Kaolin, the latter as an activating agent of the intrinsic coagulation system.[61,62] Under these circumstances, the plasma coagulation factors are maximally activated and the recalcification time performed reflects the amount of PF3 made available by the platelets. At one time, it was considered likely that PF3 was secreted from the platelet during the platelet release reaction, but studies by Sixma and Nijessen,[63] among others, have indicated a dissociation between the availability of PF3 and the release reaction under various conditions. It is highly likely that the mechanism whereby the two components are released from the platelet is different. PF3 activity increases during aggregation induced by ADP, epinephrine, and collagen-induced aggregation. PF3 activity is dependent upon the number of platelets, being low in thrombocytopenia, and is temperature dependent, i.e., more PF3 is available if the determination is performed at 37°C rather than 5°C.

PF3 availability testing seems to add little to the diagnosis of platelet function defects since it is abnormal in those conditions — thrombasthenia and thrombocytopathia — in which there is defective aggregation. It probably reflects an alteration in membrane configuration which is reflected in an abnormal aggregation pattern. This alteration may be primarily located in the membrane, as in thrombasthenia, or in a defective release mechanism which has a lack of full or second phase aggregation. PF3 activity remains associated with the platelets when disaggregation has occurred, indicating that the major source of PF3 activity is in the membrane.

Recent reports of isolated PF3 availability defects, while extremely rare, are of interest and may reawaken interest in this otherwise seldom used test.[55,62,64]

Clot Retraction

Clot retraction may be studied either in native blood or in platelet-rich plasma after recalcification, although the latter seems more appropriate in the study of platelet function. The mechanism of clot retraction depends upon the number of platelets in the sample, since clot retraction is absent in thrombocytopenia. The fibrinogen content of the plasma is also an important factor; clot retraction is absent in afibrinogenemia. Clot retraction may be delayed in samples with high fibrinogen levels, due to the high mechanical forces necessary to express serum.

The test has been of greatest value in investigating thrombasthenia, a condition in which clot retraction is absent. Clot retraction is normal in all other platelet function abnormalities, although it may be defective in uremia.

It would seem that clot retraction is a rather limited test in diagnosing platelet function defects — it is abnormal in thrombocytopenia and in thrombasthenia, two conditions which are more easily diagnosed using standard tests such as platelet counting and platelet aggregation techniques.

The rather gross nature of the test, with its limited information return, precludes its being able to discriminate in any but these two broad abnormalities. This statement seems to be true in spite of the fact that numerous attempts have been made to refine the test and give it greater sensitivity. While these have been useful in adding to our information on the mechanisms of clot retraction, they have added little to our diagnostic acumen.

The Future of Platelet Function Testing

With the exception of the bleeding time, all of the tests for measuring platelet function are studies of phenomenology: a phenomenon which occurs in a system into which a group of artifacts are introduced. If the artifacts are maintained constant, one may get an estimate of platelet function. On the other hand, if an artifact varies from laboratory to laboratory, comparable results are difficult to achieve. With the realization that one is attempting to study a group of in vivo phenomena in an artificial in vitro system, it is truly amazing that as much useful information has accrued as has been documented both through the literature and personal experience.

It seems logical that platelet function testing would be more meaningful when whole blood is used rather than anticoagulated platelet-rich plasma. Under these circumstances, the presence of red and white blood cells could influence the platelets, much as they do in vivo, as has been shown for platelet glass bead retention. Another possible advantage of utilizing whole blood rather than PRP would be avoiding the loss of a population of platelets which might be more suitable for testing than those recovered in the process of making PRP. Separation of platelets from red and white blood cells causes a loss of platelets which are different from those remaining in the PRP.[37,38,53] It may be this subpopulation of platelets which is most important in propagation of thrombosis.

The proliferation of new in vitro platelet function tests designed to test for defects in hemostasis seems to have reached a plateau. It is altogether likely that the currently available in vitro platelet function tests will continue to fulfill the need for definitive laboratory studies directed toward diagnosis of hemostatic deficiency disease states. Improvements in these tests will occur as a result of simulation of in vivo conditions, i.e., a method for detecting platelet aggregation in whole blood would more nearly simulate the in vivo situation than platelet aggregation performed in citrated PRP. It would seem that the ideal platelet function test would encompass a tool which would allow the ex vivo study of in vivo events.

The new frontier of platelet function testing is that directed toward detection of hyperfunctioning or hyperaggregable platelets. At this writing, this form of testing is in its infancy. It may be that the tests previously used have been inadvertently biased toward making a diagnosis of hypofunctioning platelets. An example of this would be the platelet glass bead retention test where it was found that increasing the weight of glass beads in the glass bead column to 2.5 g increased the glass bead retention and therefore made hyporetention and thus hypofunctional platelets more easily detectable. If the columns were to be constructed to detect platelet function which would signify thrombotic tendencies, perhaps they should contain fewer glass beads, which would decrease the normal glass bead retention, thereby making increased "adhesiveness" more prominent. Platelet glass bead retention actually may be increased in patients with diabetes mellitus and possibly thyroid disease, as has been shown for increased sensitivity to ADP in PRP as measured by aggregometry.[65,66,69] Techniques such as spontaneous platelet aggregation and circulating platelet aggregates have been reviewed and seem to show some correlation between conditions associated with thrombotic tendency and platelet hypersensitivity.[67,68,70] Increased platelet aggregation as demonstrated by increased sensitivity to the platelet aggregating agents using a log-dose relationship has been demonstrated in patients with diabetes mellitus.[69]

Increased levels of platelet factor 4 and beta-thromboglobulin have been demonstrated in myocardial infarction[61] and deep vein thrombosis. Shortened platelet survival is noted in patients with homocystinuria,[68] atherosclerosis, and metastatic carcinoma.[35] It is obvious that the conditions in which a tendency toward thrombosis are operative far outnumber those in which hemostatic defects exist. Therefore, the major thrust of future platelet function testing will probably be in the area of demonstration of reactive or hyperaggregable platelets.

Harker and Slichter[68] have demonstrated the value of platelet survival studied in thrombotic disease. Decreased survival of platelets was correlated with various forms of arterial thrombosis, probably on the basis of consumption of platelets during the formation of thrombi, as has also been shown for metastatic carcinomatosis. Aspirin therapy alone did not improve the survival of these thrombotic states, reinforcing the feeling that prostaglandin synthesis is important but not totally accountable for the increased platelet vessel wall interreaction. In contrast, the addition of dipyridamole normalizes platelet survival, although there is limited clinical evidence and experimental data to suggest that this drug, either alone or in combination with aspirin, may be useful for platelet mediated thrombotic states. Just as the template bleeding time is the only test that correlates with clinical evidence of platelet mediated bleeding, the measurement of platelet survival, either directly or indirectly by MDA production,[33] may be the only currently available technique that correlates with the clinical manifestations of platelet-mediated thrombotic disorders or with effectiveness of appropriate therapy for these disorders.

REFERENCES

1. **Holmsen, H., Day, H. J., and Stormorken, H.**, The blood platelet release reactions, *Scand. J. Haematol.*, 3, 26, 1969.
2. **Day, H. J.**, Role of platelets in hemostasis and thrombosis, *Ser. Haematol.*, 8, 3, 1976.
3. **Day, H. J. and Holmsen, H.**, Concepts of the blood platelet release reaction, *Ser. Haematol.*, 4, 3, 1971.
4. **Mustard, J. F. and Packham, M. A.**, The role of blood and platelets in atherosclerosis and complications of atherosclerosis, *Thromb. Diath. Haemorrh.*, 61, 44, 1975.
5. **Walsh, P. N.**, The role of platelets in the contact phase of blood coagulation, *Br. J. Haematol.*, 22, 237, 1972.
6. **Day, H. J., Holmsen, H., Zucker, M.**, *Platelet Function Testing*, DHEW-Pub-NIH-78-1087, 1978.
7. **O'Brien, J.**, *Platelet Function Testing*, Day, H. J., Holmsen, H., and Zucker, M. B., Eds., DHEW-Pub-NIH-78-1087, 1978, 29.
8. **Duke, W. W.**, The relation of blood platelets to hemorrhagic diseases, *JAMA*, 55, 1185, 1910.
9. **Ivy, N. C., Nelson, D., and Bucher, G. J.**, The standardization to certain factors in the cutaneous "venostasis" bleeding time technique, *J. Lab. Clin. Med.*, 26, 1812, 1941.
10. **Borchgrevink, C. F. and Waaler, P. A.**, The secondary bleeding time. A new method for the differentiation of hemorrhagic disease, *Acta Med. Scand.*, 162, 361, 1958.
11. **Mielke, C. H., Kaneshiro, M. M., Maher, I. A., Wessler, J. M., and Rapaport, S. I.**, The standardized normal Ivy bleeding time and its prolongation by aspirin, *Blood*, 34, 204, 1969.
12. **Kumar, R., Answell, J., and Deykin, D.**, Clinical trial of a new bleeding time device, in *Platelet Function Testing*, Day, H. J., Holmsen, H., and Zucker, M. B., Eds., DHEW-Pub-NIH-78-1087, 1978, 21.
13. **Pragu, R., Valentini, L., Maiorano, M., and Cortellaro, M.**, A new automatic device for the standardized Ivy bleeding time, in *Platelet Function and Thrombosis*, Mannucci, P. M. and Gorni, S., Eds., Plenum Publishing, New York, 271, 1973.
14. **Harker, L. A. and Slichter, S. J.**, The bleeding time as a screening test for the evaluation of platelet function, *N. Engl. J. Med.* 287, 155, 1972.
15. **Roth, G. J. and Majerus, P. W.**, Mechanism of the effect of aspirin on human platelets. I. Acetylation of particulate factors of protein, *J. Clin. Invest.*, 56, 624, 1975.
16. **Wright, H. P.**, The adhesiveness of blood platelets in normal subjects with varying concentrations of anticoagulants, *J. Pathol. Bacteriol.* 53, 255, 1941.
17. **Hellem, A. J.**, Platelet adhesiveness, *Ser. Haematol.*, 2, 99, 1968.
18. **Hellem, A. J.**, The adhesiveness of human blood platelets in vitro, *Scand. J. Clin. Lab. Invest.*, 12 (Suppl.51), 1, 1960.
19. **Salzman, E. W.**, Measurement of platelet adhesiveness: a simple in vitro technique demonstrating an abnormality in von Willebrand's disease, *J. Lab. Clin. Med.*, 62, 724, 1963.
20. **Bowie, E. J. W., Owen, C. A., Jr., Thompson, J. H., Jr., and Didisheim, P.**, Platelet adhesiveness in von Willebrand disease, *Am. J. Clin. Pathol.*, 52, 69, 1969.
21. **Hellem, A. J.**, Platelet adhesiveness in von Willebrand's disease: a study with a modification of the glass bead filter method, *Scand. J. Haematol.*, 7, 374, 1970.
22. **Coller, B. S. and Zucker, M. B.**, Reversible decrease in platelet retention by glass bead column (adhesiveness) induced by disturbing the blood, *Proc. Soc. Exp. Biol. Med.*, 136, 769, 1971.
23. **Weiss, H. J. and Rogers, J.**, Fibrinogen and platelets in the primary arrest of bleeding. Studies in two patients with congenital afibrinogenemia, *N. Engl. J. Med.*, 285, 369, 1971.
24. **Zucker, M. B.**, Mechanism of platelet retention in glass bead columns, in *Platelet Function Testing*, Day, H. J., Holmsen, H., and Zucker, M. B., Eds., DHEW-Pub-NIH-78-1087, 1978, 174.
25. **Zucker, M. B., Rifkin, P. L., Friedberg, N. M., and Coller, B. S.**, Mechanism of platelet function as revealed by the retention of platelets in glass bead columns, *Ann. N. Y. Acad. Sci.*, 201, 138, 1972.

26. **Bowie, E. J. W. and Owen, C. A., Jr.**, Some factors influencing platelet retention in glass bead columns including the influence of platelets, *Am. J. Clin. Pathol.*, 56, 479, 1971.
27. **Weiss, H. J.**, Platelet function tests and their interpretation (editorial), *J. Lab. Clin. Med.*, 87, 909, 1970.
28. **Smith, J. B., Ingerman, C., Hocsis, J. J., and Smith, M. J.**, Formation of an intermediate in prostaglandin biosynthesis and its association with the platelet release reaction, *J. Clin. Invest.*, 33, 1460, 1974.
29. **Hamberg, M., Svenson, J., and Samuelsson, B.**, Thromboxanes: a new group of biologically active compounds derived from prostaglandin endoperoxides, *Proc. Natl. Acad. Sci. U.S.A.*, 72, 2994, 1975.
30. **Mustard, J. F., Perry, D. W., Kinlough-Rathbone, R. L., and Packham, M. A.**, Factors responsible for ADP-induced release reaction of human platelets, *Am. J. Physiol.*, 228, 1757, 1975.
31. **Howard, M. A. and Firkin, R. G.**, Ristocetin — a new tool in the investigation of platelet aggregation, *Thromb. Diath. Haemorrh.*, 26, 362, 1971.
32. **Weiss, H. J., Rodgers, J., and Brand, H.**, Further studies on the von Willebrand factor (Factor VIII) — Ristocetin-induced platelet aggregation, *Blood*, 40, 939a, 1973.
33. **Smith, J. B., Ingerman, C. M., and Silver, M. J.**, Malondealdehyde formation as an indication of prostaglandin production by human platelets, *J. Lab. Clin. Med.*, 88, 167, 1976.
34. **Packham, M. A., Kinlough-Rathbone, R. L., Reimers, H. J., Scott, S., and Mustard, J. F.**, Mechanism of platelet aggregation independent of adenosine diphosphate, *Proc. Int. Symp. Prostaglandins Hematol.*, Philadelphia, 1976, in press.
35. **Packham, M. A., Kinlough-Rathbone, R. L., and Mustard, J. F.**, Aggregation and agglutination, in *Platelet Function Testing*, Day, H. J., Holmsen, H., and Zucker, M. B., Eds., DHEW-Pub-NIH-78-1087, 1978, 66.
36. **Born, G. V. R.**, Aggregation of blood platelets by adenosine diphosphate and its reversal, *Nature (London)*, 194, 927, 1962.
37. **Day, H. J., Holmsen, H., and Zucker, M. B.**, Methods for separating platelets from blood and plasma, *Thromb. Diath. Haemorrh.*, 33, 648, 1975.
38. **Day, H. J. and Hardisty, R. M.**, Report of the task force on platelet standards, in *Thrombosis-Pathogenesis and Clinical Trials*, Dutsch, E., Brinkhouse, K. M., Lechner, K., and Hinton, S., Eds., F. K. Schatauer Verlag, Stuttgart, 1974, 423.
39. **Born, G. V. R. and Hume, M.**, Effects of the numbers and sizes of platelet aggregation on the optical density of plasma, *Nature (London)*, 215, 1027, 1967.
40. **Mills, D. C. B., Robb, D. Q., and Roberts, G. C.**, The release of nucleotide, 5-hydroxytryptinine and enzymes from human blood platelets during aggregation, *J. Physiol.*, 195, 715, 1968.
41. **Ts'ao, C. H., Lo, R., and Raynard, J.**, Clinical importance of citrate - blood ratio on platelet aggregation studies, *Am. J. Clin. Pathol.*, 65, 518, 1976.
42. **Han, P. and Ardlie, N. G.**, The influence of pH, temperature, and calcium on platelet aggregation: maintenance of environmental pH and platelet function for in vitro studies in plasma, *Br. J. Haematol.*, 26, 373, 1974.
43. **Zucker, M. B.**, Effect of heparin on platelet function, *Thromb. Diath. Haemorrh.*, 33, 63, 1975.
44. **Day, H. J., Holmsen, H., and Zucker, M. B.**, Report of the working party on platelets, *Thromb. Haemostasis*, 1, 236, 1976.
45. **Zucker, M. B.**, Tests of platelet adhesion, aggregation and release, *Thromb. Diath. Haemorrh.*, Suppl. 42, 1, 1972.
46. **Mustard, J. F. and Packham, M. A.**, Factors influencing platelet function: adhesion, release and aggregation, *Pharmacol. Rev.*, 22, 97, 1970.
47. **Rossi, E. C. and Louis, G.**, A time-dependent increase in the responsiveness of platelet-rich plasma to epinephrine, *J. Lab. Clin. Med.*, 85, 300, 1975.
48. **Reuter, H., Podolgah, B., Hagen, I., Linker, H., Stroder, J., and Gross, R.**, Investigations on the time dependence of platelet functions, *Thromb. Res.*, 3, 307, 1973.
49. **Praga, C. A. and Pogliani, E. M.**, Effect of temperature on ADP-induced platelet aggregation, *Thromb. Diath. Haemorrh.*, 29, 183, 1973.
50. **Coller, B. S. and Gralnick, H. R.**, The effect of stir bar size and shape on quantitative platelet aggregation, *Thromb. Res.*, 8, 121, 1976.
51. **O'Brien, J. R.**, Platelet aggregation. II. Some results with a new method of study, *J. Clin. Pathol.*, 15, 452, 1962.
52. **Sixma, J. J.**, Methods of platelet aggregation, in *Platelet Function and Thrombosis*, Mannucci, P. M. and Gorini, S., Eds., Plenum Publishing, New York, 1972.
53. **Woods, B. P., Dehnnehy, A., and Clark, N.**, Some observations on the preparation of platelet-rich plasma, *Thromb. Haemostasis*, 36, 302, 1976.
54. **Levine, P. H.**, The effect of thrombocytopenia in the determination of platelet aggregation, *Am. J. Clin. Pathol.*, 65, 72, 1976.

55. Weiss, H. J., Platelet function tests and their interpretation, *J. Lab. Clin. Med.*, 87, 909, 1976.
56. Holdrinet, A., Ewals, M., Reschaft, W. J., and Haanen, C., Mathematical correlation between ADP-induced platelet aggregation and subsequent disaggregation: a parameter for the velocity of disaggregation, *Scand. J. Haematol.*, 6, 354, 1969.
57. Frojmavic, M., Quantitative parameterization of the light transmission properties of citrated, platelet-rich plasma as a function of platelet and adenosine diphosphate concentration and temperature, *J. Lab. Clin. Med.*, 82, 137, 1973.
58. Weiss, H. J., Platelet physiology and abnormalities of platelet function, *N. Engl. J. Med.*, 293 (531), 580, 1975.
59. Paretti, F. I., Day, H. J., and Mills, D. C. B., Nucleotide and serotonin metabolism in platelets with defective secondary aggregation, *Blood*, 44, 789, 1974.
60. Zahavi, J., Acquired "storage pool disease" of platelets, *Thromb. Haemostasis*, 3, 501, 1976.
61. Hardisty, R. M. and Hutton, P. A., The kaolin clotting time of platelet-rich plasma. A test of platelet factor 3 availability, *Br. J. Haematol.*, 11, 258, 1965.
62. Weiss, H. J., Platelet aggregation, adhesion and adenosine diphosphate release in thrombopathia (platelet factor 3 deficiency), *Am. J. Med.*, 43, 570, 1967.
63. Sixma, J. J. and Nijessen, J. G., Characteristics of platelet factor 3 release during ADP-induced aggregation — comparison with 5-hydroxytryptamine release, *Thromb. Diath. Haemorrh.* (Stuttgart), 24, 206, 1970.
64. Sultan, Y., Broyet, J. C., and Devergie, A., Isolated platelet factor 3 deficiency, *New Engl. J. Med.*, 294, 1121, 1976.
65. O'Malley, B. C., Timperley, W. R., Ward, J. D., Porter, N. R., and Preston, F. E., Platelet abnormalities in diabetic peripheral neuropathy, *Lancet*, 2, 1274, 1975.
66. Timperley, W. R., Ward, J. D., Preston, F. E., Duckworth, T., and O'Malley, B. C., Clinical and histological studies in diabetic neuropathy. A reassessment of vascular factors in relation to intravascular coagulation, *Diabetologica*, 12, 237, 1976.
67. Carvalho, A., Colman, R. W., and Lees, R. S., Coagulation abnormalities in hyperbetalipoproteinemia and their modification with therapy, *J. Clin. Invest.*, 53, 159, 1974.
68. Harker, L. A. Slichter, S. J., Scott, C. R., and Ross, R., Homocystininemia, vascular injury and arterial thrombosis, *N. Engl. J. Med.*, 291, 537, 1974.
69. Kwaan, H. C., Colwell, J. P., Cruz, S., Suwarwele, N., and Dobbie, J. G., Increased platelet aggregation in diabetes mellitus, *J. Lab. Clin. Med.*, 80, 236, 1972.
70. Breddin, K., Grun, H., Krzywarek, H. J., and Schremmers, W. P., The measurement of spontaneous platelet aggregation. III. The platelet aggregation test, *Thromb. Haemostasis*, 2, 666, 1976.

CONTRIBUTIONS OF PLATELETS TO INTRINSIC COAGULATION

Peter N. Walsh

Platelets function in hemostasis by carrying out a wide variety of functions including adhesion to subendothelial surfaces exposed after vascular injury, aggregation, and secretion of granular contents. Platelets also carry out essential functions by promoting intrinsic coagulation reactions. The term "platelet coagulant activities" is used to describe the multiple and complex functions of platelets in intrinsic coagulation (Figures 1 to 8). The time-honored term "platelet factor 3" has been criticized because it implies the presence in platelets of an isolable factor which promotes a specific coagulation reaction.[1,2] Although mixtures of phospholipids extracted from platelets and other tissues can substitute for platelets in some coagulation reactions, it seems likely that platelets function in intrinsic coagulation by providing a physiological surface for the optimal interaction and binding of clotting factors to form complexes with enzymatic activity resulting in proteolytic cleavage and activation of coagulation factors.[3-6]

A great deal of work has been done to define the mode of action of purified phospholipids and crude lipid extracts in coagulation reactions.[7-11] Complexes of proteins and phospholipids extracted from platelets have been shown to have far greater functional activities than phospholipids alone.[12] The recent development of methods[13] for washing platelets free of loosely adherent coagulation factors has permitted: (1) the identification of coagulation factors associated with platelets and those easily removed, and (2) the investigation of the specific coagulation reactions in which platelets are involved.

A summary of the relative affinity of various coagulation factors with platelets is presented in Table 1. The vitamin K-dependent coagulation factors, prothrombin, and factors VII, IX, and X are loosely absorbed to platelets and are readily eluted by various washing techniques.[13-15] Plasma fibrinogen is also relatively easily removed by washing, whereas intracellular fibrinogen present in platelet granules is not.[16-20] The

Table 1
ASSOCIATION OF COAGULATION FACTORS WITH PLATELETS

Characteristics	Clotting factors	Ref.
Loosely absorbed and readily eluted	Prothrombin	13—15
	Factor VII	13—15
	Factor IX	13—15
	Factor X	13—15
	Plasma fibrinogen	16—20
Less readily eluted	Factor VIII coagulant activity	13, 21—30
	Plasma factor XII	13, 25, 38—40
	Plasma factor XI	13, 25, 33, 38—43
Not eluted	Factor V	13—15, 22, 23, 31—37
	Platelet factor XI-like activity	40, 41, 43
	Platelet fibrinogen	13—15
	Factor VIII antigen	13, 21—30
Bound to platelet membranes	Thrombin	45
	Factor Xa	46
	Factor XI	43

coagulant activity of factor VIII is less readily eluted from platelets than the vitamin K-dependent factors, but the factor VIII antigen is not eluted from platelets by extensive washing, and there is contradictory evidence regarding its subcellular localization in platelet granules or plasma membranes.[13,21-30] There is general agreement that factor V remains closely associated with well-washed platelets, and recent evidence suggests that it may be present in already activated form.[13-15,22,23,31-37] Factor V has been found by some investigators in platelet plasma membranes and by others in intracellular granules.[34,36,37] Platelets possess a factor XI-like activity which is probably distinct from plasma factor XI.[13,25,33,38-43] Plasma factor XI is found in platelet membranes but is probably removed by washing, and a residual platelet factor XI-like activity can be found in platelet plasma membranes.[43] There is evidence that thrombin and factor Xa are bound to platelet membranes.[44-46]

It is well substantiated that crude lipid extracts or mixtures of purified phospholipids serve an essential function in two fundamental reactions of intrinsic coagulation.[44,47,48] It has also been demonstrated that platelets participate in these two reactions, probably by providing a phospholipoprotein surface which sequesters coagulation factors and calcium to form complexes with enzymatic (serine protease) activity (Figures 1 and 2).[3-11] As an alternative to discarding the rather unsatisfactory term "platelet factor 3" we have chosen to define it as "that activity of platelets which can be measured by shortening of the Russell's viper venom (RVV) time, for which certain phospholipids can substitute and which represents the contribution of platelets to the interaction of factor Xa, factor V, and calcium in the activation of prothrombin."[49] Platelet factor 3 activity is present in platelets in "latent" form, unavailable to participate in coagulation reactions until the platelet membrane is perturbed by various stimuli such as exposure to aggregating agents.[50] The prerequisites for and characteristics of platelet factor 3 activity are summarized in Figure 2.

It is also well substantiated that either phospholipids or platelets are required in the reaction of factor IXa with factor VIII to form factor-X activator.[44,48] The property of the platelet membrane by which it can become activated, can expose membrane

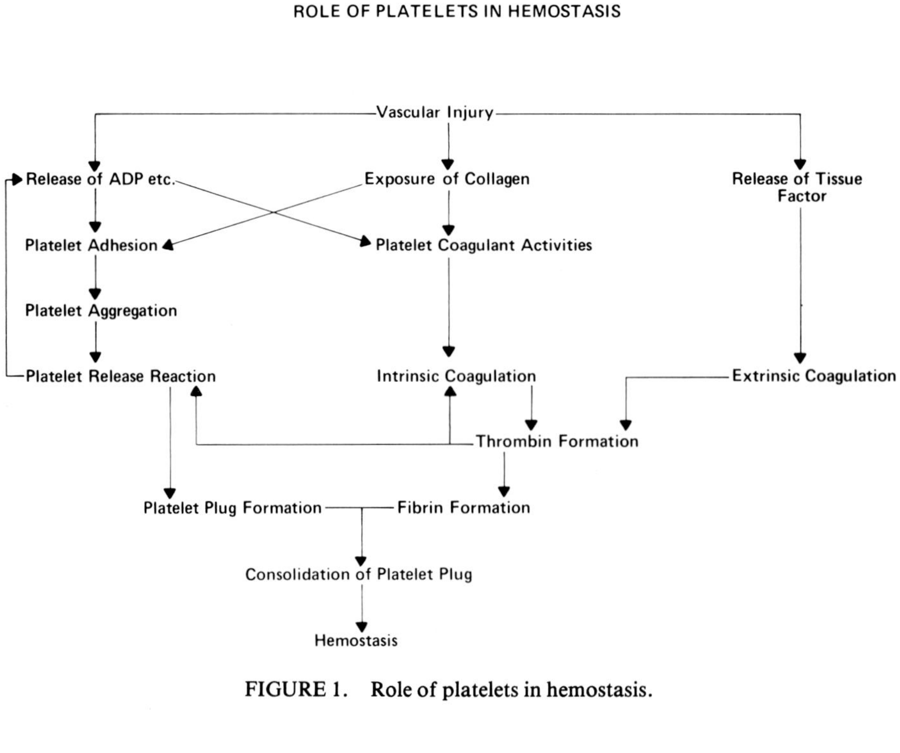

FIGURE 1. Role of platelets in hemostasis.

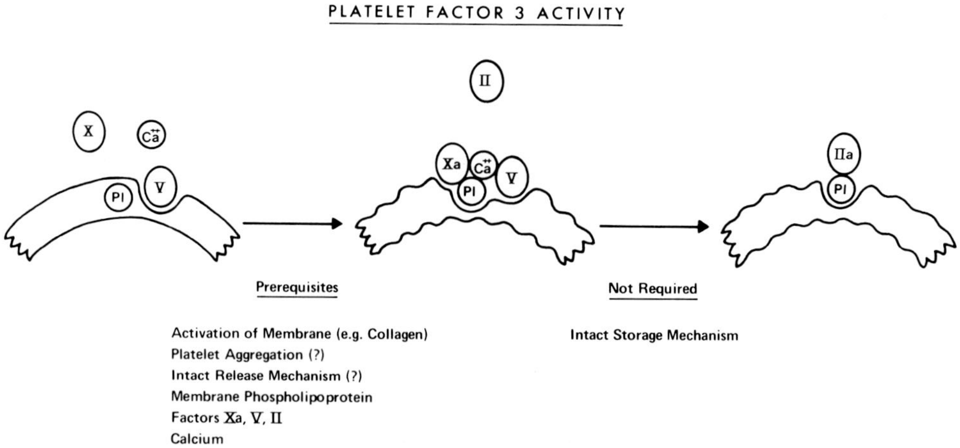

FIGURE 2. Schematic representation of platelet factor 3 activity. The platelet membrane is shown in the unactivated form as a smooth surface and in the activated form as a rough surface. Coagulation factors in the unactivated form are shown by Roman numerals and in the activated as Roman numerals with subscript "a". Pl = phospholipid, Ca^{++} = calcium, R = postulated receptor, (From Walsh, P. N., Platelet Function Testing, DHEW Publication No. (NIH) 77-108, Day, H. J., Homsen, H., and Zucker, M. B., Eds., Government Printing Office, Washington, D. C., 1977, 437—462.)

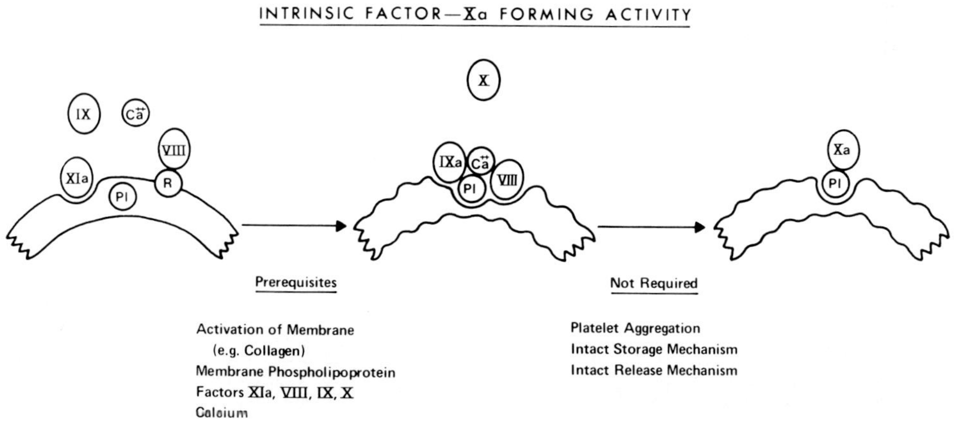

FIGURE 3. Schematic representation of intrinsic factor-Xa-forming activity. See caption to Figure 2 for explanation. (From Walsh, P. N., Platelet Function Testing, DHEW Publication No. (NIH) 77-108, Day, H. J., Homsen, H., and Zucker, M. B., Eds., Government Printing Office, Washington, D. C., 1977, 437—462.)

phospholipoproteins, and can form a complex with factor IXa, factor VIII, and calcium to activate factor X has been termed intrinsic factor-Xa forming activity (Figure 3).[44] This reaction sequence and mechanism is similar to that promoted by platelet factor 3 activity (Figure 2), but the prerequisites for and biochemical determinants of intrinsic factor-Xa forming activity would appear to be different from those for platelet factor 3 activity.[51]

Less well substantiated is the evidence suggesting that platelets have a role in the contact phase of intrinsic coagulation — a function not generally attributed to phospholipids.[40,52] It has been hypothesized that platelets can respond to ADP by a physicochemical change in the platelet surface resulting in the activation of factor XII and the initiation of intrinsic coagulation.[6,52] This hypothetical activity of platelets has been termed contact product-forming activity, the prerequisites for which are listed in Figure 4. There is also evidence for an alternative mechanism by which collagen-stimu-

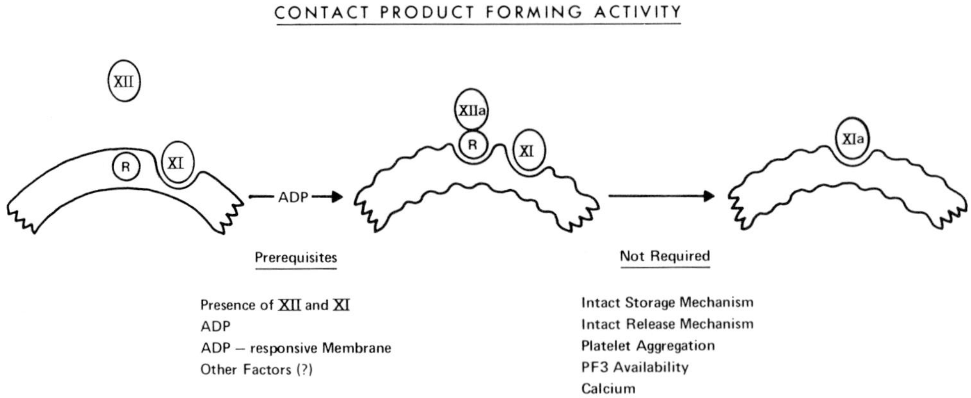

FIGURE 4. Schematic representation of contact product-forming activity. See caption to Figure 2 for explanation. (From Walsh, P. N., Platelet Function Testing, DHEW Publication No. (NIH) 77-108, Day, H. J., Homsen, H., and Zucker, M. B., Eds., Government Printing Office, Washington, D. C., 1977, 437—462.)

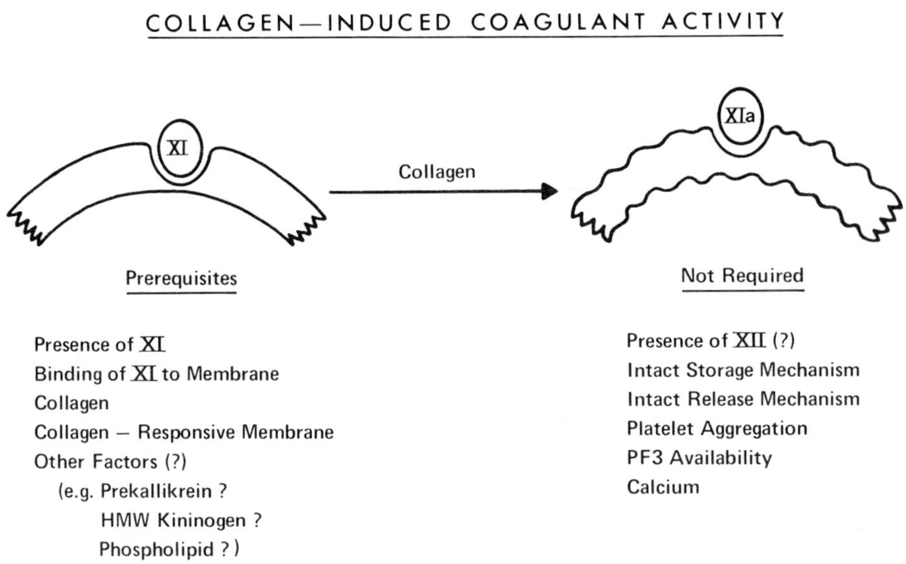

FIGURE 5. Schematic representation of collagen-induced coagulant activity. See caption to Figure 2 for explanation. (From Walsh, P. N., Platelet Function Testing, DHEW Publication No. (NIH) 77-108, Day, H. J., Homsen, H., and Zucker, M. B., Eds., Government Printing Office, Washington, D. C., 1977, 437—462.)

lated platelets can initiate intrinsic coagulation in a reaction which proceeds in factor-XII-deficient plasma.[40] The specific requirements for this platelet coagulant activity, termed collagen-induced coagulant activity, are under investigation, but it apparently requires the presence either of plasma factor XI bound to platelet membranes or the presence of factor-XI-like activity of platelets which may be distinct from plasma factor XI (Figure 5).[36,40,43,44,53] It is not known whether other factors such as prekallikrein, high molecular weight kininogen, or factor XII are required for the normal development of collagen-induced coagulant activity or what other biochemical components of platelet membranes are involved. However, it would appear that this mechanism operates independent of normal mechanisms for platelet aggregation and the storage and release of granular contents.[40,54] The activity develops under conditions not associated with the availability of platelet factor 3 activity.[40,54]

Platelets also appear to provide a protective function relative to certain activated coagulation factors.[6,44] The best documented of these protective functions is the demonstration that both platelets and phospholipids can retard the inactivation of factor Xa by antithrombin III (Figure 6).[44,55] Available evidence suggests that factor Xa is stabilized and its affinity for antithrombin III is decreased in the presence of a complex of phospholipids, factor V, and calcium.[55] Additional evidence suggests that platelets, but not crude lipid extracts, can bind factor XIa and protect it from inactivation by its natural inhibitor in plasma, probably antithrombin II or α_1-antitrypsin (Figure 7).[44]

In addition to the platelet coagulant activities described here, platelets exposed to a variety of aggregating agents can secrete the heparin-neutralizing protein, platelet factor 4, the nature and significance of which is described elsewhere in this volume. Although platelets incubated in vitro for extended periods may develop tissue factor activity, this activity may depend upon the presence of leukocytes and is not present in freshly collected platelets.[56-58] In addition, platelets incubated with endotoxin have recently been shown to develop a direct factor-X activator activity, but this observation requires confirmation.[59]

The possible importance of platelet coagulant activities in hemostasis is summarized in Figure 8.[6] Platelets may be able to trigger intrinsic coagulation reactions by two alternative mechanisms by activating contact factors, although the molecular mechanisms involved have not yet been elucidated.[40,52] If confirmed, the capacity of collagen-stimulated platelets to trigger intrinsic coagulation in factor-XII-deficient plasma may explain the lack of a hemostatic deficiency state in patients with Hageman trait.[40] Pla-

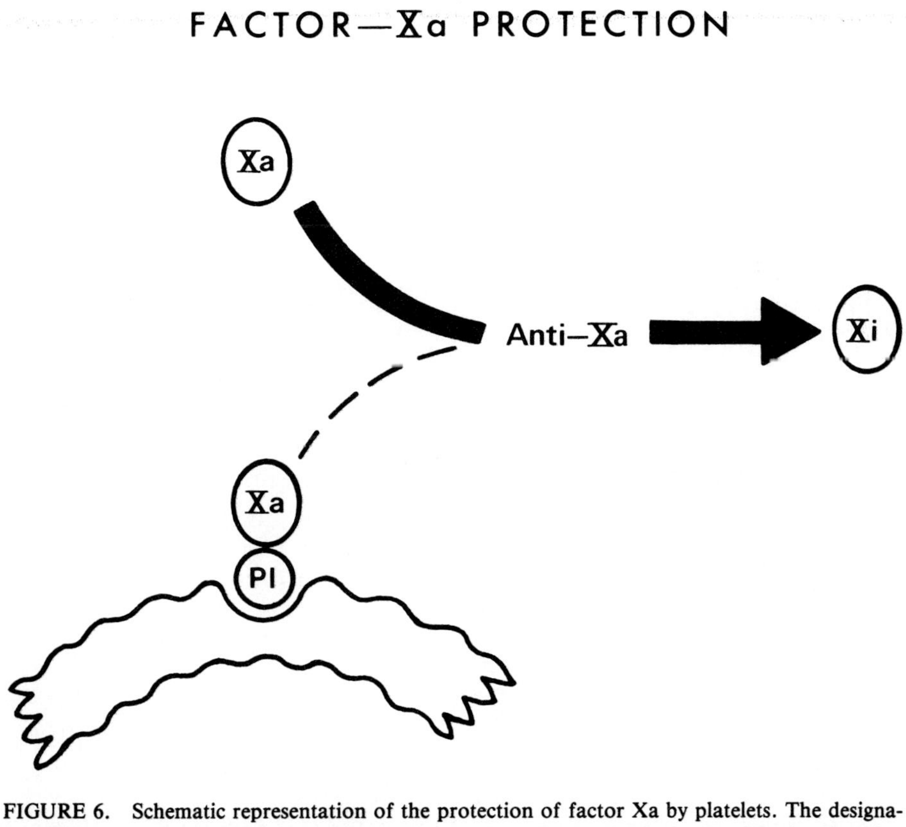

FIGURE 6. Schematic representation of the protection of factor Xa by platelets. The designation Xi represents the inactivated form of factor Xa. (From Walsh, P. N., Platelet Function Testing, DHEW Publication No. (NIH) 77-108, Day, H. J., Homsen, H., and Zucker, M. B., Eds., Government Printing Office, Washington, D.C., 1977, 437—462.)

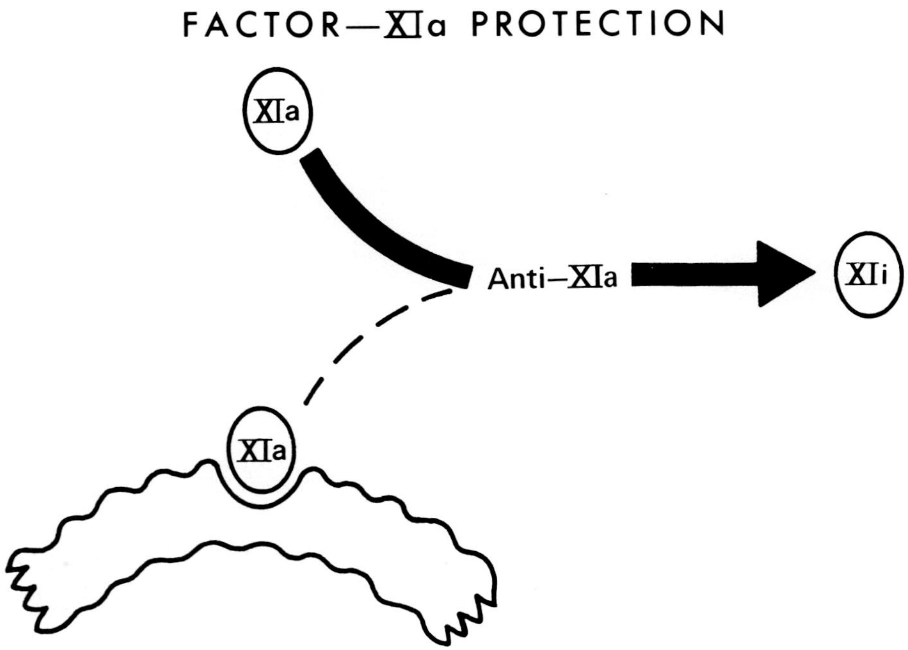

FIGURE 7. Schematic representation of the protection of factor XIa by platelets. See the captions to Figures 2 and 6 for explanations. (From Walsh, P. N., Platelet Function Testing, DHEW Publication No. (NIH) 77-108, Day, H. J., Homsen, H., and Zucker, M. B., Eds. Government Printing Office, Washington, D.C., 1977, 437—462.)

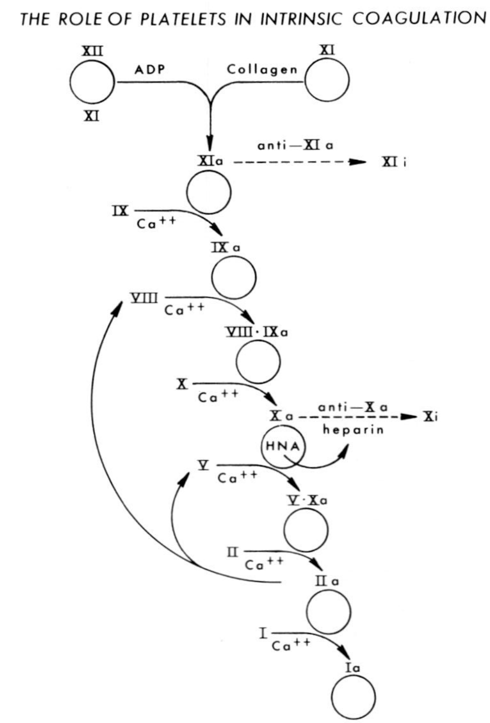

FIGURE 8. Schematic representation of the role of platelets in intrinsic coagulation. The platelets are shown as open circles with coagulation factors as Roman numerals. Ca^{++} = calcium, HNA = heparin neutralizing activity. The dotted arrows represent relative protection of activated clotting factors from inactivation by their natural inhibitors. (From Walsh, P. N., *Blood,* 43(4), 597, 1974. With permission.

telets can then provide a protective surface for the sequential formation of coagulation factor complexes resulting in the generation of activated clotting factors with serine protease activity.[44]

A summary of information relating to the possible clinical importance of platelet coagulant activities in various hemostatic deficiency states and thrombotic disorders is presented in Table 2. Generally, measurements of platelet factor 3 activity have not shown good correlations with the presence of bleeding or thrombotic conditions, whereas assays of platelet coagulant activities concerned with earlier intrinsic coagulation reactions have been deficient in patients with certain hemostatic deficiency states and have been increased in patients with selected thrombotic conditions. The significance of these observations is not clear, although they are consistent with the possibility that platelet coagulant activities, such as collagen-induced coagulant activity, are determinants of hemostatic deficiency in certain conditions and they may play a role in the pathogenesis of certain thrombotic disorders.

Table 2
PLATELET COAGULANT ACTIVITIES IN VARIOUS DISORDERS

Patient group	Collagen-induced coagulant activity	Platelet factor 3 activity	Ref.
Thrombasthenia			
Severe bleeding	Absent	Decreased	60, 61
Mild or moderate bleeding	Normal to increased	Decreased	60, 61
Hemophilia (< 1% F VIII)			
Severe bleeding	Decreased	Normal	62
Mild bleeding	Normal to increased	Normal	62
Bernard-Soulier syndrome	Absent	Increased	53
Hip surgery (1 day post-op)			
Deep vein thrombosis present	Increased	Increased	63
Deep vein thrombosis absent	Normal	Normal	63
Retinal vein occlusion			
Acute primary	Increased	Normal	64
Secondary or chronic	Normal	Normal	64
Transient cerebral ischemic attacks			
Normal serum lipids	Increased	Normal	65
Type IV hyperlipoproteinemia	Normal	Normal	65

REFERENCES

1. **Marcus, A. J.**, Platelet function, *N. Engl. J. Med.*, 280, 1213, 1969.
2. **Marcus, A. J.**, Recent advances in platelet lipid metabolism research, *Ann. N. Y. Acad. Sci.*, 201, 102, 1972.
3. **Bangham, A. D.**, A correlation between surface charge and coagulation action of phospholipids, *Nature* (London), 192, 1197, 1961.
4. **Papahadjopoulos, D., Hougie, C., and Hanahan, D. J.**, Influence of surface charge of phospholipids on their clot-promoting activity, *Proc. Soc. Exp. Biol. Med.*, 111, 412, 1962.
5. **Barton, P. G.**, Lipoproteins of blood coagulation, in *Structural and Functional Aspects of Lipoproteins in Living Systems*, Tria, E. and Scann, A. M., Eds., Academic Press, New York, 1969, 465.
6. **Walsh, P. N.**, Platelet coagulant activities and hemostasis: hypothesis, *Blood*, 43, 597, 1974.
7. **Papahadjopoulos, D. and Hanahan, D. J.**, Observations on the interaction of phospholipids and certain clotting factors in prothrombin activator formation, *Biochim. Biophys. Acta*, 90, 436, 1964.

8. **Barton, P. G., Jackson, C. M., and Hanahan, D. J.,** Relationship between factor V and activated factor X in the generation of prothrombinase, *Nature* (London), 214, 923, 1967.
9. **Hemker, H. C., Esnouf, M. P., Hemker, P. W., Swart, A. C. W., and Macfarlane, R. G.,** Formation of prothrombin converting activity, *Nature* (London, 215, 248, 1967.
10. **Hemker, H. C. and Kahn, M. J. P.,** Reaction sequence of blood coagulation, *Nature* (London), 215, 1201, 1967.
11. **Jobin, F. and Esnouf, M. P.,** Studies on the formation of the prothrombin-converting complex, *Biochem. J.,* 102, 666, 1917.
12. **Marcus, A. J., Zucker-Franklin, D., Safier, L. B., and Ullman, H. L.,** Studies on human platelet granules and membranes, *J. Clin. Invest.,* 45, 14, 1966.
13. **Walsh, P. N.,** Albumin density gradient separation and washing of platelets and the study of platelet coagulant activities, *Br. J. Haematol.,* 22, 205, 1972.
14. **Bounameaux, Y.,** Dosage des facteurs de coagulation contenus dans l'atmosphere plasmatique des plaquettes humaines, *Rev. Fr. Etud. Clin. Biol.,* 2, 52, 1957.
15. **Tangen, O., Lestrup, E. B., and Berman, H. J.,** Characterization of clotting factors associated with blood platelets after gel filtration, *Thromb. Diath. Haemorrh.,* 30, 289, 1973.
16. **Seligmann, M., Goudemand, B., Janin, A., Bernard, J., and Grabar, P.,** Etudes immunochimiques sur la presence de fibrinogene dans des extraits de plaquettes humaines lavees et dans certains extraits leucocytaires, *Rev. Hematol.,* 12, 302, 1957.
17. **Salmon, J. and Bounameaux, Y.,** Etudes des antigenes plaquettaires et, en particulier, du fibrinogene, *Thromb. Diath. Haemorrh.,* 2, 93, 1958.
18. **Gokcen, M., and Yunis, E.,** Fibrinogen as part of platelet structure, *Nature* (London), 200, 590, 1963.
19. **Nachman, R. L., Marcus, A. J., and Zucker-Franklin, D.,** Subcellular localization of platelet fibrinogen, *Blood,* 24, 853, 1964.
20. **Solum, N. O. and Lopaciuk, S.,** Bovine platelet proteins. III. Some properties of platelet fibrinogen, *Thromb. Diath. Haemorrh.,* 21, 428, 1969.
21. **Patek, A. J. and Stetson, R. P.,** Hemophilia. I. The abnormal coagulation of the blood and its relation to the blood platelets, *J. Clin. Invest.,* 15, 531, 1936.
22. **Seibert, R. H., Margolius, A., Jr., and Ratnoff, O. D.,** Observations on hemophilia, parahemophilia, and coexistent hemophilia and parahemophilia, *J. Lab. Clin. Med.,* 52, 449, 1958.
23. **Raccuglia, G.,** Factor VIII (antihemophilic factor) and factor V (proaccelerin) activity of platelets, *Proc. Soc. Exp. Biol. Med.,* 104, 309, 1960.
24. **Borchgrevink, C. F. and Owren, P. A.,** The hemostatic effect of normal platelets in hemophilia and factor V deficiency. The importance of clotting factors adsorbed on platelets for normal hemostasis, *Acta Med. Scand.,* 170, 375, 1961.
25. **Iatridis, P. G., Ferguson, J. H., and Iatridis, S. G.,** Surface factor mechanisms in relation to blood platelets: evidence that activated Hageman factor is present on the surface of platelets, *Thromb. Diath. Haemorrh.,* 11, 355, 1964.
26. **Karpatkin, M. H. and Karpatkin, S.,** In vivo and in vitro binding of factor VIII to human platelets, *Thromb. Diath. Haemorrh.,* 21, 129, 1969.
27. **Howard, M. A., Montgomery, D. C., and Hardisty, R. M.,** Factor-VIII-related antigen in platelets, *Thrombos. Res.,* 4, 617, 1974.
28. **Nachman, R. L. and Jaffe, E. A.,** Subcellular platelet factor VIII antigen and von Willebrand factor, *J. Exp. Med.,* 141, 1101, 1975.
29. **Bouma, B. N., Hordijk-Hos, J. M., de Graaf, S., Sixma, J. J., and van Mourik, J. A.,** Presence of factor VIII-related antigen in blood platelets of patients with von Willebrand's disease, *Nature* (London), 257, 510, 1975.
30. **Bouma, B. N., de Graaf, S., and Zimmerman, T. S.,** Human blood platelet factor VIII-related antigen: a glycocalicin-like protein, *Thrombos. Haemostas.,* 38, 126, 1977.
31. **Ware, A. G., Fahey, J. L., and Seegers, W. H.,** Platelet extracts, fibrin formation and interaction of purified prothrombin and thromboplastin, *Am. J. Physiol.,* 154, 140, 1948.
32. **Hjort, P. F., Rapaport, S. I., and Owren, P. A.,** Evidence that platelet accelerator (platelet factor 1) is adsorbed plasma proaccelerin, *Blood,* 10, 1139, 1955.
33. **Horowitz, H. I. and Fukimoto, M. M.,** Association of factors XI and XII with blood platelets, *Proc. Soc. Exp. Biol. Med.,* 119, 487, 1965.
34. **Breederveld, K., Giddings, J. C., Ten Cate, J. W., and Bloom, A. L.,** The localization of factor V within normal human platelets and the demonstration of a platelet-factor V antigen in congenital factor V deficiency, *Br. J. Haematol.,* 29, 405, 1975.
35. **Østerud, B., Rapaport, S. I., and Lavin, K. K.,** Factor V activity of platelets: evidence for an activated factor V molecule and for a platelet activator, *Blood,* 49, 819, 1977.
36. **Walsh, P. N. and Lipscomb, M. S.,** Collagen-induced coagulant activity (CICA) and Factor-V and -XI activities of platelets and platelet plasma membranes, *Thromb. Diath. Haemorrh.,* 34, 919, 1975.

37. **Pifer, D. D., Colman, R. W., and Chesney, C. McI.,** Subcellular localization and secretion of factor V by human platelets, *Thrombos. Haemostas.,* 38, 126, 1977.
38. **Gormsen, J.,** Hageman factor deficiency. (Demonstrated by indirect glass activation), *Thromb. Diath. Haemorrh.,* 7, 249, 1962.
39. **Iatridis, P. G. and Ferguson, J. H.,** The plasmatic atmosphere of blood platelets. Evidence that only fibrinogen, AcG and activated Hageman factor are present on the surface of platelets, *Thromb. Diath. Haemorrh.,* 13, 114, 1965.
40. **Walsh, P. N.,** The effects of collagen and kaolin on the intrinsic coagulant activity of platelets. Evidence for an alternative pathway in intrinsic coagulation not requiring factor XII, *Br. J. Haematol.,* 22, 393, 1972.
41. **Schiffman, S., Rapaport, S. I., and Chong, M. M. Y.,** Platelets and the initiation of intrinsic clotting, *Br. J. Haematol.,* 24, 633, 1973.
42. **Schiffman, S., Rimon, A., and Rapaport, S. I.,** Factor XI and platelets: evidence that platelets contain only minimal factor XI activity and antigen, *Br. J. Haematol.,* 35, 429, 1977.
43. **Lipscomb, M. S. and Walsh, P. N.,** Factor XI binding by platelet plasma membranes, *Fed. Proc.,* 36, 351, 1977.
44. **Walsh, P. N. and Biggs, R.,** The role of platelets in intrinsic factor-Xa formation, *Br. J. Haematol.,* 22, 733, 1972.
45. **Tollefson, D. M., Faegler, J. R., and Majerus, P. W.,** The binding of thrombin to the surface of human platelets, *J. Biol. Chem.,* 249, 2646, 1974.
46. **Miletich, J. P., Jackson, C. M., and Majerus, P. W.,** The interaction of coagulation factor Xa with human platelets, *Proc. Natl. Acad. Sci. U.S.A.,* in press, 1977.
47. **Milstone, J. H.,** Thrombokinase as prime activator of prothrombin: historical perspectives and present status, *Fed. Proc.,* 23, 742, 1964.
48. **Lundblad, R. L. and Davie, E. W.,** The activation of anti-hemophilic factor (factor VIII) by activated Christmas factor (activated factor IX), *Biochemistry,* 3, 1720, 1964.
49. **Walsh, P. N.,** The effect of dilution of plasma on coagulation. The significance of the dilution-activation phenomenon for the study of platelet coagulant activities, *Br. J. Haematol.,* 22, 219, 1972.
50. **Fantl, P. and Ward, H. A.,** The thromboplastic component of intact blood platelets is present in masked form, *Aust. J. Exp. Biol. Med. Sci.,* 36, 499, 1958.
51. **Walsh, P. N. and Lipscomb, M. S.,** Different requirements for intrinsic factor-Xa forming activity and platelet factor 3 activity and their relationship to platelet aggregation and release, *Thrombos. Haemostas.,* 38, 127, 1977.
52. **Walsh, P. N.,** The role of platelets in the contact phase of blood coagulation, *Br. J. Haematol.,* 22, 237, 1972.
53. **Walsh, P. N., Mills, D. C. B., Pareti, F. I., Stewart, G. J., Macfarlane, D. E., Johnson, M. M., and Egan, J. J.,** Hereditary giant platelet syndrome: absence of collagen-induced coagulant activity and deficiency of factor-XI binding to platelets, *Br. J. Haematol.,* 29, 639, 1975.
54. **Walsh, P. N.,** Effects of inhibitors of platelet aggregation on collagen-induced coagulant activity of platelets, *Fed. Proc.,* 34, 241, 1975.
55. **Marciniak, E.,** Factor-Xa inactivation by antithrombin III: evidence for biological stabilization of factor Xa by factor V-phospholipid complex, *Br. J. Haematol.,* 24, 391, 1973.
56. **Hougie, C.,** The activation of platelets by plasma, *Br. J. Haematol.,* 1, 213, 1955.
57. **Biggs, R., Denson, K. W. E., Riesenberg, D., and McIntyre, C.,** The coagulant activity of platelets, *Br. J. Haematol.,* 15, 283, 1968.
58. **Niemetz, J. and Marcus, A. J.,** The stimulatory effect of platelets and platelet membranes on the procoagulant activity of leukocytes, *J. Clin. Invest.,* 54, 1437, 1974.
59. **Semerao, N. and Vermylen, J.,** Evidence that washed human platelets possess factor-X activator activity, *Br. J. Haematol.,* 36, 107, 1977.
60. **Walsh, P. N., Rizza, C. R., and McLennan, R.,** Clinically mild thrombasthenia with normal platelet coagulant activities, *Thromb. Diath. Haemorrh.,* 28, 440, 1972.
61. **Walsh, P. N.,** Platelet coagulant activities in thrombasthenia, *Br. J. Haematol.,* 23, 553, 1972.
62. **Walsh, P. N., Rainsford, S. G., and Biggs, R.,** Platelet coagulant activities and clinical severity in haemophilia, *Thromb. Diath. Haemorrh.,* 29, 722, 1973.
63. **Walsh, P. N., Rogers, P. H., Marder, V. J., Gagnatelli, G., Escovitz, E. S., and Sherry S.,** The relationship of platelet coagulant activities to venous thrombosis following hip surgery, *Br. J. Haematol.,* 32, 423, 1976.
64. **Walsh, P. N., Goldberg, R. E., Tax, R. L., and Magargal, L. E.,** Platelet coagulant activities and retinal vein thrombosis, *Thromb. Haemostasis,* 38, 399, 1977.
65. **Walsh, P. N., Pareti, F. I., and Corbett, J. J.,** Platelet coagulant activities and serum lipids in transient cerebral ischemia, *N. Engl. J. Med.,* 295, 854, 1976.

CELL COUNTING — THE PLATELET

Richard K. Wertz

Hemocytometer Platelet Counts

Early methods of platelet counting required removal of erythrocytes and leukocytes from plasma by sedimentation, followed by direct enumeration of platelets in hemocytometer chambers.[36] Staining with brilliant cresyl blue achieved better visualization of the platelets.[43] This method, however, compromised precision and accuracy, since it was still difficult to distinguish erythrocytes, debris, and dirt from platelets. The application of phase microscopy improved recognition of platelets and demonstrated that the precision of platelet counts could approach the theoretical errors of the chamber, pipette, and field.[5] Brecher's phase contrast microscopic method used 1% ammonium oxalate both as a diluent and erythrocyte lytic agent. Evidence suggests that this agent leads to falsely low counts due to thrombolysis, and to avoid this artifact, a saline dilution-sedimentation scheme has been proposed for use with phase microscopy.[13] A formalin-acetone diluent has also been described which is used to clarify further the image of the platelets.[53] Insufficient settling time in all hemocytometer methods may be a major source of error, and a sedimentation time of 40 min may be necessary.[2] The introduction of disposable plastic capillary micropipettes with premeasured reservoirs of diluent has significantly improved diluting techniques for platelet counting. This system has not only increased the precision of pipetting, but has also provided particle-free diluent to minimize contamination by dirt. A summary of visual platelet methods appears in Table 1.

Automated and Semiautomated Platelet Counters

With the general acceptance and shrinking cost of automatic platelet counting systems, a number of new instruments are available in this field. Some instruments are designed for counting platelets only, whereas others incorporate platelet counting along with erythrocyte and leukocyte enumeration. A device that estimates platelet counts indirectly from a peripheral smear has also recently been marketed. Since there are many new instruments and a minimum amount of data on their performance, only those instruments that have been evaluated in the indexed literature will be considered in this section.

Electronic Particle Counting

The high precision and ease of operation demonstrated with electronic erythrocyte and leukocyte counting made this method an attractive alternative to visual platelet counts. It was difficult to differentiate these particles from the other formed blood elements because of their small size and adherent properties. Attempts to lyse red cells and count platelets were unsuccessful, since the erythrocyte stroma was similar in size to the platelets.[14] Therefore, the central problem in electronic particle counting of platelets has revolved around separating platelets from leukocytes and erythrocytes.[52] (Table 2.)

Early techniques of centrifugal separation of platelets from erythrocytes were not generally accepted, because the speed and duration of centrifugation were difficult to control and standardize.[14,18] Eastham proposed initial dilution of the blood specimen with saline to minimize viscosity and Bagnold forces.[11,12] These forces are electrical charges that result during sedimentation from collision and shearing and have the consequent effect of floating platelets and sinking erythrocytes. Thus sedimentation tends to concentrate platelets in the upper layers of plasma and trap platelet-poor plasma with the erythrocytes. By using gravity sedimentation in small plastic tubes, Bull noted

Table 1
HEMOCYTOMETER PLATELET COUNTING METHODS

Microscopy	Diluent	C.V. precision	Normal values	Comments	Ref.
Light	3.1% Sodium citrate 1:20 (v/v) with sedimentation of erythrocytes for 3 hr	17%[4]	241×10^9/L[24]	—	36
Light	Sodium citrate, 3.8 g; 40% formaldehyde, 0.2 mℓ; briliant cresyl blue, 0.1 g; distilled water qs ad, 100 mℓ	—	224 ± 110 (2SD) $\times 10^9$/L[42]	Errors may occur due to counting of cell debris and dirt	43
Phase	1% Ammonium oxalate as erythrocyte lysing agent	9.5—13.5%[20] 9%[22] 16.6%[8] 12.8%[15]	248 ± 110 (2SD) $\times 10^9$/L[5] 264×10^9/L[3]	This method is reported to give falsely low counts due to thrombolysis[13]	5
Phase	Blood diluted 1:100 in normal saline and erythrocytes sedimented ½ to 2 hr at room temperature	—	—	Author claims method avoids thrombolysis and erythrocytic debris	13
Phase	40% Formaldehyde, 0.5 mℓ; acetone, 2.5 mℓ; 0.9% NaCl, 20.0 mℓ; distilled water qs ad, 100 mℓ	—	265×10^9/L[53]	Platelets appear as jet black structures with phase microscopy	53

Table 2
TECHNIQUES FOR SEPARATING ERYTHROCYTES FROM PLATELETS

Method	Comment	Ref.
1. Centrifuge EDTA anticoagulated blood 60 × g and remove supernatant 2. Dilute platelet-rich plasma with 0.85% saline to give 1:5000 dilution	—	14
1. Dilute EDTA anticoagulated blood 1:125 in saline in siliconized tube 2. Sediment 2—3 hr at room temperature; redilute 50-fold and count	The initial dilution is designed to minimize charges (Bagnold forces) developed during sedimentation that would lead to falsely high platelet counts in the supernatant; the siliconized or plastic tube reduces eddy currents	11,12
1. Original method: sediment EDTA anticoagulated blood in plastic sedimentation tube for 10—50 min; cut off erythrocyte layer and dilute with saline-oxalate diluent 2. Revised method: centrifuge blood in EDTA for 25 sec at 40 × g to produce rouleaux; sediment at 1 × g for 1—2 min to produce plasma column	This author uses a correction factor to adjust for the higher concentration of platelets in the supernatant plasma as compared to visual platelet counts (see text)	8,9
1. Dilute EDTA anticoagulated blood 1:12.5 in saline (with 1% formalin and 0.1% EDTA) and centrifuge 900 r.p.m. (RCF = 130) with speed controller for 130 sec 2. Further dilute platelet-rich plasma 1:2000 and count	The authors use a special electronic speed control to obtain rapid acceleration; the 130 sec run is critical	10
1. Centrifuge EDTA anticoagulated blood 300 × g for 5 min 2. Dilute platelet-rich plasma 1:3000 in isotonic solution	This technique, although giving somewhat lower (~ 4%) values, correlated well with the sedimentation method (r = 0.9830); the authors experienced lower counts with both sedimentation and centrifugation methods than with visual counts; note that this is the opposite of the findings of Bull and Eastham	15
1. Layer EDTA anticoagulated blood on separation fluid (10 parts 32.8% Isopaque and 20 parts 6% Dextran) 2. Sediment 1 × g 30—40 min and count upper platelet-rich plasma layer	The method gives inaccurate counts at low platelet numbers, but this can be avoided by reducing the degree of dilution	4
1. Dilute blood 1:500 in 10% EDTA and sediment erythrocytes 1 × g 2. Dilute platelet-rich plasma (above) 1:10 in 1.5 mg cocaine/mℓ in water	Initial dilution with EDTA is designed to swell platelets slightly and prevent their aggregation; the secondary dilution with cocaine further swells the platelets and fixes the membranes to prevent thrombolysis	1

a similarly high platelet count in the supernatant plasma which could be corrected by adding PVP to the plasma.[8] To adjust for the higher values in the plasma, he proposed a correction factor which has been widely distributed in the form of a circular slide rule. Another investigator challenged Bull's correction factor by observing that it leads to consistently lower values than visual counts, on an average of −17% lower.[19] The correction factor was subsequently defended, which suggests that there is still considerable technical interlaboratory variability and that each laboratorian should carefully check the calibration of his counter results with visual methods.[59]

Other authors devised a modified centrifugation method for platelet separation with a special speed control to rapidly accelerate and slowly decelerate the rotor, and such centrifuges designed for platelet counting are now commercially available.[10] Later, Fry and Hoak published a centrifugal separation method in which there were somewhat lower numbers of platelets in the supernatant than with the sedimentation method, but good correlation existed between these two techniques ($r = 0.9830$).[15] Contrary to the results obtained by Bull and Eastham, these investigators obtained lower counts in the supernatant plasma than with visual counts of whole blood. More recently, Böyum published an application of his 2-phase Isopaque-Dextran cell separation technique in which anticoagulated blood is layered over a separation fluid to promote erythrocyte agglutination and settling.[4] This 2-phase method gave inaccurate results with low platelet counts, but the author claimed that this inaccuracy could be corrected by reducing the degree of dilution. More recently, Armstrong recommended a 2-step platelet separation method for using hypotonic EDTA to inhibit clumping and promote swelling, followed by cocaine to prevent thrombolysis.[1]

To increase the signal-to-noise ratio of electronic platelet counts, most workers recommend tubes with either 50- or 70-μm apertures.[8,11,14] However, other investigators have used a 100-μm aperture with apparently good results.[10,47] One advantage of the larger aperture is that clogging is diminished and the same instrument can be employed for counting leukocytes. However, if the same instrument is used for platelet and leukocyte counting, the user must scrupulously clean the aperture and carefully check the background to avoid contamination by residual erythrocyte stroma.[9]

Platelets must be counted with two electronic size thresholds: the lower to eliminate dirt and cell debris and the upper to exclude erythrocytes and leukocytes. With the single threshold devices, separate counts must be made at each setting and subtracted from one another. Therefore, electronic cell counters with a single threshold (Coulter Counter® Models A and F, Celloscope® 401) are not as convenient as those with two thresholds (Thrombocounter®, Coulter Counter® Models B and Z). (Table 3.)

Recently, there has been an evaluation of an inexpensive platelet counter that senses platelets by electrical impedence. J. T. Baker markets their MK-4S counter with a low speed centrifuge for preparing platelet-rich plasma. Its run-to-run precision at a normal platelet level is 4.6% (C.V.), and the within-run precision is 3% (C.V.). This is somewhat more precise than the Coulter Counter®, particularly when counting irregularly sized and shaped platelets. In a comparison of the MK-4S values with phase chamber counts, there was a slightly positive bias at lower levels and negative bias at higher values. The overall linear coefficient of correlation (r) was 0.982.[58]

Optical Light Scattering

Automated devices have also been developed to count platelets by optical light scattering. With the Technicon® AutoCounter system, blood is diluted in 2 *M* urea to lyse the erythrocytes. The remaining leukocytes and platelets are counted with a dark field microscope that detects the forward-scattered components of light which they diffract. The operator then subtracts the leukocyte count from the total count to produce the platelet count. The instrument is calibrated with a standard platelet suspension provided by the manufacturer. However, several workers have encountered standardization problems. (Table 4.) Handin noted that platelet counts with the optical continuous flow devices were approximately 10% lower than counts performed by visual and electronic impedance methods, and Samama noted unspecified difficulties in standardization.[22,48] A bias toward falsely elevated counts occurred with this instrument in the First College of American Pathologists Hematology Survey of platelets.[60] Whether this bias results from aggregation of the platelet reference material or the

Table 3
AUTOMATED AND SEMIAUTOMATED PLATELET COUNTING SYSTEMS

Instrument	Sensing system	Fluid counted	C.V. precision	Normal values	Calibration	Carryover
Coulter Counter® (Thrombocounter,® Model A,B,F,Z, etc.)	Electrical impedance	Platelet-rich plasma	3.8%,[8] 2.3—4%,[12] 5.4%,[15] 0.9—2.8%,[16] 4%,[22] 2—10%,[41] 1.4—7.7%,[48] 7.2%[20]	$235 \pm 70 \times 10^9/L$,[27] $260 \pm 58 \times 10^9/L$[8]	Threshold adjustments on some models	5%[9]
AutoAnalyzer® (SMA 4, AutoCounter®, Hemalog, etc.)	Optical light scatter	Whole blood	1—3%,[7] 2.95%,[17] 3.0%,[20] 4%,[22] 4%,[44] 2.2—2.9%[48]	Not reported; values correlate closely with Coulter Counter®	Count adjusted to standard platelet suspension	1—6%,[17] 3—4%[7]
HaemaCount MK-4S	Electrical impedance	Platelet-rich plasma	4—6% (run to run); 3.2% (within run)[58]	$256 \pm 144 \times 10^9/L$[58]	Precalibrated	None[58]

Table 4
SOURCES OF ERROR IN PLATELET COUNTING

	Visual light microscopy	Visual phase microscopy	Electronic particle counting	Optical light scattering
Dysproteinemias	0	0	±	+
Dirt in diluent	+	+ (var.)	+ (var.)	+ (var.)
Erythroblasts and Howell-Jolly bodies	0	0	+	+
Carryover	0	0	+	+
Leukocytosis	0	0	+	+ (var.)
Platelet clumping	+ (var.)	+ (var.)	−	+ (var.)
Large platelets	0	0	+ (var.)	0
Clotting in collection tube	−	−	−	−
Malaria parasites	0	0	+	+
Insufficient settling in chamber	−	−	0	0
Hemolysis of blood sample	+ (var.)	0	+	0
Patient on Chemotherapy	0	0	0	0 (+ or −)

light scattering effect of erythrocyte stroma adding to the platelet count has not yet been determined. To help avoid this potential for miscalibration, Technicon® has distributed a procedure by which the standard material is checked against visual counts of fresh whole blood.[64] There is good evidence that the automated optical platelet counting system offers greater precision than electronic particle counting.[7,17,20,22,44,48] Furthermore, platelets can be counted in whole blood, which eliminates the tedious and error-prone steps of separation by sedimentation or centrifugation. However, excessive variability may be found in specimens collected from patients receiving chemotherapy, especially if there is excessive delay between specimen collection and the counting procedure.

Capillary Platelet Counts

Visual platelet counts on capillary blood resulted in 2.2-fold less precision with average values registering 2½% lower than the counts on venous blood.[6] This result was attributed to the dilution of capillary blood by tissue fluid and the loss of platelets by adhesion to the wound. A modification of the phase contrast visual method used less blood in a 20-$\mu\ell$ disposable glass micropipette. Still, the normal values were about 10% lower and the coefficients of variation were 1.5-fold higher than those obtained with venous blood.[35] Bull described a finger-stick method for the Coulter Counter® using the first one or two drops of capillary blood collected by a heparin-EDTA capillary tube;[8] Hart, using an essentially similar technique, recorded precision levels from 3.9 to 15% (C.V.) depending on the levels counted.[23] Despite these results, Coulter® Instruments recommends that platelet counts on the Thrombocounter® be performed only on venous blood.[65] The automated optical counting system achieved a 2 to 6% C.V. with capillary counts, and the values were essentially the same as those with venous blood.[7] Thus it would appear that platelet counting of capillary blood with an automated optical device has many advantages over visual and electrical impedance methodologies.

REFERENCES

1. Armstrong, J. E., Electronic platelet counting: the influence of suspending fluids, *Lab. Practice,* 23, 3, 1974.
2. Ashman, B., An assessment of platelet counting methods, *Med. Lab. Sci.,* 33, 201, 1976.
3. Borchgrevink, C. F., Platelet adhesion in vivo in patients with bleeding disorders, *Acta Med. Scand.,* 170, 231, 1961.
4. Böyum, A., Stormorken, H., and Lund-Riise, A., Electronic platelet counting, *Scand. J. Clin. Lab. Invest.,* 28, 429, 1971.
5. Brecher, J. and Cronkite, E. P., Morphology and enumeration of human blood platelets, *J. Appl. Physiol.,* 3, 365, 1950.
6. Brecher, G., Schneiderman, M., and Cronkite, E. P., The reproducibility and constancy of the platelet count, *Am. J. Clin. Pathol.,* 23, 15, 1953.
7. Brittin, G. M., Dew, S. A., and Fewell, E. K., Automated optical counting of blood platelets, *Blood,* 38, 422, 1971.
8. Bull, B. S., Schneiderman, M. A., and Brecher, G., Platelet counts with the Coulter Counter®, *Am. J. Clin. Pathol.,* 44, 678, 1965.
9. Bull, B. S., Aids to electronic platelet counting, *Am. J. Clin. Pathol.,* 54, 707, 1970.
10. Davis, R. E. and Green, R. E., Automatic platelet counting with the Coulter® particle counter, *J. Clin. Pathol.,* 20, 777, 1967.
11. Eastham, R. D., Rapid whole-blood platelet counting using an electronic particle counter, *J. Clin. Pathol.,* 16, 168, 1963.
12. Eastham, R. D., Simple method for separating platelets from red cells before enumeration with an electronic counter, *J. Clin. Pathol.,* 18, 248, 1965.
13. Eastham, R. D. and Morgan, E. H., Comparison of platelet counting methods, *J. Med. Lab. Technol.,* 24, 315, 1967.
14. Eggleton, M. J. and Sharp, A. A., Platelet counting using the Coulter® electronic counter, *J. Clin. Pathol.,* 16, 164, 1963.
15. Fry, G. L. and Hoak, J. C., Improved method for electronic counting of platelets, *J. Lab. Clin. Med.,* 74, 536, 1969.
16. Gadner, H., Odenwald, E., Pluss, H. J., and Hitzig, W. H., Thrombozytenzaehlung mit elektronischem Zaehlgeraet im haematologischen Routinelabor, *Schweiz. Med. Wochenschr.,* 104, 138, 1974.
17. Gastaldi, G., Lanza, G. C., Galletti, A., and Ciampelletti, A., Evaluation of a fully automatic platelet counting technique on whole blood, *Haematologica (Pavia),* 59, 181, 1974.
18. Girling, J. H., An automatic platelet counting technique, *J. Med. Lab. Technol.,* 19, 168, 1962.
19. Gottfried, E. L., Wehman, J., and Wall, B., Electronic platelet counts with the Coulter Counter®. Reassessment of a correction factor, *Am. J. Clin. Pathol.,* 66, 506, 1976.
20. Glass, U. H., Wetherley-Mein, G., Mills, R. T., and Priest, C. J., Automated platelet counting, *Br. J. Haematol.,* 21, 529, 1971.
21. Green, A. E., Middleton, V. L., Prentis, K. G., and Signy, A. G., A report on experience with an automatic blood counting machine, *J. Clin. Pathol.,* 22, 19, 1969.
22. Handin, R. I., Lawler, K. C., and Valeri, C. R., Automated platelet counting, *Am. J. Clin. Pathol.,* 56, 661, 1971.
23. Hart, J. E., Hogue, K. A., and Hartmann, J. R., The adaptation of microtechnic to platelet counts with the Coulter Counter®, *Am. J. Clin. Pathol.,* 53, 914, 1970.
24. Hellem, A., The adhesiveness of human blood platelets in vitro, *Scand. J. Clin. Lab. Invest.,* 12 (Suppl. 51), 1, 1960.
25. Kjeldsberg, C. R. and Sherrer, C., A platelet control for use with electronic counting equipment, *Lab. Med.,* 26, 1974.
26. Lacassie, F., A rapid technic for simultaneous numeration of red blood cells and blood platelets: the complexon method, *Presse Med.,* 77, 591, 1969.
27. Le Go, A., Prudhomme, J., Finidori, N., and Le Go, R., A standard method of electronically counting blood platelets in man (100 normal subjects) and in laboratory animals, *Rev. Fr. Etud. Clin. Biol.,* 13, 531, 1968.
28. Lewis, S. M. and Coster, J. F., Standards and reference preparations, in *Quality Control in Haematology,* Academic Press, London, 1975.
29. Lindsay, R. M., Koens, F., and Linton, A. L., An evaluation of the Coulter Thrombocounter® in counting platelets before and after contact with foreign surfaces and its use in tests of platelet retention, *J. Lab. Clin. Med.,* 86, 863, 1975.
30. Maupin, B., *Blood Platelets in Man and Animals,* Vol. 1, Pergamon Press, Oxford, 1969, 37.
31. Mayer, K. and Mink, B., Slide rule calculator for platelet enumeration with the Coulter® electronic particle counter, *Am. J. Clin. Pathol.,* 49, 453, 1968.
32. Mulder, E. and Kuipers, J., Thrombocyte counting, *Ned. Tijdschr. Geneeskd.,* 112, 2222, 1968.

33. Musikhin, L. S. and Shabarov, A. A., Accuracy of calculating thrombocytes by two different methods, *Lab. Delo*, 2, 112, 1970.
34. Nakatsui, T., Sasaki, T., Yoshikuni, T., and Tsubokura, T., A standard platelet suspension: control of automatic platelet counting with the Coulter Counter®, *Am. J. Clin. Pathol.*, 53, 659, 1970.
35. Norgaard-Pedersen, B. and Siggaard-Andersen, O., Method for microscopic counting of thrombocytes and leukocytes, with special emphasis on the use of capillary blood, *Ugeskr. Laeg.*, 132, 1228, 1970.
36. Nygaard, K. K., A direct method of counting platelets in oxalated plasma, *Proc. Mayo Clin.*, 8, 365, 1933.
37. Odesskaia, T. A., Spitikova, A. S., and Papaian, L. P., Increased accuracy in the calculation of thrombocytes in peripheral blood, *Lab. Delo*, 2, 78, 1970.
38. Palumbo, F., Di Martino, G., and Branca, F., The Palumbo-Dini reagent for the direct platelet count in the phase contrast microscope, *Haematologica (Pavia)*, 52, 421, 1967.
39. Piksanov, O. N. and Shchennikova, V. P., On the magnitude of error in blood platelet counting, *Lab. Delo*, 9, 536, 1968.
40. Pliutto, A. M., On the method of calculation of thrombocytes in a chamber, *Lab. Delo*, 9, 572, 1968.
41. Price, L. W. and Gray, J. M., Experience with platelet counting by an electronic method, *Am. J. Clin. Pathol.*, 49, 606, 1968.
42. Ratto, L. A., Depiante, M. E., and Yantorno, C. E., Platelet counts: comparative statistical analysis of various methods and expression of normal values, *Sangre (Parc)*, 15, 383, 1970.
43. Rees, H. M. and Ecker, E. E., Improved method for counting blood platelets, *JAMA*, 80, 621, 1933.
44. Rowan, R. M., Allan, W., and Prescott, R. J., Evaluation of an automatic platelet counting system utilizing whole blood, *J. Clin. Pathol.*, 25, 218, 1972.
45. Rutten, W. P. F., Scholtis, R. J. H., Schmidt, N. A., and van Oers, R. J. M., Quality control in hematology by means of values from patients, *Klin. Chem. Klin. Biochem.*, 13 (Abstr.), 395, 1975.
46. Sasamoto, H. and Okuda, M., Coulter Counter® analysis of blood platelets, *Jpn. J. Clin. Pathol.*, 16, 605, 1968.
47. Samama, M., Prost, R. J., Doumenc, J., and Beuzart, A., Value of the platelet count using electronic counter, *Pathol. Biol. (Paris)*, 18 (19), 860, 1970.
48. Samama, N., Capelle, C., and Beuzart, A., Platelet counting: visual, electronic and fully automated official methods, *Adv. Exp. Med. Biol.*, 34, 221, 1972.
49. Saunders, A. M. and Scott, F., Hematologic automation by use of continuous flow systems, *J. Histochem. Cytochem.*, 22, 707, 1974.
50. Schulz, J. and Thom, R., Electrical sizing and counting of platelets in whole blood, *Med. Biol. Eng.*, 11, 447, 1973.
51. Simmons, A., Schwabbauer, M. L., and Earthart, C. A., Automated platelet counting with the AutoAnalyzer®, *J. Lab. Clin. Med.*, 77, 654, 1971.
52. Sipe, C. R. and Cronkite, E. P., Studies on the application of the Coulter® electronic counter in enumeration of platelets, *Ann. N. Y. Acad. Sci.*, 99, 262, 1962.
53. Stavem, P., Platelet count by phase contrast microscopy — new diluting fluid for better visualization, *Scand. J. Clin. Lab. Invest.*, 33, 121, 1974.
54. Terada, H., Counting of the thrombocytes, megakaryocytes and reticulocytes and phase microscope images of thrombocytes, *Jpn. J. Clin. Pathol.*, 15 (Suppl. 13), 22, 1967.
55. Truman, L. M. and Chapman, P. M., A simplified method for preparing plate-rich plasma for use with the thrombocounter C, *Med. Lab. Technol.*, 32, 239, 1975.
56. Upton, A. S., Spaet, T. H., and LaMantia, J., Automatic platelet counting with the AutoAnalyzer®, in *Automation in Analytical Chemistry*, Vol. I, Technicon Corporation, Ardsley, N. Y., 1967, 197.
57. Watanabe, T., The study on enumeration of the blood platelets, *Acta Haematol. Jpn.*, 32, 397, 1969.
58. Weisbrot, I. M. and Ewing, N. S., Evaluation of the Haema-Count MK-4S platelet counting system, *Am. J. Clin. Pathol.*, 62, 693, 1974.
59. Weisbrot, I. M., Electronic platelet counts, *Am. J. Clin. Pathol.*, 67, 313, 1977.
60. Wertz, R. K. and Koepke, J. A., A critical analysis of platelet counting methods, *Am. J. Clin. Pathol.*, 68, 195, 1977.
61. Wertz, R. K., Platelet counting: precision and quality control, *Pathologist*, 338, September 1976.
62. Widmark, R. M. and Weschler, W. A., Evaluation of a fully automatic platelet counting technique, *Technicon Quart.*, 2, 23, 1970.
63. Yasunaga, K., Katsumi, O., Terada, H., Ebata, Y., and Kuramoto, A., The normal platelet count in Japanese, *Acta Haematol. Jpn.*, 31 (2), 48, 1968.
64. Technicon® Bulletin, No. TT 3-0303-20, 1976.
65. Coulter Thrombocounter—C® Operator's Manual, 1976.

BLEEDING TIME PROCEDURES

C. H. Mielke, Jr. and Robert Rodvien

Introduction

The bleeding time (BT) measures the effectiveness of small vessel hemostasis, traditionally interpreted as being dependent on both normal platelet function and vascular integrity. Whenever blood vessels are cut or injured, several mechanisms cooperate to arrest the flow of blood. First, there is an immediate reflex vasoconstriction which temporarily impedes the flow of blood and allows the platelets to adhere to the exposed subintimal structures of the injured vessel. These platelets release adenosine disphosphate (ADP), and other platelets then aggregate to each other to form a loose plug. The platelets swell, degranulate, and release many substances, including more ADP. With aggregation, the platelets are changed so that clotting factor activation is accelerated on the platelet surface. Thrombin is rapidly generated, and fibrin is formed to stabilize the platelet plug and make it impermeable. At this point the flow of blood ceases, and the end point of the BT is reached. With time, clot retraction occurs, the vessel is repaired, and blood flow is reestablished.

The BT measures some, but not all, of the above steps; its sensitivity to individual steps is dependent on the techniques used. Until recently, the clinical utility of the BT has been limited by difficulties in standardizing the test. Various methods have been used to incise blood vessels, and some have been painful to the patient. To understand the major variations of the BT technique as it is applied today, it is necessary to review how the BT developed.

The Techniques

The BT test was first introduced by Duke[1] in 1910 in an attempt to understand why some people had a tendency to bleed. Later investigators, bothered by the lack of repeatability and information obtained by known bleeding time methods, have sought to improve these inadequacies by changing the site and frequency of incision, the temperature of the skin, the state of venous tone, the incision technique, the length and depth of the incision, and the method of blood collection. The more popular methods are described below.

The technique initially described by Duke monitors a small incision in the ear lobe at 30-sec intervals by adsorption of the blood onto a filter paper until the flow ceases. Normal individuals bleed for less than 3 min. The test has been repeatedly modified both by the use of a lancet puncture[2] and by the way in which the incision or puncture is done.[3-5] Attempts have also been made to control the depth of the puncture by the use of a spring-loaded device.[6] Despite these modifications, the method that is most commonly performed today uses a sterile lancet to puncture the ear lobe to a depth of approximately 2.5 mm.

Ivy attempted to improve the repeatability of the test by choosing the forearm as the puncture site.[7,8] He believed that the area of the forearm just distal to the antecubital fossa had the least variation in skin thickness and was rich in capillaries. In Ivy's technique, a blood pressure cuff is placed around the arm and inflated to 40 mm Hg, a maneuver designed to create uniform filling of the capillaries by impairing venous return. In addition, this maneuver prolongs the bleeding time. A puncture between 2½ and 3 mm deep is made, and the wound is blotted at regular intervals until bleeding ceases. The BT is recorded as the mean time from puncture to cessation of bleeding of the first three punctures that bleed. Frequently, punctures do not bleed. In an attempt to standardize the depth of the puncture and once again, to improve the repeatability of the test, Tocantins[9] modified a scarificator, O'Brien[10] introduced the spring lancet, and a similar spring device was produced by Owen et al.[11]

Hjort and Stormorken[12] made another modification of Ivy's BT technique by substituting a superficial incision on the forearm for the original puncture. They made three incisions, 2 to 3 mm long and 1 mm deep on the forearm. The mean time of bleeding was 6.2 min (normal range, 2.0 to 12.5 min), a substantial prolongation compared to the mean time of bleeding for the Duke technique. Borchgrevink and Waaler[13] later increased the length of the incision to approximately 12 mm and said that they were able to increase the reproducibility (mean, 7 min normal range, 3 to 11 min). They also reduced the number of incisions to two.

Copley and Lalich[14] were dissatisfied with both the lack of skin temperature control and the site of puncture. In their test, a finger is immersed in a 37.5°C saline bath for 2 min after which a blood pressure cuff is set at 40 mg Hg and the finger is removed from the bath. A puncture wound is made to a depth of 6 mm with a spring lancet. The finger is reintroduced into the saline bath and the time taken until blood flow ceases is measured. The normal range for 95% of the 174 subjects reported was 17 to 180 sec.

In 1957, Adelson and Crosby,[15] again dissatisfied with the previously chosen puncture sites, immersed the entire hand in saline at 37°C with a blood pressure cuff inflated to 40 mg Hg on the subject's upper arm. The hand is removed, a 4-mm stab wound is made in the hypothenar eminence, and the hand is then replaced in the saline and observed until the bleeding ceases. In this modification both the volume of blood loss and the time taken to stop bleeding are measured. Adelson and Crosby compared their technique with Duke's in 27 subjects. The mean BT by the Duke method was 4.54 min (range, 0.8 to 8.3 min); for the immersion method, the mean was 4 min (range, 1 to 7 min). Normal blood loss was less than 0.22 mℓ.

This first attempt to quantitate blood has led to several modifications of the BT. Willoughby and Allington[16] eluted the blood from the filter paper used to blot an Ivy puncture and measured the hemoglobin in the supernatant. DeNicola[17] used a Duke puncture and collected the blood in capillary tubes at regular intervals. Sutor et al.[18] developed an automated technique in which the blood lost from a controlled Ivy lancet puncture[11] is washed with distilled water and collected continuously in a modified AutoAnalyzer® system.[19] The hemoglobin content of the blood-water mixture is continuously measured. In this method the mean normal BT is 191 sec with a range from 100 to 260 sec, and the mean blood loss is 0.76 mg with a range from 0.25 to 1.40 mg.[20]

The template bleeding time (TBT) was introduced in 1969 by Mielke et al.[21] to improve repeatability even further. The template produces a painless incision of constant length and depth. At present a modification of the template is being evaluated.* However, the original TBT is currently the most widely used BT technique, and is therefore discussed here in detail.

Equipment

The template system** consists of a disposable plastic blade holder and a template (Figure 1). The holder has a #11 surgical blade which has been preset to make an incision exactly 1 mm deep. The transparent disposable template has a central slot exactly 9 mm long through which the blade is guided when the incision is made. Other needed materials include a sphygmomanometer, stop watch, ethyl alcohol (70%), sponge, circular porous filter paper (#40), and a "butterfly" bandage.

* Simplate, General Diagnostics, Morris Plains, N.J. 07950.

** Template Bleeding Time Device, Boston Centerless, 60 Sharon Street, Malden, MA. 02148.

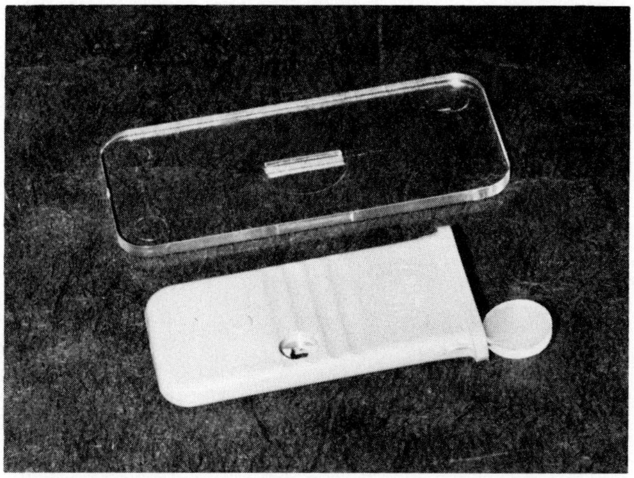

FIGURE 1. The template bleeding time device consists of a disposable plastic blade holder and a template.

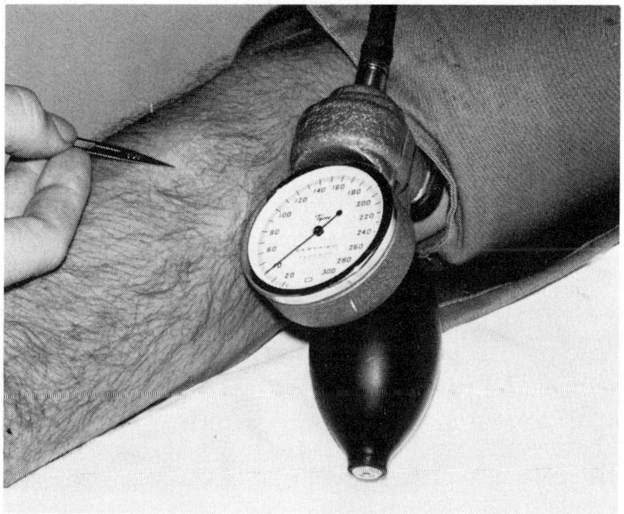

FIGURE 2. Excessive hair should be removed before the incision is made.

Procedure

The subject is seated with his forearm resting on a steady support exposing the volar surface. The forearm is thoroughly inspected for scars, small surface veins, bruises, and edematous areas which are to be avoided. The preferred site for the BT test is over the lateral aspect of the forearm, approximately 5 cm below the antecubital crease. After site selection, the blood pressure cuff is snugly wrapped around the upper arm. Patients with excessive local hair should be shaved (Figure 2). The area is gently swabbed with 70% alcohol and allowed to air dry. The cuff is then inflated to 40 mm Hg. After waiting 30 sec to allow for uniform capillary filling, the template is placed on the skin with the slot running parallel to the elbow crease. The skin surface is gently flattened (but not compressed) by firm pressure on the template (Figure 3). The blade

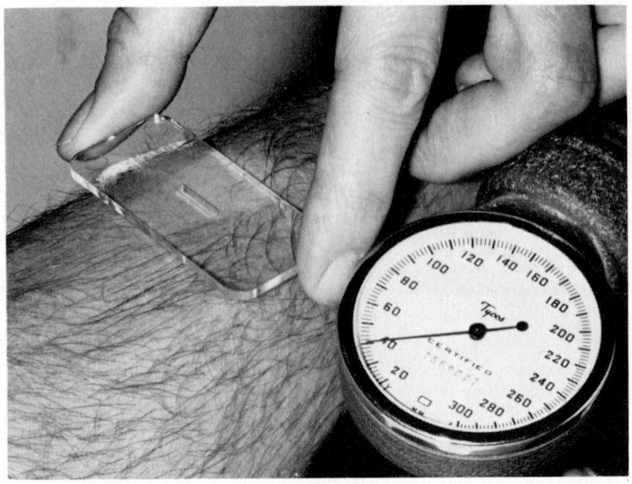

FIGURE 3. With the blood pressure cuff inflated to 40 mm Hg, the template is placed on the arm so that the skin is flattened, not compressed.

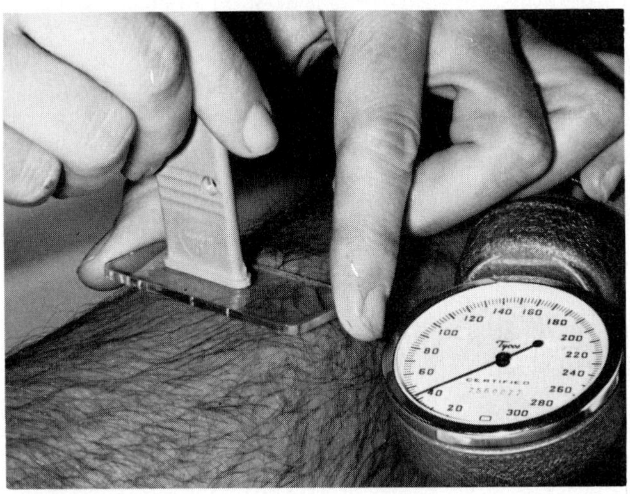

FIGURE 4. The blade is introduced into the template slot, and a smooth, rapid movement made along its entire length. (The incision should be painless.)

is introduced, and a smooth, rapid movement along the entire length of the slot is made (Figure 4). Under normal conditions the incision is painless to the patient and the first drop of blood appears between 15 and 20 sec (Figure 5). A circular filter paper is used to blot the drops of blood at 30-sec intervals (Figure 6).

The filter paper should not touch the wound edge, or the BT will be abnormally prolonged. The end point is reached when blood no longer stains the filter paper. The last drop is usually a mixture of red blood cells and serum, and has a characteristic rose color (Figure 7). The filter paper serves as a visual record of the BT. An adhesive bandage in a "butterfly" style which brings the skin edges together will minimize scarring. The bandage should be kept in place for at least 24 hr. Under most circumstances

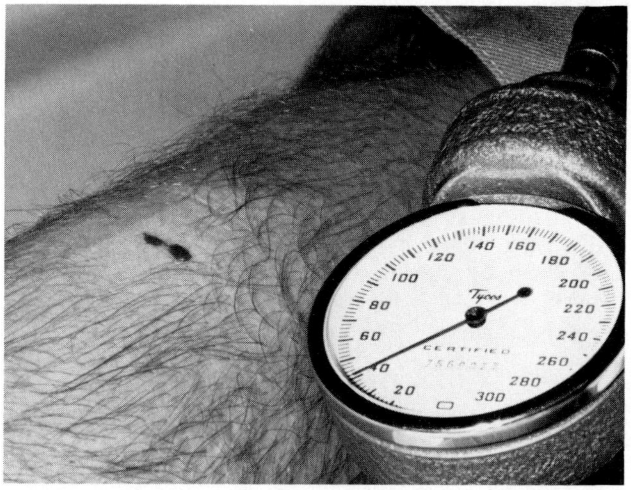

FIGURE 5. The first drop of blood appears between 15 and 20 sec after the incision.

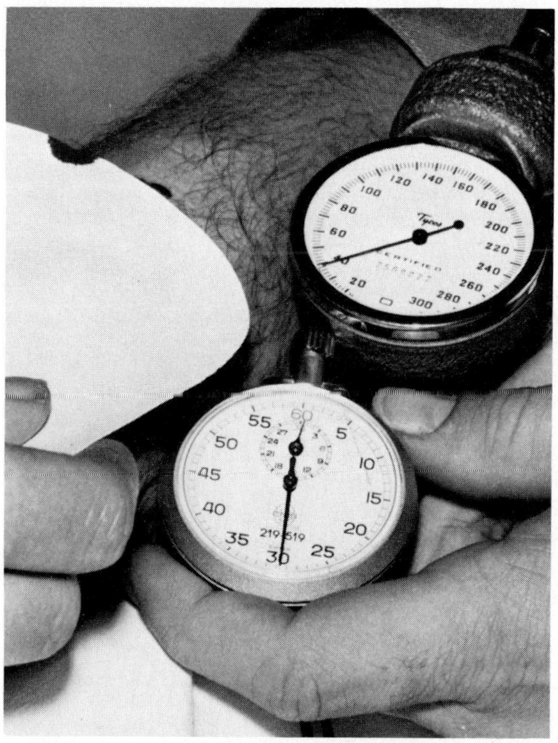

FIGURE 6. Filter paper is used to blot the drops of blood at 30-sec intervals. Note that the filter paper does not touch the incision.

when the procedure is done properly, no scarring will occur. In some individuals, however, a faint scar may occur, and patients should be warned of that possibility prior to the test.

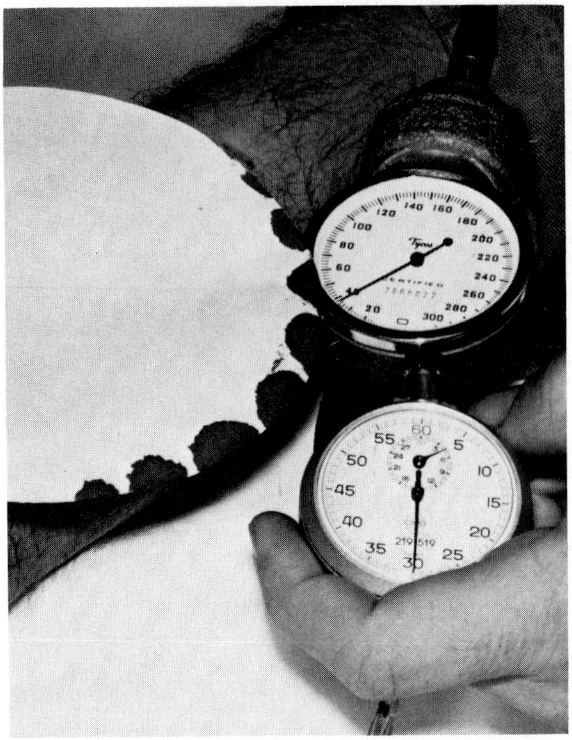

FIGURE 7. The bleeding time end point is reached when blood no longer stains the filter paper. The last drop is usually a mixture of red blood cells and serum, and has a characteristic rose color.

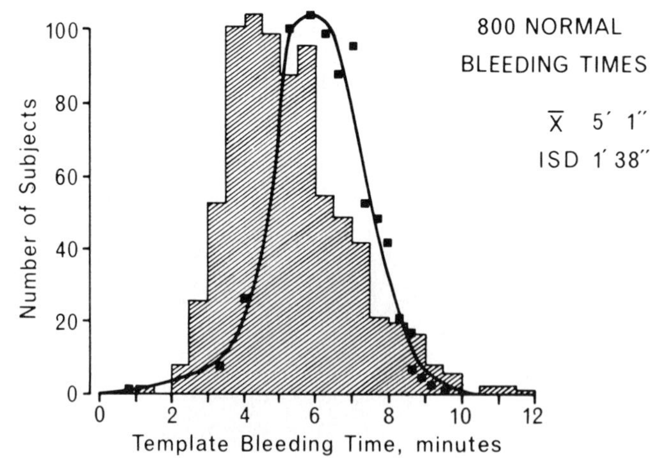

FIGURE 8. Template bleeding times performed on 800 normal individuals showed a mean time of 5 min 1 sec (range, 1'54'' to 8'18''). Note that the data exhibits a log normal distribution (■—■)

Clinical Experience in Normal Subjects

Figure 8 presents data on 800 TBT's performed on normal subjects. The mean for this group was 5 min, 1 sec (range, 1'54'' to 8'18''). These data exhibit a log normal

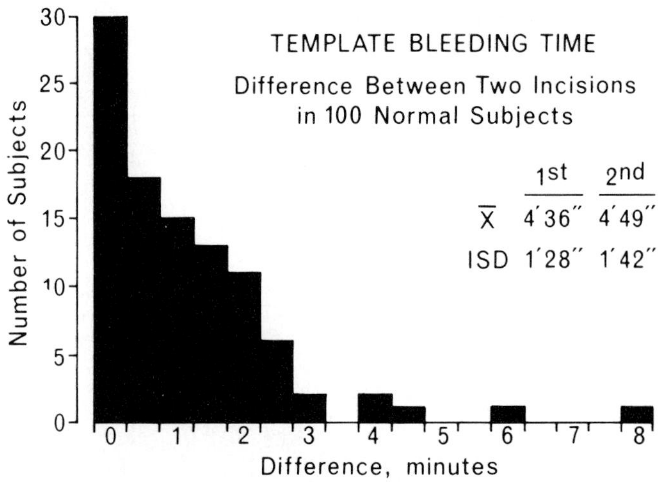

FIGURE 9. The absolute difference in template bleeding time between two studies done on each of 100 normal individuals is recorded. Note that results for 63 of the 100 individuals were within 1 min of each other, and results for 95 were within 3 min of each other.

distribution. In practice we consider a TBT less than 8'30'' to be definitely normal and suspect that the TBT is abnormal if it is between 8'30'' and 10'. A TBT longer than 10'' is definitely abnormal.

In the original Ivy technique the BT was reported as the average of the first three punctures that bled.[7] As a result, many investigators still use either three punctures or incisions. Mielke et al. tested the necessity for multiple incisions and showed that the information gained from three incisions was not different from that provided by two.[21] Recently, we have compared the results from two incisions with those from a single incision in 100 normal subjects (Figure 9). The mean value of 4'36'' for a single incision was not significantly different from the mean value of 4'49'' for a second incision done sequentially on the opposite arm. In only two instances were one of the paired results normal, while the other was abnormal. Because of the demonstrated repeatability of the template method, only one incision is necessary. If duplicate incisions are preferred, they should not be done simultaneously on the same arm since blood from one incision may run into the other and distort the end point. A second incision is performed only when there is a technical question concerning the first incision.

In order to evaluate the influence of the direction of the incision on the test results, we compared BT's made from vertical and horizontal incisions in 100 normal subjects (Figure 10). By horizontal incision we mean an incision which is parallel to the elbow crease; a vertical incision is perpendicular to the horizontal one. The mean was 5'34'' with the horizontal technique, and 4'21'' with the vertical ($p > 0.001$). This significant difference cannot be readily explained. However, the skin edges of the horizontal incision tend to separate more than those of the vertical incision, and therefore eliminate any tamponade effect.

Drugs, Diseases, and the Bleeding Time

In the interpretation of the BT, the influence of drugs, most notably aspirin, must be considered. Beaumont was the first to show that aspirin alters the bleeding time.[22] Aspirin will prolong the TBT for 5 to 7 days.[23] Other drugs, including various nonsteroidal antiinflammatory agents,[24-27] regitine,[28] antihistamines,[29] heparin,[30,31] dextran,[31] and carbenicillin[32] will also prolong the BT. A partial list of these drugs is shown in Table 1. Sulfinpyrazone and dipyridamole do not influence the BT.[33,34]

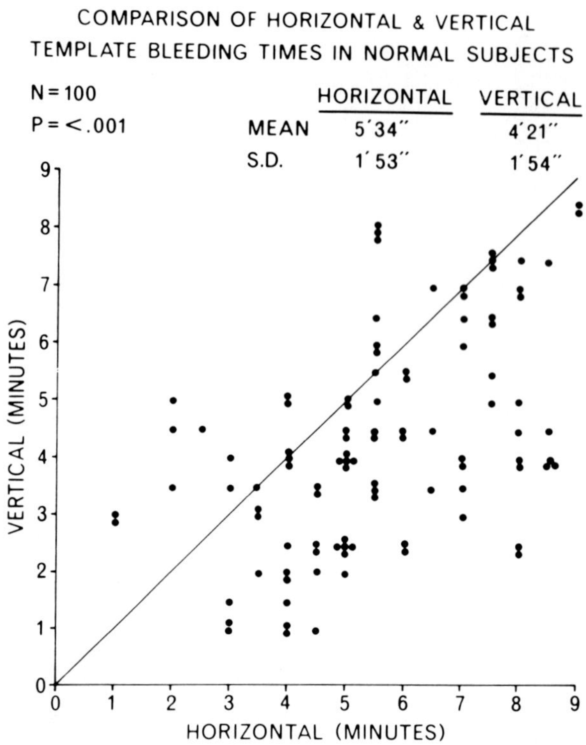

FIGURE 10. In 100 consecutive normal individuals, the horizontal TBT was consistently longer than the vertical one.

Table 1
PARTIAL LIST OF DRUGS WHICH HAVE BEEN REPORTED TO PROLONG THE BLEEDING TIME IN MAN

Trade	Generic	Company	Ref.
TOLECTIN®	Tolmetin sodium	McNeil	6
NAPROSYN®	Naproxen	Syntex	7
	Clonixin	Schering	8
INDOCIN®	Indomethacin	MSD	9
BENADRYL®	Diphenhydramine	Parke-Davis	10
REGITINE®	Phentolamine	Ciba	11
PYOPEN®	Disodium carbenicillin	Beecham	12

Of all the drugs, aspirin has the most pronounced effect. The horizontal TBT was tested in 75 normal subjects before and 2 hr after the ingestion of 10 grains of aspirin (ASA). The mean TBT prolonged from 5' to 10'22''. Figure 11 shows the distribution of the prolongation induced by ASA, and suggests the possibility that there are subgroups within the normal population. Twelve of the 75 subjects showed a change of 2' or less after ASA. Another 52, or approximately two thirds showed a moderate change from 2'30'' to 8'30'' after ASA. Several subjects had a change of 9' or longer. Notwithstanding the degree to which the bleeding time was prolonged, none of these subjects manifested any bleeding tendencies. The fact that ASA prolongs TBT does not indicate whether other drugs will affect TBT.[35]

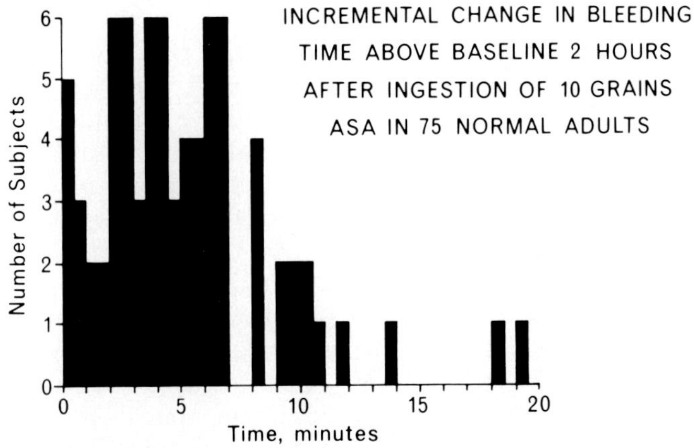

FIGURE 11. Bleeding time tests performed on 75 normal individuals before and 2 hr after ingestion of 10 grains of ASA showed that times for 60 of 75 individuals were 7 min or less. Sensitivity to ASA may define subgroups within the normal population.

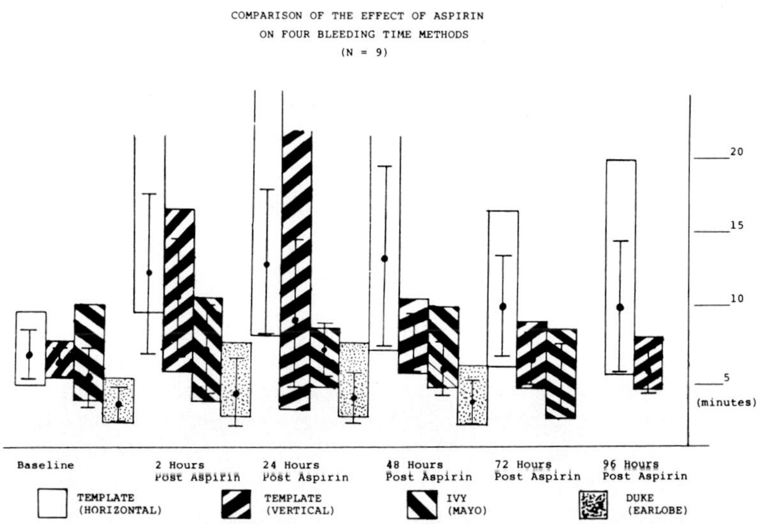

FIGURE 12. Four bleeding time techniques were compared in nine subjects before and after ingestion of 10 grains of ASA. ASA prolonged the BT to different degrees and for different periods of time depending on the technique used.

In an effort to elucidate the characteristics of the TBT, we compared the horizontal and vertical versions of this test[22] with the Ivy[11] and Duke[1] techniques. All BT tests were done simultaneously in nine normal subjects before ASA, 2 hr after the ingestion of 10 grains of ASA, and daily until the subject's bleeding time returned to base line. The results are shown in Figure 12. The template techniques showed the longest BT's and the greatest prolongation by ASA. The horizontal incision produced both a greater prolongation of the BT after ASA and a longer duration of effect than did the vertical incision. The Duke technique gave the shortest times, and apparently was not influenced by ASA. The Ivy technique showed slightly longer BT's, and the influence of ASA was moderate, returning to base line levels in 3 days. From this comparison we surmise that each BT technique measures different mechanisms and/or steps that promote hemostasis.

In 1966, Quick introduced the aspirin tolerance test for detection of mild cases of von Willebrand's disease.[36] He noted that, although patients with this disease frequently had normal bleeding times without ASA, their ingestion of the drug caused exaggerated prolongation. Recently, Stuart et al.[37] have used the TBT instead of the Duke and have found this technique to be extremely reliable in the diagnosis of von Willebrand's disease. A base line BT is obtained, the patient is given two tablets of ASA (650 mg), and the test is repeated 2 hr later. As a general rule, a normal subject will prolong his base line BT from 1 to 1½ times. This test is not specific for von Willebrand's disease; individuals with storage pool disease,[38] hemophilia A,[39] and even some normal individuals[40] may respond in a similar way.

The BT can be prolonged with thrombocytopenia. Harker and Slichter have shown that the TBT is normal with platelet counts above 100,000,[41] but that below this level, the TBT exhibits an inverse relation to the circulating platelet count. These investigators also found that patients with idiopathic thrombocytopenia or patients in a state of marrow recovery after chemotherapy had, on the basis of platelet count, bleeding times shorter than expected, even after adjustment for platelet volume. These platelets are younger and larger and presumably have enhanced hemostatic capacity as measured by the TBT.

The BT is also prolonged in the congenital qualitative platelet disorders such as thrombasthenia,[42-44] Bernard-Soulier syndrome,[45,46] "storage pool" disease,[38,47-49] aspirin-like defect,[50] and von Willebrand's disease.[51-54] The acquired platelet dysfunction abnormalities are associated with a prolonged BT; for example, the myeloproliferative disorders,[55,56] liver disease,[57] uremia,[58] and primary fibrinolysis.[59] The BT is also prolonged in patients with many of the inherited disorders of connective tissue,[60] when no platelet abnormality probably exists other than an altered platelet-connective tissue interaction. It has also been noted with exposure to cold,[6] senility,[61] and albinism.[62]

Discussion

Bleeding time techniques have been repeatedly changed to improve the test's repeatability and make it more sensitive and specific to disorders of hemostasis. The most reliable method is the TBT, but it is also sensitive to variations in technique. The sensitivity of the template method to ASA strongly suggests that the TBT is the bleeding time most sensitive to the prostaglandin mechanism of platelet recruitment.[63] Other mechanisms to promote platelet plug formation may be by independent pathways (e.g., thrombin production); this concept may explain the apparent paradox of marked prolongation of the TBT by ASA in individuals who do not have a bleeding tendency. These individuals may have a mild form of von Willebrand's disease. Thrombin's ability to bypass prostaglandin pathways is surmised because of measurements of the bleeding time in individuals with congenital coagulation defects. When both the prostaglandin-dependent mechanism and the ability to produce thrombin are impaired, as in the case of the severe hemophiliac given ASA, a highly exaggerated bleeding response is produced.[39] A similar response occurs in patients with von Willebrand's disease.[41]

These differences between BT's among normal individuals, normal individuals given ASA, and individuals with hemophilia or von Willebrand's disease given ASA, strongly suggest that there are alternative mechanisms for platelet activity in normal hemostasis.

REFERENCES

1. **Duke, W. W.**, The relation of blood platelets to hemorrhagic diseases: description of a method for determining the bleeding time and coagulation time and report of three cases of hemorrhagic disease relieved by transfusion, *JAMA*, 55, 1185, 1910.
2. **Spitz, S.**, Blutplättchenzahl and gefässfunktion, *Klin. Wochenschr.*, 2, 584, 1923.
3. **Jacobson, B. M.**, Effects of cortisone and corticotropin on prolonged bleeding time, *Am. Med. Assoc. Arch. Int. Med.*, 92, 471, 1953.
4. **Stavem, P.**, The influence of depth of the cut on the bleeding time, *Acta Med. Scand.*, 182, 389, 1967.
5. **Adelson, E., Rheingold, J. J., and Crosby, W. H.**, The platelet as a sponge: a review, *Blood*, 17, 767, 1961.
6. **Quick, A. J.**, The Duke bleeding time, *Am. J. Clin. Pathol.*, 47, 459, 1967.
7. **Ivy, A. C., Shapiro, P. F., and Melnick, P.**, The bleeding tendency in jaundice, *Surg. Gynecol., Obstet.*, 60, 781, 1935.
8. **Ivy, A. C., Nelson, D., and Bucher, G.**, The standardization of certain factors in the cutaneous "venostasis" bleeding time technique, *J. Lab. Clin. Med.*, 26, 1812, 1941.
9. **Tocantins, L. M.**, The bleeding time, *Am. J. Clin. Pathol.*, 6, 169, 1936.
10. **O'Brien, J. R.**, The bleeding time of normal and abnormal subjects, *Am. J. Clin. Pathol.*, 4, 272, 1951.
11. **Owen, C. A., Jr., Bowie, E. J. W., Didisheim, P., and Thompson, J. H., Jr.**, in *The Diagnosis of Bleeding Disorders*, Little, Brown, Boston, 1969, 78.
12. **Hjort, P. and Stormorken, H.**, A study of the *in vitro* effects of a synthetic heparin-like anticoagulant: dextran sulphate, *Scand. J. Clin. Lab. Invest.*, 9(Suppl. 29), 1, 1957.
13. **Borchgrevink, C. F. and Waaler, B. A.**, The secondary bleeding time. A new method for the differentiation of hemorrhagic disease, *Acta Med. Scand.*, 162, 361, 1958.
14. **Copley, A. L. and Lalich, J. J.**, Bleeding time, lymph time, and clot resistance in men, *J. Clin. Invest.*, 21, 145, 1941.
15. **Adelson, E. and Crosby, W. H.**, A new method to measure bleeding time. The "immersion" method, *Acta Haematol.*, 18, 281, 1957.
16. **Willoughby, M. L. N. and Allington, M. J.**, The rate of blood loss from skin punctures during the Ivy bleeding time test, *J. Clin. Pathol.*, 14, 381, 1961.
17. **De Nicola, P.**, Critical evaluation of methods for the study of blood coagulation, fibrinolysis and hemostasis, *Thromb. Diath. Haemorrh.*, 1(Suppl. 7), 325, 1962.
18. **Sutor, A. H., Bowie, E. J. W., Thompson, J. H., Jr., Didisheim, P., Mertens, B. F., and Owen, C. A., Jr.**, Bleeding from standardized skin punctures: automated technique for recording time, intensity and pattern of bleeding, *Am. J. Clin. Pathol.*, 5, 541, 1971.
19. **Bowie, E. J. W. and Owen, C. A., Jr.**, The bleeding time, in *Progress in Hemostasis and Thrombosis*, Spaet, T. H., Ed., Grune & Stratton, New York, 1969, 249.
20. **Sutor, A. H., Bowie, E. J. W., and Owen, C. A., Jr.**, Quantitative bleeding time (hemorrhagometry): a review, *Mayo Clin. Proc.*, 52, 238, 1977.
21. **Mielke, C. H., Jr., Kaneshiro, M. M., Maher, I. A., Weiner, J. M., and Rapaport, S. I.**, The standardized normal Ivy bleeding time and its prolongation by aspirin, *Blood*, 34, 204, 1969.
22. **Beaumont, J. L., Caen, J., and Bernard, J.**, Influence de l'acide acétyl salicylique dans les maladies hémorragiques, *Sang*, 27, 243, 1956.
23. **Mielke, C. H., Jr., Ramos, J. C., and Britten, A. F. H.**, Aspirin as an antiplatelet agent: template bleeding times as a monitor of therapy, *Am. J. Clin. Pathol.*, 59, 236, 1973.
24. **Mielke, C. H., Jr., Heiden, D., and Amadio, P., Jr.**, Tolmetin: hematological effects in normal subjects, in *Tolmetin: A New Non-steroidal Anti-inflammatory Agent*, Ward, J. R., Ed., Excerpta Medica, New York, 1976.
25. **Nadell, J., Bruno, J., Varady, J., and Segre, E. J.**, Effect of naproxen and of aspirin on bleeding time and platelet aggregation, *J. Clin. Pharmacol.*, 14, 176, 1974.
26. **Arkel, Y. S., Schrogie, J. J., and Williams, R.**, Effect of clonixin and aspirin on platelet aggregation in human volunteers, *J. Clin. Pharmacol.*, pp. 30-33, January 1976.
27. **DeGaetano, G., Donati, M. B., and Vermylen, J.**, Some effects of indomethacin on platelet function, blood coagulation and fibrinolysis, *Int. J. Clin. Pharmacol.*, 5, 196, 1971.
28. **O'Brien, J. R.**, Some effects of adrenaline and anti-adrenaline compounds on platelets *in vitro* and *in vivo*, *Nature (London)*, 200, 763, 1963.
29. **O'Brien, J. R.**, A comparison of platelet aggregation produced by seven compounds and a comparison of their inhibitors, *J. Clin. Pathol.*, 17, 275, 1964.
30. **Heiden, D., Mielke, C. H., Jr., and Rodvien, R.**, Impairment by heparin of primary hemostasis, *Br. J. Haematol.*, 36, 427, 1977.
31. **Borchgrevink, C. F.**, The mechanism of the prolonged bleeding time provoked by dextran sulphate or by excessive doses of heparin, *Acta Med. Scand.*, 170, 365, 1961.

32. Brown, C. H., III, Natelson, E. A., Bradshaw, M. D., Williams, T. W., and Alfrey, C. P., Jr., The hemostatic defect produced by carbenicillin. *N. Engl. J. Med.*, 291, (6), 265—270, Aug. 1974.
33. Winchester, J. F., Forbes, C. D., Courtney, J. M., and Prentice, C. R. M., Effect of sulfinpyrazone and aspirin on platelet loss induced *in vitro* by activated charcoal hemoperfusion (Abstr). VI Int. Congr. Thromb. Haematol., Philadelphia, June 26—July 2, 1977, p. 93.
34. Weston, M. J., Rubin, M. H., Langley, P. G., Westaby, S., and Williams, R., Effects of sulfinpyrazone and dipyridamole on capillary bleeding time in man, *Thromb. Res.*, 10, 833, 1977.
35. Mielke, C. H., Jr. and Rodvien, R., unpublished observation.
36. Quick, A. J., Salicylates and bleeding: the aspirin tolerance test, *Am. J. Med. Sci.*, 252, 265, 1966.
37. Stuart, M. J., Wolk, J. A., Miller, M., and Davey, F. R., The post aspirin bleeding time in the diagnosis of von Willebrand's disease (Abstr). VI Int. Congr. Thromb. Haematol., Philadelphia, June 26—July 2, 1977, p. 180.
38. Stuart, M. J., Miller, M., Wolk, J., and Davey, F., The aspirin bleeding time — a screening test for evaluation of bleeding disorders, *Pediatr. Res.*, 11(4), 482, 1977.
39. Kaneshiro, M. M., Mielke, C. H., Jr., Kasper, C. K., and Rapaport, S. I., Bleeding time after aspirin in disorders of intrinsic clotting, *N. Engl. J. Med.*, 281, 1039, 1969.
40. Mielke, C. H., Jr. and Rodvien, R., unpublished observation.
41. Harker, L. A. and Slichter, S. J., The bleeding time as a screening test for evaluation of platelet function, *N. Engl. J. Med.*, 287, 155, 1972.
42. Pittman, M. A. and Graham, J. B., Glanzmann's thrombopathy, an autosomal recessive trait in one family, *Am. J. Med. Sci.*, 247, 293, 1964.
43. Hardisty, R. M., Dormandy, K. M., and Hutton, R. A., Thrombasthenia—studies on three cases, *Br. J. Haematol.*, 10, 371, 1964.
44. Weiss, H. J., Platelet aggregation, adhesion and adenosine disphosphate release in thrombopathia (platelet factor 3 deficiency): a comparison with Glanzmann's thrombasthenia and von Willebrand's disease, *Am. J. Med.*, 43, 570, 1967.
45. Bernard, J. and Soulier, J. P., Sur une nouvelle variété de dystrophie thrombocytaire—hémorragipare congénitale, *Sem. Hop. (Paris)*, 24, 3217, 1948.
46. Howard, M. A., Hutton, R. A., and Hardisty, R. M., Hereditary giant platelet syndrome: a disorder of a new aspect of platelet function, *Br. Med. J.*, 2, 586, 1973.
47. Holmsen, H. and Weiss, H. J., Hereditary defect in the platelet release reaction caused by a deficiency in the storage pool of platelet adenosine nucleotides, *Br. J. Haematol.*, 19, 643, 1970.
48. Holmsen, H. and Weiss, H. J., Further evidence for a deficient storage pool of adenine nucleotides in platelets from some patients with thrombocytopathia — "storage pool disease," *Blood*, 39, 197, 1972.
49. Weiss, H. J., Platelet physiology and abnormalities of platelet function (two parts), *N. Engl. J. Med.*, 293, 531, 580, 1975.
50. Sahud, M. A. and Aggeler, P. M., Platelet dysfunction — differentiation of a newly recognized primary type from that produced by aspirin, *N. Engl. J. Med.*, 280, 453, 1969.
51. Cornu, P., Larrieu, M. J., Caen, J., and Bernard, J., Transfusion studies in von Willebrand's disease: effect on bleeding time and factor VIII, *Br. J. Haematol.*, 9, 189, 1963.
52. Nilsson, I. M., Magnuvvson, S., and Borchgrevink, C. F., The Duke and Ivy methods for determination of the bleeding time, *Thromb. Diath. Hemorrh.*, 10, 223, 1963.
53. Abildgaard, C. F., Simone, J. V., Honig, G. R., Forman, E. N., Johnson, C. A., and Seeler, R. A., von Willebrand's disease: a comparative study of diagnostic tests, *J. Pediatr.*, 73, 355, 1968.
54. Gralnick, H. R., Sultan, Y., and Coller, B. S., von Willebrand's disease: combined qualitative and quantitative abnormalities, *N. Engl. J. Med.*, 296, 1024, 1977.
55. Zucker, S. and Mielke, C. H., Jr., Classification of thrombocytosis based on platelet function tests: correlation with hemorrhagic and thrombotic complications, *J. Lab. Clin. Med.*, 80, 385, 1972.
56. Adams, T., Schutz, L., and Goldberg, L., Platelet function abnormalities in the myeloproliferative disorders, *Scand. J. Haematol.*, 13, 215, 1974.
57. Ivy, A. C., Shapiro, P. F., and Melnick, P., The bleeding tendency in jaundice, *Surg. Gynecol. Obster.*, 60, 781, 1935.
58. Eknoyan, G., Wacksman, S. J., Glueck, H. J., and Will, J. J., Platelet function in renal failure, *N. Engl. J. Med.*, 280, 677, 1969.
59. Kowalski, E., Fibrinogen derivatives and their biologic activities, *Semin. Hematol.*, 5, 45, 1968.
60. Kashiwagi, H., Riddle, J. M., Abraham, J. P., and Frame, B., Functional and ultra structural abnormalities of platelets in Ehlers-Danlos syndrome, *Ann. Int. Med.*, 63, 249, 1965.
61. Page, L. B. and Culver, P. J., *A Syllabus of Laboratory Examinations in Clinical Diagnosis*, Harvard University Press, Cambridge, Mass., 1960, 195.
62. Hermansky, F. and Pudlak, P., Albinism associated with hemorrhagic diathesis and unusual pigmented reticular cells in the bone marrow: report of two cases with histochemical studies, *Blood*, 14, 162, 1959.
63. Marx, J. L., Blood clotting: the role of the prostaglandins, *Science*, 196, 1072, 1977.

PLATELET AGGREGATION BY ADP, COLLAGEN AND RISTOCETIN: A CRITICAL REVIEW OF METHODOLOGY AND ANALYSIS

Barry S. Coller

Principle of Aggregometer[1,2]

A cuvette filled with platelet-rich plasma (PRP) is interposed between a light source and a light detector that is attached to a chart recorder that plots the transmission of light through the cuvette as a function of time. Initially, the platelets both absorb and reflect the light so that less light passes through the cuvette than would pass through a cuvette of platelet-poor plasma (PPP). If the platelets are stirred at 37°C and stimulated to aggregate,* then the number of "particles" will decrease (although the size of each particle will increase), and the distance between particles will increase. This will permit more light to pass and will be recorded as an increase in light transmission[3] (Figure 1). Theoretically, the maximum light transmission would occur if there were essentially no platelets. For standardization, therefore, the chart is adjusted so that the patient's PRP gives very little transmission (0 to 10%, usually) and the same patient's PPP gives essentially total transmission (90 to 100%). Thus variation between individuals in the light transmission of their PPP will not affect the results (Figure 2).

The principle is simple, but one cannot make direct correlations between a certain light transmission and the physical state of the platelets; that is, how many single platelets, small aggregates, and large aggregates exist. This results from several complicating factors:

1. The insensitivity of light transmission to changes from single platelets to very small aggregates[4]
2. The similarity in transmission curves obtained with either a decrease in the aggregation rate of all the platelets or a decrease in the total number of platelets that can enter into aggregates[3]
3. The variable presence of contaminating cells (red blood cells, primarily) in PRP that cannot aggregate and therefore will prevent ever achieving full transmission compared to PPP (from which they will be more completely removed)[3]
4. The complex kinetics of aggregation, wherein the number of particles available for collision continually declines as aggregates form[3]
5. The poorly understood phenomenon of "disaggregation"[1]
6. The contribution of platelet-aggregate contraction to the major increase in light transmission[4]

The insensitivity of the aggregometer to small aggregate formation is quite dramatic, since virtually no single platelets or even small aggregates remain when there is only a 5% change in light transmission.[2,4] Cronberg's[3] mathematical model of aggregation (based on several simplifying assumptions) is presented in Figure 3. In section A, the inverse of time is plotted as a function of the log of the percent transmittance. The slopes of the lines represent the velocity of aggregation ("stickiness") while the X intercept gives an indication of the total increase in transmission achievable if the aggregation were allowed to proceed indefinitely. Looked at in another way, the X intercept reflects the number of platelets (assuming no RBC contamination) that cannot undergo aggregation. It turns out that if 1 part of PRP is diluted with 4 parts of PPP,

* With ADP and collagen (but not epinephrine) immediately before aggregation begins, the platelets change their shape from discs to "spiny spheres." This is associated with a very small decrease in light transmission that may not be noticed unless looked for carefully.

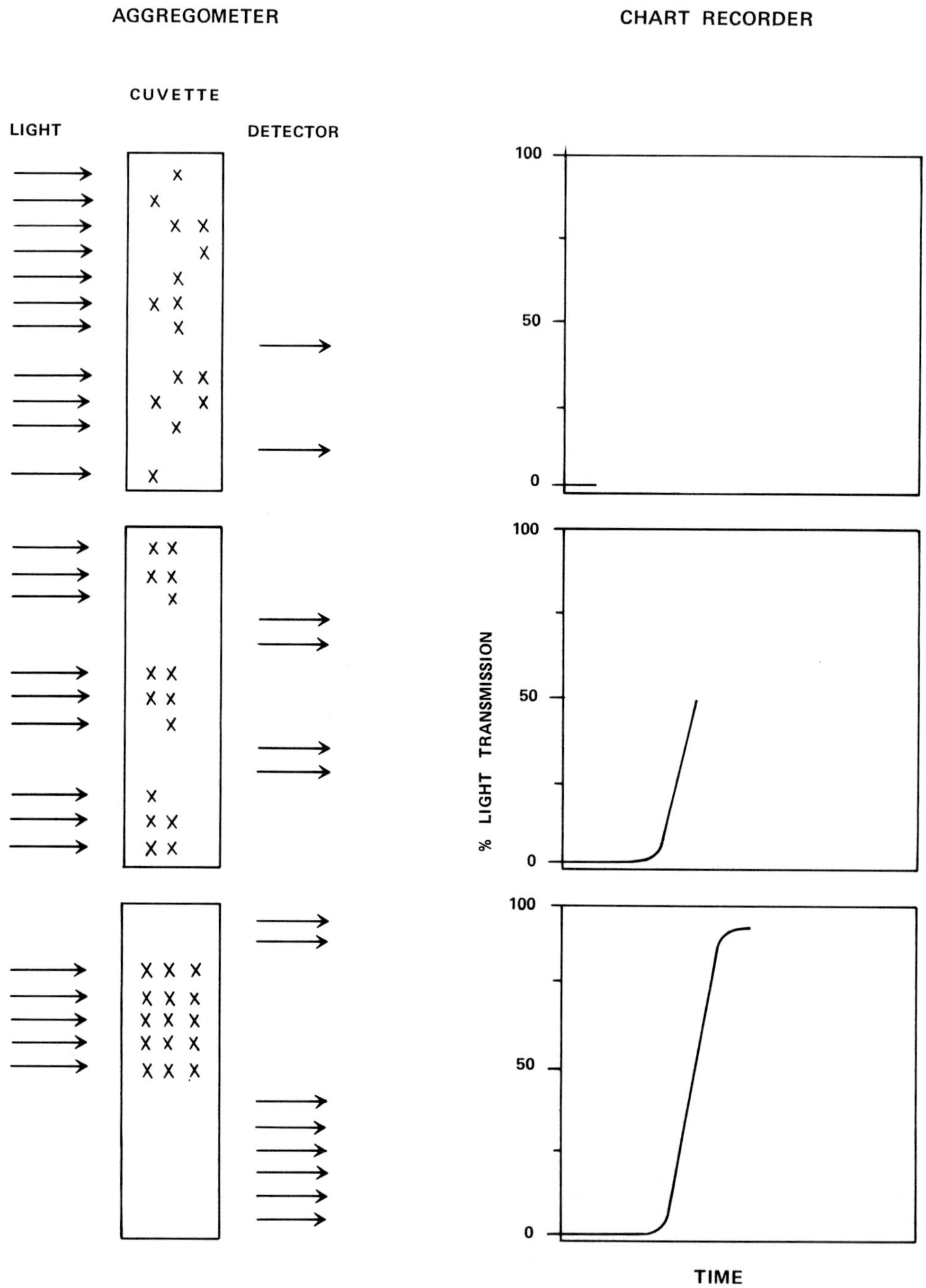

FIGURE 1. Graphic demonstration of aggregometer principle. Note that increasing amounts of light can be transmitted as aggregation proceeds.

the light transmittance will increase by about 50% and, therefore, a residual transmittance of 50% will mean that 20% of the platelets failed to enter into aggregates. In Figure 3B the aggregometer tracings corresponding to the lines in 3A are shown. Line A is taken as having a certain base-line aggregation rate with 100% of the platelets capable of aggregating. Line B has twice, and line C has half, the rate of aggregation of A; in both cases, all of the platelets can aggregate. In contrast, line D, although

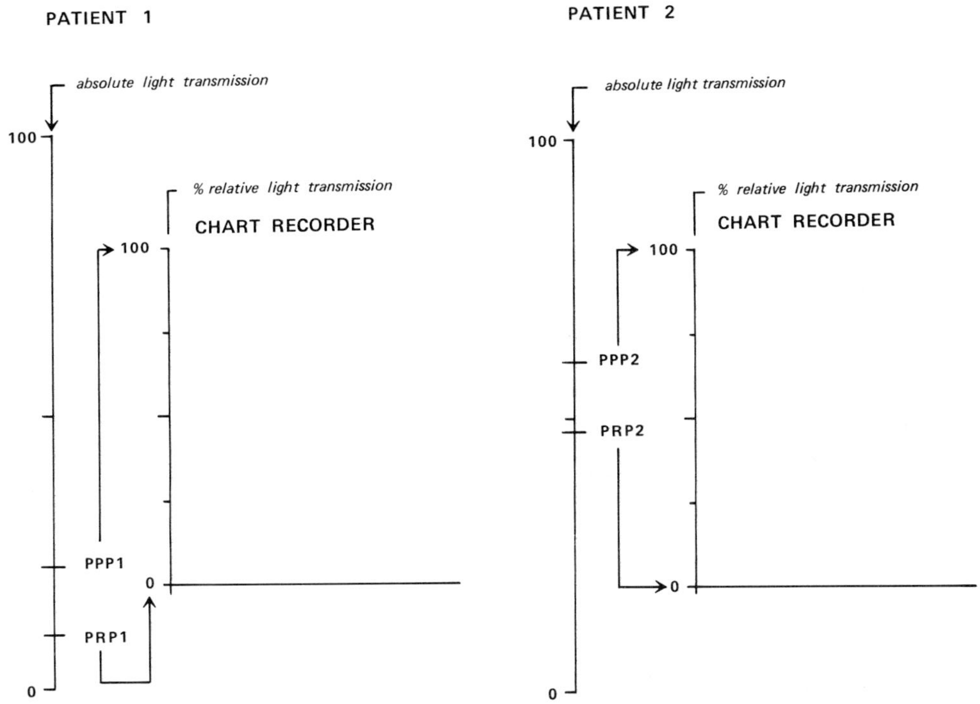

FIGURE 2. The aggregometer chart can be adjusted to give a full-scale deflection between PRP and PPP even if the absolute transmittance of the two samples is different.

having the same aggregability as A (compare slopes in Figure 3A), has a much less impressive aggregation curve because a subpopulation of platelets of about 20% does not aggregate at all. In addition, line E, although having both a decrease in aggregation rate and a reduced number of aggregatable platelets, has a curve that is difficult to differentiate from D. From a practical standpoint, these theoretical considerations require that all samples must be microscopically checked before reporting "no aggregation" and argue for caution in overinterpreting small differences in aggregometer tracings. They also emphasize the need for extremely precise and reproducible blood handling so as to avoid introducing any additional variables.

Instrumentation

The major characteristics of the four most widely used aggregometers in the U.S. are presented in Table 1. From a technical standpoint, all four instruments are capable of providing the aggregation data required to evaluate a patient, although each has its strengths and weaknesses.[5] Several important features should be investigated when evaluating or setting up an instrument.

Temperature control — Aggregation should be performed at 37 ± 0.5°C. The aggregation wells should be checked with a thermometer even if a thermistor is included in the aggregometer, since the thermistor may need adjustment. The time required for the well temperature to reach 37°C should be tested, as should the stability of the well temperature over a period of time. The time required for a sample stored at room temperature to reach 37°C after being placed in the well should be evaluated, since this will be the minimum time required for the sample to incubate in the well before an aggregating agent is added.

Stirring speed — Aggregation will vary significantly with stirring speed.[1,2] Therefore, it is crucial for aggregation studies to be done at the same speed each time. The fixed

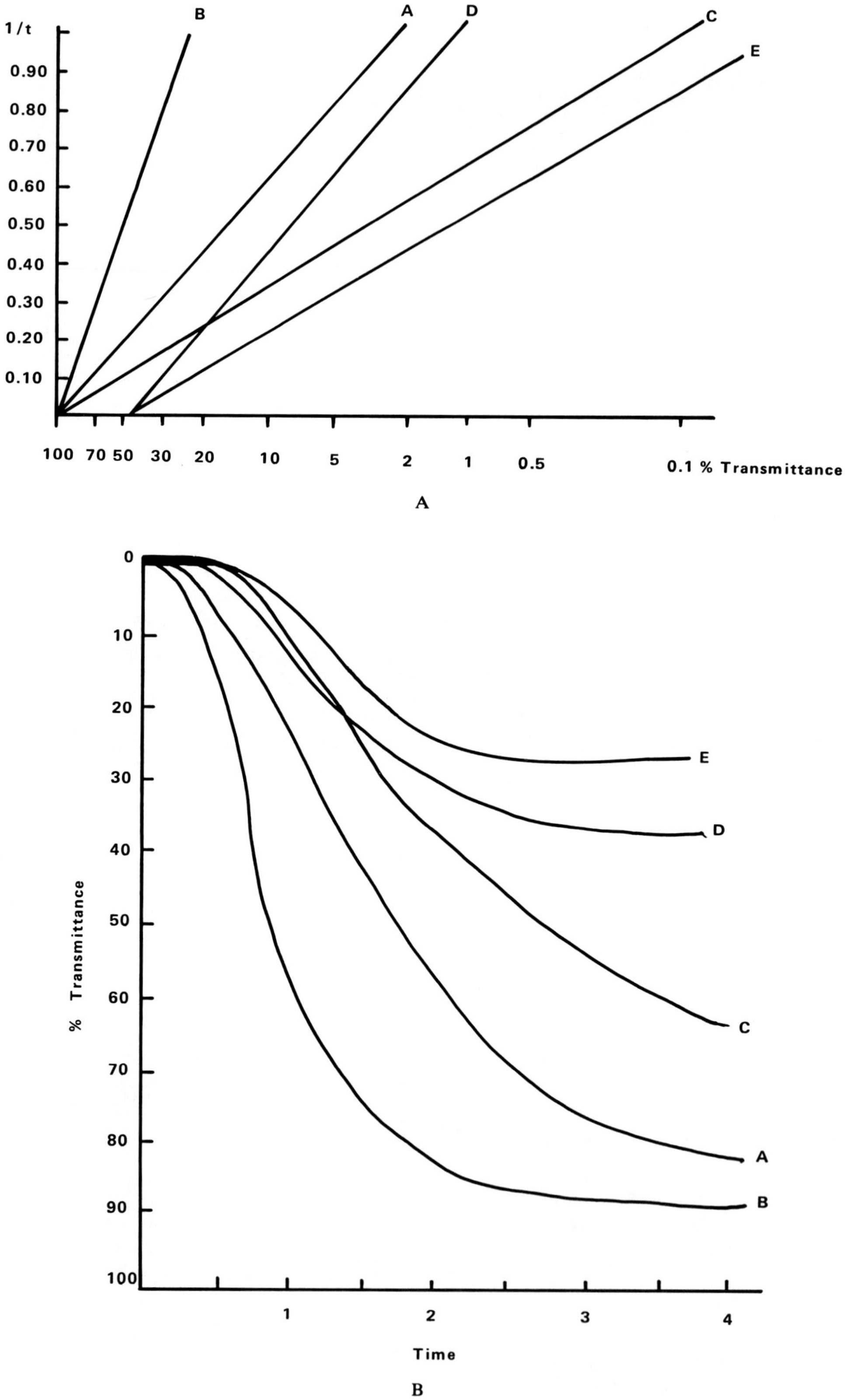

FIGURE 3. Curves constructed according to the theoretical model of platelet aggregation. (A) Semi-logarithmic representation of aggregation response. (B) Curves generated by aggregometer recorder. (From Cronberg, S., *Coagulation,* 2, 139, 1970. With permission.)

synchronous motors are usually very stable because their speed is controlled by the electrical line frequency, which is always maintained at 60 cycles per second (cps). (In Europe, where the frequency is 50 cps, these units run at 1000 rpm instead of 1200 rpm unless an adjustment is made.) The variable-speed units have the advantage of flexibility for specialized work, but one must ensure that the speed is not inadvertently changed and that there is no change in the tachometer used for adjusting the speed as the instrument ages. It is advisable to test the rate of stirring of a new aggregometer, especially the variable-speed models, with a stroboscope.

Stir bars — We found that the size and shape of the stir bar can dramatically affect aggregation.[6] In general, the more effectively a stir bar mixes the reagents, the more rapid and extensive the aggregation. The mixing ability of a stir bar is theoretically directly proportional to both its width and the square of its length. As a result, the thicker teflon-coated bars are more effective than the wire bars of comparable lengths. In addition, relatively small differences in length (1 to 2 mm) can result in significant differences in initial slope, total change in light transmission, and even the presence or absence of a second wave of aggregation.[6] Interestingly, we also noted that the rough edges created when stir bars are cut from wire may enhance the second wave of epinephrine aggregation. It is therefore crucial for studies to be performed with essentially identical stir bars. The most reliable way to achieve this, of course, is to use a single stir bar for all studies. Short of this, one should be certain that the disposable stir bars in each shipment are uniformly machined and that they are similar to previous lots. An additional caution in regard to stirring is that, by virtue of the geometry of the cuvette and stirring mechanism, filling the cuvette beyond its recommended volume can result in very poor mixing of the uppermost portion of the sample and lead to unreliable results.[7]

Instrument stability — The "drift" in the machine (and recorder) can be tested by placing a cuvette filled with PPP or water into the aggregometer and adjusting the controls so that the pen reads a light transmission value in the middle of the scale. The chart should then be allowed to run for 15 to 30 min and the amount of drift that occurs should be observed. If more than a minimal amount (1 to 2%) occurs, the machine should be checked.

Chart recorders — The recorder of the BIO/DATA® instrument is an integral part of the aggregometer. Other aggregometers can be used either with the recorders available from the manufacturer or with other compatible recorders. The curves obtained depend, in large part, on the recorder's response time and dampening; the same signal from an aggregometer may give slightly different curves on two different recorders. The speed of the recorder will also affect the curve produced. When aggregates form, their motion into and out of the light path causes oscillations of the pen; thus the extent of the oscillations reflects the size of the aggregates. The BIO/DATA® aggregometer has a dampening device that can be switched on to smooth the aggregation curves to avoid these deflections. Although the curves obtained are cleaner, information concerning the size of the aggregates is lost. Moreover, the dampening should not be employed when the aggregometer is being used to test for antiplatelet antibodies[8] since it will make it impossible to distinguish between aggregation and platelet lysis because both processes result in increased light transmission.

Sample Preparation

Patient instructions — For purposes of standardization and to avoid the optical difficulties presented by variable degrees of lipemia, studies should be performed on fasting individuals, although relatively fat-free meals are probably acceptable. The patients should not have taken any medication known to interfere with platelet function for at least 1 week.[9,10,11] While "stress" may or may not influence the results,[12,13] I know of no practicable way to avoid the immediate stress of venipuncture (e.g., as

Table 1
COMPARISON OF SOME CURRENTLY AVAILABLE AGGREGOMETERS

	Bio/Data®	Chrono-Log	Payton	Sienco®
Instruments available (channels)	Single	Single or dual[a]	Single or dual[b]	Dual only
Stirring speed (rpm)	1200[c]	1200[c]	Variable	Variable
Stir bar	Urethane-coated ceramic[d]	Teflon-coated magnet[e]	Nickel-plated steel wire[d]	Siliconized stainless steel[d]
Sample size (mℓ)	0.45	0.3—0.45; 2	0.1; 0.25 or 0.5; 1; 2—8	0.2—0.4; 1
External temperature gauge	No[f]	Yes	Yes	No[g]
External temperature adjustment	No	Yes	Yes	No
Dimensions (in.)	18×19×9	Singles: 10×9×6, 18×13×6; Duals: 13×10×6, 18×13×9	14×12×5	8×9×9
Weight (lb)	55[h]	Singles: 10 or 18; Duals: 16 or 25	20	11
Special notes	—[i,j,k,l,m,n,o,p]	—[q,r,s]	—[q,t,u,v]	—[w,x,y,z]
Recorders				
Pen	Heat	Nylon	Several available	Felt
Speed (mm/min)	25	25.4	—	Variable
Dimensions	—	17×13×5	—	18×12×7
Weight (lb)	—	15	—	18

[a] In addition to their regular single and double, Chrono-Log has single or dual instruments with:

1. Automatic full-scale adjustment
2. Warning device if PPP and PRP are insufficiently different in transmission
3. Infra-red light source (no filter required)

They have recently marketed a new aggregometer which simultaneously reads light transmission and ATP release (Lumi-Aggregometer)

[b] In addition to their regular single and dual, Payton has:

1. Dual with automatic full-scale adjustment and built-in recorder
2. Small single with automatic full-scale adjustment

[c] Fixed stirring rate
[d] Disposable
[e] Reusable
[f] Sign lights when 37°C, but no meter
[g] Low temperature indicator plus ready indicator
[h] Includes recorder
[i] Measures PPP and PRP simultaneously and automatically adjusts full scale deflections
[j] Warns if "too few" or "too many" platelets in PRP (based on light transmission)
[k] Reads out percent aggregation numerically on a continuous basis
[l] Trace can be "filtered" to average oscillations of pen
[m] Indicates if stir bar not present
[n] Automatic shut-off feature
[o] Built-in timer
[p] Event hold button
[q] Visual ports for viewing aggregation
[r] Recorder zero pushbutton
[s] Differentiator available
[t] Accommodates wide range of light transmissions
[u] Accessories available for measuring scattered light and UV light induction of aggregation
[v] Narrow portion of cuvette scanned to enhance shape-change measurements
[w] Outputs from both channels can be multiplexed into a single recorder
[x] Water temperature control of aggregometer well available
[y] Light-emitting diode light source, photo diode sensor, and solid state circuitry
[z] DC motor on stirrer controlled by servofeedback

with an indwelling catheter) without introducing other variables that may be more important. Cigarette smoking[12] may also produce acute effects and so should be avoided.

Venipuncture — Although there is some controversy about the importance of avoiding venous stasis and "unclean" venipunctures,[13] a clean venipuncture with an adequately large bore needle (I use a 19 gauge) firmly attached to a plastic syringe (to avoid bubbling of the sample) is the standard technique. The syringe plunger should be "cracked" before venipuncture by moving it up and down and any residual air expelled. It is probably a good idea to avoid excessive suction on the syringe during blood drawing. There seems to be no advantage to a 2-syringe technique if a clean venipuncture is performed,[13] and the manipulations involved in the former may produce their own problems. "Butterfly" needles have the theoretical disadvantage of exposing the blood to another plastic surface in the tubing, but are often more convenient and seem to work equally well. It is probably a good idea to avoid drawing blood for a large number of other tests into the same syringe, since this will lengthen the time between blood drawing and anticoagulation.

Anticoagulation — Sodium citrate is the anticoagulant of choice for aggregation studies. Solutions between 3.2 and 3.8% (note that because sodium citrate comes as the dihydrate, in fact, these solutions are 0.11 to 0.13 M) have been recommended. Usually 9 parts of blood are added to 1 part citrate solution. I have also used 1/100 volume of 40% sodium citrate to minimize dilution effects and find that it also yields reproducible results. Since citrate is distributed exclusively in the plasma space, variations in patient hematocrits will result in differences in citrate concentrations in the PRP which, in turn, will affect the unbound, ionized calcium concentration in the PRP. Whereas aggregation (with the exception of ristocetin) depends on the presence of at least low levels of calcium, the increased plasma citrate concentrations seen with higher hematocrits will necessitate use of higher concentrations of reagents to induce full aggregation.[14,15] A chart showing the volume of 3.8% citrate needed to be added to 9 mℓ of whole blood of various hematocrits to yield constant plasma concentrations of citrate is shown in Figure 4.[16] Moreover, unless pH is controlled (see below), as samples of PRP become more alkaline, the binding affinity of citrate for calcium becomes greater, resulting in a decrease in the ionized calcium concentration.[15] Finally, there is some evidence that the second wave of ADP-induced aggregation seen in the aggregometer is dependent on the ionic environment produced by citrate or, perhaps, the presence of citrate itself,[17-19] although this subject is still controversial.[20]

Transfer and storage — Only plastic pipettes and test tubes should be used. Some workers siliconize their aggregometer cuvettes and stirring wires; others do not.

Centrifugation — Various combinations of centrifugal force and time will produce good yields of platelets in PRP. One rule of thumb is that the product of the average centrifugal force (i.e., the force in the center of the column of blood being centrifuged) and the time in minutes should be between 1750 and 2400.[21] Red blood cell contamination should be avoided by removing only as much PRP as is necessary. All centrifugation should be at room temperature. Although it is quite likely that a subpopulation of the densest platelets is selectively lost in the centrifugation process,[22] this doesn't seem to be of consequence for routine aggregation studies.[23] The remaining blood sample should be centrifuged at room temperature at a higher centrifugal force and for a longer period of time for PPP.

Platelet count adjustment — While there remains some controversy,[23] I believe the evidence is strongly in favor of adjusting the platelet count with PPP to a predetermined level (I use 300,000 because it is just about the highest achievable without discarding too many samples because their levels are too low). While Levine has reported reproducible aggregation results with ADP and collagen at platelet counts as low as

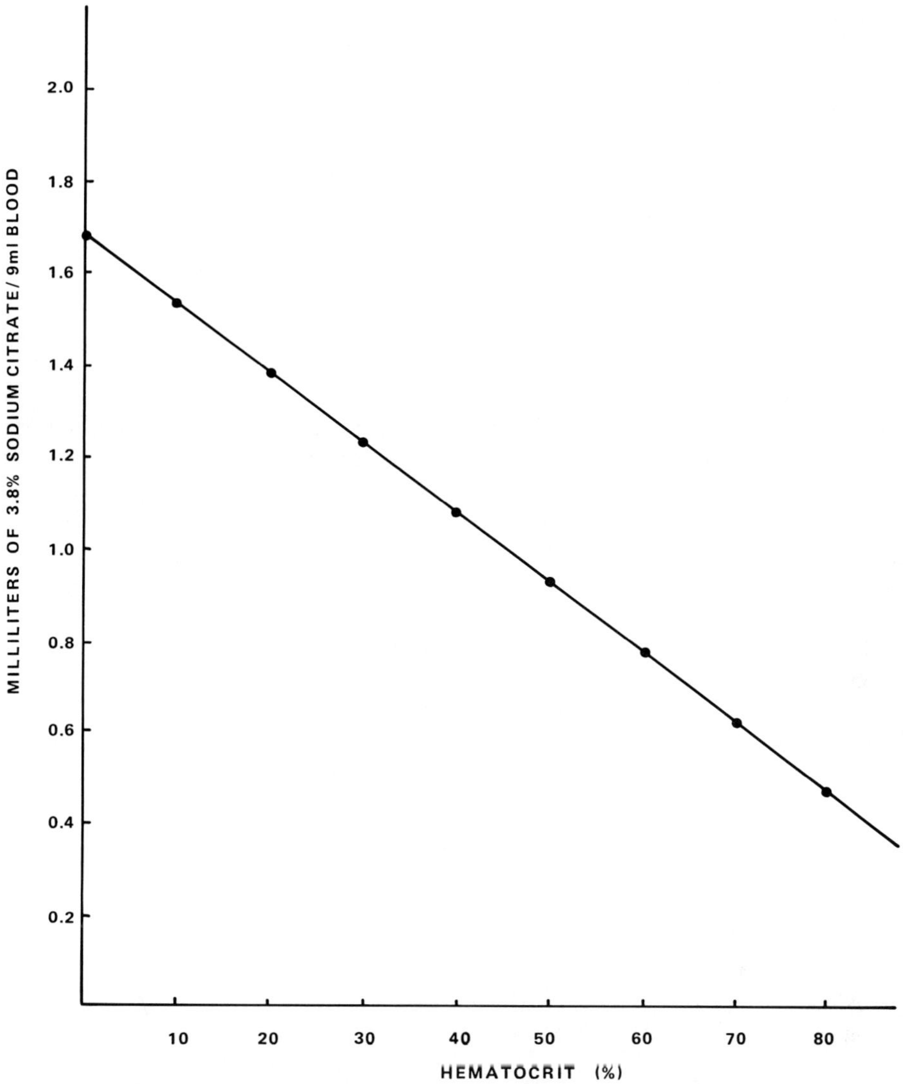

FIGURE 4. Amount of 3.8% citrate required per 9 m*ℓ* of blood with varying hematocrits to obtain a final concentration of 0.64% citrate in the plasma. (Courtesy of Newhouse, P. and Clark, C., *Platelet Function: Laboratory Evaluation and Clinical Application,* Triplett, D. A., Ed., American Society of Clinical Pathologists, Chicago, 1978. Used by permission.)

50,000/mm,[3,24] I have not been able to get consistent results with these reagents at counts below 100,000 to 200,000/mm.[3] Therefore, I do not perform studies unless the count is equal to or greater than 200,000/mm.[3] With ristocetin we found that even minor differences in platelet count (50,000/mm^3) would result in significant differences in initial slope.[25] Moreover, if one considers platelet aggregation analogous to a chemical reaction, it is difficult to justify inconsistently varying the concentration of one of the reactants (the platelets) when one is attempting to compare responses.

Temperature of storage — It is agreed that platelets should not be stored at 4°C because this tends to produce spontaneous aggregation,[26,27] although with a precise rewarming schedule, this may be less of a problem.[28] There is less agreement about whether it is preferable to maintain platelets at 37°C or room temperature. With short-term storage at 37°C, platelets require a higher concentration of ADP to induce second-wave aggregation, and there is greater variation in sensitivity to aggregating agents among individuals; these features are apparently considered virtues by some investigators,[15] although one may question this interpretation. On the other hand, 37°C storage is less convenient, will facilitate pH change if this is not carefully regulated, and will shorten the time interval between blood drawing and deterioration in aggregation response. Thus, until further studies suggest additional advantages to 37°C storage, I believe PRP should be stored at room temperature.

pH of storage — PRP, in contrast to whole blood, has little buffering capacity. Moreover, since PRP has a high pCO_2 and the surrounding air has a very low pCO_2, the CO_2 will diffuse out of the PRP and the pH will rise. The rate of CO_2 loss, and thus pH rise, is quite variable and will depend on many factors, including the surface area-to-volume relationship, temperature, capping, and mixing.[29] Aggregation by ADP, epinephrine, collagen, and ristocetin are all pH dependent,[15,30-32] and thus this parameter must be carefully controlled. Among the methods employed to accomplish this are replacing the air over the PRP with 5% CO_2 in air,[15,30] incubation under mineral oil,[31] collection into citrate buffer,[33] or addition of concentrated base immediately before testing.[34] To overcome the limitations of each of these techniques, we devised a simple apparatus for controlling and maintaining PRP pH by adjusting the ambient pCO_2 (Figure 5).[29] The choice of the proper pH at which to store PRP and perform aggregation studies is still unsettled. ADP- and epinephrine-induced aggregation are maximal at pH 7.7 to 8.0,[30-32,34] while ristocetin-induced aggregation is maximal at pH 7.3 and decreases sharply above pH 7.7.[29] Changes in pH between 7.0 and 8.0 have little effect on "particulate" collagen-induced aggregation, but will dramatically affect the lag phase (although not the extent) of soluble collagen-induced aggregation.[35] The shortened lag phase results from the increased rate of collagen fibril formation that occurs at higher pH.[36] Another consideration in choosing a pH for platelet storage is that the length of time between blood drawing and the onset of the deterioration of aggregation response is shorter when platelets are kept at a higher pH, since the release reaction is more labile in an alkaline environment.[37] After considering all these factors, we chose to store and test all samples at pH 7.7.[29]

Duration of PRP storage — Aggregation responses to ADP, epinephrine, collagen, and ristocetin all vary as a function of time after venipuncture.[5,29,38,39] With ristocetin,

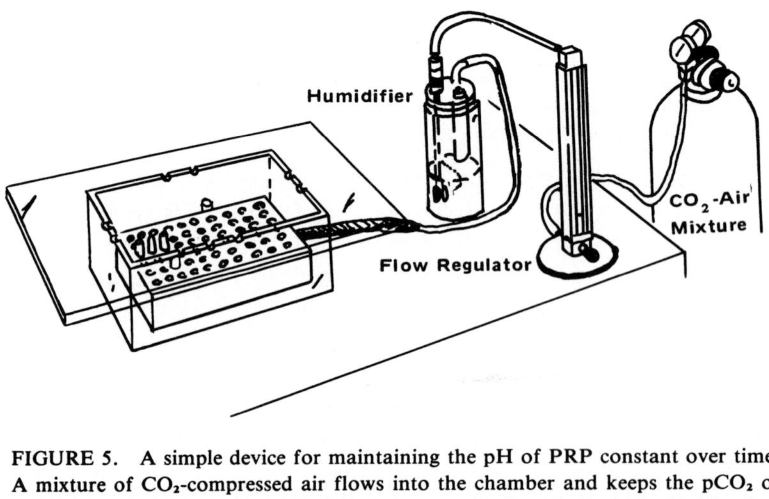

FIGURE 5. A simple device for maintaining the pH of PRP constant over time. A mixture of CO_2-compressed air flows into the chamber and keeps the pCO_2 of the surrounding air equivalent to the pCO_2 of the PRP at the desired pH. The flow regulator allows for fine control and the humidifier prevents evaporation of samples. (From Coller, B. S., Franza, B. R., Jr., and Gralnick, H. R., *Blood*, 47, 841, 1976. By permission.)

this variability is caused exclusively by changes in pH, since ristocetin-induced aggregation remains constant for at least 6 hr if the pH is controlled.[29] The changes in epinephrine aggregation (first an increase and then a decrease) occur even if the pH is kept constant.[39,40] The results with collagen and ADP are less clear. Although there is some suggestion that despite a constant pH they aggregate less well immediately after preparation than a short time later,[41] the effect seems to be less significant than with epinephrine. The poorly understood "refractory" period of platelets, wherein platelets exposed to ADP or epinephrine without stirring have a reduced ability to aggregate in response to these same agents for a short period of time,[42-44] may be partially responsible for some of these findings. Since the red blood cell is a rich source of ADP, precautions (such as adequate bore needle and gentle suction) should be taken to avoid red blood cell trauma (hemolysis) in blood drawing.[45] After a variable period of time, aggregation responses to ADP, epinephrine, and collagen will begin to deteriorate. I have found that these reagents produce relatively consistent patterns for 90 min after PRP is prepared if the pH is maintained at 7.7. Storage at a lower pH might conceivably prolong the useful time span, since the release reaction is less labile at lower pH. From a practical standpoint, several recommendations can be made:

1. The time of blood drawing, PRP preparation, and aggregation with each agent should be recorded.
2. It is advantageous to have as many aggregometer channels as possible since this will narrow the time it takes to complete the studies.
3. If a poor response is obtained with epinephrine, ADP, or collagen early in a study, the aggregation should be repeated in approximately ½ hr.
4. The extreme variability with epinephrine has led some laboratories to abandon it as an aggregating agent. I believe it still has a place if the studies are well controlled, since it can give information regarding the release reaction, and may correlate with hemorrhage in some disease states.[46]

Technical Considerations

Reagent additions — To ensure prompt mixing, one should ensure that the reagent is forcefully introduced into the cuvette. I have found that microliter syringes (Hamilton®), which can be dedicated to a single reagent, are very useful for ADP, epinephrine, and ristocetin. Soluble collagen solutions are more viscous and blow-out Lang-Levy type pipettes work better with this reagent.

pH measurements — The pH of the PRP in the cuvette should be determined just before aggregation is initiated and the result recorded on the chart paper. A combination electrode with a very small bulb (Beckman® #39505 or equivalent) is required to obtain this measurement.

Reagent preparations — ADP and ristocetin can be made up in saline or any convenient buffer (which should not contain sodium azide) to any convenient concentration. I have always tried to minimize the volume of reagent added so that there is little dilution of the sample, and thus, little change in the base line. Therefore, I use ADP at 20 to 100 μM and ristocetin at 50 mg/mℓ. A stock solution of ADP can be prepared, aliquoted, and frozen so that a fresh sample is thawed and diluted each day. Ristocetin is stable (if not in an alkaline buffer) at 4°C for at least 1 to 2 weeks and probably longer. While epinephrine is available as a powder, the stability of stock solutions seems to be somewhat less reliable than for ADP and ristocetin. For this reason, we open a new vial of 1/1000 (5.46 mM) epinephrine (Parke-Davis) at the beginning of each day's aggregation and dilute it 1/50 in saline to achieve a final concentration of 110 μM. Collagen preparations have more serious problems. There are basically two different preparations available: (1) a particulate suspension extracted from connective tissue or partially purified collagen that is composed of fully formed collagen fibrils along with mucopolysaccharides and other contaminants.[47,48] These suspensions are easy to prepare, but are usually poorly characterized chemically and (2) acid-soluble collagen, which is not in fibrillar form but is better characterized chemically. Since collagen must exist in the fibrillar form in order to induce aggregation,[49-51] the major portion of the lag phase with soluble collagen is due to the time required for fibrils to form. The ideal reagent would be chemically well-characterized collagen preparation stabilized in a precisely defined fibrillar form.[52] Such a reagent does not exist. Our approach is to use the commercially available acid-soluble collagen, which is kept on ice and used directly from the bottle. In this way, the increased temperature and pH of the PRP (both of which are kept constant) compared to the soluble collagen preparation facilitates fibril formation in a reproducible way. Others prefer to dilute the collagen first and let it form fibrils before adding it to the PRP. Poor responses with this reagent should be confirmed with the particulate collagen to see if the decreased response is due to impaired fibril formation or to an abnormality in the platelet response. All preparations of collagen should be tested to determine the minimum dose that produces aggregation in several normal individuals.

Analysis of Aggregation Results

Quantitation

The patterns generated by the aggregometer are complex. Although curves produced by all the reagents have superficial similarities, each reagent, in fact, produces a characteristic type of pattern. Thus choosing a single parameter and employing it alone for analysis of curves produced by different reagents is unlikely to be successful. Several approaches to quantitation have been attempted and they fall into three general categories: (1) analysis of patterns produced by a single concentration of reagents in terms of slopes, changes in transmission, lag times, or other measurable parameters (Figure 6),[53] (2) dose response curves with analysis of the above parameters at different reagent concentrations, and (3) derived functions, based on mathematical models conceived of exclusively for the aggregometer[3] or based on classical kinetic theory.[54] This last group, while of major theoretical interest, is not yet sufficiently developed for use in a routine laboratory. The first two approaches are more widespread and will be discussed for each of the aggregating agents.

ADP — At low concentrations of ADP, a pattern of an initial increase in transmission (1° aggregation) followed by a return toward the baseline (disaggregation) is obtained. At high concentrations, a single large increase in transmission occurs. At a critical dose in between these, a 1° wave of aggregation is followed by a plateau and then a 2° wave. While there are probably some exceptions, the PRP's from almost all normals should have a concentration (usually 1 ± 0.5 μM) at which this double wave pattern occurs.[14] However, it may take some time to find the correct dose, and the secondary wave may be quite subtle. This is in contrast to epinephrine where double waves occur over a very wide range of concentrations and where the second wave is almost always more prominent than the first. It should be stressed that drugs that interfere with the release reaction (e.g., aspirin and indomethacin) will have no effect on primary ADP aggregation.[54,55] Thus it is very misleading to interpret a single, full wave of aggregation produced by a high dose of ADP as "normal ADP aggregation." In fact, if performed in this way, only the very rare disorder "thrombasthenia" will give an abnormal result. Thus from a practical standpoint, if a dose of ADP produces only a single, small wave, then the dose should be increased until either a double wave appears or alternatively, a very large single wave is obtained that is essentially full scale. Each wave should be interpreted separately and the concentration required to achieve the double wave (if present) recorded.

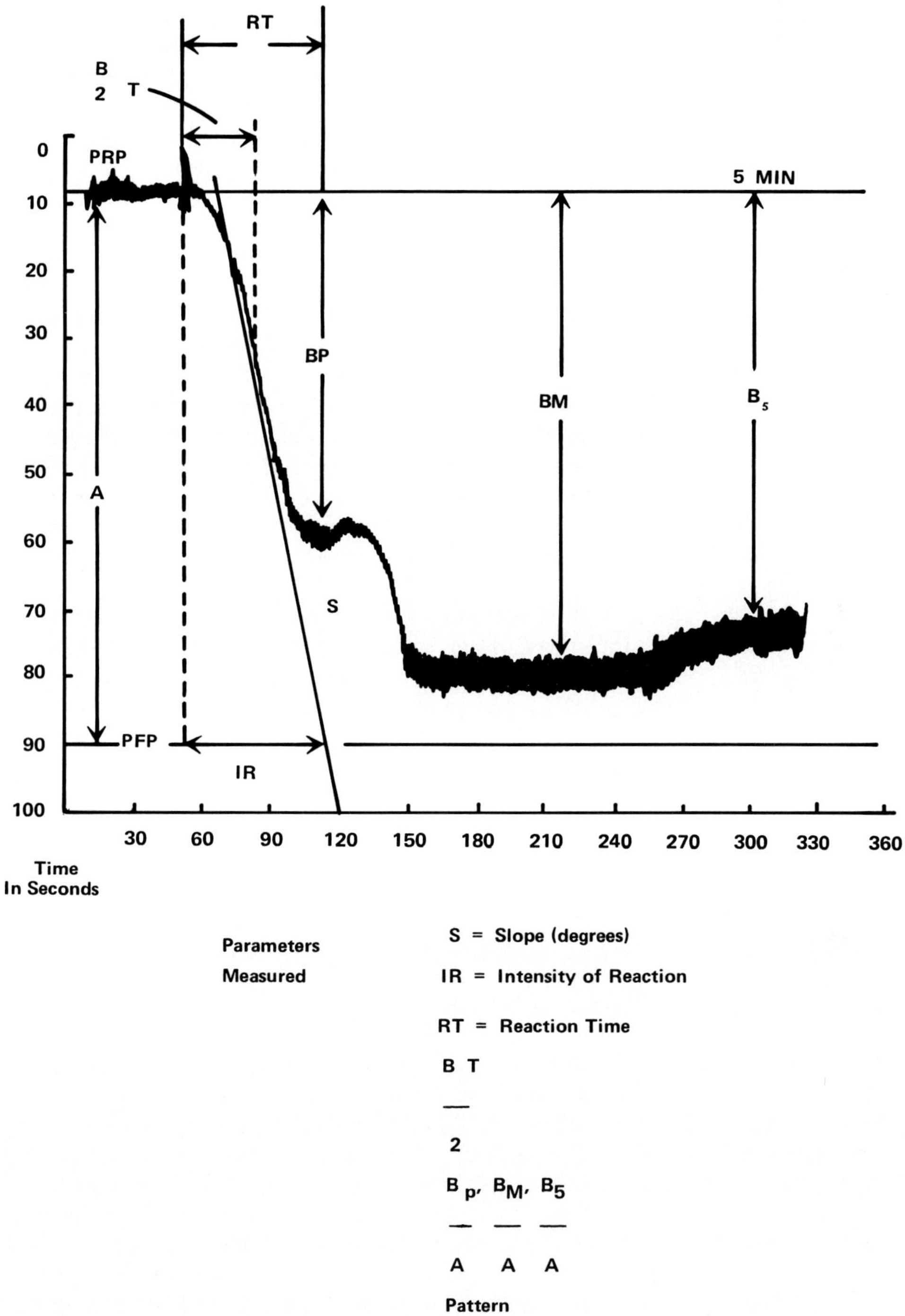

FIGURE 6. Variables used to measure platelet aggregation. (From Yamazaki, H., Takahashi, T., and San,T., *Thromb. Diath. Haemorrh.*, 34, 44, 1975. With permission.)

Connective tissue ("collagen") — This reagent produces a single wave of aggregation after an initial lag. While defects in adhesion to collagen[56] or lack of response to ADP (thrombasthenia) may theoretically give abnormal results, in the vast majority of cases, collagen-induced aggregation measures the integrity of the platelet release reaction. It must be emphasized that defects in the release reaction do not usually result in complete absence of collagen-induced aggregation, since increasing the dose often gives essentially "normal" patterns.[54] Thus each batch of collagen reagent must be tested against a large number of normal individuals to define the lowest dose that produces full aggregation. A patient's response should then be interpreted with respect to the normal range and the dose required to produce full aggregation recorded. If one uses only a single, high concentration of collagen and reports the response as "normal," then one will miss many subtle defects that may be clinically significant, e.g., aspirin ingestion or storage pool disease.[57] We now know that much of the lag phase before aggregation begins is related to the time for collagen fibrils to form. Shortened lag times may therefore reflect either the need for fewer collagen fibrils to initiate aggregation, or alternatively, differences in the plasma that facilitates fibril formation.

Ristocetin — Aggregation by ristocetin requires the presence of the von Willebrand factor in the patient's plasma[58] and a platelet factor that is missing from the platelets of patients with the Bernard-Soulier syndrome.[59] Aggregation does not require divalent cations or platelet energy metabolism and so it is more akin to agglutination than aggregation. At low concentrations (1.2 mg/mℓ), aggregation occurs in two waves with the first phase independent but the second phase dependent on the release reaction. At high concentrations (1.5 to 1.8) only a single phase occurs that is independent of the release reaction. The two most common ways to quantitate aggregation are to measure the initial slope or the extent of aggregation. Note that if one uses the extent of aggregation as the measure of response while employing a low dose, then one is also measuring the integrity of the release reaction. This is undesirable since one wants this test to reflect the level of von Willebrand factor in the patient's plasma (or the patient's platelet membrane abnormality) and not the release reaction, which can be studied by other techniques. For these reasons I recommend measuring the initial slope of aggregation while using a relatively high concentration of ristocetin. All slope measurements are highly subjective, especially when they are changing rapidly, as in ADP and collagen-induced aggregation. The initial slopes with ristocetin tend to be more easily defined. An alternative method for quantitation is to determine the concentration of ristocetin required to give a certain percent increase in light transmission.[60]

Quality Control and Establishment of Normal Range

Platelet aggregation is a rapidly evolving technique that is useful for evaluating platelet function. It requires meticulous technical attention for reproducible, meaningful results. One cannot rely on published values for comparison, since the many variables that have been discussed above will differ slightly from laboratory to laboratory. The most important thing, I believe, is to perform as many tests as is practicable on normal individuals so as to develop an idea of the range of normal responses. It is not acceptable to compare a patient's response with the response of just the one control drawn on that same day. If the control's response is particularly brisk (compared to other normals) then that does not mean that a patient with a slightly less brisk response is "abnormal." Where quantitation is achievable, as with the range of initial slopes for ristocetin aggregation, means and standard deviations for the normal population should be determined. The daily control then functions as a test of reagent integrity, while the patient's response should be compared to responses of the entire normal population.

REFERENCES

1. Born, G. V. R. and Cross, J., The aggregation of blood platelets, *J. Physiol.*, 168, 178, 1963.
2. O'Brien, J. R., Platelet aggregation. II. Some results with a new method of study, *J. Clin. Pathol.*, 15, 452, 1962.
3. Cronberg, S., Evaluation of platelet aggregation, *Coagulation*, 2, 139, 1970.
4. Born, G. V. R. and Hume, M., Effects of the numbers and sizes of platelet aggregates on the optical density of plasma, *Nature (London)*, 215, 1027, 1967.
5. Clark, C. A., Newhouse, P. A., and Triplett, D. A., A comparative study of three aggregometers: Bio/Data®, Chronolog®, and Sienco®, *Am. J. Clin. Pathol.*, 67, 205, 1977.
6. Coller, B. S. and Gralnick, H. R., The effect of stir bar size and shape on quantitative platelet aggregation, *Thromb. Res.*, 8, 121, 1976.
7. Coller, B. S., unpublished observation.
8. Deykin, D. and Hellerstein, L. J., The assessment of drug-dependent and isoimmune antiplatelet antibodies by the use of aggregometry, *J. Clin. Invest.*, 51, 3142, 1972.
9. Leist, E. R. and Banwell, J. G., Products containing aspirin, *N. Engl. J. Med.*, 291, 710, 1974.
10. Selner, J., More aspirin-containing medicines, *N. Engl. J. Med.*, 292, 372, 1975.
11. Weiss, H. J., The pharmacology of platelet inhibition, in *Progress in Hemostasis*, Vol. 1, Spaet, T. H., Ed., Grune & Stratton, 1972, 199.
12. Levine, P. H., An acute effect of cigarette smoking on platelet function. A possible link between smoking and arterial thrombosis, *Circulation*, 48, 619, 1973.
13. Harrison, M. J. G., Emmons, P. R., and Mitchell, J. R. A., The variability of human platelet aggregation, *Atherosclerosis Res.*, 7, 197, 1967.
14. Hardisty, R. M., Hutton, R. A., Montgomery, D., Rickard, S., and Trebilcock, H., Secondary platelet aggregation: a quantitative study, *Br. J. Haematol.*, 19, 307, 1970.
15. Han, P. and Ardlie, N. G., The influence of pH, temperature, and calcium on platelet aggregation: maintenance of environmental pH and platelet function for in vitro studies in plasma, *Br. J. Haematol.*, 26, 373, 1974.
16. Newhouse, P. and Clark, C., Variability of platelet aggregation, in *Platelet Function: Laboratory Evaluation and Clinical Application*, Triplett, D. A., Ed., American Society of Clinical Pathologists, Chicago, 1978.
17. Mustard, J. F., Perry, D. W., Kinlough-Rathbone, R. L., and Packham, M. L., Factors responsible for ADP-induced release reaction of human platelets, *Am. J. Physiol.*, 228, 1757, 1975.
18. Macfarlane, D. E., Walsh, P. N., Mills, D. C. B., Holmsen, H., and Day, H. J., The role of thrombin in ADP-induced platelet aggregation and release: a critical evaluation, *Br. J. Haematol.*, 30, 457, 1975.
19. Lages, B. A. and Weiss, H. J., Platelet aggregation and secretion: effects of anticoagulants and divalent cation chelators, *Thromb. Haemostasis*, 38 (Abstr.), 123, 1977.
20. Ardlie, N. G. and Huzoor-Akhbar, Further evidence of the involvement of thrombin in platelet release by ADP and other agents, *Thromb. Haemostasis*, 38 (Abstr.), 36, 1977.
21. Woods, B. P., Dennehy, A., and Clarke, N., Some observations on the preparation of platelet-rich plasma, *Thromb. Haemostasis*, 36, 302, 1976.
22. Corash, L., Tan, H., and Gralnick, H. R., The heterogeniety of human whole blood platelet subpopulations. I. Relationship between buoyant density, cell volume and ultrastructure, *Blood*, 49, 71, 1977.
23. O'Brien, J. R., Factors influencing the optical platelet aggregation test, *Acta Med. Scand. Suppl.*, 525, 43, 1971.
24. Levine, P. H., The effect of thrombocytopenia on the determination of platelet aggregation, *Am. J. Clin. Pathol.*, 65, 79, 1976.
25. Coller, B. S. and Gralnick, H. R., unpublished observations.
26. Zucker, M. B. and Borelli, J., Reversible alterations in platelet morphology produced by anticoagulants and by cold, *Blood*, 9, 602, 1954.
27. Kattlove, H. E. and Alexander, B., The effect of cold on platelets. I. Cold induced platelet aggregation, *Blood*, 38, 39, 1971.
28. Kattlove, H. E., Alexander, B., and White, F., The effect of cold on platelets. II. Platelet function after short-term storage at cold temperatures, *Blood*, 40, 688, 1972.
29. Coller, B. S., Franza, B. R., Jr., and Gralnick, H. R., The pH dependence of quantitative ristocetin-induced platelet aggregation: theoretical and practical implications. A new device for maintenance of platelet-rich plasma pH, *Blood*, 47, 841, 1976.
30. Rogers, A. B., The effect of pH on human platelet aggregation induced by epinephrine and ADP, *Proc. Soc. Exp. Biol. Med.*, 139, 1100, 1972.

31. **Rodman, N. F. and Penick, G. D.,** The effect of pH on platelet aggregation responses, *Blood,* 40, 953, 1972.
32. **Skoza, L., Zucker, M. D., Jerushalmy, Z., and Grant, R.,** Kinetic studies of platelet aggregation induced by adenosine diphosphate and its inhibition by chelating agents, guanidino compounds, and adenosine, *Thromb. Diath. Haemorrh.,* 18, 713, 1967.
33. **Zimmerman, T. S., Ratnoff, O. D., and Powell, A. E.,** Immunologic differentiation of classic hemophilia (factor VIII deficiency) and von Willebrand's disease, *J. Clin. Invest.,* 50, 244, 1971.
34. **Shattil, S. J., Annayo-Gilindo, R., Bennett, J., Colman, R. W., and Cooper, R. A.,** Platelet hypersensitivity induced by cholesterol incorporation, *J. Clin. Invest.,* 55, 636, 1975.
35. **Coller, B. S.,** unpublished observations.
36. **Coller, B. S., Jaffe, R., Tan, H., and Gralnick, H. R.,** unpublished observations.
37. **Zucker, M. B.,** Proteolytic inhibitors, contact and other variables in the release reaction of human platelets, *Thromb. Diath. Haemorrh.,* 28, 393, 1972.
38. **Rossi, E. C. and Gerlinde, L.,** A time-dependent increase in the responsiveness of platelet-rich plasma to epinephrine, *J. Lab. Clin. Med.,* 85, 300, 1975.
39. **Warlow, C., Corina, A., Ogston, D., and Douglas, A. S.,** The relationship between platelet aggregation and time after venipuncture, *Thromb. Diath. Haemorrh.,* 31, 133, 1974.
40. **Coller, B. S.,** unpublished observation.
41. **Joist, J. H. and Kay, D.,** Reversible Inhibition of Platelet Function in Normal Platelet Rich Plasma, (Abstr.), American Society of Hematology, Boston, 1976, 200.
42. **O'Brien, J. R.,** Changes in platelet membranes possibly associated with platelet stickiness, *Nature (London),* 212, 1057, 1966.
43. **Harbury, C. B. and Schrier, S. L.,** The effect of a partial release reaction on subsequent platelet function, *J. Lab. Clin. Med.,* 83, 977, 1974.
44. **Holme, S. and Holmsen, H.,** ADP-induced refractory state of platelets in vitro. I. Methodological studies on aggregation in platelet-rich plasma, *Scand. J. Haematol.,* 15, 96, 1975.
45. **Haslam, R. J. and Mills, D. C. B.,** The adenylate kinase of human plasma, erythrocytes and platelets in relation to degradation of adenosine dephosphate in plasma, *Biochem. J.,* 103, 773, 1967.
46. **Zucker, S. and Mielke, C. H.,** Classification of thrombocytosis based on platelet function tests: correlation with hemorrhagic and thrombotic complications, *J. Lab. Clin. Med.,* 80, 385, 1972.
47. **Zucker, M. B. and Borelli, J.,** Platelet clumping produced by connective tissue suspensions and by collagen, *Proc. Soc. Exp. Biol. Med.,* 109, 779, 1962.
48. **Hovig, T.,** Aggregation of rabbit blood platelets produced in vitro by saline "extracts" of tendons, *Thromb. Diath. Haemorrh.,* 9, 248, 1963.
49. **Jaffe, R. and Deykin, D.,** Evidence for a structural requirement for the aggregation of platelets by collagen, *J. Clin. Invest.,* 53, 875, 1974.
50. **Muggli, R. and Baumgartner, H. R.,** Collagen induced platelet aggregation: requirement for tropocologen multimers, *Thromb. Res.,* 3, 715, 1974.
51. **Brass, L. F. and Bensusan, H. B.,** The role of collagen quarteruary structure in the platelet: collagen interaction, *J. Clin. Invest.,* 54, 1480, 1974.
52. **Day, H. J., Holmsen, H., and Zucker, M. B.,** Report of the working party on platelets, *Thromb. Haemostasis,* 36, 263, 1976.
53. **Yamazaki, H., Takahashi, T., and San, T.,** Hyperaggregability of platelets in thromboembolic disorders, *Thromb. Diath. Haemorrh.,* 34, 44, 1975.
54. **Rossi, E. C. and Gerlinde, L.,** Kinetic parameters of platelet aggregation as an expression of platelet responsiveness, *Thromb. Haemostasis,* 37, 283, 1977.
55. **Zucker, M. B. and Peterson, J.,** Inhibition of adenosine diphosphate-induced secondary aggregation and other platelet functions by acetylsalicylic acid ingestion, *Proc. Soc. Exp. Biol. Med.,* 127, 547, 1968.
56. **Caen, J. and Legrand, Y.,** Abnormalities in the platelet collagen reaction, *Ann. N. Y. Acad. Sci.,* 201, 194, 1972.
57. **Holmsen, H. and Weiss, H. J.,** Further evidence for a deficient storage pool of adenine nucleotides in platelets from some patients with thrombocytopathia — "storage pool disease," *Blood,* 39, 197, 1972.
58. **Weiss, H. J., Rogers, J., and Brand, H.,** Defective ristocetin-induced platelet aggregation in von Willebrand's disease and its correction by factor VIII, *J. Clin. Invest.,* 52, 2697, 1973.
59. **Jenkins, C. S. P., Philips, D. R., Clemeston, K. J., Meyer, D., Larrien, M.-J., and Luscher, E. F.,** Platelet membrane glycoprotein implicated in ristocetin-induced aggregation. Studies of the proteins on platelets from patients with Bernard-Soulier syndrome and von Willebrand's disease, *J. Clin. Invest.,* 57, 112, 1976.
60. **Italian Working Group,** The spectrum of von Willebrand's disease, *Br. J. Haematol.,* 35, 101, 1977.

PLATELET RETENTION PROCEDURES

E. J. Walter Bowie and Charles A. Owen, Jr.

The tests to be described in this chapter have been devised to give some measure of platelet adhesion, and they fall into two groups: tests that measure platelet adhesion only and tests that measure platelet aggregation in addition to platelet adhesion.

A number of tests have been devised to measure platelet adhesion alone. These include immersion of glass slides and cover slips in blood or platelet-rich plasma,[1-4] the adhesion of platelets to tanned red cells,[5] and the use of rotating glass tubes[6-8] or glass rods[9] that have been coated with collagen or other proteins. It is also possible to adapt the platelet aggregometer to measure mainly platelet adhesion.[10-13] The measurement of adhesion-aggregation can be done by the in vivo method of Borchgrevink[14-16] or by in vitro methods using glass wool braid,[17] the Wright rotating glass bulb technique,[18-20] and the passage of blood through columns filled with small glass beads.[21-32]

The glass bead column methods are the most popular despite the fact that they are difficult to standardize. It is possible, however, to standardize them if a number of variables are taken into account. These variables include the presence or absence of red cells, temperature, the anticoagulant, the contact time of the blood with the glass beads, "disturbing" the blood, and the type of plastic used for construction of the column.[33,34]

Numerous studies have been carried out in both bleeding and thrombosing states using tests of platelet adhesion-aggregation.[35-37] The literature is replete with contradictions, largely because the methods used are different and are not comparable. There is suggestive evidence that the glass bead column test measures the primary phase of hemostasis and has much the same significance as the bleeding time.[38] It has, in fact, been suggested that it is a sensitive test of bleeding time.[39] Because the test measures both adhesion and aggregation of platelets, it is usually called the platelet "retention test" because results are expressed as the percentage of platelets retained in the glass bead column. The platelet retention test is not diagnostic of any specific disease. Its main application has been in von Willebrand's disease and in qualitative platelet diseases.[16,17,37,40-49] The test at one time played a very important role in the diagnosis of von Willebrand's disease, but it has recently been superseded by other tests such as the measurement of factor VIII antigen and of the Willebrand factor.

If the test were commercially available, it could be used as a screening test of platelet function and would be particularly useful in laboratories that are not specialized in the more sophisticated tests of hemostasis. It is of particular use in patients who have von Willebrand's disease but in whom the diagnosis has been obscured as a result of transfusions, pregnancy, or birth control pills. In these three conditions, the level of factor VIII coagulant activity, factor VIII antigen, and the Willebrand factor may approach normal, but platelet retention, although it may increase, usually remains in the abnormal range.[37]

The In Vivo Method of Didisheim and Bunting[16]

The method is modified from the original description of the test by Borchgrevink.[14,15] An area on the volar surface of the forearm is cleaned with 70% alcohol and allowed to dry. The area selected should be free of visible blood vessels. The pressure in the capillaries is standardized by inflating a blood pressure cuff to a pressure of 40 mm Hg. An incision 5 mm deep is made with a no. 11 Bard-Parker blade. Blood is collected starting at 1 min and the collection is continued at 2-min intervals until the 9th min or until bleeding stops. On each sample a platelet count is

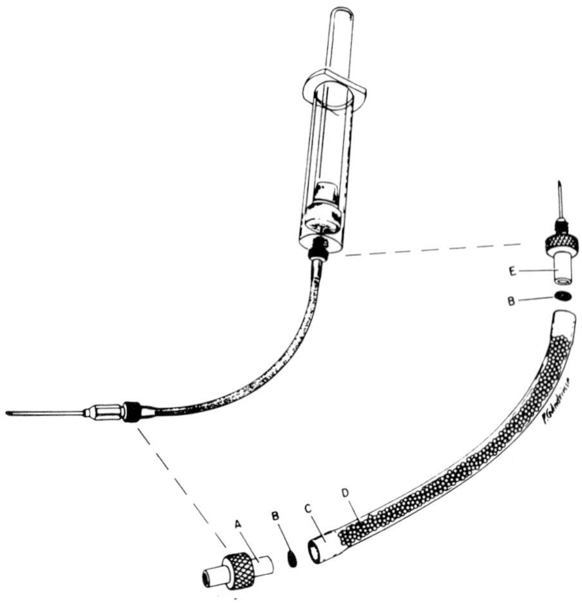

FIGURE 1. Salzman glass bead column for test of platelet adhesiveness. Polyvinyl tubing (C), internal diameter 0.113 in., is filled with 1.3 g of soda-lime-silica glass beads (D), 0.0185-in. average diameter. Siliconized nylon mesh (B) is glued with Duco cement to the ends of the metal adapters (A, E). Adapter A accepts hub of 20-gauge needle for venipuncture; adapter E accepts needle to puncture seal of Vacutainer tube (#3204Q, Becton-Dickinson). (From Salzman, E. W., *J. Lab. Clin. Med.*, 62, 724—735, 1963. By permission of The C. V. Mosby Company.)

performed. Half a minute before each collection, the wound is gently wiped with dry gauze in order to make sure that the sample of blood is fresh. All the platelet counts from the blood exuding from the wound are averaged, and the mean is subtracted from the venous platelet count. The difference, as the percentage of the venous platelet count, is a measure of platelet adhesiveness.

The Salzman Test[22]

The blood is drawn by venipuncture directly from the vein through a glass bead column that is attached to a 7-mℓ Vacutainer tube (Becton-Dickinson, Rutherford, N.J.). The glass bead column contains 1.3 g of glass beads; the details of its construction are shown in Figure 1. Another sample of blood is obtained after the glass bead column has been disconnected. The platelets in the two blood samples are counted, and the difference between the two counts is expressed as a percentage of the venous count. This value is called "platelet retention". The column is discarded after use. In our laboratory the normal range is 27 to 83%. Vacutainers may have a variable vacuum, and special ones have been made for the performance of this test.

The Platelet Retention Test of Bowie [24]

This is the test that we perform in our laboratory, and it will be presented in detail.

Equipment

1. Polycarbonate plastic tube (6.5 cm long by 2.6 cm inside diameter)

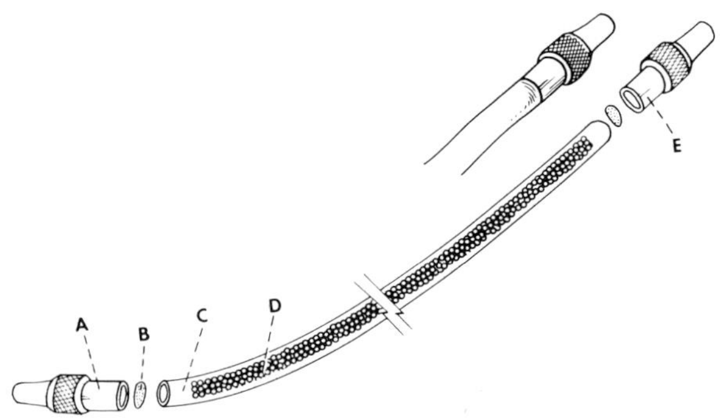

FIGURE 2. Details of glass bead column used for platelet retention: Metal adapter (A) for attaching to needle; siliconized nylon mesh (B) to prevent beads from leaving column, glued to (A) and (C); plastic tube (C) (polyvinyl, internal diameter 0.113 in.) in which is deposited 2.6 g of beads (D) (soda-lime-silica beads, 0.0185-in. average diameter); adapter (E) for connecting to syringe. (From Owen, C. A., Jr., Bowie, E. J. W., and Thompson, J. H., Jr., *The Diagnosis of Bleeding Disorders,* 2nd ed., Little, Brown & Company, Boston, 1975, 102. By permission.)

2. Plastic snap-cap tubes in which 0.1 mℓ of 2% dipotassium ethylenediaminetetra-cetate (EDTA) has been allowed to dry
3. Plastic syringes, 20 mℓ
4. Infusion pump (Model 975, Harvard Apparatus Co.)
5. Glass bead column (constructed according to the method of Salzman)[22] but containing 2.6 g of glass beads with Becton-Dickinson ML/ML adapter at each end (Figure 2). The glass bead column is packed by the vibrations of an electric engraving pen (the tip of the pen is passed once down the length of the column)

Reagents

1. Sodium heparin for injection (Panheprin®, 1000 U/mℓ, Abbott Laboratories)
2. K_2EDTA, 2% in water

Procedure

A sample of 15 mℓ of blood is drawn into a plastic syringe by a clean venipuncture. Of this, 3.5 mℓ is transferred to a Vacutainer tube containing EDTA, and a platelet count is done — "initial platelet count". A 10-mℓ portion of the remaining blood is dispensed into a polycarbonate plastic tube by allowing it to flow gently down the side of the tube. The tube contains 0.04 mℓ of sodium heparin solution (40 U) as an anticoagulant. The blood is mixed gently with the heparin by inverting it six times. The heparinized blood is drawn gently into a plastic 20-mℓ syringe, which is clipped into the infusion pump. The column is then attached to the end of the syringe by a ½-in. length of polyvinyl tubing. The pump is started at a flow rate of 5.7 mℓ/min, which gives a contact time with the beads of 12 sec. As the blood exudes from the end of the column, it is collected in 1-mℓ aliquots in the EDTA collection tubes. The "final platelet count" is calculated by averaging the platelet counts in the fourth and fifth milliliters. The percentage of platelets remaining in the column, called "platelet retention", is calculated by:

$$\text{Platelet retention (\%)} = \frac{\text{initial platelet count} - \text{final platelet count}}{\text{initial platelet count}} \times 100$$

where normal = >65

Test Materials

Glass beads:

Microbeads Division
Cataphote Corporation
Box 2369
Jackson, MS 39205
Paul R. Schmersey

Mr. F. J. Brackenbury
Manager Customer Service
Potters Industries, Inc.
Industrial Road, P. O. Box 14
Carlstad, N.J. 07072

Becton-Dickinson adapter, #3113 ML/ML:
V. Mueller & Co.
6600 W. Touhy Ave.
Chicago, IL 60748

Polyvinyl (Tygon®) tubing, internal diameter 0.113 inch:
U.S. Stoneware Division
Box 350
Akron, OH 44309

Multifilament nylon, #20XX 172 by 184 mesh;
aperture opening, 0.0028":
Tobler, Ernset & Traber, Inc.
420 Saw Mill River Road, P. O. Box 112
Elmsford, NY 10523

Disposable syringe, 20-mℓ (Stylex®):
Pharmaseal Laboratories
Stendale, CA

Beaded plastic vials with snap-on caps 2" by 5/8", Jolite treated:
Lermer Plastic, Inc.
502 South Avenue
Garwood, NJ 07027

Heparin (Panheprin®), 10,000 USP units per vial:
Abbott Laboratories
North Chicago, IL 60064

I. E. C. Autoclear polycarbonate tubes, 30-mℓ capacity, #1697; caps #16, #1518:
Scientific Products Co.
McGaw Park
Waukegan, IL 60085

Infusion pump, model no. 975:
Harvard Apparatus Co., Inc.
Dover, MA 02030

Tips on Performing the Test

1. Use a column made of polyvinyl plastic.
2. Pack the glass beads with a vibrator before use to ensure even flow.
3. Perform a careful venipuncture to obtain an immediate free flow of blood. "Disturbed" blood yields low values.
4. Add the blood to the heparin gently and invert the tube very gently. (Alternatively, the heparin can be placed in the collecting syringe.)

5. The flow rate of blood through the column, and hence the contact time of the blood with the glass beads, must be rapid enough to allow discrimination between normal and von Willebrand's disease yet slow enough for normal platelets to be retained. We find 5.7 mℓ/min to be optimal.
6. The hematocrit should be more than 30%.
7. Collect the blood in 1-mℓ aliquots and use the average of the fourth and fifth milliliters in calculating the platelet retention.

REFERENCES

1. **Mason, R. G. and Gilkey, J. M.**, A simple test for quantitation of platelet adhesion to glass: studies in bleeder and nonbleeder subjects, *Thromb. Diath. Haemorrh.*, 25, 21, 1971.
2. **Zucker, M. B. and Vroman, L.**, Platelet adhesion induced by fibrinogen absorbed onto glass, *Proc. Soc. Exp. Biol. Med.*, 131, 318, 1969.
3. **Breddin, K.**, Zur Messung der Thrombozytenadhäsivitat, *Thromb. Diath. Haemorrh.*, 12, 269, 1964.
4. **George, J. N.**, Direct assessment of platelet adhesion to glass: a study of the forces of interaction and the effects of plasma and serum factors, platelet function, and modification of the glass surface, *Blood,* 40, 862, 1972.
5. **Zbinden, G. and Tomlin, S.**, Effect of heparin on platelet adhesiveness, *Acta Haematol.*, 41, 264, 1969.
6. **Packham, M. A., Evans, G., Glynn, M. F., and Mustard, J. F.**, The effect of plasma proteins on the interaction of platelets with glass surfaces, *J. Lab. Clin. Med.*, 73, 686, 1969.
7. **Jenkins, C. S. P., Packham, M. A., Guccione, M. A., and Mustard, J. F.**, Modification of platelet adherence to protein-coated surfaces, *J. Lab. Clin. Med.*, 81, 280, 1973.
8. **Cazenave, J.-P., Packham, M. A., and Mustard, J. F.**, Adherence of platelets to a collagen-coated surface: development of a quantitative method, *J. Lab. Clin. Med.*, 82, 978, 1973.
9. **Cazenave, J.-P., Reimers, H.-J., Kinlough-Rathbone, R. L., Packham, M. A., and Mustard, J. F.**, Effects of sodium periodate on platelet functions, *Lab. Invest.*, 34, 471, 1976.
10. **Spaet, T. H. and Lejnieks, I.**, A technique for estimation of platelet-collagen adhesion, *Proc. Soc. Exp. Biol. Med.*, 132, 1038, 1969.
11. **Mustard, J. F., Hegardt, B., Rowsell, H. C., and MacMillan, R. L.**, Effect of adenosine nucleotides on platelet aggregation and clotting time, *J. Lab. Clin. Med.*, 64, 548, 1964.
12. **Hovig, T., Jørgensen, L., Packham, M. A., and Mustard, J. F.**, Platelet adherence to fibrin and collagen, *J. Lab. Clin. Med.*, 71, 29, 1968.
13. **Hirsh, J., McBride, J. A., and Dacie, J. V.**, Thromboembolism and increased platelet adhesiveness in post-splenectomy thrombocytosis, *Aust. Ann. Med.*, 15, 122, 1966.
14. **Borchgrevink, C. F.**, A method for measuring platelet adhesiveness in vivo, *Acta Med. Scand.*, 168, 157, 1960.
15. **Borchgrevink, C. F.**, Platelet adhesion in vivo in patients with bleeding disorders, *Acta Med. Scand.*, 170, 231, 1961.
16. **Didisheim, P. and Bunting, D.**, Abnormal platelet function in myelofibrosis, *Am. J. Clin. Pathol.*, 45, 566, 1966.
17. **Moolten, S. E. and Vroman, L.**, The adhesiveness of blood platelets in thromboembolism and hemorrhagic disorders. I. Measurement of adhesiveness by the glass-wool filter, *Am. J. Clin. Pathol.*, 19, 701, 1949.
18. **Wright, H. P.**, The adhesiveness of blood platelets in normal subjects with varying concentrations of anticoagulants, *J. Pathol. Bacteriol.*, 53, 255, 1941.
19. **Wright, H. P.**, The adhesiveness of blood platelets in rabbits treated with dicoumarol, *J. Pathol. Bacteriol.*, 57, 382, 1945.
20. **Wright, H. M. P.**, Adhesiveness of blood-platelets in haemophilia, *Lancet,* 1, 306, 1946.
21. **Hellem, A. J.**, The adhesiveness of human blood platelets in vitro, *Scand. J. Clin. Lab. Invest.*, 12 (Suppl. 51), 12, 1960.
22. **Salzman, E. W.**, Measurement of platelet adhesiveness: a simple in vitro technique demonstrating an abnormality in von Willebrand's disease, *J. Lab. Clin. Med.*, 62, 724, 1963.
23. **O'Brien, J. R.**, The adhesiveness of native platelets and its prevention, *J. Clin. Pathol.*, 14, 140, 1961.

24. **Bowie, E. J. W., Owen, C. A., Jr., Thompson, J. H., Jr., and Didisheim, P.**, Platelet adhesiveness in von Willebrand's disease, *Am. J. Clin. Pathol.*, 52, 69, 1969.
25. **Bowie, E. J. W., Owen, C. A., Jr., Thompson, J. H., Jr., and Didisheim, P.**, A Test of platelet adhesiveness, *Mayo Clin. Proc.*, 44, 306, 1969.
26. **Hellem, A. J.**, Platelet adhesiveness in von Willebrand's disease: a study with a new modification of the glass bead filter method, *Scand. J. Haematol.*, 7, 374, 1970.
27. **Maschouf, C., Robinson, R. W., and LeBeau, R. J.**, Evaluation of nialamide on the coagulation of blood: introduction of a new technic for measuring adhesiveness of the platelets, *Blood*, 24, 289, 1964.
28. **Sharp, A. A.**, Platelets in multiple sclerosis (letter to the editor), *Lancet*, 2, 1296, 1965.
29. **Hirsh, J., McBride, J. A., and Wright, H. P.**, Platelet adhesiveness: a comparison of the rotating bulb and glass-bead column methods, *Thromb. Diath. Haemorrh.*, 16, 100, 1966.
30. **Rossi, E. C. and Green, D.**, A study of platelet retention by glass bead columns ("platelet adhesiveness" in normal subjects), *Br. J. Haematol.*, 23, 47, 1972.
31. **Rosner, P., Bouvier, C. A., and Berthoud, S.**, Mesure de l'adhésivité plaquettaire au verre (modification de la méthode de Hellem), *Nouv. Rev. Fr. Hematol.*, 7, 185, 1967.
32. **Hume, M.**, Platelet adhesiveness and other coagulation factors in thrombophlebitis, *Surgery*, 59, 110, 1966.
33. **Bowie, E. J. W. and Owen, C. A., Jr.**, Some factors influencing platelet retention in glass bead columns including the influence of plastics, *Am. J. Clin. Pathol.*, 56, 479, 1971.
34. **Coller, B. S. and Zucker, M. B.**, Reversible decrease in platelet retention by glass bead columns (adhesiveness) induced by disturbing the blood, *Proc. Soc. Exp. Biol. Med.*, 136, 769, 1971.
35. **Meyer, D.**, In vitro platelet adhesiveness: methods of study and clinical significance, in *Advances in Experimental Medicine and Biology*, Vol. 34, Mannucci, P. M. and Gorini, S., Eds., Plenum Press, New York, 1972, 123.
36. **Hellem, A. J. and Stormorken, H.**, Platelet adhesion-aggregation reaction and its clinical significance, in *Recent Advances in Blood Coagulation*, Poller, L., Ed., Little, Brown & Company, Boston, 1969, 69.
37. **Bowie, E. J. W. and Owen, C. A., Jr.**, The value of measuring platelet "adhesiveness" in the diagnosis of bleeding diseases, *Am. J. Clin. Pathol.*, 60, 302, 1973.
38. **Bowie, E. J. W. and Owen, C. A., Jr.**, unpublished data.
39. **Weiss, H. J.**, Platelet function tests and their interpretation (editorial), *J. Lab. Clin. Med.*, 87, 909, 1976.
40. **Neemeh, J. A., Bowie, E. J. W., Thompson, J. H., Jr., Didisheim, P., and Owen, C. A., Jr.**, Quantitation of platelet aggregation in myeloproliferative disorders, *Am. J. Clin. Pathol.*, 57, 336, 1972.
41. **Gilchrist, G. S., Fine, R. N., and Donnell, G. N.**, The hemostatic defect in glycogen storage disease, type I, *Acta Paediatr. Scand.*, 57, 205, 1968.
42. **Goudemand, M. and Parquet-Gernez, A.**, Les anomalies de l'hémostase dans les thrombocytémies, *Nouv. Rev. Fr. Hematol.*, 6, 570, 1966.
43. **Hardisty, R. M. and Hutton, R. A.**, Bleeding tendency associated with "new" abnormality of platelet behaviour, *Lancet*, 1, 983, 1967.
44. **Caen, J. P., Castaldi, P. A., Leclerc, J. C., Inceman, S., Larrieu, M. J., Probst, M., and Bernard, J.**, Congenital bleeding disorders with long bleeding time and normal platelet count. I. Glanzmann's thrombasthenia (report of fifteen patients), *Am. J. Med.*, 41, 4, 1966.
45. **Caen, J. P., Sultan, Y., and Larrieu, M.-J.**, A new familial platelet disease (letter to the editor), *Lancet*, 1, 203, 1968.
46. **Cronberg, S., Nilsson, I. M., and Gydell, K.**, Haemorrhagic thrombocythaemia due to defect platelet adhesiveness, *Scand. J. Haematol.*, 2, 208, 1965.
47. **Salzman, E. W. and Neri, L. L.**, Adhesiveness of blood platelets in uremia, *Thromb. Diath. Haemorrh.*, 15, 84, 1966.
48. **Spaet, T. H., Lejnieks, I., Gaynor, E., and Goldstein, M. L.**, Defective platelets in essential thrombocythemia, *Arch. Intern. Med.*, 124, 135, 1969.
49. **De Vries, S. I., ten Cate, J. W., den Hartog-Veerman, M. E., and van Dooren, M. M.**, Quelques remarques sur la thrombocytopathie acquise chez les malades urémiques, *Schweiz. Med. Wochenschr.*, 98, 1658, 1968.

LABORATORY EVALUATION OF PLATELET COAGULANT ACTIVITIES

Peter N. Walsh

The laboratory methods employed for measuring platelet coagulant activities are summarized in Table 1. These methods have used either platelets washed by a variety of techniques or platelet-rich plasma. Most of them probably measure what is commonly referred to as "platelet factor 3 activity." Many tests for platelet coagulant activities have been designed to detect deficiencies in the capacity of platelets to contribute to intrinsic coagulation reactions. Since the thrombocytopathies characterized by deficiencies in platelet factor 3 activity are relatively rare, the utility of many tests for platelet coagulant activities has been limited. However, more recently developed techniques have been designed to quantitate platelet coagulant activities relative to normal platelets, and these assays permit quantitation of platelet coagulant hyperactivity as well as deficiency states.[1]

A number of tests provide qualitative assessments of the contribution of platelets to intrinsic coagulation (Table 1). The prothrombin consumption test provides an assessment of the efficiency of prothrombin consumption during clotting by comparing measurements of prothrombin in serum and in plasma obtained simultaneously.[2] The amount of prothrombin in serum is abnormally high, indicating inadequate consumption, when intrinsic clotting factor deficiencies are present or the platelets are deficient in their contribution to clotting. Thus if clotting factor deficiencies can be ruled out, an abnormal prothrombin consumption test suggests a deficiency of platelet coagulant activity. The thromboplastin generation test is generally used to detect intrinsic coagulation factor deficiencies, but if the patient's platelets are washed and compared with normal washed platelets, an abnormal result suggests a deficiency in platelet coagulant activity.[3] The kaolin clotting time of platelet-rich plasma can be used to compare a patient's platelets with normal platelets by testing mixtures of platelet-rich plasma and platelet-poor plasma.[4] Platelet factor 3 activity (i.e., the contribution of platelets to the interaction of factor Xa, factor V, and calcium in the activation of prothrombin) can be measured either qualitatively or quantitatively in either platelet-rich plasma or washed platelets by testing the platelets after an appropriate stimulus in a test system containing plasma to which Russell's viper venom is added as a direct activator of factor X (Figure 1).[5] Quantitative results can be obtained by comparing the clotting times of platelets obtained from a patient and a normal donor at various known concentrations of platelets.[1] The logarithm of clotting time is plotted against the logarithm of platelet concentration, and the platelet factor 3 activity of the patient's platelets is expressed as a percentage of the activity of normal platelets.[1]

Platelets have recently been shown to participate in coagulation reactions in the contact phase and early stages of intrinsic coagulation. Assays for these platelet coagulant activities can be carried out in either platelet-rich plasma or washed platelets and the results expressed quantitatively as described above for the assay for platelet factor 3 activity. Contact-forming activity, the capacity of ADP-stimulated platelets to activate factor XII, can be assayed in platelet-rich plasma, incubated with ADP, and tested in plastic tubes with minimal dilution of plasma (Figure 2).[6] Collagen-induced coagulant activity, the capacity of collagen-stimulated platelets to activate platelet-associated factor XI and thereby initiate intrinsic coagulation, can be assayed in washed platelets in a test system involving the use of partially purified coagulation factors (Figure 3).[7] Intrinsic factor-Xa forming activity, the capacity of collagen-activated platelets to promote the activation of factor X by a complex of factors IXa and VIII with calcium and platelets, can be assayed in washed platelets in a similar test system (Figure 4).[8]

Table 1
METHODS FOR MEASURING PLATELET COAGULANT ACTIVITIES

Test system	Sample tested	Stimulus to platelets	Purpose of assay	Ref.
Prothrombin consumption	Serum and plasma	Clotting	Qualitative test of platelet contribution to clotting	2
Thromboplastin generation test	Washed platelets	Washing of platelets	Qualitative test of platelet contribution to clotting	3
Kaolin clotting time	PRP and PPP	Kaolin	Qualitative test of platelet contribution to clotting	4
Stypven (RVV) time	PRP or washed platelets	Kaolin, collagen, freezing and thawing	Qualitative or quantitative test of platelet contribution (PF3) to prothrombin activation by factors Xa and V	1, 5
Contact product forming activity assay	PRP	ADP	Quantitative assay of factor XII-activation by ADP-treated platelets	1, 6
Collagen-induced coagulant activity assay	Washed platelets	Collagen	Quantitative assay of factor XI-activation by collagen-treated platelets	1, 7
Intrinsic factor-Xa forming activity assay	Washed platelets	Collagen	Quantitative assay of platelet contribution to factor-X activation by factors VIII and IX	1, 8

ASSAY OF PLATELET FACTOR 3 ACTIVITY

STAGE	COMPONENTS	EVENTS
I	Washed Platelets or PRP Aggregated with Collagen or Incubated with Kaolin or Frozen and Thawed	Membrane Phospholipids (PI*) Made Available
II	Aliquot of I Russell's Viper Venom (RVV) Plasma Calcium	X → (RVV) Xa · V · Ca^{++} · PI* II → IIa I → Ia

* Component Assayed

FIGURE 1. Assay of platelet factor 3 activity. (From Walsh, P. N., Platelet Function Testing, DHEW Publication No. (NIH) 77-108, Day, H. J., Homsen, H., and Zucker, M. B., Eds., Government Printing Office, Washington, D. C. 1977, 437—462.)

ASSAY OF CONTACT PRODUCT FORMING ACTIVITY

STAGE	COMPONENTS AND CONDITIONS		EVENTS
I	PRP ADP Phospholipid	Non Contacted Undiluted Plasma	XII / XI → (ADP) XIIa / XI → XIa
II	Addition of Calcium		Measurement of F XIa

FIGURE 2. Assay of contact product-forming activity. (From Walsh, P. N., Platelet Function Testing, DHEW Publication No. (NIH) 77-108, Day, H. J., Homsen, H., and Zucker, M. B., Eds., Government Printing Office, Washington, D. C. 1977, 437—462.)

ASSAY OF COLLAGEN–INDUCED COAGULANT ACTIVITY

STAGE	COMPONENTS	EVENTS
I	Washed Platelets Collagen	XI —Collagen→ XIa
II	Aliquot of I Factors VIII, IX, X Calcium	F–X Activation
III	Aliquot of II F–X Deficient Plasma Phospholipid Calcium	Measurement of F Xa

FIGURE 3. Assay of collagen-induced coagulant activity. (From Walsh, P. N., Platelet Function Testing, DHEW Publication No. (NIH) 77-108, Day, H. J., Homsen, H., and Zucker, M. B., Eds., Government Printing Office, Washington, D. C. 1977, 437—462.)

ASSAY OF INTRINSIC FACTOR–Xa FORMING ACTIVITY

STAGE	COMPONENTS	EVENTS
I	Washed Platelets (Pl*) Factors XIa, VIII, IX, X Calcium	IX —XIa→ IXa · VIII · Ca^{++} · Pl* X → Xa
II	Aliquot of I F–X Deficient Plasma Phospholipid Calcium	Measurement of F Xa

* Phospholipid: Component Assayed

FIGURE 4. Assay of intrinsic factor-Xa-forming activity. (From Walsh, P. N., Platelet Function Testing, DHEW Publication No. (NIH) 77-108, Day, H. J., Homsen, H., and Zucker, M. B., Eds., Government Printing Office, Washington, D. C. 1977, 437—462.)

REFERENCES

1. **Walsh, P. N.,** Platelet coagulant activities in thrombasthenia, *Br. J. Haematol.,* 23, 553, 1972.
2. **Biggs, R.,** *Human Blood Coagulation, Haemostasis and Thrombosis,* Blackwell Scientific Publications, Oxford, England, 1972, 290.
3. **Biggs, R. and Douglas, A. S.,** Thromboplastin generation test, *J. Clin. Pathol.,* 6, 23, 1953.
4. **Hardisty, R. M. and Hutton, R. A.,** The kaolin clotting time of platelet-rich plasma: a test of platelet factor-3 availability, *Br. J. Haematol.,* 11, 258, 1965.
5. **Spaet, T. H. and Cintron, J.,** Studies on platelet factor-3 availability, *Br. J. Haematol.,* 11, 269, 1965.
6. **Walsh, P. N.,** The role of platelets in the contact phase of blood coagulation, *Br. J. Haematol.,* 22, 237, 1972.
7. **Walsh, P. N.,** The effects of collagen and kaolin on the intrinsic coagulant activity of platelets. Evidence for an alternative pathway in intrinsic coagulation not requiring factor XII, *Br. J. Haematol.,* 22, 393, 1972.
8. **Walsh, P. N. and Biggs, R.,** The role of platelets in intrinsic factor-Xa formation, *Br. J. Haematol.,* 22, 743, 1972.

PLATELET SIZING*

Simon Karpatkin

Techniques

Platelet size and/or volume can be measured directly under visual observation on peripheral smears or indirectly via either electronic particle size counting or packed cell volume/platelet counts.

The direct method involves the preparation of a stained blood smear from EDTA-anticoagulated blood. The platelet diameter is measured with a calibrated ocular micrometer, under oil immersion at 1000 × magnification with or without the presence of polystyrene reference spheres (Figure 1);[1-11] or the platelet surface area can be measured by planimetry techniques.[12] The platelet surface area measurement is probably more reliable than diameter measurement, since platelets on EDTA smears are not always round, but may also be elipsoidal. The EDTA anticoagulant, 3.7 mM in whole blood, changes the shape[13-16] and possibly volume[13-15] of platelets from discoid to

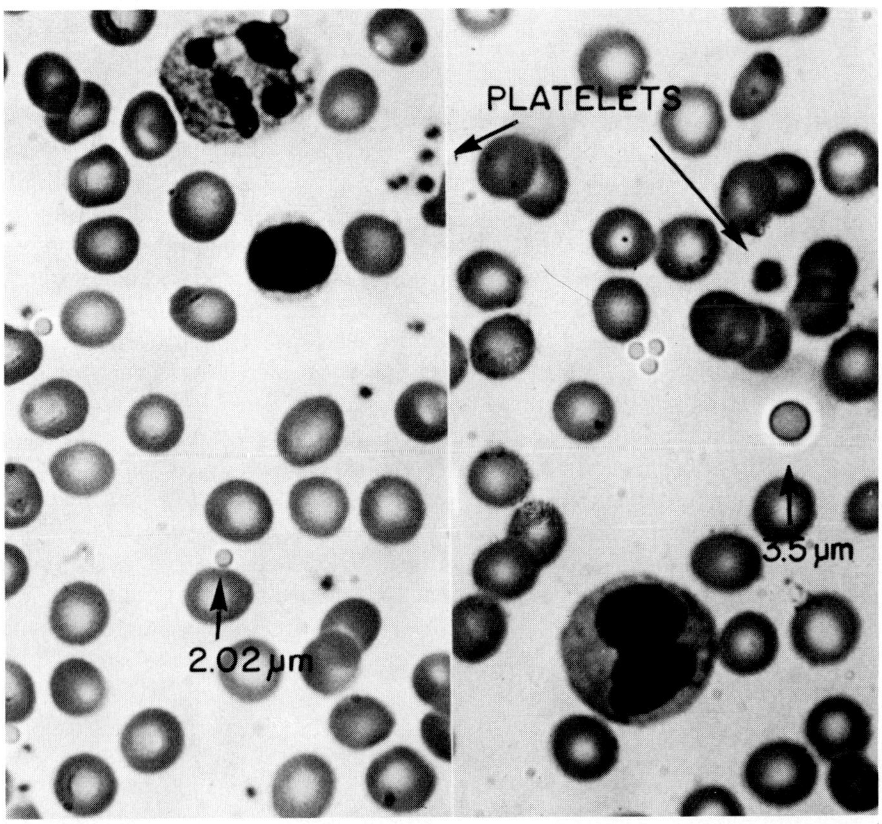

FIGURE 1. Wright-stained EDTA-anticoagulated peripheral blood smears. A mixture of the standard-sized spheres has been applied over the stained smears. (From Rivard, G. E. and Lazerson, J., A simple method for platelet sizing, *J. Lab. Clin. Med.*, 86, 547, 1975. With permission.)

Supported by Grant HL-13336-09 National Heart and Lung Institute and Contract DADA 17-68-C-8163 U.S. Army Research and Development Command.

spherical. Since EDTA-treated platelets do not spread or aggregate on glass slides as native platelets would, reasonable measurements can be obtained. The time of slide preparation is critical. It has been recommended that platelet smears be made in the 10- to 60-min interval following collection into EDTA anticoagulant, since this is an interval of time during which platelet diameters remain constant following smearing of platelets on glass.[11] The area of the slide employed for measurements is also critical, since the periphery of the slide tends to accumulate large platelets, presumably via the centrifugal effect of making the smear. It is therefore important to measure cell size in the area of the slide generally used to observe cell morphology, i.e., where red blood cells barely overlap and the red blood cell central "pallor" is observable. The smear method for evaluation of platelet size has three advantages: (1) it is simple, rapid, and economical, (2) one observes the cell that is being measured and artifacts are not spuriously enumerated, and (3) the entire platelet population can be observed, since whole blood, rather than platelet-rich plasma, is employed. The disadvantages are (1) it is conceivable that in some pathological conditions, platelets that have a "normal" size (volume) in vivo may have an abnormal size following smearing and (2) the measurement is subjective; an observer must select the area of the slide that is to be measured and determine whether the diameter of the cell is greater than an arbitrarily defined value (i.e., >2.5 μ^3).[1]

The indirect methods entail electronic particle size enumeration or packed cell volume/platelet count determination. Electronic particle size counting has been performed with various equipment.[1,8,13-15,17-20] Our experience is with a transistorized Coulter Counter®, Model B, with a 70-micron aperture tube, attached to a P64-channel Analyzer with an electronic recording device. The technique is based on the principle that particles passing through an electric current create a resistance that is proportional to the particle volume. Thus platelets with an approximate volume of 5 μ^3 are drawn through a 70-μ aperture tube via suction and impede a current that is applied between a platinum electrode and the aperture tube. The equipment is designed to interpret the different resistance signals in terms of the various platelet volumes. The equipment contains window thresholds, which register platelets with different volumes. These windows can be calibrated with latex particles, or other known inert or biologic (red blood cells) materials. With our equipment, one window is calibrated to equal 0.25 μ^3. Thus windows 1 to 100 measure a range of 0.25 to 25 μ^3, excluding large cells such as red or white blood cells. The distribution of the platelet volume is recorded electronically on graph paper. The distribution curve that is obtained is skewed to the right on an arithmetic axis plot (Figure 2), and has been shown to be log normal.[8]

The advantage of this technique is that it is objective and avoids the in vitro artifact(s) of the smear method. Platelets tend to swell on standing in EDTA at room temperature or in the cold and should be measured within 2 hr of collection in EDTA. Coulter Counter® measurements of EDTA blood are slightly larger than identical blood collected in citrate.[13-16] The disadvantages of this technique are several:

1. The procedure is blind, so all particles of a certain size, regardless of origin, are enumerated. Thus fragmented red blood cells or broken white blood cells would be included.
2. The entire platelet population is not being measured, since platelet-rich plasma is employed. The preparation of platelet-rich plasma eliminates 15 to 25% of the total platelet population, as well as a population enriched with large platelets (see below,[15-20]).
3. Coincidence counting can take place; i.e., if the platelet concentration is too high, more than one platelet can be pulled across the "resistance-measuring" device. If this occurs, the volume of two or more platelets will be recorded as one.
4. The path in which the platelets are drawn through the current is critical. If they

bounce off the sides of the aperture tube, this can lead to measurement artifacts in the electronic pulse heights.

5. Coincidence counting of large platelet volume tends to spuriously shift the curve towards the right (larger platelets) more than coincidence counting of smaller platelet volume.
6. The lower threshold of the machine which measures small particle size is not very accurate on most available equipment. Machine noise, with consequent spurious counts, can be introduced in this area.
7. Although the proponents of electronic particle counting claim that the electrical resistance is proportional to the particle volume, others have claimed that changes of cell shape (in the absence of changes in volume) can be spuriously recorded as volume changes on the Coulter Counter®.[16] However, the contribution of shape change to volume change appears to be minor at best.

Another indirect method entails the centrifugation of platelet-rich plasma in a capillary tube to determine the total platelet volume. If this is divided by the total platelet count in this volume, an indirect measurement of mean platelet volume can be obtained.[16,21] However, this has to be corrected for extracellular space entrapped within the packed platelet volume. The advantage of this technique is its relative simplicity. The disadvantages are (1) it is performed blind, so red blood cells, white blood cells, or other particles are measured in the packed cell volume, (2) the extracellular space

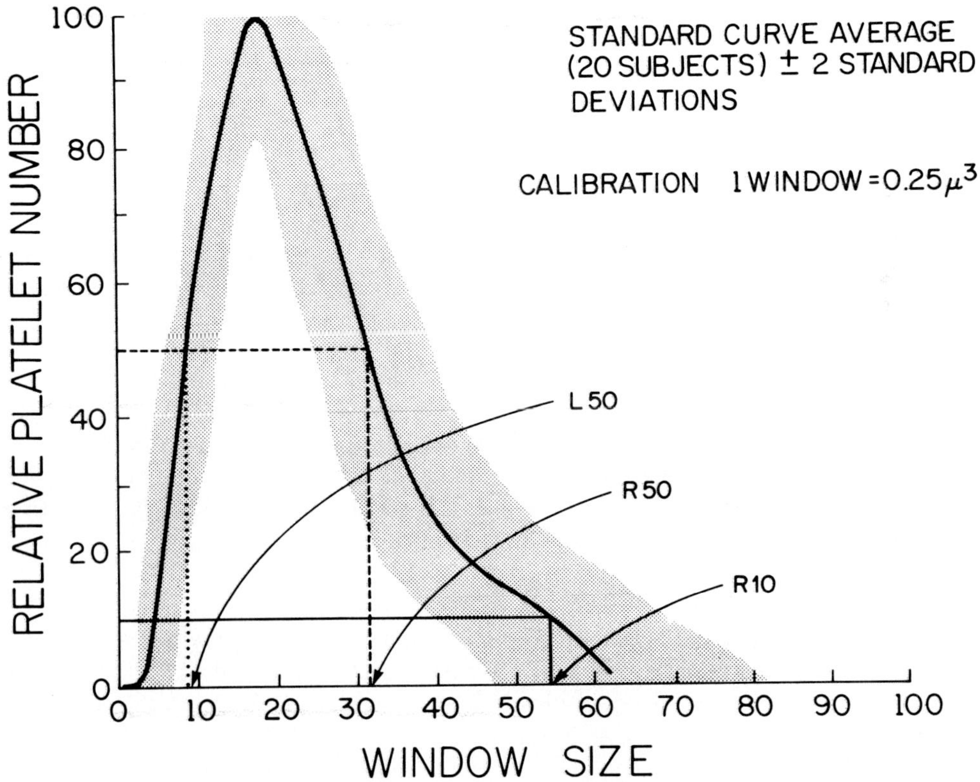

FIGURE 2. Mean platelet volume distribution curve and platelet volume parameters obtained from EDTA-anticoagulated platelet-rich plasma of 20 normal subjects. Shaded area represents ± 2 SD's. (From Karpatkin, S., *Blood*, 51, 307, 1978. With permission of Grune & Stratton.)

must be carefully measured and subtracted from the packed cell volume. This requires either spectrophotometric or isotopic monitoring equipment, (3) packing of centrifuged cells may conceivably alter their volume, and (4) the total platelet population is not isolated with the preparation of platelet-rich plasma. The platelets retained in the buffy coat and red blood cells could represent 15 to 25% of the total platelet population that is enriched with large platelets.

Parameters Employed with Electronic Particle Size Counters

Figure 2 depicts an "arithmetic" platelet volume distribution curve. This represents the mean curve obtained from platelet-rich plasma, anticoagulated with EDTA, of 20 normal subjects ± 2 SD. One window is calibrated to equal 0.25 μ^3. The mode is obtained from the coordinate on the horizontal axis where a line drawn from the peak of the platelet volume distribution curve transects the horizontal axis as a perpendicular and is found to be 17.5 ± 5.6 or 4.4 ± 1.4 μ^3 (2 SD). The R50 coordinate of the horizontal axis is obtained from the 50th percentile of the vertical axis where it transects the descending limb (right side) of the platelet volume distribution curve and is found to be 31.2 ± 3.2 or 7.8 ± 0.9 μ^3. The L50 coordinate of the horizontal axis is similarly obtained from the ascending limb (left side) of the platelet volume distribution curve and is found to be 8.38 ± 3.2 or 2.10 ± 0.65 μ^3. The mean platelet volume is estimated by averaging the R50 and L50 coordinates and is found to be 19.8 ± 2.6 or 5.0 ± 0.65 μ^3. A megathrombocyte (large platelet) index of "R10" is arbitrarily defined on the coordinate of the horizontal axis where the 10th percentile on the vertical axis transects the descending limb (right side) of the platelet volume distribution curve. The above five platelet volume parameters therefore measure gradations of platelet size, with the R10 representing the largest platelet size parameter for a given platelet-rich plasma, the R50 representing an intermediate platelet size parameter, the mean and mode representing relatively smaller platelet size parameters, and the L50 representing the smallest platelet size parameter.

Percent megathrombocytes has also been employed with Coulter Counter® measurements. This is obtained by dividing the number of platelets having a volume greater than 13.5 μ^3 by the total number of platelets counted and multiplying by 100. The percent megathrombocytes of 100 normal subjects is 4.7 ± 5.7 μ^3 (2 SD). Percent megathrombocytes can also be obtained by the peripheral smear method. It is obtained by dividing the number of platelets having a diameter greater than 2.5 μ^3 by the total number of platelets counted and multiplying by 100. The percent obtained from 67 normal subjects is 10.8 ± 6.2. Both methods correlate reasonably well with each other (Figure 3).

Table 1 details the various platelet parameters obtained by different investigators, employing all of the above techniques, in humans and animals. These include measurements of platelet diameter, surface area, mean platelet volume, L50, R50, R10 (megathrombocyte index), and percent megathrombocytes.

Relationship between Platelet Volume and Platelet Number

The mean platelet volume or megathrombocyte index has been shown to be inversely proportional to platelet count (Figure 4), within the normal range of 150 to 350,000 platelets/mm^3.[8,15,19,22] Thus normal individuals with lower platelet counts tend to have an increased percent of larger platelets, whereas patients with higher platelet counts tend to have a decreased percent of larger platelets. Thus the absolute number of larger platelets per individual tends to be more constant than the number of total platelets per individual.

Interestingly enough, this inverse proportionality also applies to different mammalian species (Figure 5). Thus the mouse, which has the highest mean platelet count of the four species studied, has the smallest platelets of the four species studied.

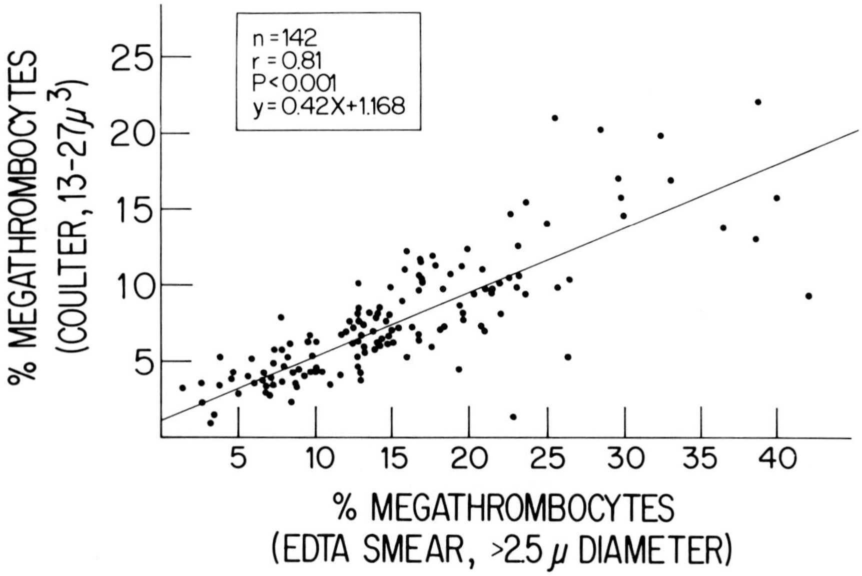

FIGURE 3. Correlation between the percentage of megathrombocytes measured by EDTA-anticoagulated smear (>2.5 μ in diameter) and the percentage of megathrombocytes measured by the Coulter Counter© (13 to 27 μ^3) in patients with various clinical disorders and normal platelet counts. The straight line was determined by the method of least squares and is given by the formula y = 0.42 × + 1.168. The correlation coefficient, r, was equal to 0.81, with a P value less than 0.001. (From Karpatkin, S., Garg, S. K., and Siskind, G. W., *Am. J. Med.*, 51, 1, 1971. With permission.)

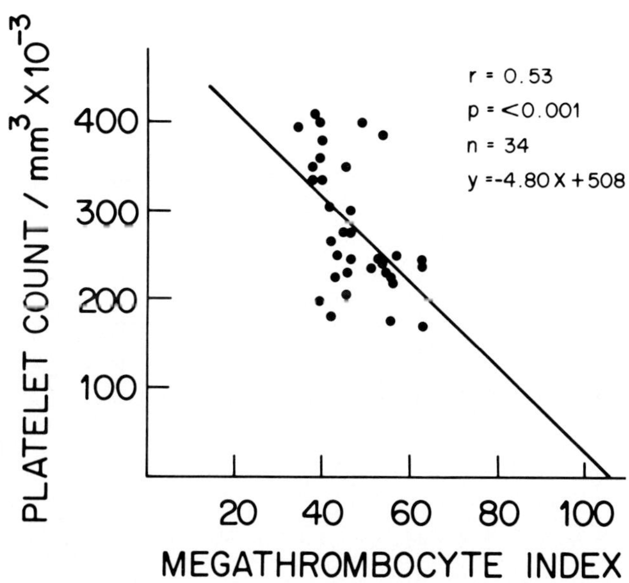

FIGURE 4. Correlation between whole blood platelet count and megathrombocyte index. The regression line was determined by the method of least squares and is given by the formula y = 4.8 × + 508. The correlation coefficient, r = −0.53 has a P value less than 0.001. (From Karpatkin, S., *Blood,* 51, 307, 1978. With permission of Grune & Stratton.)

Table 1
VARIOUS PLATELET PARAMETERS[a] OBTAINED BY DIFFERENT INVESTIGATORS IN MAN AND ANIMALS

Anticoagulant	Species	MPV	Mode	Diameter	Surface area	L50	R50	R10	MPV via PCV	Megas(%)	Ref.
EDTA	Man	5.0	4.4	—	—	2.1	7.8	13.8	7.5	4.7	1,15
Citrate	Man	4.0	3.3	—	—	1.9	6.0	11.8	—	—	15
Citrate	Man	7.1	—	—	—	—	—	—	—	—	13
EDTA	Man	9.1	—	—	—	—	—	—	—	—	13
EDTA	Man	7.7	—	—	—	—	—	—	—	—	17
EDTA	Man	6.6	3.7	—	—	—	—	—	—	—	8
EDTA	Man	10.8	8.2	—	—	—	—	—	—	—	19
Citrate	Man	5.2	—	—	—	—	—	—	—	—	20
Citrate	Man	8.0	4.9	—	—	—	—	—	—	—	14
Citrate	Man	7.1	—	3.6	22.2	—	—	—	—	—	10
EDTA	Dog	7.2	—	—	—	—	—	—	—	—	17
Citrate	Dog	9.2	—	2.6	5.3	—	—	—	—	—	12
Citrate	Rabbit	—	—	—	—	—	—	6.6	—	—	16
Citrate	Rabbit	3.1	—	3.1	15.8	—	—	—	—	—	10
EDTA	Rat	5.4	—	—	—	—	—	—	—	—	17
EDTA	Mouse	4.0	—	—	—	—	—	—	—	—	17

[a] These values were generally derived from electronic particle volume counters at room temperature, except for Reference 14 at 37°; and equipment calibrated with inert spheres, except for Reference 19, calibrated with red blood cells. Reference 10 refers to values derived from diameter and thickness measurements. MPV via PCV refers to values obtained indirectly via packed cell volume and platelet count measurements. Diameter and surface area measurements were obtained from stained, fixed smears.

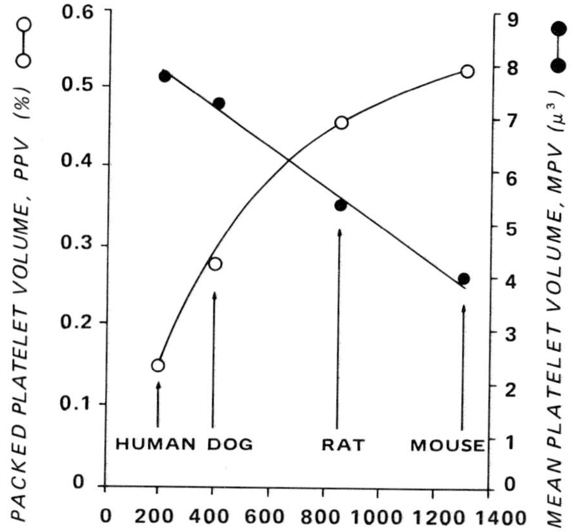

FIGURE 5. Relationship between platelet count, mean platelet volume (MPV), and packed platelet volume (PPV) for four species studied. (From Nakeff, A. and Ingram, M., *J. Appl. Phys.*, 28, 530, 1970. With permission.)

Relationship between Platelet Volume and Platelet Density

A platelet population is heterogeneous for density in humans,[18,20,21] dogs,[23] rabbits,[6,24] and rats.[25] Platelets have been separated into heavy and light fractions by employing various density gradients as well as centrifugal forces: inert lipid oils,[21] albumin,[6] silicone oil,[23] polyvinylpyrollidone,[25] arabino-galactan polymers,[20] and platelet-poor plasma.[18,24] These studies have demonstrated that heavy platelets are enriched with large platelets and light platelets are enriched with small platelets (Figure 6).

Relationship between Platelet Volume and Platelet Function

Heavy human platelets, enriched with large platelets, have been shown to function better than lighter platelets.[26] Following platelet aggregation of human platelets with aggregating agents, large platelets appear to be entrapped within the platelet aggregate, whereas smaller platelets tend to remain unaggregated in the "residual" platelet-rich plasma (i.e., after removal of the aggregates).[15,27] When canine platelets are passed through a column of glass beads, the larger platelets are preferentially retained[12] (i.e., aggregated). Recent studies have revealed a direct linear proportional relationship between megathrombocyte index and platelet aggregation velocity (employing platelet aggregometry) with the aggregating agents ADP, collagen, or epinephrine (Figure 7). Thus platelet-rich plasma containing a greater number of megathrombocytes aggregates more rapidly than platelet-rich plasma containing fewer megathrombocytes. Excellent correlation coefficients were obtained when the megathrombocyte index parameter was employed. Poorer correlations were obtained when smaller platelet volume parameters were employed (Table 2).

Relationship between Platelet Volume and Splenic Sequestration

Large platelets, like reticulocytes (large red blood cells), have been shown to be preferentially sequestered by the spleen.[28,29] The spleen normally contains 35 to 40% of

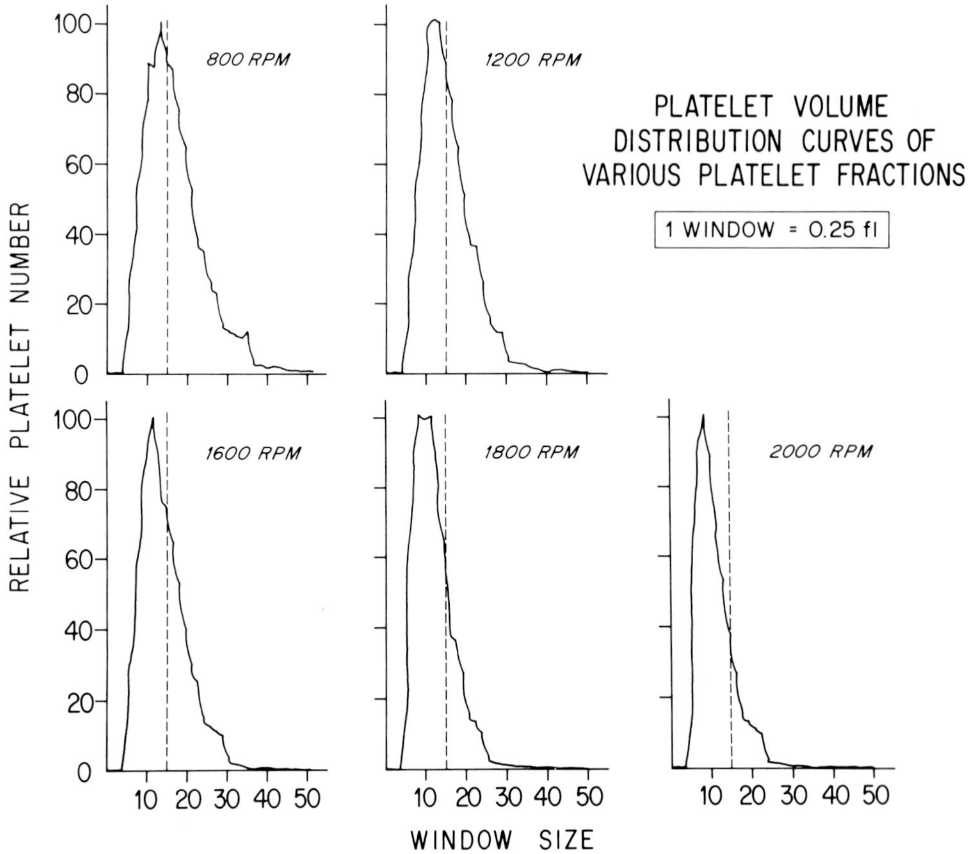

FIGURE 6. Platelet volume distribution curves from subpopulations obtained following centrifugation of rabbit platelet-rich plasma (PRP) successively at 800 RPM (196 g), 1200 RPM (420 g), 1600 RPM (728 g), 1800 RPM (924 g) and 2000 RPM (1120 g), respectively, for 20 min at 4°C. The respective platelet sediments were resuspended in 1 mℓ of human Ringer-2mm EDTA, pH 7.1. An aliquot of this suspension was utilized for platelet volume distribution analysis on a Coulter Counter© Model B attached to a P-64 Channel Analyzer with electronic recorder. The data is representative of 66 different rabbits. (From Karpatkin, S., *Br. J. Haematol.*, 39, 459, 1978. With permission.)

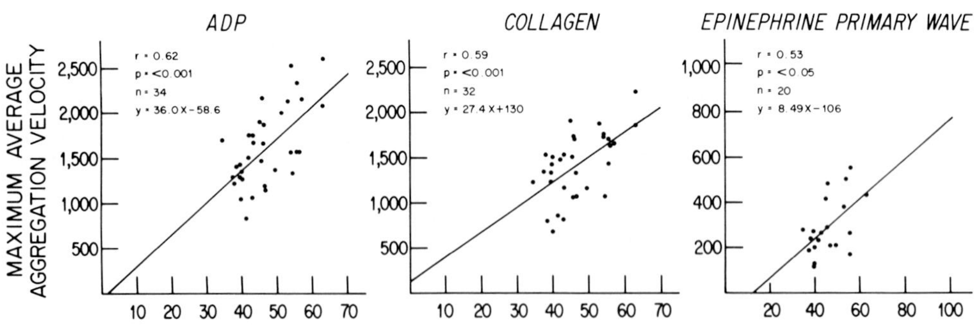

FIGURE 7. Correlation between maximum average aggregation velocity and megathrombocyte index. (A) ADP-induced aggregation (maximum average of 2.6×10^{-5}M and 2.6×10^{-6}M). Formula for regression line, y = 34.74x. The correlation coefficient, r = 0.62 has a P value less than 0.001. (B) Collagen-induced aggregation (maximum average of 1:18,000 and 1:36,000 dilution). Formula for regression line, y = 30.24x. The correlation coefficient r = 0.59 has a P value less than 0.001. (C) Epinephrine-induced primary wave aggregation (maximum average of 5×10^{-5}M and 5×10^{-6}M. Formula for regression line, y = 6.26x. The correlation coefficient r = 0.53 has a P value less than 0.02. (From Karpatkin, S., ***Blood,*** 51, 307, 1978. With permission of Grune & Stratton.)

Table 2
CORRELATION COEFFICIENTS OF PLATELET COUNT, VOLUME, AND AGGREGATION VELOCITY[a]

	Platelet count (34)	ADP (34)	Collagen (32)	Epinephrine (20)
Megathrombocyte index (R10)	r = −0.53	r = 0.62	r = 0.59	r = 0.53
	P < 0.001	P < 0.001	P < 0.001	P < 0.02
R50	r = −0.43	r = 0.43	r = 0.34	r = 0.51
	P = 0.01	P < 0.02	P < 0.05	P < 0.02
Mean	r = −0.36	r = 0.27	r = 0.40	r = 0.38
	P < 0.05	NS[b]	P < 0.01	P < 0.1
Mode	r = −0.33	r = 0.22	r = 0.39	r = 0.46
	P < 0.05	NS[b]	P < 0.05	P < 0.05

[a] Correlation coefficients of maximum average platelet aggregation velocity and aggregating agent are given in Columns 2 through 4 (number of pairs is given in parentheses). Correlation coefficients of platelet count and volume parameters are given in Column 1 and were obtained from blood anticoagulated with sodium citrate.

[b] NS: P > 0.1.

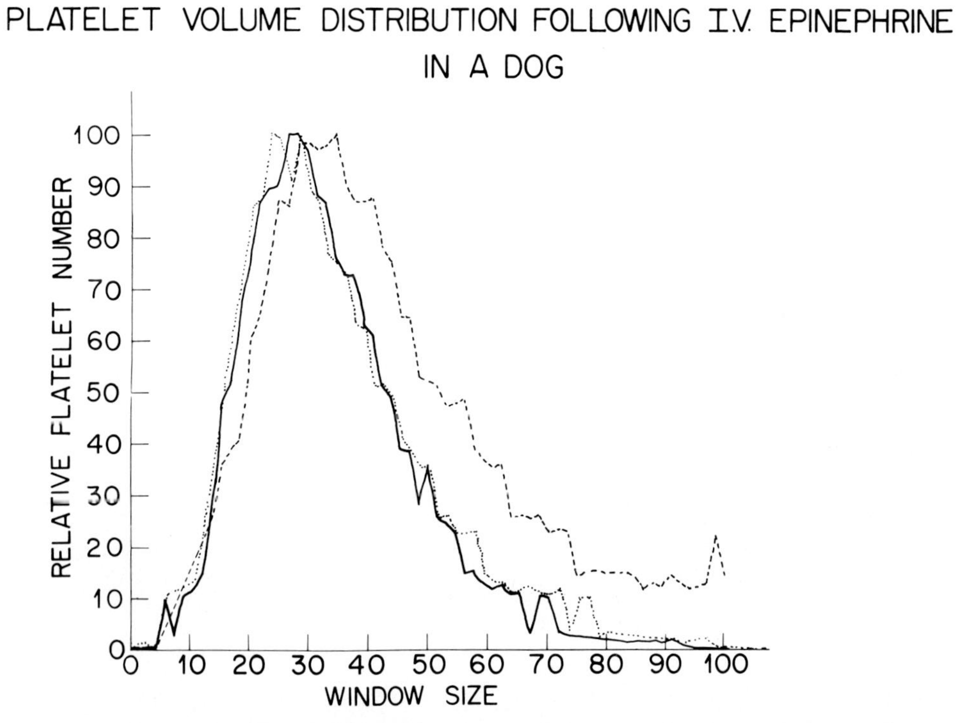

FIGURE 8. Effect of 1 μg/kgm adrenaline given intravenously on the platelet volume distribution curve of a dog. The solid line refers to preadrenaline infusion, the interrupted line to postadrenaline infusion at 1 min, and the dotted line to postadrenaline infusion at 8 min. (From Freedman, M. L. and Karpatkin, S., *Br. J. Haematol.*, 31, 255, 1975. With permission.)

the total platelet pool and preferentially sequesters 54% of the total megathrombocyte pool. This pool is rapidly mobilizable with epinephrine and/or exercise in man, rabbit, and dog (Figures 8 and 9). Thus large platelets with greater functional capacity are routinely sequestered by the spleen.

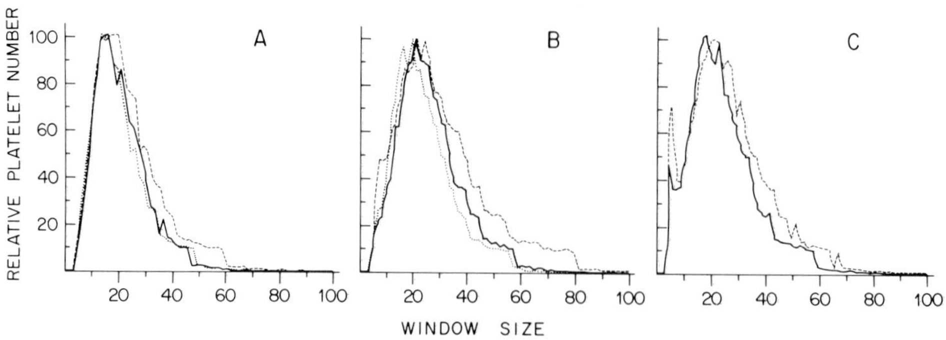

FIGURE 9. Effect of exercise on platelet volume distribution in three different subjects, A, B, and C. One window is equivalent to 0.25 μ^3. Solid line, preexercise values; broken line, values after 8 min of exercise for A, 11 min of exercise for B, and 4 min of exercise for C; dotted line, post exercise values following 11 min of rest for A and B. Exercise was bicycle pedaling on an ergometer with weight adjusted to give heart rates of greater than 150/min for 11 min. (From Freedman, M., Altszuler, N., and Karpatkin, S., *Blood*, 50, 419, 1977. With permission of Grune & Stratton.)

Table 3
EFFECT OF CENTRIFUGATION AND SUCCESSIVE WASHES IN THE PREPARATION OF PLATELET-RICH PLASMA ON PLATELET YIELD

RPM	Initial PRP (%)	First wash (%)	Second wash (%)	Third wash (%)	Total (%)
500[a] (69)	59.4	4.8	5.3	—	69.5
1000 (280)	61.2	15.0	2.4	—	78.6
1000	68.7	15.0	3.0	1.5	88.2
1000	55.4	8.1	1.0	0.4	64.9
1000	78.0	20.0	3.5	1.0	102.5
1000	34.6	30.7	9.6	3.8	78.7
1000	45.1	5.6	9.0	2.4	62.0
1250 (455)	49.3	25.3	6.8	2.0	83.4
1250	41.2	28.6	6.6	1.5	77.9
Average	54.8	15.0	5.2	1.8	78.4

[a] Whole rabbit blood was anticoagulated with EDTA and centrifuged at either 500, 1000, or 1250 RPM for 20 min at 4°C in a calibrated test tube. The volume of the PRP and the platelet count were determined. The remaining red blood cells, white blood cells, and "trapped" platelets were then resuspended in Isoton to the same volume as the original whole blood and recentrifuged at the same RPM for 20 min for the first wash. The second and third washes were similarly treated. The g force is given in parentheses.

Relationship between Platelet Volume and Recovery from Whole Blood by Differential Centrifugation Techniques

Most methods for preparation of platelet-rich plasma entail centrifugation of whole blood collected into an anticoagulant. The yield of platelets by this procedure is no better than 75 to 85%.[20,30] The lost platelets are enriched with heavy-large platelets which are entrapped in the buffy coat (Table 3; Figure 10). Thus a significant number of large platelets with greater functional capacity are routinely trapped within the buffy coat with conventional methods of preparation of platelet-rich plasma.

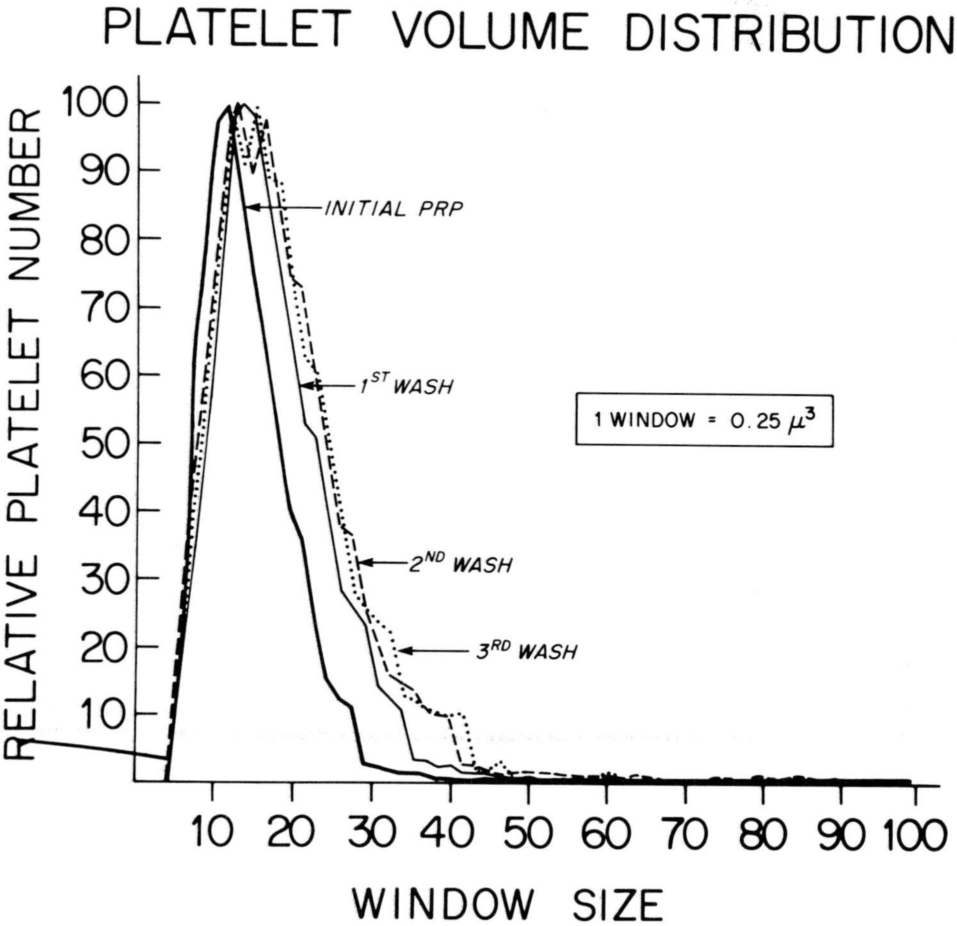

FIGURE 10. Effect of centrifugation and successive washes in the preparation of rabbit platelet-rich plasma (PRP) anticoagulated with EDTA on the platelet volume distribution curve. The platelet volume distribution curve of initial PRP (———) and that of residual platelets 'trapped' in the remaining buffy coat and red blood cell mass are compared after the first wash (———), second wash (– – –), and third wash (. . .) of the remaining blood cells (see Table 3 for further details). (From Karpatkin, S., Khan, I., and Freedman, M. L., *Am. J. Med.*, 64, 542, 1978. With permission.)

Relationship between Platelet Volume and Platelet Senescence

Early studies on the heterogeneity of human platelets led to the isolation of two extreme density populations via differential centrifugation techniques employing various suspending media.[6,21,26,31-33] The heavy population that was enriched with large platelets was more metabolically active, more resistant to osmotic stress,[21] and more resistant to lipid peroxidation.[33] These data led to the suggestion that the heavy fraction was enriched with younger-large platelets that became smaller-lighter with age. This was supported by kinetic studies performed in human volunteeers with the in vivo cohort label, Se^{75}-selenomethionine, which does not appreciably label circulating platelets but does label megakaryocytes.[31] A critical concentration of injected isotope leads to its complete removal from the circulation by platelet precursors, other protein-synthesizing tissue, and excretion. There is insignificant in vitro incorporation of isotope into peripheral platelets (young platelets). The isotope is thought to be an irreversible label (although some reutilization does appear to take place). These properties make it possible to follow a platelet from birth to death. A theoretical senescent curve should provide an ascending limb, plateau, and descending limb. The approximation

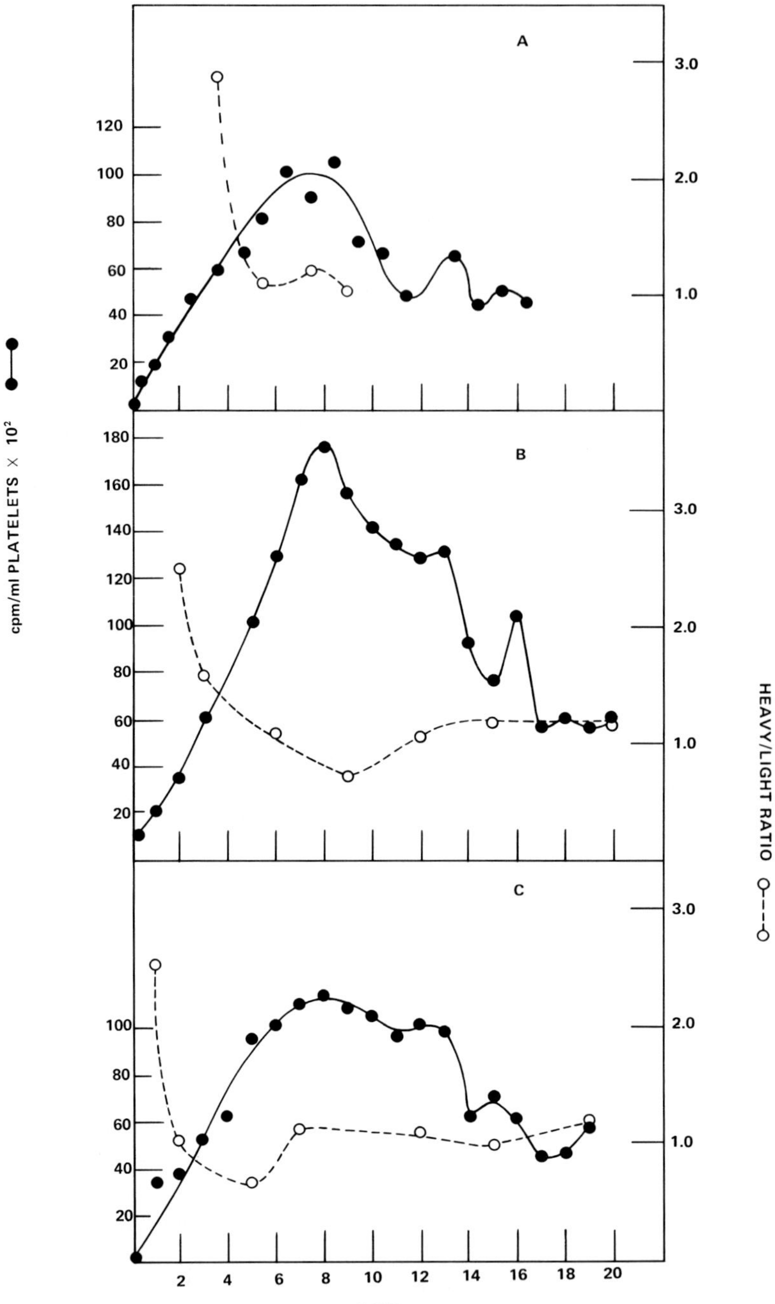

FIGURE 11. In vivo Se[75]-selenomethionine platelet survival curves on subjects A, B, and C. Data are expressed as cpm/mℓ packed platelets (●) At varying time intervals, one unit of platelet-rich plasma was removed from the subject, processed into "heavy" and "light" platelet populations, and assayed for radioactivity and packed cell volume. Data are expressed as above. The heavy/light ratio is plotted as 0. (From Amorosi, E., Garg, S. K., and Karpatkin, S., *Br. J. Haematol.*, 21, 227, 1971. With permission.)

obtained in vivo is depicted in Figure 11. The time interval between the 50% ascending limb and 50% descending limb is equivalent to the platelet survival, 10 to 12 days. Following injection of the cohort label, platelets were harvested at various time inter-

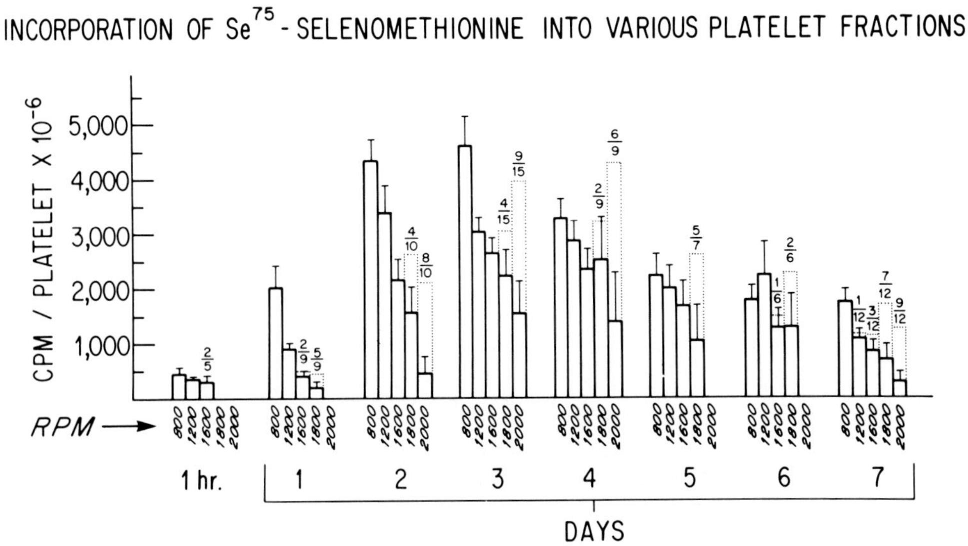

FIGURE 12. Specific activity of various rabbit platelet subpopulations obtained by differential centrifugation of rabbit PRP on days 0 through 7 following the intravenous injection of 44 microcuries of Se^{75}-selenomethionine. Specific activity is expressed as cpm/platelet × 10^{-6}. SEM is given for the mean of all experiments including zero values. Interrupted bars refer to the mean of all experiments including the zero values. The fraction over some of the bars refers to the number of zero value experiments divided by the total number of experiments. (From Karpatkin, S., *Br. J. Haematol.*, 39, 459, 1978. With permission.)

vals during the platelet survival (red blood cells, white blood cells, and residual plasma returned to the subject) and separated into heavy-large and light-small populations via centrifugation in inert density oils. An increase in the heavy/light specific activity ratio on early days of the survival, followed by a decrease in this ratio on late days, is consistent with the concept that heavy-large platelets are young platelets that progress with age to lighter-smaller platelets. Similar observations were obtained in rabbits[6] by using a discontinuous albumin gradient to separate extreme heavy and light platelet populations.

The relationship between platelet density, volume, and cohort labeling has recently been further examined by isolating five different platelet density populations[24] rather than two, as described previously. This was made possible by the recent demonstration that platelet populations could be further resolved by repetitive centrifugation of platelet-rich plasma at increasing centrifugal forces, with harvesting of the successive platelet sediments obtained.[18]

Figure 4 demonstrates a typical platelet volume distribution of the platelet sediments obtained at 800, 1200, 1600, 1800, and 2000 RPM. Approximately 65% of the platelets were in fractions obtained at 800, 1200, and 1600 RPM and approximately 35% of the platelets in fractions 1800 and 2000 RPM.

Figure 12 depicts the specific activity and SEM (cpm/platelet × 10^{-6}) for each of the different platelet sediments obtained at 1 hr and days 1 through 7 after injection of Se^{75}-selenomethionine.[24] The ratios of the specific activity of the 800 RPM platelet sediment (heavy-large platelets) to the specific activities of the platelets sedimented at higher g forces (lighter-smaller platelets) are given in Table 4. As can be noted, the heavy/light ratio increases when increasing RPM (lighter platelets) is employed as denominator (note horizontal lines of Table 4). Furthermore, the heavy/light ratio decreases on each day (except 7, where reutilization of isotope is suspected to have occurred). The individual components of this ratio are depicted in Figure 12. Thus, as

Table 4
SPECIFIC ACTIVITY RATIOS OF 800 RPM PLATELET SEDIMENT FRACTIONS TO OTHER RPM PLATELET SEDIMENT FRACTIONS ON DAYS 1 THROUGH 7 FOLLOWING SE^{75}-SELENOMETHIONINE INJECTION[a]

	Ratio of 800 RPM platelet fraction to:				
Day	1200	1600	1800	2000	N
1	2.24	4.96	9.63	—	(9)
2	1.28	1.99	2.74	10.3	(10)
3	1.40	1.74	2.06	2.94	(15)
4	1.13	1.41	1.30	2.30	(9)
5	1.10	1.31	2.06	—	(7)
6	0.79	1.38	1.37	—	(6)
7	1.61	2.03	2.45	5.51	(12)

[a] Forty-four microcuries of Se^{75}-selenomethionine was injected into eight rabbits for each experiment (1 hr sample not shown). Each rabbit served as an experimental point in the kinetic analysis. Forty mℓ of whole blood was removed from one rabbit and the PRP harvested at 600 RPM for 20 min at 4°. Platelet sediments were then obtained at increasing RPM from the original PRP, and processed for platelet count and radioactivity. The specific activity obtained from the 800 RPM sediments (cpm/platelet × 10^{-6}) was divided by the specific activities obtained at 1200, 1600, 1800, and 2000 RPM, respectively, to obtain the ratios. N refers to number of rabbits employed for each time point.

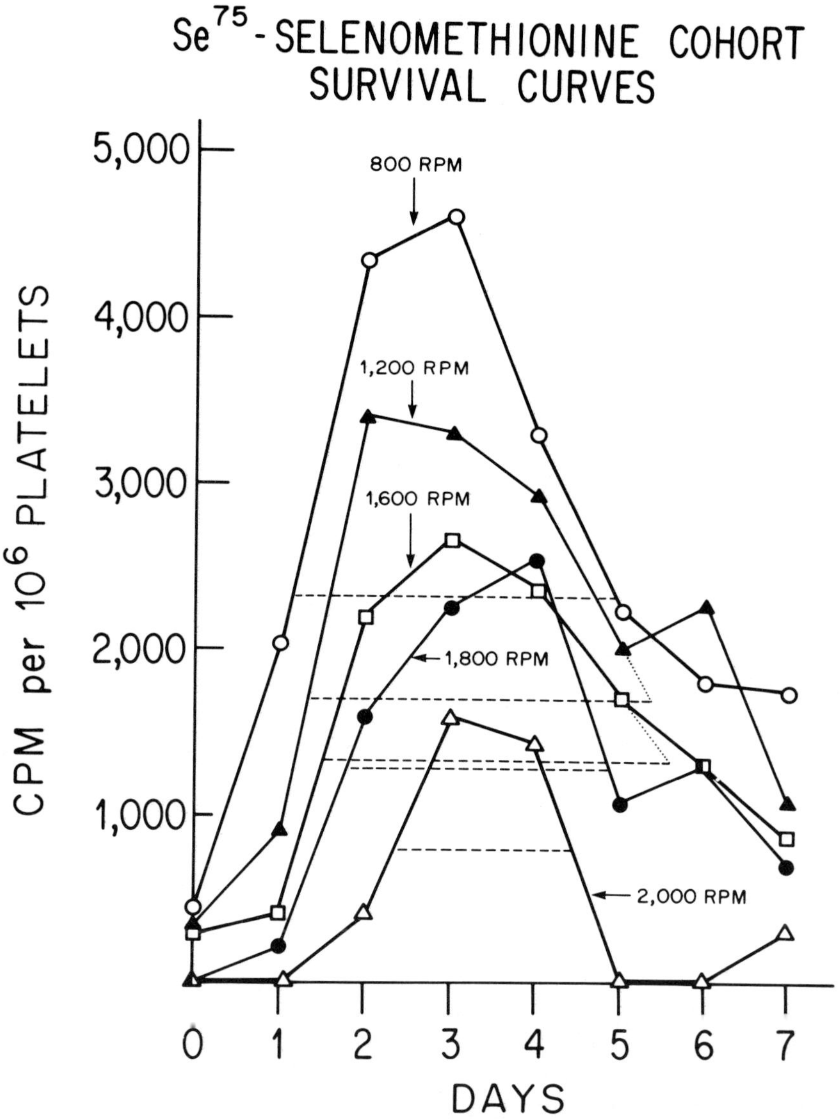

FIGURE 13. Cohort Se^{75}-selenomethionine platelet survival curves obtained from the various platelet subpopulations is isolated as in Figures 6 and 12 following injection of 44 microcuries of isotope. Platelet survival was determined from the time interval between the 50% ascending limb and 50% descending limb of the cohort curve (interrupted horizontal line). Platelet survival curves for the 800, 1200, 1600, 1800, and 2000 RPM fractions were 3.8, 4.0, 4.1, 3.1, and 2.1 days, respectively. (From Karpatkin, S., *Br. J. Haematol.*, 39, 459, 1978. With permission.)

the specific activity of heavier (800 RPM) platelets declined on days 3 to 4, the specific activity of lighter platelets (1600, 1800, and 2000 RPM) remained the same, suggesting a transition of heavy to light platelets.

Figure 13 depicts the entire cohort curve obtained for each RPM platelet sediment. Of particular interest is the lag period noted before radioactivity appears in the platelets that sediment at and above 1200 RPM. This is associated with a progressive decrease in the slope of the ascending limb of the cohort survival curve obtained from 1200 to 2000 RPM samples. Of further interest is the shorter platelet survival of the 1800 and 2000 RPM samples (3.1 and 2.1 days, respectively) compared to the 800, 1200, and 1600 RPM samples (3.8, 4.0, and 4.1 days, respectively), $P < 0.001$.

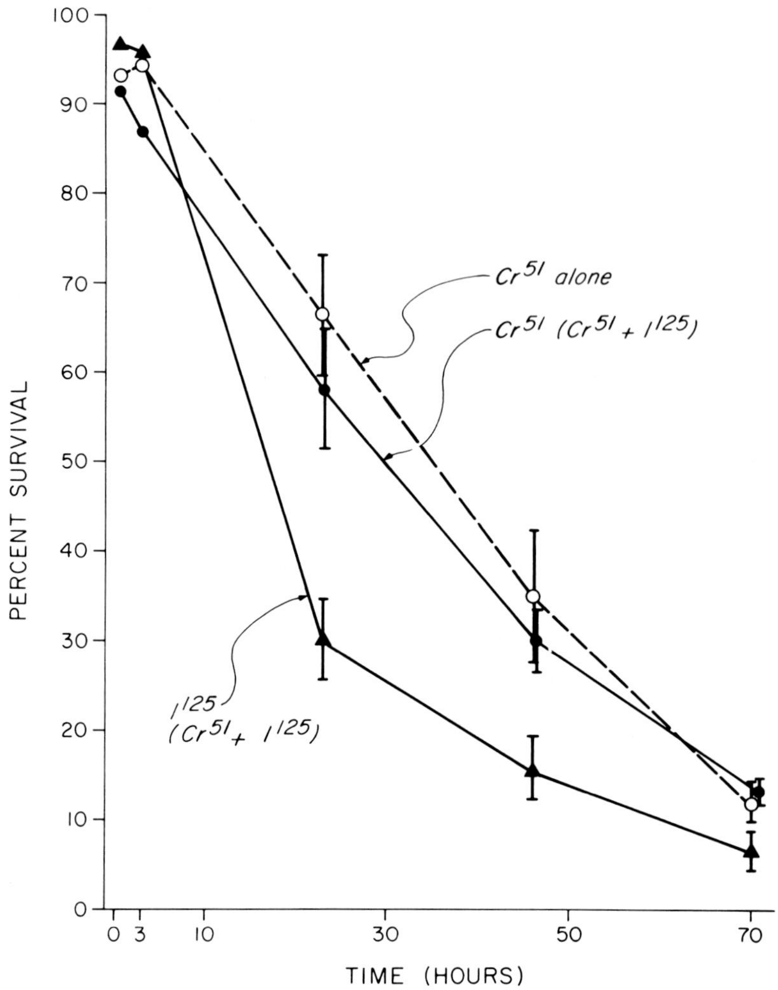

FIGURE 14. In vivo survival of singly and doubly labeled platelets. Data from 11 rabbits are shown, four studied with platelets labeled by Cr^{51} alone and seven studied with platelets labeled simultaneously by Cr^{51} and $DD^{125}ISA$. The point of maximal in vivo recovery of each isotope, which occurred at 30 min or 3 hr after injection, was assigned a value of 100%. Mean values ± SE are plotted. There was no difference among any of the values at 30 min and 3 hr and no difference between the rate of subsequent disappearance of Cr^{51} of singly labeled platelets (open circles) and doubly labeled platelets (solid circles) ($P > 0.2$). The differences between the Cr^{51} (solid circle) and $DD^{125}ISA$ (solid triangles) disappearance from the doubly labeled platelets were significant at 23 hr ($p < 0.002$), 46 hr ($p < 0.02$), and 70 hr ($p < 0.05$). (From George, J. N., Lewis, P. C., and Sears, D. A., Studies on platelet plasma membranes. II. Characterization of surface proteins of rabbit platelets in vitro and during circulation in vivo using diazotized (^{125}I)-diiodosulfanilic acid as a label, *J. Lab. Clin. Med.*, 88, 247, 1976. With permission.)

The hypothesis that platelets get smaller with time is supported by studies performed on rabbit platelets, in which the cell interior was labeled with Cr^{51} and the cell membrane glycopeptides labeled with I^{125}.[34] These studies revealed a selective loss of iodinated platelet membrane-glycopeptide during in vivo circulation, but not following in vitro incubation (Figure 14). More recent work strengthens the hypothesis that platelets get lighter with time. Rabbit platelets were labeled with the cohort isotope S^{35} and separated by density with a stractan (arabino-galactan polymer) gradient.[35] Heavy platelets incorporated four times more isotope per mg protein than light platelets. Platelets were also labeled with Cr^{51} in vitro, injected into rabbits, and followed in vivo. Following 48 hr of in vivo circulation, heavy platelets lost 50% of their isotope, whereas light platelets "gained" 2.5-fold more Cr^{51} per mg protein. Removal of sialic acid from rabbit platelets shortens their in vivo survival. The sialic acid distribution has been examined in heavy vs. light platelets. Heavy platelets contain 25% more sialic acid per mg protein than light platelets. Thus, as platelets circulate in vivo, they may lose their sialic acid, possibly as sialo-glycopeptides.

The above kinetic considerations, however, do not indicate that heavy-large platelets are the only young platelets. The data are also consistent with the concept that all platelets, regardless of initial size, become lighter and smaller with age.

Alternatively, it is also conceivable that large-heavy platelets might be derived from specific megakaryocytes that are more metabolically active with respect to incorporation of the cohort label and thus produce platelets that appear preferentially labeled on days 1 to 2 in the peripheral circulation.[25,36] This has been proposed by a group that suggests that heavy-large platelets are released independently of lighter-smaller platelets by different bone marrow megakaryocytes and that heavy platelets do not become lighter platelets.[25] The decline in heavy/light ratio with time is explained by suggesting that heavy platelets selectively lose protein and not density with time, compared to lighter-smaller platelets. However, this group does believe that platelets become smaller with age and that megathrombocytes, on the average, are younger platelets. Needless to say, both hypotheses are not mutually exclusive. Specific megakaryocytes could give rise to specific density-size platelets, which could become lighter and smaller with time, regardless of their density-size at birth.

Clinical Significance of Platelet Size Measurements

Regardless of the above arguments, megathrombocytes can be conveniently employed to predict megakaryocyte number, and hence, platelet turnover.[1] An excellent correlation has been found between the number of megakaryocytes in the bone marrow and the percent megathrombocytes in the peripheral blood in most clinical situations with normal or low platelet counts, $r = 0.70$, $P < 0.001$ (Figure 15). In disorders of increased peripheral destruction or utilization of platelets, such as autoimmune thrombocytopenic purpura (ATP/ITP), drug-induced immunologic thrombocytopenic purpura, systemic lupus erythematosus (SLE), and disseminated intravascular coagulation (DIC), percent megathrombocytes was increased 2.6- to 3.6-fold over basal levels. This was associated with a 2.3- to 4.2-fold increase in megakaryocyte number. In aplastic anaemia, percent megathrombocytes and megakaryocyte number were decreased to 0.15- and 0.29-fold, respectively.

A compensated thrombocytolytic state could be postulated in patients with increased megathrombocytes in the peripheral blood and a normal platelet count.[1,3] This was demonstrated with in vivo DFP^{32} platelet survival studies in seven patients: one with a history of easy bruising, five with SLE, and one (A) subject screened from 105 healthy volunteers with a persistent elevation of megathrombocyte number (Figure 16). The possibility of a compensated thrombocytolytic state was further explored in several other clinical disorders with normal platelet counts, where this might be predicted:[4] (1) chronic autoimmune thrombocytopenic purpura (ATP) in "remission", (2) increased utilization of platelets, such as disseminated intravascular coagulation (DIC), and (3) increased mechanical destruction such as rheumatic heart disease (RHD) with abnormal heart valves and/or prosthetic devices, or small vessel angiopathies such as diabetes mellitus and retinitis or vasculitis. Megathrombocyte elevation was noted in 47% of patients with ATP in apparent "remission," 48% of patients with severe RHD, 20% of patients with RHD and prosthetic valves, 52% of patients with DIC, and 30% of patients with diabetes mellitus and retinopathy (Figure 17).

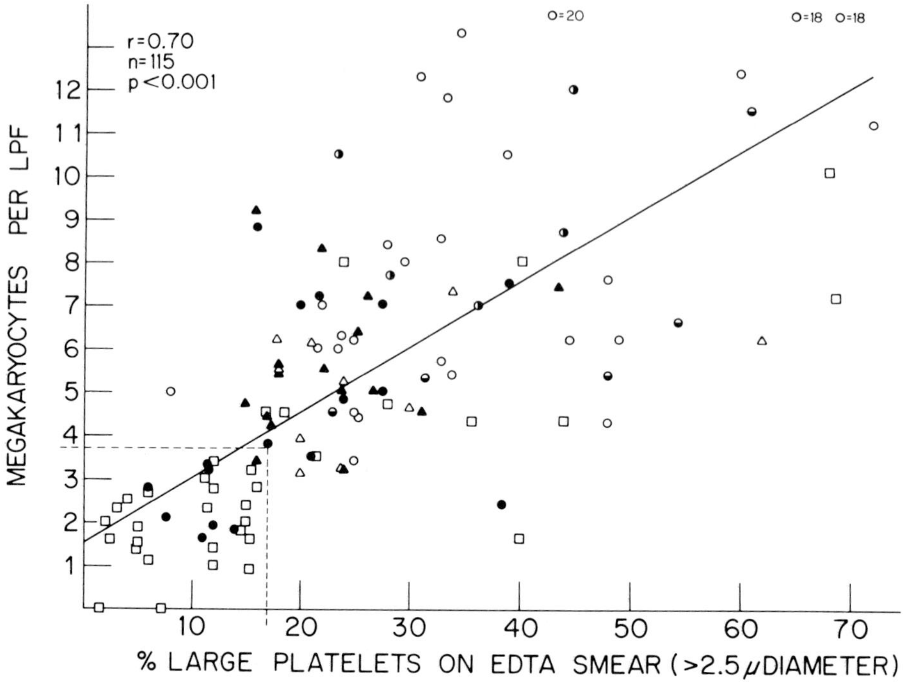

FIGURE 15. Correlation between the percentage of large platelets on EDTA peripheral smear (diameter > 2.5 μ) and the number of megakaryocytes per low power field (magnified 100 ×). The open circles refer to ATP, the closed circles to SLE, the horizontal half-closed circles to DIC, the vertical half-closed circles to drug-induced thrombocytopenia, the open triangles to hypersplenism, the closed triangles to iron-deficiency anemia (normal or low platelet count), and the open boxes to other disorders. The interrupted lines include +2 SD of the control mean. (Reprinted by permission from Garg, S. K., Amorosi, E. L., and Karpatkin, S., *The New England Journal of Medicine,* 284, 11, 1971.)

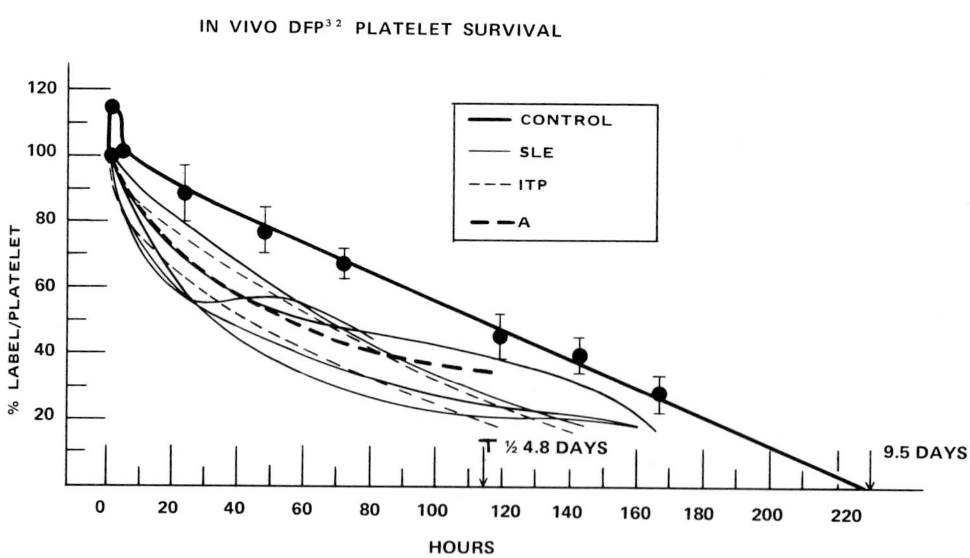

FIGURE 16. In vivo DFP³² platelet survival studies in ten control subjects compared with eight subjects having increased numbers of megathrombocytes and normal platelet counts. (From Karpatkin, S., Garg, S. K., and Siskind, G. W., *Am. J. Med.,* 51, 1, 1971. With permission.)

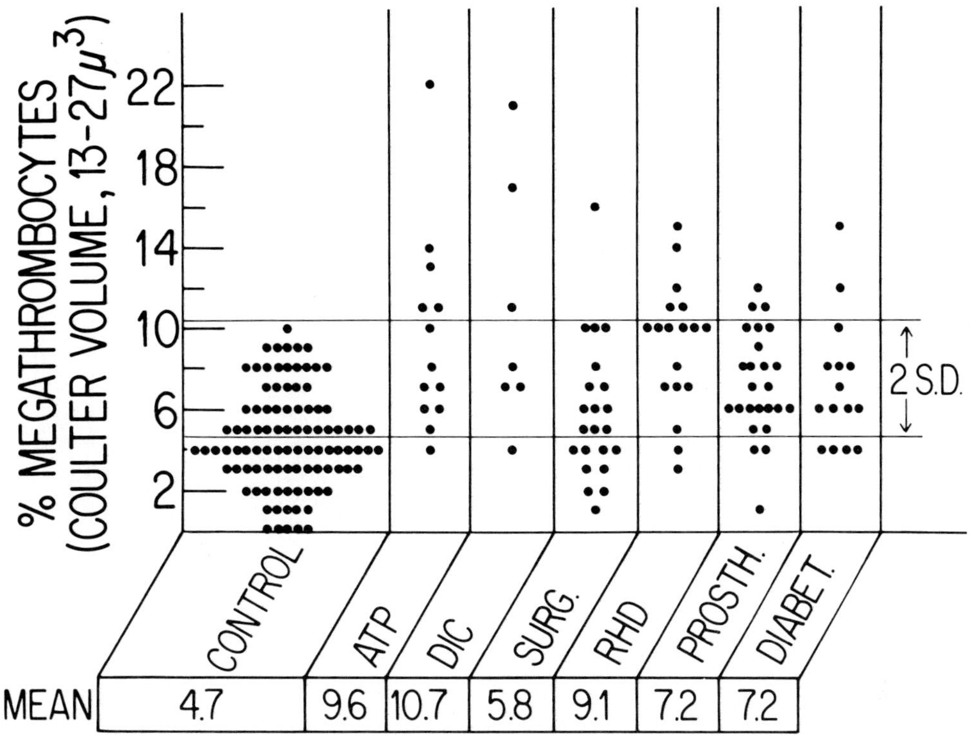

FIGURE 17. Distribution of the percent megathrombocytes as measured by Coulter Counter®, in 96 control subjects and 101 patients with normal platelet counts. These included 13 patients with autoimmune thrombocytopenic purpura (ATP), 7 patients with disseminated intravascular coagulation (DIC), 22 patients studied two hours after surgery, 19 patients with rheumatic heart disease (RHD), 25 patients with rheumatic heart disease and prostheses (PROSTH), and 15 patients with diabetes mellitus and retinopathy (DIABET). The two thin horizontal lines refer to the mean control measurement + 2 SD. (From Garg, S. K., Lackner, H., and Karpatkin, S., *Ann. Intern. Med.*, 77, 361, 1972. With permission.)

Patients with ATP in apparent remission are of particular interest in illustrating the compensated thrombocytolytic state. Twelve such patients with previous histories of thrombocytopenia were studied during an apparent spontaneous recovery phase or an apparent recovery while on steroids. Figure 18 illustrates the marked shift to the right in their platelet volume distribution curve (dashed line) compared to the normal curve, indicating increased megathrombocytes as well as other large platelets. The platelet volume distribution curves eventually shifted to normal patterns (solid line, Figure 18) for eight of these twelve patients. A negative linear relationship has recently been demonstrated for platelet count and platelet volume in normal subjects (Figure 4) as well as patients with various clinical disorders. This "normal physiologic pattern" could not explain the marked shift in platelet volume distribution for patients A, B, F, G where no significant change in platelet count was noted.

Decreased Platelet Volume in Peripheral Blood of Patients with Hypersplenism

Since the spleen preferentially sequesters large platelets, it was of interest to examine platelet volume distribution in patients with hypersplenism.[37] Platelet volume distribution was measured in 16 patients with hepatosplenomegaly and platelet counts of 45 to 90,000/mm^3, 12 patients with autoimmune thrombocytopenic purpura (ATP) randomly matched for similar platelet counts, and 20 normal subjects. Several platelet volume parameters were determined: L50, mean, mode, R50, and R10. Patients with

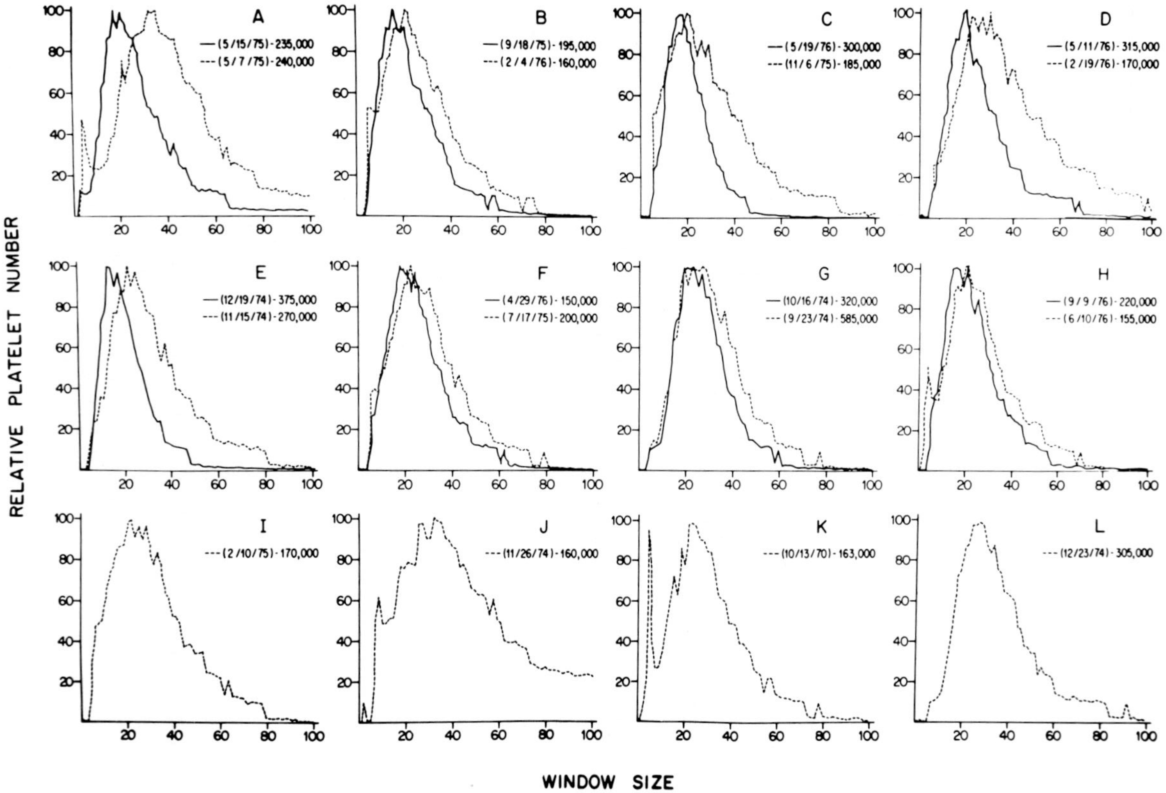

FIGURE 18. Platelet volume distribution curves from twelve patients with autoimmune thrombocytopenic purpura in remission following a spontaneous recovery phase or recovery following treatment. (——) refers to a transient shift of the platelet volume distribution curve toward the right suggesting a compensated thrombocytolytic state. (———) refers to a return of the platelet volume distribution curve toward normal.

hypersplenism have decreased volume parameters of 78 to 87% (mean 83%) of the average normal population. Patients with ATP have values significantly greater than the normal population by 124 to 149% (mean 134%). Patients with ATP, when compared to hypersplenic patients, have significantly greater values ranging from 154 to 174% (mean 161%). Thus patients with hypersplenism, a thrombocytopenic disorder of increased platelet production in the absence of increased platelet destruction, can be distinguished from patients with ATP, a thrombocytopenic disorder of increased platelet production in the presence of increased platelet destruction. A typical platelet volume distribution curve from a patient with hypersplenism has skewing to the left, a narrow distribution range, and a relatively straight border to the ascending (left) limb of the curve. A typical ATP patient has skewing to the right, a wide distribution range, and a relatively less steep slope of the ascending limb of the curve.

Detection of Red Blood Cell and Platelet Fragments with Electronic Particle Size Counting in Patients with Autoimmune Thrombocytopenic Purpura

Red blood cells as well as platelet fragments were found in the 27,000 g plasma sediment of 15 patients with severe autoimmune thrombocytopenic purpura (ATP) (Figure 19), but not in 12 normal subjects, two healthy asplenic subjects, three patients with thrombocytopenia of nonimmunologic origin, or in two patients with ATP in remission.[38] This was discovered because of the presence of a "small particle" Coulter® particle volume spike in the platelet-rich plasma of the patients affected (Figure 20). The distribution curves reveal a shift of the distribution to the left, i.e., smaller L50 value, as well as to the right, i.e., increased R10 (megathrombocytes).[39] The shift to the left with smaller particles presents either a separate peak distinguishable from the remainder of the platelet volume distribution (D, E—H) or as a shift of the entire curve to the left (B, C). The data from 82 measurements on 21 patients with ATP are shown in Figure 21, where the L50 and mode are compared to the control curve ± 2 SD. Of the 21 patients, 86% demonstrated a pronounced shift to the left (i.e., L50 less than 2 SD from the control curve), on one or more occasions. At least 50% of the 82 measurements were similarly shifted.

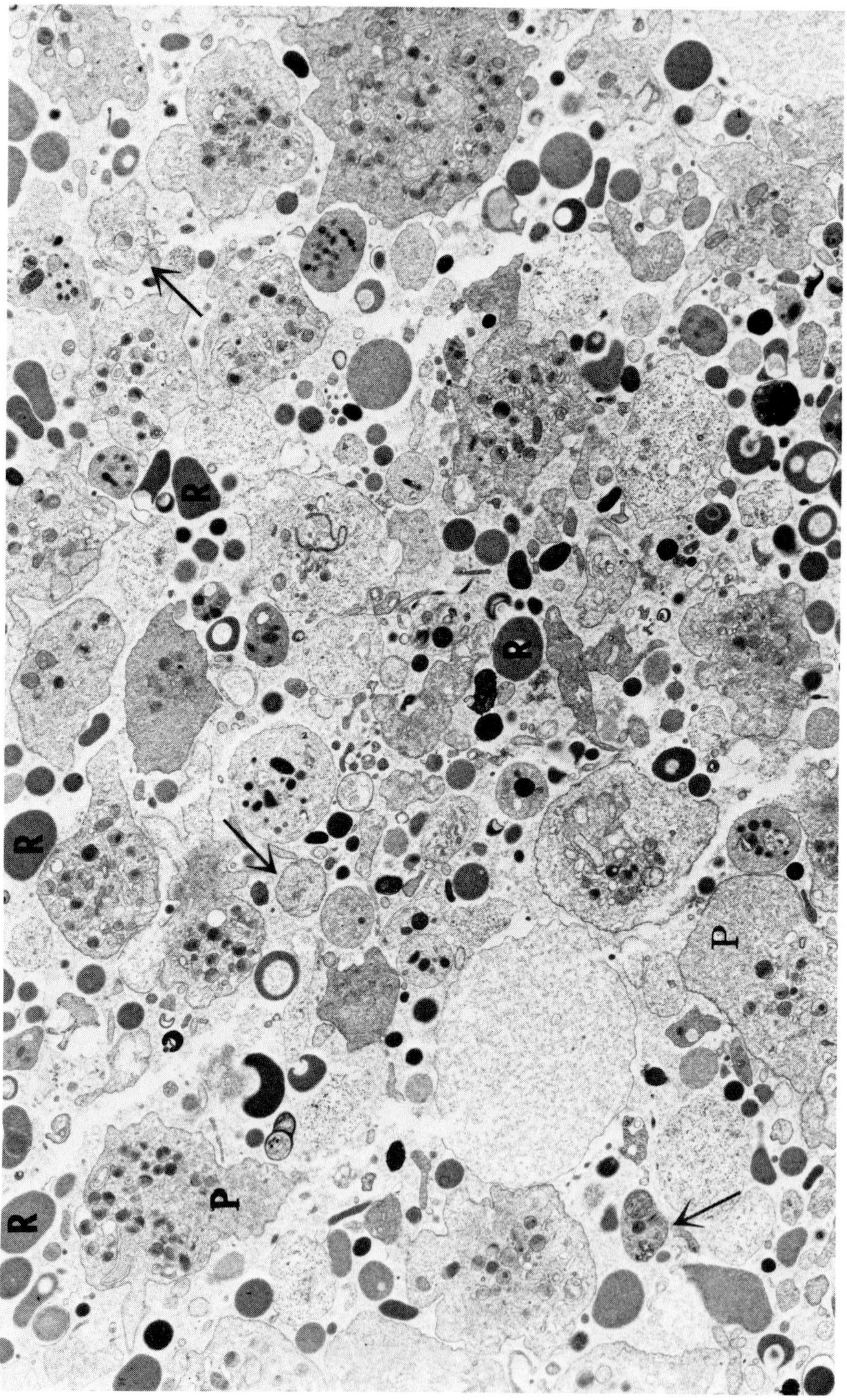

FIGURE 19. Characteristic survey electron micrograph of plasma sediment from a patient with IATP. The electron-dense erythrocyte fragments (R) are particularly striking. Several intact large platelets (P) are recognizable. Smaller cytoplasmic fragments (arrows) are probably derived from platelets. Magnification × 7,000.

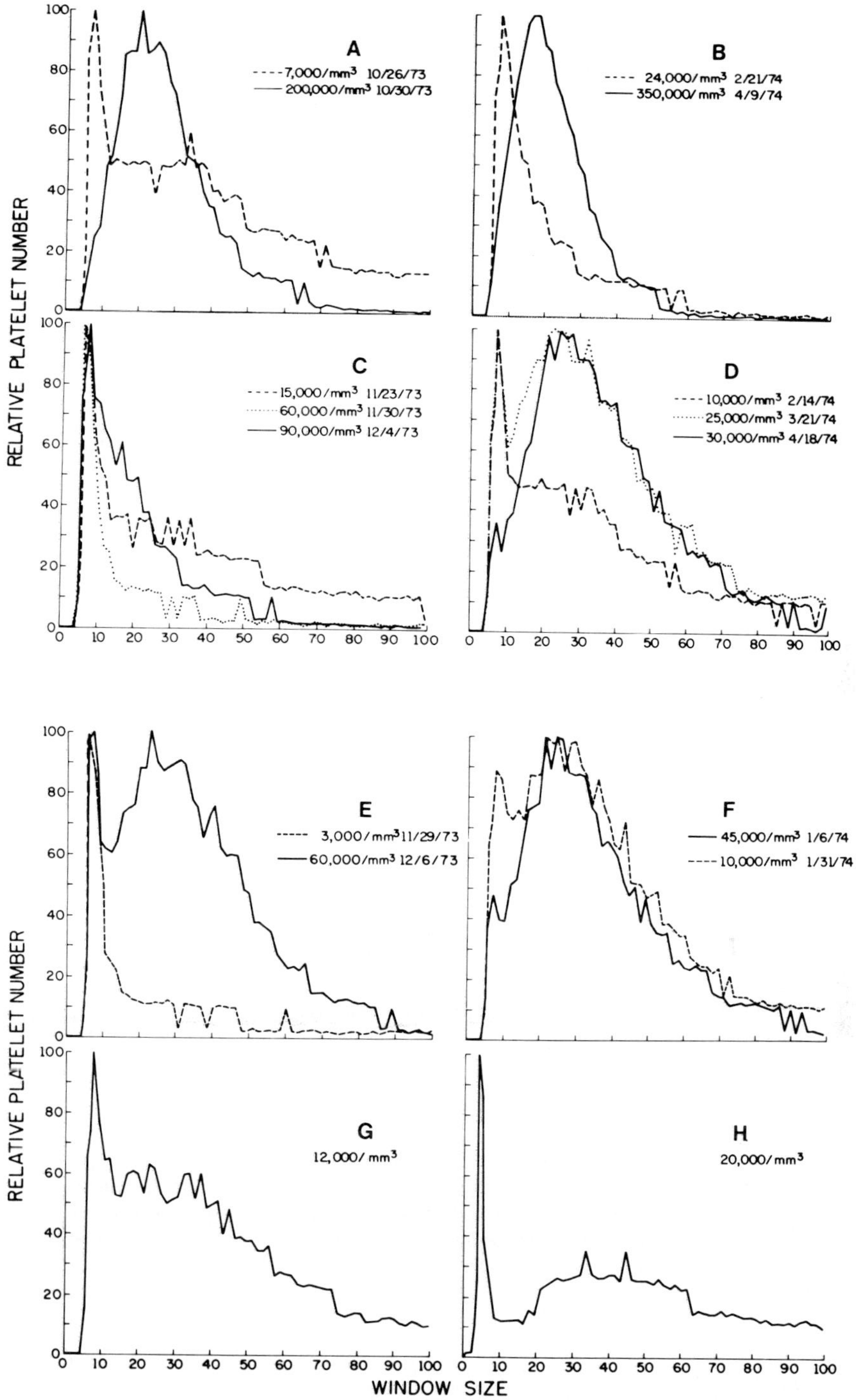

FIGURE 20. Platelet volume distribution obtained in eight patients with autoimmune thrombocytopenic purpura at different time intervals, with varying platelet counts. (From Khan, I., Zucker-Franklin, D., and Karpatkin, S., *Br. J. Haematol.*, 31, 449, 1975. With permission.)

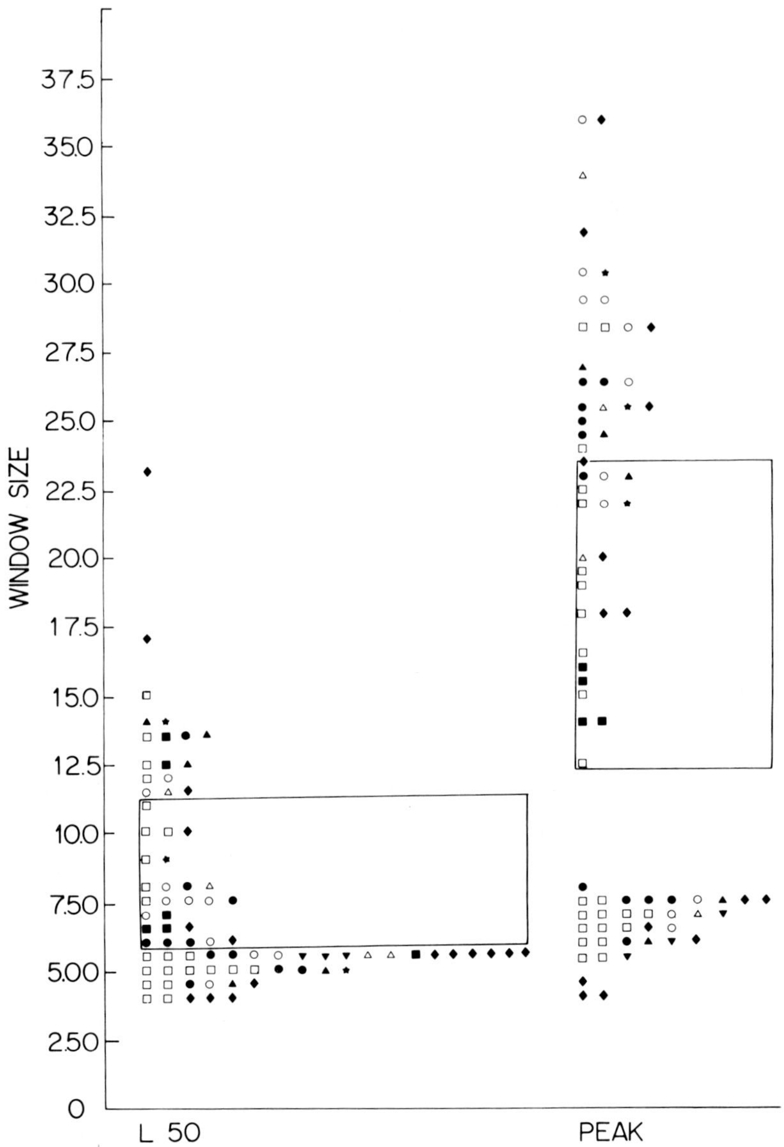

FIGURE 21. Scattergram of L50 and mode windows of 21 different patients studied on 82 different occasions. Each symbol refers to a different patient studied on one or more occasions. The area within the two boxes refers to ± 2 SD's. (From Kahn, I., Zucker-Franklin, D., and Karpatkin, S., *Br. J. Haematol.*, 31, 449, 1975. With permission.)

REFERENCES

1. **Garg, S. K., Amorosi, E. L., and Karpatkin, S.**, Use of the megathrombocyte as an index of megakaryocyte number, *N. Engl. J. Med.*, 284, 11, 1971.
2. **Sahud, M. A.**, Platelet size and number in alcoholic thrombocytopenia, *N. Engl., J. Med.*, 286, 355, 1972.
3. **Karpatkin, S., Garg, S. K., and Siskind, G. W.**, Autoimmune thrombocytopenic purpura and the compensated thrombocytolytic state, *Am. J. Med.*, 51, 1, 1971.
4. **Garg, S. K., Lackner, H., and Karpatkin, S.**, The increased percentage of megathrombocytes in various clinical disorders, *Ann. Intern. Med.*, 77, 361, 1972.
5. **Murphy, S., Oski, F. A., Naiman, L., and Gardner, F.**, Platelet size and kinetics in hereditary and acquired thrombocytopenia, *N. Engl. J. Med.*, 286, 499, 1972.
6. **Charmatz, A. and Karpatkin, S.**, Heterogeneity of rabbit platelets. I. Employment of an albumin density gradient for separation of a young platelet population identified with Se^{75}-selenomethionine, *Thromb. Diath. Haemorrh.*, 31, 485, 1974.
7. **Rivard, G. E. and Lazerson, J.**, A simple method for platelet sizing, *J. Lab. Clin. Med.*, 86, 547, 1975.
8. **Paulus, J-M.**, Platelet size in man, *Blood*, 46, 321, 1975.
9. **Lackner, H. and Karpatkin, S.**, On the easy bruising syndrome with normal platelet count. A study of 75 patients, *Ann. Int. Med.*, 83, 190, 1975.
10. **Frojmovic, M. M. and Panjwani, R.**, The geometry of normal mammalian platelets by quantitative microscopic studies, *Biophys. J.*, 16, 1071, 1976.
11. **Zeigler, Z., Murphy, S., and Gardner, F.**, Microscopic platelet size and morphology in various hematologic disorders, *Blood*, 51, 479, 1978.
12. **Kraytman, M.**, Platelet size in thrombocytopenias and thrombocytosis of various origin, *Blood*, 41, 587, 1973.
13. **Bull, B. S. and Zucker, M. B.**, Changes in platelet volume produced by temperature, metabolic inhibitors and aggregating agents, *Proc. Soc. Exp. Biol. Med.*, 120, 296, 1965.
14. **Salzman, E. W., Ashford, T. P., Chambers, D. A., Neri, L. L., and Dempster, A. P.**, Platelet volume: effect of temperature and agents affecting platelet aggregation, *Am. J. Phys.*, 217, 1330, 1969.
15. **Karpatkin, S.**, Heterogeneity of human platelets. VI. Correlation of platelet function with platelet volume, *Blood*, 51, 307, 1978.
16. **Born, G. V. R.**, Observations on the change in shape of blood platelets brought about by adenosine diphosphate, *J. Phys.*, 209, 487, 1970.
17. **Nakeff, A. and Ingram, M.**, Platelet count: volume relationships in four mammalian species, *J. Appl. Phys.*, 28, 530, 1970.
18. **Khan, I., Zucker-Franklin, D., and Karpatkin, S.**, Microthrombocytosis and platelet fragmentation associated with idiopathic/autoimmune thrombocytopenic purpura, *Br. J. Haematol.*, 31, 449, 1975.
19. **Von Behrens, W. E.**, Mediterranean macrothrombocytopenia, *Blood*, 46, 199, 1975.
20. **Corash, L., Tan, H., and Gralnick, H. R.**, Heterogeneity of human whole blood platelet subpopulations. I. Relationship between buoyant density, cell volume and ultrastructure, *Blood*, 49, 71, 1977.
21. **Karpatkin, S.**, Heterogeneity of human platelets. I. Metabolic and kinetic evidence suggestive of young and old platelets, *J. Clin. Invest.*, 48, 1073, 1969.
22. **O'Brien, J. R.**, A relationship between platelet volume and platelet number, *Thromb. Diath. Haemorrh.*, 31, 363, 1974.
23. **Minter, F. M. and Ingram, M.**, Platelet volume: density relationships in normal and acutely bled dogs, *Br. J. Haematol.*, 20, 55, 1971.
24. **Karpatkin, S.**, Heterogeneity of rabbit platelets. VI. Further resolution of changes in platelet density, volume and radioactivity following cohort labeling with Se^{75}- selenomethionine, *Br. J. Haematol.*, 39, 459, 1978.
25. **Penington, D. G., Lee, N. Y. T., Roxburgh, A. E., and McGready, J. E.**, Platelet density and size: the interpretation of heterogeneity, *Br. J. Haematol.*, 34, 365, 1976.
26. **Karpatkin, S.**, Heterogeneity of human platelets. II. Functional evidence suggestive of young and old platelets, *J. Clin. Invest.*, 48, 1083, 1969.
27. **Manucci, P. M. and Sharp, A. A.**, Platelet volume and shape in relation to aggregation and adhesion, *Br. J. Haematol.*, 13, 604, 1967.
28. **Freedman, M. L. and Karpatkin, S.**, Heterogeneity of rabbit platelets. V. Preferential splenic sequestration of megathrombocytes, *Br. J. Haematol.*, 31, 255, 1975.
29. **Freedman, M. L., Altszuler, N., and Karpatkin, S.**, Presence of a nonsplenic platelet pool, *Blood*, 50, 419, 1977.
30. **Karpatkin, S., Khan, I., and Freedman, M. L.**, Heterogeneity of platelet function: correlation with platelet volume, *Am. J. Med.*, 64, 542, 1978.

31. **Amorosi, E., Garg, S. K., and Karpatkin, S.**, Heterogeneity of human platelets. IV. Identification of a young platelet population with Se^{75}-selenomethionine, *Br. J. Haematol.*, 21, 227, 1971.
32. **Karpatkin, S. and Charmatz, A.**, Heterogeneity of human platelets. III. Glycogen metabolism in platelets of different sizes, *Br. J. Haematol.*, 19, 135, 1970.
33. **Karpatkin, S. and Strick, N.**, Heterogeneity of human platelets. V. Glycolytic and related enzymes with possible relation to platelet age, *J. Clin. Invest.*, 51, 1235, 1972.
34. **George, J. N., Lewis, P. C., and Sears, D. A.**, Studies on platelet plasma membranes. II. Characterization of surface proteins of rabbit platelets in vitro and during circulation in vivo using diazotized I^{125}-diiodosulfanilic acid as a label, *J. Lab. Clin. Med.*, 88, 247, 1976.
35. **Greenberg, J. P., Rand, M. L., and Packham, M. A.**, Relation of platelet age to platelet sialic acid, *Fed. Proc.*, 36, 966A, 1977; Packham, personal communication.
36. **Penington, D. G., Streatfield, K., and Roxburgh, A. E.**, Megakaryocytes and the heterogeneity of circulating platelets, *Br. J. Haematol.*, 34, 639, 1976.
37. **Karpatkin, S. and Freedman, M. L.**, Hypersplenic thrombocytopenia differentiated from increased peripheral destruction by platelet volume, *Ann. Intern. Med.*, 89, 200, 1978.
38. **Zucker-Franklin, D. and Karpatkin, S.**, Red blood cell and platelet fragmentation in idiopathic autoimmune thrombocytopenic purpura, *N. Engl. J. Med.*, 297, 517, 1977.
39. **Khan, I., Zucker-Franklin, D., and Karpatkin, S.**, Microthrombocytosis and platelet fragmentation associated with idiopathic/autoimmune thrombocytopenic purpura, *Br. J. Haematol.*, 31, 449, 1975.

CHARACTERIZATION AND ASSAY OF PLATELET SECRETORY PROTEINS

Stefan Niewiarowski and Shirley P. Levine

Introduction

Adhesion, aggregation, and secretion are thought to be the most important functions of platelets. There is now good evidence that proteins secreted by the platelets participate in hemostasis, inflammation, and cell growth. In 1962, Grette[1] demonstrated that thrombin, in addition to liberating serotonin, also caused rapid release of adenine nucleotides and fibrinogen from pig platelets. Since this early observation, a multitude of other proteins that are stored and secreted by platelets have been described. Davey and Lüscher[2] determined that 10^9 platelets contain approximately 1.6 mg protein that can be solubilized after platelet homogenization with digitonin and Triton X-100, and by repeated freezing and thawing. Thrombin releases approximately one tenth of the total platelet proteins. This observation is in agreement with the data obtained in our laboratory.

In the past few years, extensive studies on platelet-secreted proteins have been carried out in many laboratories. It is obvious that by studying these proteins, normal platelet physiology can be better defined. Sensitive assays for these proteins may also permit measurements of the platelet release reaction in vivo. Until recently, the only method available for studying platelet stimulation in vivo was that of platelet survival time. Rabbit platelets that have been degranulated by thrombin, however, have normal survival times.[3] Therefore, the measurement of platelet survival in humans may not reflect platelet stimulation either. Many difficulties were encountered in the study of the release of serotonin or ADP by platelets in vivo, because these substances are rapidly metabolized. In the last few years, several platelet secretory proteins have been purified, and at least three of these platelet proteins — platelet factor 4, low affinity platelet factor 4 (LA-PF_4), and β-thromboglobulin (βTG) — have been shown to be immunologically specific for platelets.[4,5,6] Therefore, these platelet proteins could be considered as platelet markers, and their elevation in carefully prepared platelet-poor plasma (PPP) may indicate platelet secretion in vivo.

In this chapter we will briefly review these platelet-secreted proteins and the methods for their determination and discuss the possible clinical significance of these tests.

Characterization of Platelet Secretory Proteins

Proteins secreted by platelets can be tentatively classified into three groups (Table 1): (1) proteins identical or similar to plasma proteins, (2) lysosomal enzymes, and (3) platelet specific proteins.

According to Davey and Lüscher,[2] protein material secreted by thrombin-stimulated platelets contained 35% albumin, 20% β_2-globulin, 15% β_1-globulin, 10% fibrinogen, and smaller quantities of γ- and α-globulins. Platelet and plasma albumin appear to be identical proteins,[8] although some of the α- and β-globulins secreted by the platelets do not cross-react with antisera to plasma proteins.[2]

The level of platelet fibrinogen varies from 50 to 200 μg/10^9 platelets,[7,33,34] and the ratio of plasma fibrinogen to platelet fibrinogen is 1:30.[7] James et al.[35] observed differences between plasma fibrinogen and platelet fibrinogen. Doolittle et al.[36] state that these differences depend on degradation of platelet fibrinogen in vivo or in vitro, and Lopaciuk et al.[7] hold that they may depend on the variable content of carbohydrate components. Fibrinogen occurs in platelets both as an intracellular component associated with α-granules[37] and as material bound to platelet membranes.[38] Intracellular

Table 1
PROTEINS SECRETED BY THE PLATELETS

	Ref.
Proteins identical or similar to plasma proteins	
Fibrinogen	17
Albumin	8
Factor V	9
α_1-Antitrypsin	10
Enzymes (lysosomal hydrolases)	
β-Glucuronidase	11
β-N-acetylglucosaminidase	
β-Galactosidase	
Aryl sulphatase	
Cathepsins	11,12
Elastase	13
Collagenase	14
Endogluconidase degrading heparan sulfate	15
Cyclic 3′:5′-nucleotide phosphodiesterase	16
Platelet specific proteins	
Vascular permeability factor	17
Chemotactic factor	18
Bactericidal factor	19
Platelet growth factors	20—22
Platelet factor 4 (high affinity antiheparin factor, high affinity platelet factor 4, PF_4)	23—26
Low affinity platelet factor 4, LA-PF_4	7, 28
β-thromboglobulin	29, 30
Thrombin-specific protein	31
Platelet antiplasmin	32

fibrinogen is released during platelet aggregation induced by collagen,[7] thrombin,[33] and plasmin.[34] James et al.[39] suggested that extruded platelet fibrinogen may contribute to the stability of thrombus. It is difficult to understand, however, the physiological significance of fibrinogen secretion by the platelets, since an excess of fibrinogen occurs in PPP.

Østerud et al.[9] discovered that Factor V and its activator are released from gel-filtered platelets after freezing and thawing or after platelet aggregation by collagen but not by ADP. Pifer et al.[40] confirmed this observation and demonstrated that platelet Factor V is primarily associated with platelet granules. Platelet Factor V is missing in platelets of patients with congenital Factor V deficiency; and in platelets from normal subjects, it is neutralized by anti-Factor V antibody.[9] The presence of plasma Factor V on the surface of platelets, as observed by earlier investigators,[41] is probably due to the damage of platelets during preparative procedures. Factor V is not present on the surface of intact platelets obtained by gel filtration or albumin density centrifugation.[9] Release of an activated Factor V by platelets exposed to collagen may be of great significance in hemostasis. It may bypass the need for an initial trace of thrombin in the extrinsic clotting reaction for the initial activation of plasma Factor V. The possibility that "collagen-induced platelet coagulant activity"[42] is due to the release of activated Factor V from the platelets should be considered.

Although platelets contain and secrete low quantities of α_1-antitrypsin, which is identical with plasma α_1-antitrypsin,[10] the significance of this phenomenon is not clear. A number of hydrolases secreted by stimulated platelets have been described, including β-glucuronidase,[11] βN-acetyl glucosaminidase, β-galactosidase, aryl sulphatase,[11] the cathepsins,[11,12] elastase,[13] collagenase,[14] endoglucosidase-degrading heparan sulphate, and cyclic 3′:5′-nucleotide phosphodiesterase.[16] Platelet secretion of enzymes that can degrade various components of the vessel wall (collagen, elastin, and heparan sulphate) may have a pathophysiological significance.

Marcus et al.[43] and Day et al.[44] concluded that platelet hydrolases occur in the α-granules, which were considered to be the platelet lysosomes. This opinion has been questioned by Siegel and Lüscher[45] and by Broekman et al.[46] In both of these studies, only low levels of acid hydrolases could be demonstrated in the α-granule fraction, whereas fractions with high activities of these enzymes were morphologically heterogenous and therefore difficult to interpret. Bentfeld and Bainton,[47] applying cytochemical staining to rat platelets and megakaryocytes, differentiated vesicles containing arylsulfatase and acid phosphatase from α-granules, which are probably a reservoir of other proteins secreted by the platelet.

The list of platelet specific proteins also includes proteins that are either biologically or immunologically characteristic for platelets.

Platelets secrete vascular permeability factor,[17] bactericidal factor,[19] chemotactic factor,[18] and platelet growth factor.[20-22] The first three of these factors resemble some cationic proteins of human polymorphonuclear leukocytes. Chemotactic factor may be identical with the protease cleaving C_5 component of complement.[18] Platelet growth factor (PGF) stimulates DNA synthesis and cell division in confluent populations of various cells, but it has little effect on transformed cells.

Antoniades et al.[22,48] obtained a highly purified PGF from human serum and platelets. This protein was homogenous in SDS polyacrylamide gel electrophoresis and had an approximate molecular weight of 13,700 and an isoelectric point at pH 9.7. These researchers also developed a radioimmunoassay for PGF. The values of PGF in serum obtained from platelet-rich plasma (PRP) are of the order of magnitude of 50 ng/mℓ, i.e., approximately 160 times less than the level of PF_4. PGF is a heterogenous protein. Heldin et al.[49] isolated two anionic and one cationic cell multiplication factors from platelets.

PGF is released from human platelets stimulated by ADP, thrombin, collagen, and epinephrine.[50,51] It is probably localized in platelet granules. PGF differs from other serum factors that stimulate cell proliferation, including insulin, steroid hormones, and lipoproteins.[22] Recent evidence indicates that PGF might play a significant role in the pathogenesis of atherosclerosis by stimulating proliferation of arterial smooth muscle cells.[52]

Antiheparin proteins secreted by human platelets: PF_4, $LAPF_4$, and βTG are immunologically distinct from proteins produced by other cells. Ludlam and Anderton[5] found that the level of βTG antigen in various tissues is at least 10,000-fold less than in platelets. LA-PF_4[5] and PF_4 antigen[6] were not detected in leukocytes and red cells. βTG and PF_4 are not cationic proteins. Two other platelet secretory proteins — thrombin-sensitive protein[31] and platelet antiplasmin, described by Joist et al.[32] — may also be platelet specific. However, these proteins must be further studied if they are to be further characterized.

There is no doubt that PF_4 is, at present, the best characterized platelet protein. PF_4 is released from platelets complexed with a proteoglycan carrier molecule, and the calculated molecular weight is approximately 350,000.[53] This complex can be eluted close to the void volume by filtration on a Sephadex G-200 or Biogel®-A column. The dissociation of PF_4 and the proteoglycan carrier molecule occurs at high ionic strength or acidic pH.

Several methods have been used to purify human PF_4 including precipitation with $ZnSO_4$[28] and ethanol,[26] gel filtration,[23,24] chromatography on SP-Sephadex,[54] and affinity chromatography with heparin-agarose.[25] The PF_4 subunit is composed of a single chain containing 70 amino acids, and has a molecular weight of 7800 daltons. The primary structure of human PF_4 has been established independently in four different laboratories.[54-57] Evidence has been obtained that lysine is a main constituent of the PF_4 reacting site with heparin.[26] This site is probably located in the C-terminal domaine of the molecule, which is rich in lysine, leucine, and isoleucine. Evidence obtained by ultracentrifuge measurements[23,24] indicates that the PF_4 molecule is composed of four subunits, apparently linked by noncovalent bonds. Thus its molecular weight would be 31,200. Barber et al.[53] determined that the carrier molecule is composed of four chondroitin sulfate chains of molecular weight 12,000 and a polypeptide backbone of molecular weight 11,000, giving a total molecular weight for the carrier of 59,000. Each chondroitin sulfate chain binds one molecule of PF_4. The entire complex occurs as a dimer of a molecular weight of approximately 350,000. Heparin interacts with PF_4 by displacing chondroitin sulfate.[53] Recent evidence indicates that platelet factor 4 is a potent inhibitor of collagenase in connective tissue.[58]

βTG is a protein released by platelets after stimulation by thrombin. It was isolated by gel filtration[29] and more recently by affinity chromatography on heparin-agarose.[30] βTG has a molecular weight of 36,000, as estimated by gel filtration and sedimentation velocity. At pH 3.2, it dissociates into six subunits. Originally it was thought that this protein might inhibit urokinase, but in their later studies, Moore and Pepper[30] could not ascribe any definitive function to this protein. Recently, Begg et al.[59] established the complete covalent structure of βTG. It consists of identical subunits of 81 amino acids, each with a molecular weight of 8851. Forty two of the 81 residues of βTG are identical with those of PF_4.

In recent studies, platelet factor 4 (PF_4) and low-affinity PF_4 (LA-PF_4) were purified to homogeneity from washed human platelets by $ZnSO_4$ precipitation and affinity chromatography on heparinagarose columns.[28,60,61] As shown by double immunodiffusion and specific radioimmunoassays, LA-PF_4 and PF_4 were immunologically distinct. The levels of PF_4 and LA-PF_4 and PF_4 were immunologically distinct. The levels of PF_4 and LA-PF_4 antigens in intact platelets were 12.4 and 24.2 $\mu g/10^9$ platelets, respectively. Heparin-neutralizing activity was assayed by measuring the degree of hydrolysis of the chromogenic substrate Bz-Ile-Glu-Gly-Arg-pNA in the presence of antithrombin III and heparin; 1 mg each of PF_4 and LA-PF_4 neutralized 17.0 and 2.6 units of beef lung heparin, respectively. Both proteins accounted for 28% of the total heparin neutralizing activity of the platelets. The molecular weight of LA-PF_4 as calculated by amino acid analysis and SDS polyacrylamide gel electrophoresis was 9070 and 7800 daltons, respectively. LA-PF_4 shared common antigenic determinants with β-thromboglobulin (βTG) and connective tissue-activating peptide III. The difference between LA-PF_4 and βTG was shown by electrophoresis on cellulose acetate at pH 8.6 LA-PF_4 migrated in the γ-globulin region, in contrast to βTG, which migrated in the β globulin region. The NH_2 terminal amino acids of LA-PF_4 and βTG were asparagine and glycine, respectively. Partial amino acid sequencing of LA-PF_4 showed differences between this protein and βTG. At the NH_2 terminal end LA-PF_4 had four additional amino acids (Asn-Leu-Ala-Lys); however, residues 5—12 of LA-PF_4 and 1—8 of βTG were identical. LA-PF_4 and βTG were identified and measured by a combination of isoelectric focusing (LKB-ampholine column; pH gradient, 3.6—10.9, in sucrose) and radioimmunoassay.[62] The isoelectric points of βTG and LA-PF_4 were at pH 7.0 and pH 8.0, respectively. Ionophore A23187 was used to aggregate washed human platelets. The proportions of LA-PF_4 and βTG released were 75% and 14%, respectively. The remaining 16% corresponded to a basic protein (isoelectric point 10.9) which cross-reacted immunologically with βTG and LA-PF_4. Incubation of supernate after platelet aggregation at 37°C for 60 min resulted in a decrease of LA-PF_4 and accumulation of βTG as demonstrated by a shift of the isoelectric point of antigens from 8.0 to 7.0, by disappearance of N-terminal asparagine and appearance of N-terminal glycine. These changes were prevented by heating the platelet supernate for 5 min at

100°C or 30 min at 56°C. LA-PF_4 appears to be a protein originally secreted by human platelets and converted to βTG by a heat labile protease associated with the platelets. LA-PF_4 was also prepared from human platelets by $ZnSO_4$ precipitation and DEAE-cellulose chromatography according to Nath et al.[27] We have demonstrated the immunological identity of LA-PF_4 and connective tissue activating peptide III (CATP III) isolated from human platelets by Castor et al.[64] CATP III stimulates the biosynthesis of DNA, RNA, and of glucosaminoglycans in synovial cells and human skin fibroblasts. More recently we found that βTG, LA-PF_4, and platelet basic protein separated by isoelectric focusing initiate DNA synthesis in 3T3 cells. The activity of platelet basic protein was observed below 1 ng/mℓ and was saturated at 50 ng/mℓ. LA-PF_4 and βTG were 10 and 40 times less active, respectively.[103]

Assay of Platelet Secretory Proteins

All proteins secreted by platelets can be assayed by using various biological or immunological tests. Certainly, the assay of those proteins which either have very specific functions or which can be considered as platelet markers have the greatest potential in clinical and laboratory medicine. The assay of platelet proteins which are identical or similar to plasma proteins is of less value from this point of view. Platelet lysosomal enzymes have not yet been sufficiently purified and characterized; however, there is evidence that platelet elastase is immunologically distinct from leukocyte elastase.[65] If this is so, the immunoassay of this enzyme may be of further significance.

In the last few years, a lot of work has been done to elaborate methods of measuring PF_4 (LA-PF_4) and βTG. It is still difficult, however, to evaluate the clinical significance of these methods. These factors can be measured by biological assay (neutralization of heparin activity) and by immunoassay. The clotting assays of heparin-neutralizing activity in plasma are usually based on the measurements of a heparin thrombin time.[66-70] These assays have low sensitivity, and they are nonspecific since erythrocytes[68,71] and leukocytes[72] also contain antiheparin activity. Moreover, the sensitivity of plasma to heparin may depend on variations in the level of fibrinogen, antithrombin III, α_2-macroglobulin, albumin, α_1 acid glycoprotein, γ globulin, and the lipoproteins.[74-76] Walsh et al.[77] proposed an assay of platelet antiheparin activity based on the neutralization of heparin by platelet extracts and subsequent measurement of the ability of residual heparin to inactivate Factor Xa in the presence of antithrombin III. This test is at least ten times more sensitive than the heparin-thrombin time, but it lacks specificity, and it has not been adopted for measurements of PF_4 in PPP. More recently, we have elaborated an assay of antiheparin activity in a similar system in which Factor Xa activity is measured by hydrolysis of the chromogenic substrate S-2222.[28] In our hands, this method is more reproducible and much more rapid than the original test proposed by Walsh et al.[77] Because of its limited specificity, however, it cannot be recommended for measurements of the level of platelet antiheparin factors in plasma. It is useful in evaluating the antiheparin activity of platelet lysates and purified fractions.

In 1962, Niewiarowski et al.[78] described an increased antiheparin activity in the plasma of some patients with thrombocythemia and suggested that this factor may be derived from the circulating platelets. Farbiszewski et al.[69] and Fuster et al.[79] suggested that antiheparin activity in PPP increases after thrombin has been injected into rabbits[69] and thromboplastin into dogs,[79] and suggested that this is due to platelet release of PF_4. An increase in antiheparin activity of PPP has also been noted in patients with coronary thrombosis, thromboembolic complications, and disseminated intravascular coagulation.[69,70] More recently, O'Brien et al.[80] observed increasing heparin-neutralizing activity in patients with myocardial infarction and suggested that in some situations, their test measures PF_4 derived from activated platelets. According to these au-

Table 2
RADIOIMMUNOASSAY OF PF_4

Method of separating antigen-antibody complex	Time required to perform the assay (days)	The lowest quantity of antigen detectable	Normal values of PF_4 antigen: Platelets in PRP ($\mu g/10^9$)	Serum from whole blood ($\mu g/m\ell$)	PPP ($ng/m\ell$)	Ref.
Double antibody	2	2 ng/mℓ	—	8.14 ± 2.33	13 ± 5.5	90
Ammonium sulfate	1	250 pg/mℓ	7.6	—	16 ± 4	91
Ammonium sulfate	1	1.5 ng/mℓ	—	13.2 ± 3.2	4.7 ± 2.5	89
Double antibody	—	1.6 ng/mℓ	—	8.14 ± 19.2	7.4	92
Ammonium sulfate	1	1 ng/mℓ	12.4 ± 3.1	—	—	28
Sodium sulfate	1	179 pg per sample	—	—	< 2.5	93

thors, determination of heparin-neutralizing activity in patients with myocardial infarction may be of clinical significance. We believe, however, that few conclusions can be drawn from these experiments. The level of PF_4 LA-PF_4 per 10^9 platelets is 12.4 μg and 24.2 μg,[28] respectively. The minimal amounts of PF_4 and LA-PF_4 detectable by the the heparin thrombin time method are 1 μg and 10 μg, respectively. Experiments with radioimmunoassays demonstrated that in PPP obtained from adequately collected blood, the level of PF_4 and βTG antigens is well below 50 ng/mℓ. For instance, Handin[82] found normal values of PF_4 in PPP to be 16 ng/mℓ and in patients with myocardial infarction, 100 ng/mℓ. Obviously, this elevation of PF_4 level in PPP cannot be detected by clotting assays.

Laurel's immunoelectrophoresis[82] and Mancini's radialimmunodiffusion[4] have been applied for measuring the level of platelet-specific proteins in platelets and in plasma, but these methods are much less sensitive than radioimmunoassay; the minimum measured is 0.5 μg antigen per mℓ.

LA-PF_4 measured by radialimmunodiffusion appeared to be an excellent marker of the platelet release reaction induced by ionophores,[83] thrombin,[4] collagen,[4] ADP,[4] antigen-antibody complexes,[4] endotoxin,[84] thrombocytin — a thrombin-like snake venom protease,[85] and following contact of platelets with a silicone rubber surface during extracorporeal circulation.[86,87] Measuring low affinity antiheparin antigen by radialimmunodiffusion seems to be useful in evaluating the platelet release reaction in vitro, however, this method is not sufficiently sensitive to measure the release of LA-PF_4 from platelets in vivo.

In the radioimmunoassay of antiheparin factors in PPP, the most crucial procedure is the preparation of plasma devoid of platelets. It has been found that both antigens rapidly leak from platelets during routine preparation of platelet-rich plasma (PRP) and PPP from citrate or ACD blood. We found that incubating PRP at room temperature for 3 hr results in the leakage of about 15 to 20% of total low affinity antiheparin factor (βTG) into ambient fluids.[60] Adding PGE_1 inhibited this process. Blood for radioimmunoassay is carefully collected by venipuncture and immediately added to a cocktail containing EDTA, theophyline, PGE_1,[88] or EDTA, PGE_1, and dibutyryl cyclic AMP.[89] This blood is then kept in ice and centrifuged at specific times to prepare PPP. Details for preparing PPP are enclosed in the addendum.

The various methods of determining PF_4 and βTG-LA-PF_4 antigens by radioimmunoassay are summarized in Tables 2 and 3. These methods usually detect as little as 1 ng of antigen per mℓ. The levels of PF_4 and βTG-LA-PF_4 antigens per mℓ of serum, per 10^9 platelets, and per mℓ of PFP are also shown in these tables. The level of LA-PF_4 appears to be at least twice as high as the level of PF_4.

Table 3
RADIOIMMUNOASSAY OF βTG AND LA-PF_4

Method of separating antigen-antibody complex	Time required to perform the assay	The lowest quantity of antigen detectable	Normal values of βTG antigen: Platelets in PRP (μg/mℓ)	Serum from whole blood(μg/mℓ)	PPP (ng/mℓ)	Ref.
Double antibody	3—6 days	1 ng/mℓ	—	17.4 ± 6.3	1.3 ± 7.5	94
Antiserum coupled covalently to sepharose	2¼ hr	0.5 ng	—	—	38.7 ± 9.1	88
Double antibody	2 days	2.5 ng/mℓ	—	—	30.5 ± 12.8	5
Sodium sulfate	24 hr	14 pg per sample	—	—	18.1 ± 1.93 (SEM)	93
Ammonium sulfate	24 hr	0.1 ng/mℓ	24.2 ± 4.3	—	31.9 ± 2.8	81

Clinical conditions in which the values of PF_4 and LA-PF_4-βTG antigens in PPP are elevated are summarized in Table 4. Although these data are still preliminary, it appears that increased levels of both antigens in PPP may indicate platelet stimulation in vivo. According to Ludlam and Anderton,[5] there was no correlation between platelet turnover and βTG antigen level in the plasma of normal individuals. There was a good correlation, however, between both parameters in patients with such conditions as leukemia, polycythemia, and thrombocythemia.

According to Chesterman et al.[92] plasma PF_4 levels are markedly increased during cardiopulmonary bypass surgery with shortened ^{51}Cr labeled survival times and during arterial thrombosis. However, despite similarly shortened platelet survival times, the plasma level of PF_4 was normal in immune thrombocytopenia.

The clearance of βTG and PF_4 have been studied in normal individuals infused with human serum or platelet concentrates. Dawes et al.[99] found that βTG was cleared from circulation with a half-life time of 100 min but the clearance of PF_4 was so rapid that its half-life could not be estimated. Both proteins appeared to be excreted, at least in part, in urine. Recent observations on the elevation of LA-PF_4 in PPP of patients with chronic renal failure and its increased urinary secretion suggest a significant role of kidney in the metabolism of platelet specific secretory proteins.[100]

Addendum: Preparing PPP for the Assay of Platelet Secretory Proteins

Blood must be collected in "anticoagulant cocktails" to prevent release of platelet secretory proteins. The most satisfactory results were obtained with EDTA-dibutyryl-cyclic AMP-prostaglandin E_1 cocktail[89] or EDTA-theophylline-prostaglandin E_1 cocktail.[88]

Cocktail I
- 10% EDTA — 5 mℓ
- N^6O^2 dibutyrylcyclic AMP — 50 mM
- Prostaglandin E_1 (2.9 μM) — 50 $\mu\ell$

Cocktail II
- 10% EDTA — 5 mℓ
- Theophylline — 27.0 mg
- Prostaglandin E_1 — 50 $\mu\ell$

Table 4
ELEVATION OF PF_4 OR LA-PF_4-βTG ANTIGENS IN PPP IN VARIOUS PATHOLOGICAL CONDITIONS

	Protein elevated	Ref.
Venous thrombosis	βTG	95
Rising platelet count after splenectomy	βTG	5
Stroke	βTG	5
Renal failure	βTG,LA-PF_4	5,100
Transplant rejection	βTG	5
Myocardial infarction	PF_4	91,92
Artificial heart valves	βTG	5
Disseminated intravascular coagulation	PF_4	92
Myeloproliferative syndromes	βTG	96
Diabetes	βTG	97,98
Coronary artery disease	PF_4	101,102

Aliquots of 0.5 mℓ of the cocktail are added to centrifuge tubes and kept on ice. Blood is collected by venipuncture, using a 19-gauge butterfly needle. The tourniquet is left in place, the first five drops are discarded, and the blood sample is dropped directly into the chilled tube to 5.0 mℓ marker. The blood is immediately centrifuged at 4°C at 2400 gravities for 60 min or 12,000 gravities for 10 min. The PPP is transferred to another tube and deep frozen until ready for use. Samples may be mailed for radioimmunoassay either on dry ice or in lyophilized form.

REFERENCES

1. **Grette, K.**, Studies on the mechanism of thrombin catalyzed hemostatic reactions in blood platelets, *Acta Physiol. Scand.*, 56 (Suppl. 195), 1962.
2. **Davey, M. G. and Lüscher, E. F.**, Release reactions of human platelets induced by thrombin and other agents, *Biochim. Biophys. Acta*, 165, 490, 1968.
3. **Reimers, H. J., Packham, M. A., Kinlough-Rathbone, R. L., and Mustard, J. F.**, Effect of repeated treatment of rabbit platelets with low concentrations of thrombin on their function, metabolism and survival, *Br. J. Haematol.*, 25, 675, 1973.
4. **Niewiarowski, S., Lowery, C. T., Hawiger, J., Millman, M., and Timmons, S.**, Immunoassay of human platelet factor 4 (PF_4, antiheparin factor) by radial immunodiffusion, *J. Lab. Clin. Med.*, 87, 120, 1976.
5. **Ludlam, C. A. and Anderton, J. L.**, Platelet β thromboglobulin, in Platelet Function Tests — Proceedings from the Workshop on Platelets, Philadelphia, 1976, Day, H. J., Holmsen, H., and Zucker, M. B., Eds., U.S. Government Printing Office, Washington, D.C., 1977.
6. **Kaplan, K. L., Drillings, M., Nossel, H. L., and Lesznik, G.**, Radioimmunoassay of β thromboglobulin (βTG) and platelet factor 4 (PF_4), in Platelet Function Tests — Proceedings from the Workshop on Platelets, Philadelphia, 1976, Day, H. J., Holmsen, H., and Zucker, M. B., Eds., U.S. Government Printing Office, Washington, D.C., 1977.
7. **Lopaciuk, S., Lovette, K. M., McDonagh, J., Chuang, H. Y. K., and McDonagh, R. P.**, Subcellular distribution of fibrinogen and factor XIII in human blood platelets, *Thromb. Res.*, 8, 453, 1976.
8. **Ganguly, P.**, Studies on platelet proteins. III. The identity of platelet and serum albumins, *Biochim. Biophys. Acta*, 188, 78, 1969.
9. **Østerud, B., Rapaport, S. I., and Lavine, K. K.**, Factor V activity of platelets: evidence for an activated factor V molecule and for a platelet activator, *Blood*, 49, 819, 1977.
10. **Bagdasarian, A. and Colman, R. W.**, Subcellular localization and purification of platelet α_1 antitrypsin, *Blood*, 51, 139, 1978.

11. Holmsen, H. and Day, H. J., The selectivity of the thrombin-induced platelet release reaction: subcellular localization of released and retained constituents, *J. Lab. Clin. Med.*, 75, 849, 1970.
12. Nachman, R. L. and Ferris, B., Studies of human platelet protease activity, *J. Clin. Invest.*, 47, 2530, 1968.
13. Robert, B. Y., Legrand, G., Pignand, J., Caen, J., and Robert, L., Activité élastinolytique associée aux plaquettes sanguines, *Pathol. Biol.*, 17, 615, 1969.
14. Chesney, C. McI., Harper, E., and Colman, R. W., Human platelet collagenase, *J. Clin. Invest.*, 53, 1647, 1974.
15. Wasteson, Å., Hook, M., and Westermark, B., Demonstration of a platelet enzyme degrading heparan sulphate, *FEBS Lett.*, 64, 218, 1976.
16. Hidaka, H. and Asano, T., Platelet cyclic 3′:5′-nucleotide phosphodiesterase released by thrombin and calcium ionophore, *J. Biol. Chem.*, 252, 7508, 1976.
17. Nachman, R. L., Weksler, B., and Ferris, B., Increased vascular permeability produced by human platelet granule cationic extract, *J. Clin. Invest.*, 49, 274, 1970.
18. Weksler, B. B. and Coupal, C. E., Platelet-dependent generation of chemotactic activity in serum, *J. Exp. Med.*, 137, 1419, 1973.
19. Roberts, R. R., Tew, J. G., and Donaldson, D. M., Release of β-lysin from platelets caused by antigen-antibody complexes, purified enzymes and platelet-aggregating substances, *Infect. Immun.*, 15, 485, 1977.
20. Ross, R., Glomset, J., Kariya, B., and Harker, L., A platelet-dependent serum factor that stimulates the proliferation of arterial smooth muscle cells in vitro, *Proc. Natl. Acad. Sci. U.S.A.*, 71, 1207, 1974.
21. Westermark, B. and Wasteson, Å., A platelet factor stimulating human normal glial cells, *Exp. Cell Res.*, 98, 170, 1976.
22. Antoniades, H. N., Stathakos, D., and Scher, C. D., Isolation of a cationic polypeptide from human serum that stimulates proliferation of 3T3 cells, *Proc. Natl. Acad. Sci. U.S.A.*, 72, 2635, 1975.
23. Käser-Glanzmann, R., Jakabova, M., and Lüscher, E. F., Heparin-neutralizing factor (platelet factor 4) from human blood platelets and its reactivity with fibrinogen and soluble fibrin monomer complexes, *Haemostasis*, 1, 136, 1972-1973.
24. Moore, S., Pepper, D., and Cash, J., Platelet antiheparin activity: the isolation and characterization of platelet factor 4 released from thrombin-aggregated washed human platelets and its dissociation into subunits and the isolation of membrane-bound antiheparin activity, *Biochim. Biophys. Acta*, 379, 370, 1975.
25. Levine, S. P. and Wohl, H., Human platelet factor 4 (PF_4) purification and characterization by affinity chromatography, *J. Biol. Chem.*, 251, 324, 1976.
26. Handin, R. I. and Cohen, H. J., Purification and binding properties of human platelet factor four, *J. Biol. Chem.*, 251, 4273, 1976.
27. Nath, N., Lowery, C. T., and Niewiarowski, S., Antigenic and antiheparin properties of human platelet factor 4 (PF_4), *Blood*, 45, 537, 1975.
28. Rucinski, B., Niewiarowski, S., James, P., Walz, D. A., Budzynski, A. Z., Antiheparin proteins secreted by human platelets. Purification, characterization and radioimmunoassay, *Blood*, 53, 47, 1979.
29. Moore, S., Pepper, D. S., and Cash, J. D., The isolation and characterization of a platelet specific β-globulin (β-thromboglobulin) and the detection of antiurokinase and antiplasmin released from thrombin-aggregated washed human platelets, *Biochim. Biophys. Acta*, 379, 360, 1975.
30. Moore, S. and Pepper, D. S., Identification of a platelet specific release product β thromboglobulin, in *Platelet Physiology*, Gordon, J. L., Ed., Elsevier/North Holland, Biomedical Press, Amsterdam, 1976, 293.
31. Baenziger, N. L., Brodie, G. N., and Majerus, P. W., A thrombin-sensitive protein of human platelet, *Proc. Natl. Acad. Sci. U.S.A.*, 68, 240, 1971.
32. Joist, H. J., Niewiarowski, S., Nath, N., and Mustard, J. F., Platelet antiplasmin: its extrusion during the release reaction, subcellular localization, characterization and relationship to antiheparin in pig platelets, *J. Lab. Clin. Med.*, 87, 659, 1976.
33. Keenan, J. P. and Solum, N. O., Quantitative studies on the release of platelet fibrinogen by thrombin, *Br. J. Haematol.*, 23, 461, 1972.
34. Niewiarowski, S., Senyi, A. F., and Gillies, P., Plasmin-induced platelet aggregation and platelet release reaction, *J. Clin. Invest.*, 52, 1647, 1973.
35. James, H. L., Bradford, H. R., and Ganguly, P., Platelet fibrinogen. Identity and initial observations on the mode of its degradation by plasmin, *Biochim. Biophys. Acta*, 386, 209, 1975.
36. Doolittle, R. F., Takagi, T., and Cottrell, B. A., Platelet and plasma fibrinogens are identical gene products, *Science*, 185, 368, 1974.
37. Nachman, R. L., Marcus, A. J., and Zucker-Franklin, D., Immunological studies of protein associated with subcellular fractions of normal human platelets, *J. Lab. Clin. Med.*, 69, 651, 1967.

38. Tollefsen, D. M. and Majerus, P. W., Inhibition of human platelet aggregation by monovalent antibody fragments, *J. Clin. Invest.*, 55, 1259, 1975.
39. James, H. L., Ganguly, P., and Jackson, C. W., Characterization and origin of fibrinogen in blood platelets. A review, *Thromb. Haemostasis,* 38, 939, 1977.
40. Pifer, D. D., Cogman, R. W., and Chesney, C. Mc.I., Subcellular localization and secretion of factor V by human platelets, *Thromb. Haemostasis,* 38 (Abstr.), 126, 1977.
41. Hjort, P., Rapaport, S. I., and Owren, P. A., Evidence that platelet accelerator (platelet factor 1) is adsorbed plasma proaccelerin, *Blood,* 10, 1139, 1955.
42. Walsh, P. N., The effect of collagen and kaolin on the intrinsic coagulant activity of platelets. Evidence for an alternative pathway in intrinsic coagulation not requiring factor XII, *Br. J. Haematol.,* 22, 393, 1972.
43. Marcus, A. J., Zucker-Franklin, D., Safier, L. B., and Ullman, H. L., Studies on human platelet granules and membranes, *J. Clin. Invest.,* 45, 14, 1966.
44. Day, H. J., Holmsen, H., and Hovig, T., Subcellular particles of human platelets. A biochemical and electromicroscopic study with particular reference to the influence of fractionation techniques, *Scand. J. Haematol. Suppl.,* 7, 1969.
45. Siegel, A. and Lüscher, E. F., Nonidentity of the α-granules of human blood platelets with typical lysosomes, *Nature (London),* 215, 745, 1967.
46. Broekman, M. J., Westmoreland, N. P., and Cohen, P., An improved method for isolating alpha granules and mitochondria from human platelets, *J. Cell Biol.,* 60, 507, 1974.
47. Bentfeld, M. E. and Bainton, D. F., Cytochemical localization of lysosomal enzymes in rat megakaryocytes and platelets, *J. Clin. Invest.,* 56, 1635, 1975.
48. Antoniades, H. N. and Scher, C. D., Radioimmunoassay of a human serum growth factor for Balb lc-3T3 cells: derivation from platelets, *Proc. Natl. Acad. Sci. U.S.A.,* 74, 1973, 1977.
49. Heldin, C. A., Wasteson, Å., and Westermark, B., Partial purification and characterization of platelet factors stimulating the multiplication of normal human glial cells, *Exp. Cell Res.,* 109, 429, 1977.
50. Busch, C., Wasteson, Å., and Westermark, B., Release of a cell growth promoting factor from human platelet, *Thromb. Res.,* 8, 493, 1976.
51. Ihnatowycz, I. O., Moore, S., and Mustard, J. F., Platelet growth factor (PGF) stimulation of DNA synthesis in smooth muscle cells (SMC) in vitro, *Fed. Proc. Abstr.,* 36, 430, 1977.
52. Ross, R. and Glomset, J. A., The pathogenesis of atherosclerosis, *N. Engl. J. Med.,* 295, 369, 1976.
53. Barber, A. G., Käser-Glanzmann, R., Jakabova, M., and Lüscher, E. F., Characterization of chondroitin sulfate proteoglycan carrier for heparin neutralizing activity — (PF_4) released from human blood platelets, *Biochim. Biophys. Acta,* 286, 312, 1972.
54. Hermodson, M., Schmer, G., and Kurachi, K., Isolation, characterization and primary aminoacid sequence of human platelet factor 4, *J. Biol. Chem.,* 252, 6276, 1977.
55. Deuel, T. F., Keim, P. S., Farmer, M., and Heinrikson, R. L., Platelet factor 4: complete aminoacid sequence, *Proc. Natl. Acad. Sci. U.S.A.,* 74, 2256, 1977.
56. Morgan, F. J., Begg, G. S., and Chesterman, C. N., Primary structure of human platelet factor 4, *Thromb. Haemostasis,* 38 (Abstr.), 231, 1977b.
57. Walz, D. A., Wu, V. Y., De Lamo, R., and McCoy, L. E., Primary structure of human platelet factor 4, *Thromb. Res.,* 11, 893, 1977.
58. Hiti-Harper, J., Wohl, H., and Harper, E., Platelet factor 4: an inhibitor of collagenase, *Blood,* 50 (Abstr.), Suppl. 241, 1977.
59. Begg, S., Pepper, D. S., Chesterman, C. N., and Morgan, F. J., Complete covalent structure of human β thromboglobulin, *Biochemistry,* 17, 1739, 1978.
60. Niewiarowski, S., Rucinski, B., Millman, M., and Hawiger, J., Immunoassay of human platelet factor 4 (antiheparin factor) and its significance for evaluation of the platelet function, in Platelet Function Tests — Proceedings from the Workshop on Platelets, Philadelphia, 1976, Day, H. J., Holmsen, H., and Zucker, M. B., Eds., U.S. Government Printing Office, Washington, D.C., 1977.
61. Niewiarowski, S., Proteins secreted by the platelets, *Thromb. Haemostasis,* 38, 294, 1977.
62. Niewiarowski, S., James, P., Rucinski, B., Varma, K. G., Kueppers, F., and Watz, D. A., Separation of low affinity platelet factor 4 and β-thromboglobulin by isoelectric focusing, *Fed. Proc.,* in press.
63. Niewiarowski, S., Castor, C. W., Rucinski, B., Ritchie, J. C., and Scott, M. E., Identity of low affinity platelet factor 4 and connective tissue activating peptide III, *Fed. Proc.,* 37(Abstr.), 260, 1978.
64. Castor, C. W., Ritchie, J. C., Scott, M. E., and Whitney, S. L., Connective tissue activation. XI. Stimulation of glycosaminoglycans and DNA formation by a platelet factor, *Arthritis Rheum.,* 20, 859, 1977.
65. Legrand, Y., Caen, J. P., Robert, L., and Wautier, J. L., Platelet elastase and leukocyte elastase are two different entities, *Thromb. Haemostasis,* 37, 580, 1977.

66. **Deutsch, E., Wawersich, E., and Franke, G.,** Uber das Vorkommen eines Antiheparin-Faktors in Thrombozyten and Geweben. I. Mitteilung. Antiheparin Aktivitat der Thrombozyten, *Thromb. Diath. Haemorrh.,* 1, 3, 1957.
67. **Harada, K. and Zucker, M. B.,** Simultaneous development of platelet factor 4 activity and release of ^{14}C-serotonin, *Thromb. Diath. Haemorrh.,* 25, 41, 1971.
68. **Poplawski, A. and Niewiarowski, S.,** Method for determining antiheparin activity of platelets and erythrocytes, *Thromb. Diath. Haemorrh.,* 13, 149, 1965.
69. **Farbiszewski, R., Niewiarowski, S., Worowski, K., and Lipinski, B.,** Release of platelet factor 4 in vivo during intravascular coagulation and in thrombotic states, *Thromb. Diath. Haemorrh.,* 19, 578, 1968.
70. **Fuster, V., Kazmier, F. J., Cash, J. D., Bowie, E. J. W., and Owen, C. A., Jr.,** Assay of platelet factor 4 in plasma, *Mayo Clin. Proc.,* 48, 103, 1974.
71. **Rapaport, S. I. and Ames, S. B.,** Antiheparin activity of erythrocyte hemolysate, *Proc. Soc. Exp. Biol. Med.,* 95, 158, 1957.
72. **Saba, H. J., Roberts, H. R., and Merion, J. C.,** Antiheparin activity of lysosomal cationic proteins from polymorphonuclear leukocytes, *Blood,* 31, 369, 1968.
73. **Godal, H. C.,** The assay of heparin in thrombin systems, *Scand. J. Clin. Lab. Invest.,* 13, 153, 1961.
74. **Godal, H. C.,** Heparin tolerance and the plasma protein, *Scand. J. Clin. Lab. Invest.,* 13, 314, 1961.
75. **Cotton, R. C. and Johnson, F. L.,** Plasma antiheparin activity and the heparin precipitable fraction of plasma in rheumatoid arthritis, *Ann. Rheum. Dis.,* 27, 425, 1968.
76. **Beaumont, J. L. and Lemort, N.,** Les immunoglobulines antiheparine. Un facteur de thromboses, d'hyperlipidemies et d'atherosclerose, *Pathol. Biol.,* 22, 67, 1973.
77. **Walsh, P. N., Biggs, R., and Gagnatelli, G.,** Platelet antiheparin activity. Assay based on factor-Xa inactivation by heparin and antifactor Xa, *Br. J. Haematol.,* 26, 405, 1974.
78. **Niewiarowski, S., Zywicka, H., and Latallo, Z.,** Coagulation disorders in thrombocythaemia. A study of seven cases, *Thromb. Diath. Haemorrh.,* 7, 114, 1962.
79. **Fuster, V., Bowie, E. J. W., Kazmier, F. J., and Owen, C. A., Jr.,** Plasma platelet factor 4 like activity reflecting rate of platelet consumption in chronically induced intravascular coagulation in dog, *Thromb. Res.,* 4, 274, 1974.
80. **O'Brien, J. R., Etherington, M., Jamieson, S., Lawford, P., Sussex, J., and Lincoln, S. V.,** Heparin neutralizing activity — test in the diagnosis of acute myocardial infarction, *J. Clin. Pathol.,* 28, 975, 1975.
81. **Handin, R. I.,** Clinical application of a radioimmunoassay for platelet factor 4, in Platelet Function Tests — Proceedings from the Workshop on Platelets, Philadelphia, 1976, Day, H. J., Holmsen, H., and Zucker, M. B., Eds., U.S. Government Printing Office, Washington, D.C., 1977.
82. **Gjesdahl, K.,** Platelet factor 4 (PF_4): an electroimmunoassay for PF_4 in human plasma, *Scand. J. Haematol.,* 13, 232, 1974.
83. **Mürer, E. H., Davenport, K., and Day, H. J.,** Metabolic aspects of the secretion of stored compounds from blood platelets. IV. Effects of ionophore X537A on washed platelets, *Biochim. Biophys. Acta,* 428, 369, 1976.
84. **Hawiger, J. and Niewiarowski, S.,** Antiheparin factor of human platelets (platelet factor 4, PF_4). immunological detection in plasma, serum and during endotoxin induced release reaction in vitro, *Blood,* 46 (Abstr.), 1020, 1975.
85. **Niewiarowski, S., Kirby, E., and Stocker, K.,** Thrombocytin — a novel platelet activating enzyme from Bothrops atrox venom, *Thromb. Res.,* 10, 863, 1977.
86. **Hennesy, V. L., Jr., Hicks, R. F., Niewiarowski, S., Edmunds, L. H., and Colman, R. W.,** Function of human platelet during extracorporeal circulation, *Am. J. Physiol.,* 1977.
87. **Addomizio, V. P., Macarek, E. J., Niewiarowski, S., Colman, R. W., and Edmunds, L. H., Jr.,** Preservation of human platelets with prostaglandin E_1 during in vitro cardiopulmonary bypass, *Circ. Res.,* in press, 1979.
88. **Ludlam, C. A. and Cash, J. D.,** Studies on the liberation of β-thromboglobulin from human platelets in vitro, *Br. J. Haematol.,* 33, 239, 1976.
89. **Levine, S. P. and Krentz, L. S.,** Development of a radioimmunoassay for human platelet factor 4, *Thromb. Res.,* 11, 673, 1977.
90. **Bolton, A. E., Ludlam, C. A., Pepper, D. S., Moore, S., and Cash, J. D.,** A radioimmunoassay for platelet factor 4, *Thromb. Res.,* 8, 51, 1976.
91. **Handin, R. I., McDonough, M. and Lesch, M.,** Elevation of platelet factor 4 in acute myocardial infarction: measurement by radioimmunoassay, *J. Lab. Clin. Med.,* 91, 340, 1978.
92. **Chesterman, C. N., McGready, J. R., Doyle, D. J., and Morgan, F. J.,** Plasma levels of platelet factor 4 measured by radioimmunoassay, *Br. J. Haematol.,* 40, 489, 1978.
93. **Kaplan, K. L., Nossel, H. L., Drilling, M., and Lesznik, G.,** Radioimmunoassay of platelet factor 4 and β thromboglobulin — development and application to studies of platelet release in relation to fibrinopeptide A generation, *Br. J. Haematol.,* 39, 129, 1978.

94. **Ludlam, C. A., Moore, S., Bolton, A. E., Pepper, D. S., and Cash, J. D.**, The release of a human platelet specific protein measured by a radioimmunoassay, *Thromb. Res.*, 6, 543, 1975.
95. **Ludlam, C. A., Bolton, A. E., Moore, S., and Cash, J. D.**, New rapid method for diagnosis of deep venous thrombosis, *Lancet*, 3, 259, 1975.
96. **Boughton, B. J., Allington, M. J., and King, A.**, Platelet and plasma β thromboglobulin in myeloproliferative syndromes and secondary thrombocytosis, *Br. J. Haematol.*, 40, 125, 1978.
97. **Burrows, A. W., Chavin, S. I., and Hockaday, T. D. R.**, Plasma thromboglobulin concentrations in diabetes mellitus, *Lancet*, 1, 235, 1978.
98. **Preston, F. E., Ward, J. D., Marcola, B. H., Porter, N. R., and Timperley, W. R.**, Elevated β thromboglobulin levels and circulating platelet aggregates in diabetic microangiopathy, *Lancet*, 1, 238, 1978.
99. **Dawes, J., Smith, R. C., and Pepper, D. S.**, The release, distribution and clearance of human β thromboglobulin and platelet factor 4, *Thromb. Res.*, 12, 851, 1978.
100. **Guzzo, J., Reo, A. K., Berman, I., James, P., and Niewiarowski, S.**, Increased levels of platelet specific protein in plasma and urine of patients with chronic renal failure, *Clin. Res.*, in press, 1979.
101. **Ellis, J. B., Krentz, L. S., and Levine, S. P.**, Increased plasma platelet factor 4 (PF4) in patients with coronary artery disease, *Circulation*, 57—58 (Abstr.), Suppl. 2, 116, 1978.
102. **Levine, S. P., Lindenfeld, J., Raymond, N. M., and Krentz, L. S.**, Plasma platelet factor 4 in angiographically defined coronary artery disease, *Clin. Res.*, (Abstr.), in press, 1979.
103. **Paul, D. and Niewiarowski, S.**, unpublished observations.

QUALITATIVE ABNORMALITIES OF PLATELET FUNCTION HEREDITARY

Douglas A. Triplett

The interest in disorders of hemostasis caused by qualitative platelet abnormalities has been stimulated by the development of various in vitro methods of studying platelet function. Many different techniques have been utilized, including platelet aggregation, platelet retention in glass bead columns, platelet sizing, and the ultrastructural study of the platelet anatomy by electron microscopy.

Disorders of platelet function are difficult to classify because of the rarity of many forms, incompletely studied cases, and nosologic confusion. In the past, the terms "thrombocytopathia" or "thrombopathia" were used to identify any bleeding disorder in which a defect in platelet function was found other than the type of defect seen in Glanzmann's disease. Both of these terms have also been used to refer to patients who had abnormalities in platelet factor 3. The popularity of these terms was due to a lack of specific tests of platelet function, such as aggregation and retention, with which such patients could be more accurately characterized and classified as to their functional abnormality. Prior to 1967, the majority of patients described in the literature were diagnosed by demonstrating a decreased availability or content of platelet factor 3. These patients typically had normal platelet counts with a long bleeding time and abnormalities in platelet factor 3 content or availability. The clinical picture was extremely variable.

With the use of the newer procedures available in the hemostasis laboratory, such patients can be more comprehensively evaluated and better classified as to the underlying functional abnormality. Therefore, the terms "thrombopathia" and "thrombocytopathia" should be discarded, because of their past association and identification with abnormalities of platelet factor 3. Recent work in this field has indicated that isolated abnormalities of platelet factor 3 are indeed quite rare.

Although inherited disorders of platelet function are relatively rare and are usually associated with histories of mild bleeding, they can be responsible for serious bleeding at the time of surgery. Several reviews of qualitative platelet functional disorders have appeared, the most recent being those of Stuart[1] and Weiss.[2]

Platelet functional abnormalities can be logically classified on the basis of the various processes that occur during the platelet participation in hemostasis, ie., adhesion, release, and aggregation (Tables 1 and 2).*

The initial step in the evaluation of a patient with a history of easy bruising or bleeding is to attempt to distinguish a deficiency of a plasma coagulation protein from a platelet defect. A good clinical history is invaluable. In platelet dysfunctional states, the bleeding is usually superficial, in contrast to bleeding into joints and large muscle masses, which is quite typical of coagulation protein defects such as hemophilia A (Table 3).

The usual screening tests in the laboratory, such as a partial thromboplastin time, prothrombin time, template bleeding time, platelet count, and an examination of the peripheral smear for platelet morphology, will generally be adequate for the primary classification of the patient (Figures 1 and 2).

Occasionally, hereditary qualitative abnormalities of platelet function are associated with thrombocytopenia. Therefore, it is necessary to consider platelet dysfunctional syndromes in all patients with histories of chronic thrombocytopenic purpura. The clinical history should include the age at which the first evidence of bruising and bleeding manifested itself as well as an extensive family history.

* All figures and tables for this chapter follow text.

Platelet sizing has been useful in the classification of thrombocytopenic states, since large platelets generally signify young platelets and suggest accelerated platelet destruction as a mechanism for the reduced platelet count. This only holds true in acquired conditions. In the hereditary platelet dysfunctional states, platelet size is determined more by the nature of the intrinsic defect than by the mean cell age.

In patients with thrombocytopenia, additional studies may be necessary, such as bone marrow aspiration, platelet kinetic studies, tests for platelet antibodies, and electron microscopic examination of the platelets (Table 4).

Differentiation from acquired states of platelet dysfunction must also be made. The most important acquired platelet dysfunctional states are those related to drug ingestion. Therefore, an extensive history regarding prescription drugs as well as proprietary medications must be taken.

Once it is established that the defect lies in the platelets and is inherited, additional tests of platelet function should be utilized to appropriately characterize and define the nature of the defect.

Table 1
CLASSIFICATION OF HEREDITARY QUALITATIVE PLATELET DISORDERS

	Ref.
Abnormalities of Platelet Adhesiveness	
von Willebrand's syndrome	3—10
Bernard-Soulier syndrome	11—14
Impaired adhesion to collagen	—
Platelet membrane abnormality	15, 16
Intrinsic collagen abnormality	17
Abnormalities of Primary Aggregation	
Glanzmann's thrombasthenia	18—22
Essential athrombia	23—25
Abnormalities of Secondary Aggregation	
Storage pool disease	26—29
Hermansky-Pudlak syndrome	30, 31
Wiskott-Aldrich syndrome	32, 33
Thrombocytopenia with absent radii	34
Chediak-Higashi syndrome	35, 36
"Aspirin-like" defect	37
Cyclooxygenase deficiency	38
Thromboxane synthetase deficiency	39
Phospholipase A_2 deficiency	—
Other hereditary diseases with platelet "release" abnormalities	—
May Hegglin anomaly	40
Marfan's syndrome	41
Ehlers Danlos syndrome	42
Pseudoxanthoma elasticum	43
Osteogenesis imperfecta	43
Hurlers syndrome	43
Hunters syndrome	43
Glycogen storage disease (Type 1)	44, 45
Isolated Deficiency of Platelet Factor 3	
	46
Glucose-6 — phosphate dehydrogenase deficiency	47

Table 1 (Continued)
CLASSIFICATION OF HEREDITARY QUALITATIVE PLATELET DISORDERS

Disorders of Platelet Function Associated with Plasma Coagulation	
Factor deficiency	—
Afibrinogenemia	48
Factor VIII deficiency	49, 50
Factor IX deficiency	51
Miscellaneous	
Macrothrombocytopenia, nephritis, deafness	52, 53
Gray platelet syndrome	54
Swiss cheese platelet	55
Down's syndrome	56
Complement (C_2 component) deficiency	57
Cronberg-Nilsson syndrome	58
Progressive muscular dystrophy	59

Table 2
CLINICAL AND LABORATORY FEATURES OF HEREDITARY FUNCTIONAL PLATELET DISORDERS

	Platelet							Platelet function tests										
	Heredity	Platelet count	Platelet size	Membrane	Storage pool	Prostaglandin	Release reaction	Bleeding time	Platelet retention	ADP aggregation	Epinephrine aggregation	Collagen aggregation	Ristocetin	Platelet factor 3	Clot retraction	Baumgartner-adhesion	Baumgartner-aggregation	Remarks
Abnormalities of adhesion																		
von Willebrand's syndrome	AD	N	N	N	N	N	N	P	D	N	N	N	D	N	N	D	N	Factor VIII decreased, characteristic transfusion response
Bernard-Soulier	AR	D	L	(D-GP),I	N	N	N	P	D	N	N	N	D	N	N	D	N	Membrane glycoprotein I is decreased, decreased sialic acid
Abnormalities primary aggregation																		
Glantzmann's	AR	N	N	(D-GP),II-III	N	N	N	P	D	A	A	A	D-N	D	A	N	A	Membrane glycoprotein II, III decreased, decreased sialic acid and fibrinogen
Essential athrombia	AR	N	N	?	N	N	N	P	D	A	A	A	N	D	D	N	A	Detectable clot retraction
Abnormalities secondary aggregation																		
Storage pool deficiency	AD-V	N	N	N	D	N	D	P	D	D, 2nd	D, 2nd	D	V	D	N	N	D	Absent dense bodies on EM
Wiskott-Aldrich	SL	D	Sm	N	D	?	N	P	D	D, 2nd	D, 2nd	D	N	D	N	N	D	Eczema, decreased IgM, infections
Hermansky-Pudlak	AR	N	N	N	D	N	N	P	D	D, 2nd	D, 2nd	D	N	V	N	N	D	Albinism, ceroid storage cells in bone marrow

Table 2 (continued)
CLINICAL AND LABORATORY FEATURES OF HEREDITARY FUNCTIONAL PLATELET DISORDERS

		Platelet			Platelet function tests													
	Heredity	Platelet count	Platelet size	Membrane	Storage pool	Prostaglandin	Release reaction	Bleeding time	Platelet retention	ADP aggregation	Epinephrine aggregation	Collagen aggregation	Ristocetin	Platelet factor 3	Clot retraction	Baumgartner-adhesion	Baumgartner-aggregation	Remarks
					Abnormalities secondary aggregation													
Thrombocytopenia absent radii	AR	D	N	N	D	N	N	P	D	D, 2nd	D, 2nd	D	N	V	N	N	D	Multiple congenital abnormalities
Chediak-Higashi	AR	N	N	N	D	N	N	N-P	D	D, 2nd	D, 2nd	D	N	V	N	N	D	Albinism, giant granules in leukocytes
"Aspirin-like deficiency																		
Cyclooxygenase deficiency	?	N	N	N	N	D	D	N-P	D	D, 2nd	D, 2nd	D	N	V	N	N	D	Mimics defect of aspirin ingestion
Thromboxane synthesis deficiency	?	N	N	N	N	D	D	N-P	D	D, 2nd	D, 2nd	D	N	V	N	N	D	—
Other "release" abnormalities																		
May-Hegglin	AD	D-N	L	?	N-D	?	N	P	?	N	?	D	N	N	N	?	?	Döhle bodies in granulocytes
Glycogen storage disease, Type I	AR	N	N	?	?	?	N	P	D	D, 2nd	D, 2nd	D	N	N	N	?	?	Defect corrected by treating metabolic disorder
Ehlers Danlos	AD	N	L	N	N	?	D	P	N	D, 2nd	D, 2nd	D	N	D	N	?	?	"Cigarette paper" scars, abnormal elastic tissue
Other connective tissue disorders	AR	N	L	N	N	?	D	P	N	D, 2nd	D, 2nd	D	N	?	N	?	?	Marfans, pseudoxanthoma, osteogenesis imperfecta, etc.
Deficiency of PF-3	AR	N	N	N	N	N	N	N-P	N	N	N	N	N	D	N	N	N	Rare abnormality
Afibrinogenemia	AR	N	N	N	N	N	D*	P	D	D*	D*	D*	N	D*	N	D*	D*	*Corrected by fibrinogen

Table 2 (continued)
CLINICAL AND LABORATORY FEATURES OF HEREDITARY FUNCTIONAL PLATELET DISORDERS

		Platelet						Platelet function tests										
	Heredity	Platelet count	Platelet size	Membrane	Storage pool	Prostaglandin	Release reaction	Bleeding time	Platelet retention	ADP aggregation	Epinephrine aggregation	Collagen aggregation	Ristocetin	Platelet factor 3	Clot retraction	Baumgartner-adhesion	Baumgartner-aggregation	Remarks
Abnormalities secondary aggregation																		
Factor VIII deficiency, release abnormality	V	N-D	N	?	D	?	?	P	D	D, 2nd	D, 2nd	D	N	D	N	N	D	May mimic von Willebrand's Syndrome
Macrothrombocytopenia nephritis, deafness	AD	D	L	D-S	?	?	?	P	D	D	D	D	N	D	N	?	?	Foam cells in renal interstitial tissue
Miscellaneous																		
Gray platelet syndrome																		
	?	D	L	N	N	N	N	P	N	N	N	N	N	?	N	?	?	

Note:

AD — Autosomal dominant
AR — Autosomal recessive
SL — Sex-linked recessive
V — Variable
N — Normal

D — Decreased
P — Prolonged
L — Large
GP — Glycoprotein
S — Sialic acid

A — Absent
? — Not known
Sm — Small

From Triplett, D. A., "Qualitative, or Functional, Disorders of Platelets," in Triplett, D. A., et al: *Platelet Function: Laboratory Evaluation and Clinical Application* (Chicago: American Society of Clinical Pathologists, 1978). Used by permission.

Table 3
CLINICAL MANIFESTATIONS IN PATIENTS WITH HEREDITARY COAGULATION AND PLATELET DISORDERS

Findings	Disorders of coagulation	Disorders of platelets or vessels ("purpuric" disorders)
Petechiae	Rare	Characteristic
Deep dissecting hematomas	Characteristic	Rare
Superficial ecchymoses	Common; usually large and solitary	Characteristic; usually small and multiple
Hemarthrosis	Characteristic	Rare
Delayed bleeding	Common (eg., following tooth extraction, often 1—4 hr later)	Rare, usually starts immediately
Bleeding from superficial cuts and scratches	Minimal	Persistent; can be profuse
Sex of patient	80—90% of hereditary forms occur in males (only)	More common in females
Mucosal bleeding	Minimal	Usual clinical picture (epistaxis, gingival bleeding, menorrhagia, etc.)
Bleeding increased by aspirin, and other antiinflammatory drugs	Yes	Yes
Positive family history	Common	Unusual

Table 4
ULTRASTRUCTURAL FEATURES OF HEREDITARY QUALITATIVE PLATELET DISORDERS

Ultrastructural divisions with associated platelet disorders	Dense bodies	Other organelles, granules, and mitochondria	Nonmetabolic adenine nucleotides	Serotonin	Calcium	Enzymes and biosynthesis	Tubular system	Cytoplasm	Surface membrane
Organelle Zone — associated diseases									
Hermansky-Pudlak syndrome	Reduced number or absent; reduced ADP[a] and serotonin content		Reduced pool; insufficient ADP for irreversible aggregation	Very low levels; normal uptake; quickly saturated; discharged as metabolites	Reduced concentration in dense bodies	Defective synthesis or degradation of prostaglandins			
Storage Pool disease	Reduced number		Very deficient storage pool; ADP more reduced than ATP	Reduced level in proportion to ATP reduction; normal uptake; quickly saturated; discharged as metabolites; released slowly		Very deficient ability to synthesize intermediates of prostaglandins biosynthesis			
Chediak-Higashi syndrome	Normal number	Acid phosphatase in one type of granule	Decreased level	Low or absent level					

Table 4 (Continued)
ULTRASTRUCTURAL FEATURES OF HEREDITARY QUALITATIVE PLATELET DISORDERS

Ultrastructural divisions with associated platelet disorders	Dense bodies	Other organelles, granules, and mitochondria	Nonmetabolic adenine nucleotides	Serotonin	Calcium	Enzymes and biosynthesis	Tubular system	Cytoplasm	Surface membrane
Organelle Zone — associated diseases									
Hereditary macrothrombocytopenia nephritis and deafness		Uneven distribution of granules							
Other storage pool diseases: Wiskott-Aldrich syndrome, thrombocytopenia with absent radii (TAR baby syndrome)	Normal number; deficient structure	Normal number; 20% bizarre structure	Decreased level	Normal uptake; discharge amine rapidly; reduced release		Synthesize prostaglandin endoperoxides normally			
Gray platelet syndrome	Normal number	Numerous mitochondria; few granules						Giant bags of cytoplasm with no organelles; large vacuoles	
May-Hegglin anomaly		Increased number of giant granules							

Table 4 (Continued)
ULTRASTRUCTURAL FEATURES OF HEREDITARY QUALITATIVE PLATELET DISORDERS

Ultrastructural divisions with associated platelet disorders	Dense bodies	Other organelles, granules, and mitochondria	Nonmetabolic adenine nucleotides	Serotonin	Calcium	Enzymes and biosynthesis	Tubular system	Cytoplasm	Surface membrane
Primary release defects			Normal level; unable to secrete	Normal level; unable to secrete		Deficient in enzymes for prostaglandin biosynthesis	Increase and dilation of surface connected canalicular system; increased dense tubular system		
Cyclooxygenase deficiency									
Thromboxane synthetase deficiency									
Phospholipase deficiency									

Sol-Gel Zone — no diseases clearly documented as associated with this zone

Peripheral Zone — associated diseases

Thrombasthenia	Normal granules	Normal concentration; normal secretion	Normal concentration; normal secretion	Normal hydrolytic enzyme concentration; some deficient in enzymes for glycolysis Deficiency of glyceraldehyde 3-PO_4 dehydrogenase Other enzymes		No abnormal vacuoles	Deficient, absent, or altered glycoproteins; deficient contractile protein
Bernard-Soulier syndrome	Variation in number of granules				Prominence and hypertrophy of surface connected canalicular system and dense tubular system	Vacuolization	Lack a specific glycoprotein I

[a] ADP is adenosine diphosphate; ATP, adenosine triphosphate.

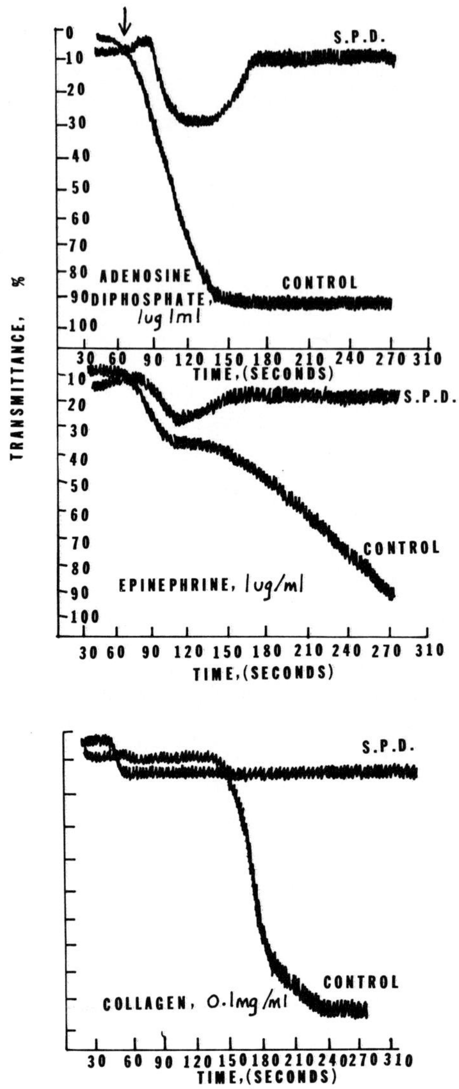

FIGURE 1. Representative aggregation tracings from a patient with storage pool disease (S.P.D.).

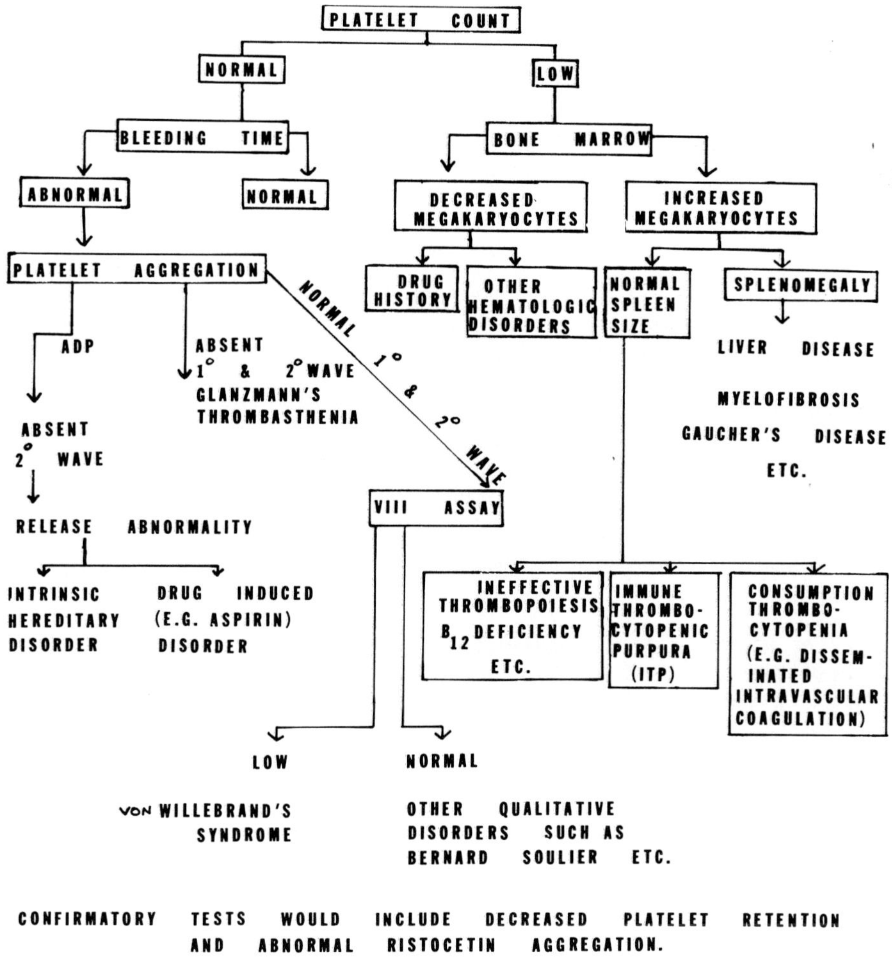

FIGURE 2. Flow diagram for diagnosis of platelet disorders.[60]

REFERENCES

1. **Stuart, M. J.,** Inherited defects of platelet function, *Semin. Hematol.,* 12, 233, 1975.
2. **Weiss, H.J.,** Platelet physiology and abnormalities of platelet function, *N. Engl. J. Med.,* 293, 580, 1975.
3. **Zimmerman, T. S., Ratnoff, O. D., and Powell, A. E.,** Immunologic differentiation of classic hemophilia (factor VIII deficiency) and von Willebrand's disease, with observations on combined deficiencies of antihemophiliac factor and proaccelerin (factor V) and an acquired circulating anticoagulant against antihemophiliac factor, *J. Clin. Invest.,* 50, 244, 1971.
4. **Howard, M. A. and Firkin, B. G.,** Ristocetin: a new tool in the investigation of platelet aggregation, *Thromb. Diath. Haemorrh.,* 26, 362, 1971.
5. **Weiss, H. J., Hoyer, L. W., Rickles, F. R., Armd, J., and Rogers, J.,** Quantitative assay of a plasma factor, deficient in von Willebrand's disease, that is necessary for platelet aggregation. Relationship to factor VIII procoagulant activity and antigen content, *J. Clin. Invest.,* 52, 2708, 1973.
6. **Tschopp, T. B., Weiss, H. J., and Baumgartner, H. R.,** Decreased adhesion of platelets to subendothelium in von Willebrand's disease, *J. Lab. Clin. Med.,* 83, 296, 1974.
7. **Jaffe, E. A.,** Endothelial cells and the biology of factor VIII, *N. Engl. J. Med.,* 296, 377, 1977.
8. **Hoyer, L. W.,** von Willebrand's disease, *Prog. Hemostasis Thromb.,* 3, 231, 1976.
9. **Gralnick, H. R., Coller, B. S., and Sultan, Y.,** Carbohydrate deficiency of the factor VIII/von Willebrand factor protein in von Willebrand's disease variants, *Science,* 192, 56, 1976.
10. **Bowie, E. J. W., Fass, D. N., Olson, J. D., and Owen, C. A., Jr.,** The spectrum of von Willebrand's disease revisited, *Mayo Clin. Proc.,* 51, 35, 1976.
11. **Bernard, J. and Soulier, J. P.,** Sur une nouvelle variete de dystrophie thrombocytaire hemorragipare congenitale, *Semin. Paris,* 24, 3217, 1948.
12. **Howard, M. A., Hutton, R. A., and Hardisty, R. M.,** Hereditary giant platelet syndrome: a new disorder of platelet function, *Br. Med. J.,* 2, 586, 1973.
13. **Caen, J. P., Michel, H., Tobelem, G., Bodevin, E., and Levy-Toledano, S.,** Adhesion and aggregation of human platelets to rabbit subendothelium. A new approach for investigation: specific antibodies, *Experientia (Basle),* 33, 91, 1977.
14. **Walsh, P., Mills, D. C., Pareti, F. I., Stewart, G. J., MacFarlane, D. E., Johnson, M. M., and Egan, J. J.,** Hereditary giant platelet syndrome: absence of collagen induced coagulant activity and deficiency of factor XI binding to platelets, *Br. J. Haematol.,* 29, 639, 1975.
15. **Hirsh, J., Castelan, D. J., and Loder, P. B.,** Spontaneous bruising associated with a defect in the interaction of platelets and connective tissue, *Lancet,* 2, 18, 1967.
16. **Papyanis, A. G., Watson-Williams, E. J., and Israels, M. C. G.,** Platelet functional abnormalities: a report of two familial defects and the interaction between collagen and platelets and ADP release, *Blood,* 38, 745, 1971.
17. **Caen, J. and Legrand, Y.,** Abnormalities in the platelet collagen reaction, *Ann. N.Y. Acad. Sci.,* 201, 194, 1972.
18. **Glanzmann, E.,** Hereditäre hämorrhagische thrombasthenie: ein beitrag zür pathologic der blütlattchen, *Jahrb. Kinderheilk.,* 88, 113, 1918.
19. **Caen, J.,** Glanzmann thrombasthenia, *Clin. Haematol.,* 1, 383, 1972.
20. **Karpatkin, S. and Weiss, H. J.,** Deficiency of glutathione peroxidase associated with high levels of reduced glutathione in Glanzmann's thrombasthenia, *N. Engl. J. Med.,* 287, 1062, 1972.
21. **Moser, K., Lechner, K., and Vinazzer, H.,** A hitherto not described enzyme defect in thrombasthenia: glutathione reductase, *Thromb. Diath. Haemorrh.,* 19, 46, 1968.
22. **Nurden, A. T. and Caen, J. P.,** An abnormal platelet glycoprotein pattern in three cases of Glanzmann's thrombasthenia, *Br. J. Haematol.,* 28, 253, 1974.
23. **Inceman, S., Unuger, A., and Aran, M.,** Essential athrombia, *Thromb. Diath. Haemorrh.,* 8, 502, 1962.
24. **Ulutin, O. N.,** Qualitative platelet disorders: classification and pathogenesis, *Ann. N.Y. Acad. Sci.,* 201, 174, 1972.
25. **Inceman, S. and Tangün, Y.,** Essential athrombia, *Thromb. Diath. Haemorrh.,* 33, 278, 1975.
26. **Weiss, H. J.,** Platelet aggregation, adhesion and adenosine diphosphate release in thrombopathia (platelet factor-3 deficiency): a comparison with Glanzmann's thrombasthenia and von Willebrand's disease, *Am. J. Med.,* 43, 570, 1967.
27. **Hardisty, R. M. and Hutton, R. A.,** Bleeding tendency associated with "new" abnormality of platelet behavior, *Lancet,* 1, 983, 1967.
28. **Pareti, F. I., Day, H. J., and Mills, D. C. B.,** Nucleotide and serotonin metabolism in patients with defective secondary aggregation, *Blood,* 44, 789, 1974.
29. **Holmsen, H. and Weiss, H. J.,** Further evidence for a deficient storage pool of adenine nucleotides in platelets from some patients with thrombocytopathia, "Storage-Pool Disease", *Blood,* 39, 197, 1972.

30. White, J. G. and Witkop, C. J., Effects of normal and aspirin platelets on defective secondary aggregation in the Hermansky-Pudlak syndrome: a test for storage pool deficient platelets, *Am. J. Pathol.*, 68, 57, 1972.
31. Witkop, C. J., White, J. G., Gerritsen, S. M., Townsend, D., and King, R. A., Hermansky-Pudlak syndrome (HPS): a proposed block in glutathione peroxidase, *Oral Surg.*, 35, 740, 1973.
32. Baldini, M. G., Nature of the platelet defect in the Wiskott-Aldrich Syndrome, *Ann. N.Y. Acad. Sci.*, 201, 437, 1972.
33. Kuramoto, A., Steiner, M., and Baldini, M. G., Lack of platelet response to stimulation in the Wiskott-Aldrich syndrome, *N. Engl. J. Med.*, 282, 475, 1970.
34. Day, H. J. and Holmsen, H., Platelet adenine nucleotide "storage pool deficiency" in thrombocytopenia absent radii syndrome, *JAMA*, 221, 1053, 1972.
35. Bell, T. G., Meyers, K. M., Prieur, D. J., Fauci, A. S., Wolff, S. M., and Padgett, G. A., Deceased nucleotide and serotonin storage associated with defective function in Chediak-Higashi syndrome cattle and human platelets, *Blood*, 48, 175, 1976.
36. Costa, J. L., Fauci, A. S., and Wolff, S. M., A platelet abnormality in the Chediak-Higashi syndrome of man, *Blood*, 48, 517, 1976.
37. Weiss, H. J., Abnormalities in platelet function due to defects in the release reaction, *Ann. N. Y. Acad. Sci.*, 201, 161, 1972.
38. Malmsten, C., Hamberg, M., Svensson, J., and Samuelsson, B., Physiological role of an endoperoxide in human platelets: hemostatic defect due to platelet cyclo-oxygenase deficiency, *Proc. Natl. Acad. Sci. U.S.A.*, 72, 1446, 1975.
39. Weiss, H. J. and Lages, B. A., Possible congenital defect in platelet thromboxane synthetase, *Lancet*, 1, 760, 1977.
40. Lüsher, J. M., Schneider, J., Mizukami, I., and Evans, R. K., The May-Hegglin anomaly: platelet function, ultrastructure and chromosome studies, *Blood*, 32, 950, 1968.
41. Estes, J. W., Carey, R. J., and Desai, R. G., Marfan syndrome: hematologic abnormalities in a family, *Arch. Intern. Med.*, 116, 889, 1965.
42. Hedner, U. and Nilsson, I. M., Platelet aggregating properties of Ehlers-Danlos Syndrome "Collagen", *Thromb. Diath. Haemorrh.*, 33, 380, 1975.
43. Estes, J. W., Platelet size and function in the inheritable disorders of connective tissue, *Ann. Intern. Med.*, 68, 1237, 1968.
44. Czapek, E., Deykin, D., and Salzman, E. W., Platelet dysfunction in glycogen storage disease type I, *Blood*, 41, 235, 1973.
45. Gilchrist, G. S., Fine, R., and Donnell, G. N., The hemostatic defect in glycogen storage disease type I, *Acta Paediatr. Scand.*, 56, 205, 1968.
46. Sultan, Y., Brouet, J. C., and Devergie, A., Isolated platelet factor 3 deficiency, *N. Engl. J. Med.*, 294, 1121, 1976.
47. Schwartz, J. P., Cooperberg, A. A., and Rosenberg, A., Platelet-function studies in patients with glucose-6-phosphate dehydrogenase deficiency, *Br. J. Haematol.*, 27, 273, 1974.
48. Inceman, S., Caen, J., and Bernard, J., Aggregation, adhesion and viscous metamorphosis of platelets in congenital fibrinogen deficiencies, *J. Lab. Clin. Med.*, 68, 21, 1966.
49. Weiss, H. J., Abnormalities of factor VIII and platelet aggregation: use of ristocetin in diagnosing the von Willebrand's syndrome, *Blood*, 45, 403, 1975.
50. Chesney, C., Colman, R. W., and Pechet, L., A syndrome of platelet release abnormality in mild hemophilia, *Blood*, 43, 821, 1974.
51. Bowie, E. J. W. and Owen, C. A., Thrombopathy, *Semin. Hematol.*, 5, 73, 1968.
52. Epstein, C. L., Sahud, M. A., Piel, C. F., Goodman, J. R., Bernfield, M. R., Kushner, J. H., and Ablin, A. R., Hereditary macrothrombocytopathia, nephritis, and deafness, *Am. J. Med.*, 52, 299, 1972.
53. Eckstein, J. D., Filip, D. J., and Watts, J. C., Hereditary thrombocytopenia, deafness and renal disease, *Ann. Intern. Med.*, 82, 639, 1975.
54. Raccuglia, G., Gray platelet syndrome — a variety of qualitative platelet disorders, *Am. J. Med.*, 51, 818, 1971.
55. Smith, T. P., Dodds, J. W., and Tartaglia, A. P., Thrombasthenic thrombopathic thrombocytopenia with giant "Swiss-cheese" platelets, *Am. J. Intern. Med.*, 79, 828, 1973.
56. Lott, I. T., Chase, T. N., and Murphy, D. L., Down's Syndrome: transport, storage and metabolism of serotonin in blood platelets, *Pediatr. Res.*, 6, 730, 1972.
57. Tobelem, G., Wautier, J. L., and Peltier, A. P., C_2 deficiency, platelet aggregation reduction and Lobstein's disease in the same family, *BioMed.*, 21, 190, 1974.
58. Cronberg, S. and Nilsson, I. M., Investigation of patients with mild thrombasthenia: a haemorrhagic disorder with prolonged bleeding time probably due to a primay platelet defect, *Acta Med. Scand.*, 183, 163, 1968.

59. **Démos, J.**, Platelet diphenol oxidases in progressive muscular dystrophy (P.M.D.), *Clin. Genet.*, 4, 79, 1973.
60. **Triplett, D. A.**, Qualitative platelet disorders, in *Platelet Function: Laboratory Evaluation and Clinical Application,* American Society of Clinical Pathologists Press, Triplett, D. A., Ed., Chicago, 1978.

ACQUIRED QUALITATIVE ABNORMALITIES OF PLATELET FUNCTION

J. Roger Edson

Introduction

The following discussion will be limited to acquired platelet disorders that may cause a bleeding tendency. After many years, methods of studying platelet function are still inexact. It is only in a relatively few disorders that the abnormality has been characterized on a biochemical basis, e.g., the inherited disorder called storage pool deficiency, where there is a deficiency of "storage pool" adenine nucleotides and serotonin normally found in the electron dense bodies. The tests of platelet function that can be applied more or less readily to clinical situations are not specific for a particular biochemical defect.

Platelet counts done by particle counting methods may occasionally grossly overestimate the true platelet count by counting particles of the same size and density as the platelets, most commonly blast cell fragments found in acute nonlymphocytic leukemias. Phase-contrast counts and careful estimates from blood films are less precise, but are not subject to this gross error. In the most commonly used platelet adhesiveness test (glass bead retention test), freshly drawn heparinized blood is passed through a plastic tube containing a large number of tiny glass beads. Normally, after the first 2 or 3 mℓ of blood have passed through the tube, most of the platelets are retained in the glass beads, so the platelet count on the effluent blood is much less than it was before the blood was passed through the glass beads. Platelet adhesiveness may be reduced in diverse inherited and acquired platelet disorders.

Platelet aggregation tests are now commonly done with one of several different commercially available "aggregometers". The test is usually set up so that one gets biphasic aggregation with epinephrine and norepinephrine, and sometimes with ADP and thrombin. Collagen characteristically gives a single phase of aggregation equivalent to the secondary aggregation with the other reagents. Tests for platelet factor 3 (platelet phospholipid) availability were commonly used 8 to 10 years ago, but in recent years they seem to have fallen out of fashion. Our own experience has been that the test usually does not distinguish normals from abnormals. In the last few years, we have used a prothrombin consumption test (one-stage assay of prothrombin in citrated plasma and anticoagulated serum from the same patient). If the plasma coagulation factors are normal, prothrombin consumption can be used as a test of platelet function. With normal plasma coagulation factor levels, prothrombin consumption may be incomplete in thrombocytopenia and in a number of platelet functional disorders. Tests of platelet factor 4 (platelet antiheparin factor) have been developed, but have not seen wide clinical application. At the present time, assay of factor VIII antigen and von Willebrand ristocetin cofactor are considered essential to the evaluation of many inherited disorders, but are not generally applicable to acquired abnormalities of platelet function.

Of all the tests of platelet function, the template modification of the Ivy bleeding time is the single most useful test. The bleeding time will be prolonged when there is "an insufficient number" of normally functioning platelets. The test nevertheless has its limitations. Some patients with significant platelet functional abnormalities (von Willebrand's syndrome, myeloproliferative disorders, hypothyroidism) may have normal bleeding times at least part of the time. Conversely, individuals whose hemostatic systems are otherwise perfectly normal may have a prolonged bleeding time because they have recently taken aspirin. In spite of their prolonged bleeding time, however, there is no evidence that such individuals have significantly increased bleeding upon operation. Finally, an examination of platelet morphology on blood films is generally worthwhile. In order to see the platelet cytoplasm adequately, smears have to be overstained with the usual Wright-Giemsa stains. In blood films made from carefully collected EDTA-anticoagulated blood, normal platelets have a mean diameter of a little over 2 μm. Morphologic abnormalities may be seen in both inherited and acquired platelet disorders. One must use great care in interpreting platelet morphology, because poor blood collection or processing technique may result in platelet activation and consequent pseudopod formation, centralization of granules, and even degranulation.

Drug-Induced Platelet Dysfunction

A large number of drugs have been reported to impair platelet function in vitro. The excellent review by Weiss in 1972 is still pertinent.[1] Of these drugs, a smaller number have been studied in vivo. Of those shown to have an in vivo effect on platelet function, only a few have clearly been shown to be associated with a bleeding tendency. Of the drugs that impair platelet function, aspirin has probably been the most widely studied. Aspirin inhibits the secondary phase of aggregation and prolongs the bleeding time. It may affect prothrombin consumption, but does not alter platelet adhesiveness. Among all the drugs that impair platelet function, aspirin stands alone in that it permanently damages the platelet population with which it comes in contact. In healthy people, the average bleeding time (5½ min) is, on the average, prolonged to over 13 min 3 hr after the ingestion of three aspirin tablets.[2] It takes several days for the bleeding time to come back to the base-line value after the single dose of aspirin. Abnormalities of secondary aggregation and collagen-induced aggregation may persist for 8 to 10 days after administration of a single dose of aspirin.

It has been postulated that the effect of aspirin is mediated through acetylation of sites on the platelet membrane, since acetic anhydride produces a similar effect, while salicylic acid does not. The final common pathway for all drugs that prevent the "release reaction" and the secondary phase of platelet aggregation appears to be through inhibition of prostaglandin synthesis. The effect of aspirin on the bleeding time of normals is grossly exaggerated when aspirin is given to an individual who already has an abnormal bleeding time. The late Dr. Armand Quick utilized this principle in the aspirin tolerance test,[3] and thought that the exaggerated prolongation of the bleeding time was specific for von Willebrand's syndrome. We now know that this is not so and that exaggerated prolongations of the bleeding time after aspirin can occur with a variety of underlying hemostatic abnormalities. Aspirin not only causes abnormal platelet aggregation in vitro and prolongs the bleeding time, it also clearly exacerbates any underlying bleeding tendency. A worse clinical bleeding tendency has been observed after aspirin ingestion in such diverse disorders as inherited factor VII deficiency, hemophilia, von Willebrand's syndrome, hypothyroidism, and myeloproliferative syndromes.

Antihistamines have repeatedly been reported to impair secondary aggregation and collagen-induced aggregation in vitro.[4] Our own studies and other studies have shown similar effects in vivo after oral administration of diphenhydramine (Benadryl). Results of studies on the effect of antihistamines on the bleeding time have not been reported. We have, however, seen clear cases of exacerbation of the bleeding tendency in hemophilia, thrombocytopenia, and uremia following administration of diphenhydramine. In contrast to the effect of aspirin, the effect of antihistamines on platelet function is reversible when the drug has been metabolized.

The large number of other drugs reported to impair platelet function includes adenosine, dipyridamole, methol xanthines, nonsteroidal antiinflammatory drugs, local anesthetics, phenothiazines, tricyclic antidepressants, sympathetic blocking agents, Colchicine, Vincristine, reserpine, and Carbenicillin. Of these, indomethacin and phenothiazines have been associated with clinical bleeding. Dilantin® has been reported to impair platelet function in vitro,[5] but hemophiliacs taking Dilantin® for seizure disorders that we have studied have had perfectly normal platelet function tests.

The foregoing discussion should indicate that, although a large number of drugs may alter platelet aggregation in vitro, not all of these are of clinical significance. The practical problem one faces is in interpretation of an abnormal set of platelet aggregation tracings. Are these due to an intrinsic platelet defect or to a drug or drugs? One cannot interpret results of platelet aggregation tests without a very careful drug history from the patient.

Uremia

Uremic bleeding was the subject of another review in 1972[6] that has not been improved upon. In uremia, the bleeding time may be prolonged, platelet adhesiveness and prothrombin consumption low, (prothrombin consumption time short), ADP-induced platelet aggregation and platelet factor 3 availability reduced, and clot retraction poor. The best evidence suggests that uremic platelet dysfunction is caused by retention of five-guanidinosuccinic acid (an abnormal urea metabolite), phenol, and hydroxyphenolic acids. It is quite clear from a number of studies that uremic platelet dysfunction and uremic bleeding can be controlled by hemodialysis; thus, whatever the substances are which are responsible for uremic platelet dysfunction, they are dialyzable. Horowitz et al. showed that guanidinosuccinic acid produced defective ADP-induced platelet factor 3 activation after 1 hr incubation with normal platelet-rich plasma.[7] Other studies have shown that phenolic acids require 2 or 3 hr of preincubation in order to impair platelet function. Guanidinosuccinic acid and phenols and hydroxyphenolic acids apparently operate by different mechanisms. Since most authors report no correlation between serum urea levels and uremic platelet dysfunction, there is no easy test or combination of tests that is diagnostic of uremic platelet dysfunction.

Patients on hemodialysis or after renal transplantation who develop bleeding complications tend to have multiple hemostatic abnormalities. We generally do not perform platelet function tests on these patients because of the high risk of contaminating the laboratory equipment with hepatitis B virus. On the hemodialysis and renal transplant services, the practice is to dialyze the bleeding patient with a serum urea nitrogen over 80 mg/dℓ, in spite of the lack of correlation between urea concentration and platelet functional abnormalities. If platelet function tests are found to be abnormal in uremia, the abnormalities can only be attributed to uremia if other causes of abnor mal platelet function can be excluded. Two final points should be made: because inhibition of normal platelet function occurs within 1 hr of incubation with quanidinosuccinic acid, platelet transfusions to the bleeding uremic patient make no sense whatsoever. To quote the last sentence of Dr. Rabiner's review, "When bleeding occurs, either spontaneously or owing to trauma, prompt, thorough dialysis is the treatment of choice."[6]

Myeloproliferative Syndromes

The chronic myeloproliferative disorders include myeloid metaplasia, chronic myelogenous leukemia, essential thrombocythemia, and polycythemia vera. While these four disorders have long been classified as more or less distinct entities, it is well recognized that individual patients may show features of more than one disorder. For example, a recent patient seen at the University of Minnesota clinically behaved as if he had essential thrombocythemia, with a platelet count that was constantly over 1.5 million per mm^3 from the time of diagnosis. His white blood count was only slightly elevated and his hemoglobin was normal. Nevertheless, because he was Philadelphia chromosome positive, he was classified as having chronic myelogenous leukemia.

With that preface, one can state that in myeloproliferative disorders, the platelet morphology is generally abnormal. Except sometimes in end-stage disease, the platelet count is usually elevated and often markedly so. Increased absolute numbers of large platelets, hypogranular and agranular platelets, platelets without pseudopods, platelets with abnormal blunted pseudopods, and abnormal giant granules may all be observed. The later the course of the disease, the more profound the platelet morphologic abnormalities are likely to be. Generally, even in fairly early disease it is not difficult to find platelets as large as red cells in blood films. With advanced disease, platelets up to 30 μm across may be observed in peripheral blood films; abnormal megakaryocytes may also be present in the peripheral blood. Early in the course of myeloproliferative syndromes, normal appearing small platelets may have centralization of granules and pseudopod formation, while hypogranular or agranular platelets of various sizes may either have abnormal pseudopods or no pseudopods at all. Platelet function abnormalities in chronic myeloproliferative disorders have been the subject of a number of reports.[8,9] Abnormalities of the bleeding time, platelet aggregation, platelet adhesiveness, platelet factor 3 availability, and prothrombin consumption have been observed. There is a tendency for catecholamine-induced aggregation to be quite abnormal in patients with polycythemia vera, essential thrombocythemia, and myeloid metaplasia. We have observed a number of such individuals who had absolutely no platelet aggregation response, either primary or secondary, to epinephrine, norepinephrine, or serotonin. There is not a consensus that the severity of abnormality of the platelet function tests in these patients correlates very well with their clinical bleeding tendency. In spite of this, at the University of Minnesota, we feel that patients with myeloproliferative syndromes who have grossly abnormal platelet function tests do have a bleeding tendency. In these cases, bleeding that is either spontaneous or due to operation or dental extraction can usually be controlled by transfusion with normal platelets.

The major points to be made here are that (1) platelet function is abnormal in chronic myeloproliferative disorders, (2) the patients may have a bleeding tendency which can be controlled by transfusion of normal platelets, and (3) the diagnosis, in an emergency, can be inferred from examination of a peripheral blood film.

It should be noted that some cases of acute nonlymphocytic leukemia have been reported to have abnormal platelet function,[9] although many patients with acute nonlymphocytic leukemia have platelet counts too low for platelet function to be adequately studied.

Dysproteinemias and Abnormally High Concentrations of Fibrinogen

A variety of hemostatic abnormalities have been reported in patients with dysproteinemias in multiple myeloma and Waldenstrom's macroglobulinemia. These abnormalities include antithrombin activity, antithromboplastin activity, inhibition of fibrin monomer polymerization, and anti-factor VIII antibody activity. Interference with platelet function has been manifested by long bleeding times, decreased platelet adhesiveness, abnormal aggregation with connective tissue, ADP, and thrombin, abnormal platelet factor 3 availability, and abnormal clot retraction.[10,11] Vigliano and Horowitz reported a single patient in whom an IgA myeloma protein interacting with connective tissue appeared to account for the patient's prolonged bleeding time.[12] Perkins et al.[11] found normal platelet adhesiveness with IgG paraproteins. Two patients with an IgA paraprotein and three patients with an IgM paraprotein who were clinical bleeders had abnormal platelet adhesiveness. Three of four patients with IgM paraproteins who were nonbleeders had low platelet adhesiveness. Perkins et al. found that 8 of 32 patients with total serum proteins over 8 g/dℓ had bleeding, whereas only one out of twelve with total serum proteins less than 8 g/dℓ had hemorrhage. Penny et al.[10] found that clinical bleeding was prevalent only in patients with levels of paraprotein in excess of 5 g/dℓ, essentially consonant with the results of Perkins et al.

In summary, abnormal proteins in macroglobulinemia and multiple myeloma may have very specific activities, including in some cases specific activities that impair hemostasis. The majority of patients with dysproteinemias, however, will have interference with fibrin monomer polymerization and platelet function when paraprotein concentrations are over 5 g/dℓ. Thus evaluation of the bleeding patient should include examination of the blood film (for rouleaux formation), serum protein electrophoresis, and sometimes urine protein immunoelectrophoresis. If an abnormal protein is found to be present, an extensive investigation may be necessary to define the nature of its effect on hemostasis, if any. It is important to note that a number of reports indicate that plasmapheresis is effective in improving or totally correcting hemostasis in these patients.

Abnormal platelet function in patients with hemophilia who had marked hyperfibrinogenemia after repeated transfusions with cyroprecipitate was reported by Hathaway et al.[13] Tests reported to be abnormal included bleeding time, platelet adhesiveness, platelet aggregation to ADP, and platelet factor 3 release. Hathaway et al. cite the fibrinogen concentration in only one of their patients: 1.30 g/dℓ. Several years ago at the University of Minnesota, we observed abnormal platelet function tests in hemophiliacs who had received large amounts of cryoprecipitate or in hemophiliacs with inhibitors that had received excessively large amounts of glycine-precipitated concentrate. Our patients with abnormal platelet function all had fibrinogen concentrations substantially over 1.0 g/dℓ. In contrast, we have studied two other hemophiliac patients who had been treated with commercial concentrate and who had peak fibrinogen concentrations of approximately 0.80 g/dℓ: their platelet function tests were normal. It should be pointed out that the cryoprecipitated fibrinogen in cryoprecipitate is not really a normal fibrinogen. Patients transfused with cryoprecipitate, as noted by Hathaway et al., develop elevated fibrinogen/fibrin split product levels in serum and prolonged thrombin times as well as abnormal platelet function. Thus, in the hemophiliac patient receiving repeated doses of cryoprecipitate, there is a minimum concentration of fibrinogen associated with platelet dysfunction — a situation analogous to that in the dysproteinemias.

Hypothyroidism

In hypothyroidism, deficiencies of factors VII, VIII, and IX and XI have been reported. In 1975, we reported a series of 17 patients with hypothyroidism in whom the most consistent hemostatic abnormality was low platelet adhesiveness, found in three fourths of the patients.[14] In patients who did not have intercurrent disease, the bleeding time was also prolonged. Several of the patients with hypothyroidism clearly had a bleeding tendency in association with their abnormal hemostatic profile. Since that report was published, we have studied a few other patients, with similar findings. Although we have not done factor VIII antigen or ristocetin cofactor assays on patients with severe hypothyroidism, in some respects, the disorder appears to be similar to an acquired von Willebrand's syndrome. The platelet aggregation tests are normal, and we have found bleeding to stop in two patients with hypothyroidism who were transfused with cryoprecipitate. The matter clearly deserves further investigation. The importance of this entity lies in the fact that patients may have significant hemostatic abnormalities without exhibiting any of the more classical signs and symptoms of hypothyroidism. One must think of the entity and do the appropriate thyroid function tests in order to rule it out.

Morphologic Abnormalities of Platelets That May be Associated With Abnormal Platelet Function

In megaloblastic anemias, all three myeloid cell lines are usually involved: platelets, granulocytes, and erythrocytes. Since the turnover of granulocytes and platelets is more rapid than that of erythrocytes, the morphologic abnormalities are more likely to appear in these two cell lines first. In megaloblastic anemias, there is generally a pancytopenia. The platelets are generally somewhat larger than normal and usually average over 3 μm in diameter on Wright-stained EDTA blood films. The platelets tend to be more uniformly large, rather than showing the marked anisocytosis common in myeloproliferative syndromes. In common with myeloproliferative syndromes, however, the platelets are likely to be hypogranular to agranular and occasionally have abnormally large granules. There tend to be no pseudopods, and if they are present, they are blunted instead of the normal thread-like type. We have observed this constellation of morphologic findings in a number of patients documented to have folate deficiency. The patients that we have seen had all been on bizarre weight-reducing diets, so unfortunately it is not even clear that the morphologic abnormalities were due to folate deficiency alone. To my knowledge, platelet function in megaloblastic anemias has not been the subject of any report.

In iron deficiency, there may be either a thrombocytopenia or thrombocytosis, but thrombocytosis is more common.[15] The platelets are uniformly small, and the mean platelet diameter on Wright-stained EDTA blood films may be less than 1.5 μm. We have studied a few patients who have had intrinsic platelet defects and iron deficiency in whom the platelet function improved but did not normalize after treatment with iron. No reports on platelet function in uncomplicated iron deficiency have been published.

Patients with autoimmune thrombocytopenic purpura have been reported to have normal bleeding times even when the platelet counts were quite low.[16] In contrast, we have observed a few patients with autoimmune thrombocytopenic purpura and with lupus erythematosis and thrombocytopenia on an immune basis in whom platelet function was abnormal and in whom no explanation other than immune damage could be postulated. In autoimmune thrombocytopenic purpura, the mean platelet diameter is usually markedly increased (the more severe the thrombocytopenia, the larger the remaining platelets), and the platelets are generally well granulated. The normal morphologic appearance (abnormal in size only) is more in keeping with the observations of Harker and Slichter[16] than with our own.

This heterogenous group of disorders clearly deserves more investigation. In patients with megaloblastic anemias or iron deficiency in whom there is uncontrollable bleeding, platelet transfusions should be considered on the basis of the morphologic abnormalities alone, pending availability of further information.

Scurvy

Abnormal platelet adhesiveness has been reported in scorbutic guinea pigs,[17] and abnormal bleeding is one of the features of scurvy. Vitamin C deficiency uncomplicated by other vitamin deficiencies is unlikely to be observed in the U.S. at the present time. Nevertheless, the possibility of vitamin C deficiency contributing to a hemorrhagic diathesis should be kept in mind.

Liver Disease

I have purposely left the discussion of liver disease for the end of this section. Hemostatic alterations in liver disease may be extremely complex. Multiple plasma coagulation factor abnormalities may be present. Thrombocytopenia may have several causes: splenic sequestration, accelerated consumption in low grade intravascular coagulation, and deficient production due to generalized marrow suppression, acute alcohol toxicity, or folate and possible other dietary deficiencies. Horowitz[7] reported abnormal ADP-induced platelet factor 3 availability in 17 of 17 patients with liver disease, although the types of liver disease were not specified. The possibility that the morphologically abnormal platelets in megaloblastic anemias may be functionally abnormal was suggested above. Abnormal platelet function due to bilirubin has been reported.[17] Abnormal function in the thromboplastin generation test was found when platelets had been exposed to bilirubin concentrations greater than 15 mg/dℓ for 1 hr. Platelets from four of eight infants with bilirubin over 18 mg/dℓ functioned abnormally in the thromboplastin generation test. ADP-induced platelet factor 3 activation was inhibited by exposure to bilirubin concentrations over 10 mg/dℓ for 1 hr. Some inhibition of clot retraction with bilirubin concentrations greater than 15 mg.dℓ was also observed. Thus, in liver disease, both intrinsic platelet abnormalities and inhibition of platelet function by bilirubin may be present.

Summary

No effort has been made to present a comprehensive bibliography. I have touched on the major acquired qualitative abnormalities of platelet function. From a clinical standpoint, it is important to note that this group of entities exists. In patients with unexplained bleeding, or in patients with serious bleeding that seems difficult to control, the possibility that one or more of these entities might be present should always be considered.

REFERENCES

1. Weiss, H. J., The pharmacology of platelet inhibition, in *Progress in Hemostasis and Thrombosis,* Vol. 1, Spaet, T. H., Ed., Grune & Stratton, New York, 1972, 199.
2. Mielke, C. H., Jr., Kaneshiro, M. M., Maher, I. A., Weiner, J. M., and Rapaport, S. I., The standardized normal Ivy bleeding time and its prolongation by aspirin, *Blood,* 34, 204, 1969.
3. Quick, A. J., *Bleeding Problems in Clinical Medicine,* W. B. Saunders, Philadelphia, 1970, 40.
4. Warlow, C., Ogston, D., and Douglas, A. S., The effect of chlorpromazine and antihistamines on human blood platelets in vivo and in vitro, *Bibl. Anat.,* 12, 249, 1973.
5. Rodman, N. F., McDevitt, N. B., and Almond, J. R., Platelet function inhibition by diphenylhydantoin, *Fed. Proc.,* 30(Abstr.), 285, 1971.
6. Rabiner, S. F., Uremic bleeding, in *Progress in Hemostasis and Thrombosis,* Vol. 1, Spaet, T. H., Ed., Grune & Stratton, New York, 1972, 233.
7. Horowitz, H. I., Cohen, B. D., Martinez, P., and Papoyoanou, M. F., Defective ADP-induced platelet factor 3 activation in uremia, *Blood,* 30, 331, 1967.
8. Neemeh, J. A., Bowie, E. J. W., Thompson, J. H., Didishiem, P., and Owen, C. A., Quantitation of platelet aggregation in myeloproliferative disorders, *Am. J. Clin. Path.,* 57, 336, 1972.
9. Cardamone, J. M., Edson, J. R., McArthur, J. R., and Jacob, H. S., Abnormalities of platelet function in myeloproliferative disorders, *JAMA,* 221, 270, 1972.
10. Penny, R., Castaldi, P. A., and Whitsed, H. M., Inflammation and hemostasis in paraproteinemias, *Br. J. Haematol,* 20, 35, 1971.
11. Perkins, H. A., MacKenzie, M. R., and Fudenberg, H. H., Hemostatic defects in dysproteinemias, *Blood,* 35, 695, 1970.
12. Vigliano, E. M. and Horowitz, H. I., Bleeding syndrome in a patient with IgA myeloma: interaction of protein and connective tissue, *Blood,* 29, 823, 1967.
13. Hathaway, W. E., Mahasandana, C., Clarke, J., and Humbert, J. R., Paradoxical bleeding in intensively transfused hemophiliacs: alteration of platelet function, *Transfusion,* 13, 6, 1973.
14. Edson, J. R., Fecher, D. R., and Doe, R. P., Low platelet adhesiveness and other hemostatic abnormalities in hypothyroidism, *Ann. Intern. Med.,* 82, 342, 1975.
15. Choi, S. I. and Simone, J. V., Platelet production in experimental iron deficiency anemia, *Blood,* 42, 219, 1973.
16. Harker, L. A. and Slichter, S. J., The bleeding time as a screening test for evaluation of platelet function, *New Engl. J. Med.,* 287, 155, 1972.
17. Born, G. V. R. and Wright, H. P., Platelet adhesiveness in experimental scurvy, *Lancet,* 1, 477, 1967.
18. Suvansri, U., Cheung, W. H., and Sawitsky, A., The effect of bilirubin on the human platelet, *J. Pediatr.,* 74, 240, 1969.

VON WILLEBRAND'S DISEASE

E. J. W. Bowie and C. A. Owen, Jr.

Von Willebrand's disease has always been a puzzling disorder, but in recent years a number of discoveries have been helpful in integrating its diverse clinical and laboratory manifestations. This chapter will attempt to clarify these involved and interdependent developments.

In 1926, the Finnish internist Erik von Willebrand reported a family of bleeders in the Åland Islands in the Gulf of Bothnia.[1,2] He initially studied a 5-year-old girl, four of whose seven sisters had bled to death. The affected islanders had a history of bleeding, mainly from the skin and mucous membranes. Epistaxis, particularly early in life, was a common symptom. Frequently there was bleeding from the gums, and the shedding of deciduous teeth was often associated with hemorrhage. Menorrhagia was extremely common. Some of the patients who had a more severe form of the disease experienced gastrointestinal bleeding, hematuria, and hemarthroses. The disease was autosomal and its expressivity was quite variable. It was inherited directly by the child from the parents and occurred equally in both sexes.

In most patients, von Willebrand found that the bleeding time was prolonged, and he suspected that the prolongation was due to an abnormality of the platelets and capillaries. Since that time a decrease in the level of factor VIII (antihemophilic factor) has been described.[3-5] Recent developments relating to these various abnormalities will be discussed in detail below. They include prolongation of the bleeding time, abnormalities of platelet function, and altered plasmatic coagulation.

Prolongation of the Bleeding Time

In the severe forms of von Willebrand's disease, both the Duke and the Ivy bleeding time is prolonged. It has been suggested that the absence of a plasmatic factor may cause the prolongation of bleeding time in the same way that the absence of a plasmatic factor may cause platelet dysfunction. It was shown, for example, that transfusing blood or fresh frozen plasma would shorten the Duke bleeding time.[6,7] A subfraction (I-O) of Cohn fraction I from normal subjects or even from patients with classic hemophilia corrected or at least shortened the Duke bleeding time for more than 24 hr.[8-17] This fraction produced no corrective effect of the bleeding time when it was made from patients with von Willebrand's disease.

The Ivy bleeding time has been corrected by a fraction of Cohn fraction I made by precipitation with 3% alcohol,[18] and Perkins[19] found that a similar correction could be obtained by using a transfusion of cryoprecipitate. With the use of a method in which the amount of blood from the bleeding time incision was quantitated,[20] the effect of transfusions on a patient with von Willebrand's disease was measured and the amount of blood flowing from the wound was found to be decreased. The work of Bowie and Owen[21] suggests that the response to plasma or cyroprecipitate may result in normalization of the bleeding time or platelet adhesiveness, but that the response is unpredictable.

After the ingestion of aspirin, an increased rate of bleeding can be demonstrated by the quantitative bleeding time test.[22] It has been suggested by Quick[23] that such an aspirin tolerance test is a diagnostic procedure in von Willebrand's disease, although it has now been shown that some patients with mild von Willebrand's disease have negative responses to aspirin tolerance tests.[24-26]

In addition to the possibility that the long bleeding time is due to decrease of a "bleeding time factor", it has also been proposed that the defect in bleeding time is due to impaired platelet-vessel wall interaction. In support of this contention, Tschopp and associates[27] found that the platelets of patients with von Willebrand's disease adhered less well than did normal platelets to the subendothelium of rabbit aortas. It is of interest in this connection that the Willebrand factor (see below) is made in the endothelial cell[28,29] and that in semiconfluent endothelial cell cultures it appears as an extracellular fibrillar protein.[30] The interaction of platelets with fibrils in these cultures can be abolished by treatment with an antibody to Willebrand factor.[30]

Platelet Abnormalities

The initial suggestion that bleeding in these patients is due to a platelet abnormality was made by von Willebrand himself, who said that the bleeding was due to "disturbance of function in the thrombocytes and general alteration of the capillary walls". Morawitz and Jürgens[31] made the first experimental observation that suggested platelet dysfunction with an instrument known as a capillary thrombometer. They found that the time it took for blood to stop streaming through a capillary tube was strikingly prolonged in von Willebrand's disease, although in hemophilia it was apparently normal.[32,33] It was then shown by Borchgrevink[34] that the concentration of platelets in blood flowing from a standardized incision was approximately the same as the concentration of platelets in the circulating blood. This is in sharp contrast to the situation in normal blood, in which the platelet count falls rapidly as the blood exudes. These observations have been confirmed by other workers.[35-42]

The situation is different, however, regarding in vitro tests of platelet dysfunction, about which there is considerable disagreement.[21] Results with the Wright rotating-tube technique were found to be abnormal in the Åland Islands patients,[38] but Bowie and co-workers,[42] using a modified technique, were unable to find any abnormality in their patients.

Subsequently, numerous studies of platelets have been made by passing blood through columns filled with small glass beads. The test measures both platelet adhesion (sticking to nonplatelet surfaces) and platelet aggregation (adhering to each other), and nowadays it is usually called a test of "platelet retention." Hellem[43] was the first to use the test and he found that platelet "adhesiveness" was abnormal in von Willebrand's disease, but he attributed his abnormal results to the low hematocrit and concluded that the platelet "adhesiveness" was actually normal in this disease. Zucker[44] found decreased platelet retention in glass bead columns, but when she changed the type of glass beads, the results could not be reproduced. Salzman[45] introduced a modification of the test in which blood was drawn directly from a vein through the glass bead column into a vacuum tube. He showed that platelet retention was decreased in 10 of 11 patients with von Willebrand's disease. Meyer and associates[46] found that it was a sensitive test in the diagnosis of von Willebrand's disease, although it was not specific. A cooperative international study confirmed that the Salzman test was abnormal in von Willebrand's disease, although there was some spread into the normal range.[47]

It was then shown that the flow rate of blood through the column was important in discriminating between normal persons and patients with von Willebrand's disease, because if the rate was too slow, the platelet retention in von Willebrand's disease became normal;[48] if it was too fast, retention of normal platelets was limited. Subsequently, many of the variables have been identified, and a reproducible method has been introduced by Bowie and co-workers.[49]

The abnormal platelet retention in von Willebrand's disease appears to be due to the absence of a normal plasmatic factor. In 1969, Bowie et al.[49] showed that the addition of factor VIII-containing fractions of plasma to the glass beads before passage of the blood produced correction of the abnormal platelet retention. This finding has been confirmed by other workers, who have also shown that cryoprecipitate or factor VIII fractions from hemophilic plasma but not from von Willebrand's plasma will correct the abnormality.[12,50,51] Bouma et al.[52] further showed that the material correcting abnormal platelet retention had the same antigenic determinants as did factor VIII, as shown by the fact that anti-factor VIII serum decreased the platelet retention of normal blood and inhibited the corrective effects of purified factor VIII. This has also been observed by other workers.[53,54] The mechanism of this interaction has been studied by McPherson and Zucker,[55] who described several steps in the process of glass bead retention.

The platelet retention test is not specific for von Willebrand's disease. Results are abnormal in a number of qualitative platelet diseases, valvular heart disease, disseminated intravascular coagulation, myeloproliferative disorders,[56] and afibrinogenemia.[57] The platelet retention test, if carefully done and properly standardized, may actually be a good screening test for the qualitative platelet disorders.[58]

The functional platelet defect found in von Willebrand's disease has been further investigated by the use of ristocetin. Ristocetin is an antibiotic that was removed from the market when it was found to cause thrombocytopenia. It was subsequently shown that ristocetin caused platelet aggregation in vitro.[59] Howard and associates [60,61] then made the observation that ristocetin-induced platelet aggregation was absent or impaired in the platelet-rich plasma from patients with von Willebrand's disease. They also showed that the addition of normal platelet-poor plasma to platelet-rich von Willebrand plasma caused a normal platelet aggregation; this finding suggested that the plasmatic defect was responsible for the abnormality.[61,62] Several other workers have confirmed these observations[63-66] and have shown that patients with von Willebrand's disease are more easily differentiated from normal persons at low ristocetin concentrations (between 1 and 1.2 mg/mℓ).[67] Ristocetin-induced platelet aggregation does not require energy, and it has been suggested that the phenomenon be called "agglutination" rather than "aggregation". In fact, the reaction can be produced with platelets fixed in formaldehyde.[68,69] The plasmatic factor necessary for the support of ristocetin-induced platelet aggregation is present in normal plasma, normal serum, hemophilic plasma, and hemophilic serum.[61,66,67,70] Cryoprecipitate and partially purified fractions of factor VIII are also effective.[65-67,71] The material has antigenic determinants similar to those of factor VIII as shown by the fact that heterologous rabbit antibodies against human factor VIII will abolish ristocetin-induced platelet aggregation.[54,66,67,70,72]

Weiss and co-workers[73] have shown that the degree of platelet aggregation of multiply washed platelets could be used as an assay for the plasmatic factor. This has been confirmed by other workers.[66,74] Olson and associates'[63] modification of the assay uses gel filtration of platelets, after which only a single wash is necessary. The assay can also be performed by using formaldehyde-fixed, washed platelets and measuring the interval between the addition of ristocetin to the platelet suspension and the production of a visible "snow storm" aggregation.[75] The time interval is inversely related to the amount of plasmatic factor.

Ristocetin-induced platelet aggregation is also absent in patients with the Bernard-Soulier syndrome.[76,77] In this instance, the abnormality is apparently due to a platelet defect, for the level of von Willebrand factor in the plasma of these patients is normal. Mild abnormalities of ristocetin-induced platelet aggregation have been found in patients with thrombasthenia, storage pool disease, idiopathic thrombocytopenic purpura, infectious mononucleosis, and acute leukemia. [61]

Decreased Factor VIII

In 1953, three groups of investigators reported that patients with von Willebrand's disease had reduced factor VIII coagulant activity.[3-5] Patients in the Åland Islands were subsequently studied by Nilsson et al.[15] and by Jürgens et al.[78] and were found to have factor VIII deficiency also. This was an intriguing observation because it had been thought that factor VIII deficiency was inherited only as an X-linked recessive trait (classic hemophilia), but surprisingly in von Willebrand's disease, it appeared to be inherited autosomally.

In 1959, Nilsson et al.[79] made an even more intriguing observation when they reported that the increase of factor VIII coagulant activity after transfusion was greater than could be explained from the amount of factor VIII coagulant activity transfused. Furthermore, unlike the situation in hemophilia, in patients with von Willebrand's disease the peak increase of factor VIII after transfusion is delayed for several hours and stays elevated several hours before returning to the previous low levels.[42,80-82] This unusual response could also be produced by the transfusion of plasma from the patient with classic hemophilia,[42,82] serum, and even absorbed serum.[42,80,83] In the porcine model of von Willebrand's disease, it was shown that stimulated factor VIII overresponse was present in the fraction of plasma or serum that contained factor VIII.[84]

The next important advance in relation to factor VIII came from immunologic studies. It was reported that the protein immunologically related to factor VIII was present in normal amounts in patients with classic hemophilia despite their lack of factor VIII coagulant activity.[85,86] In von Willebrand's disease, on the other hand, the factor VIII-related antigen level was reduced — a finding that has been subsequently reported by many other laboratories.[30,54,73,87-92]

Bennett and co-workers[93] reported that after transfusion, factor VIII-related antigen decreased to low levels more quickly than did the factor VIII coagulant activity. A less rapid decrease has been noted by other workers.[94,95] The Willebrand factor measured by ristocetin-induced platelet aggregation decreases in parallel with the factor VIII-related antigen.[70,95-97]

An increase in both the factor VIII coagulant activity and the factor VIII-related antigen occurs during pregnancy,[17,56,98-100] in women taking oral contraceptives,[56,101,102] after vigorous exercise, and after epinephrine[103] and 1-diamino 8-arginine vasopressin[101] infusion. The vasopressin derivative produces an increase in factor VIII coagulant activity with less of an increase in factor VIII-related antigen. The material has been used to permit operations to be performed on patients with hemophilia and von Willebrand's disease.[104]

Diagnosis of von Willebrand's Disease

The patient with the classic form of von Willebrand's disease has the following abnormalities: long bleeding time, decreased platelet retention, decreased factor VIII coagulant activity, "overresponse" of factor VIII coagulant activity to transfusion, decreased factor VIII-related antigen, and decreased or absent platelet aggregation with ristocetin. The findings in von Willebrand's disease and hemophilia are compared in Table 1.

It was suggested a number of years ago that von Willebrand's disease formed a spectrum of abnormalities.[42] With the advent of the test for the factor VIII-related antigen and the ristocetin-Willebrand factor, the spectrum has been broadened.[105] The factor VIII coagulant activity, the factor VIII-related antigen, and the ristocetin-Willebrand factor are usually equally depressed in patients with the classic form of von Willebrand's disease. A number of patients have now been described in whom these activities are not congruent. These patients are said to have variant forms of von Willebrand's disease. Table 1 indicates the variant patterns that have been reported. Table 2 lists the variant patients who have been reported in the literature.

Holmberg and Nilsson[106-108] recently reported that 20 of 77 patients with von Willebrand's disease had low levels of factor VIII coagulant activity but normal amounts of factor VIII-related protein. This is the usual pattern in patients with hemophilia A.

Table 1
CLASSIC PATTERNS OF HEMOPHILIA A AND VON WILLEBRAND'S DISEASE

	Hemophilia A	von Willebrand's disease[a]
Inheritance	Sex-linked	Autosomal
Bleeding time	Normal	Long
Platelet retention	Normal	Decreased
Factor VIII	Decreased	Decreased
Overresponse of factor VIII to transfusion	No	Yes
Factor VIII antigen	Normal	Decreased
Ristocetin-Willebrand factor	Normal	Decreased
Ristocetin aggregation of platelet-rich plasma	Normal	Decreased

[a] Variants in every attribute have been reported in patients presumed to have von Willebrand's disease.

From Bowie, E. J. W., Fass, D. N., Olson, J. D., and Owen, C. A., Jr., *Mayo Clin. Proc.*, 51, 35, 1976. With permission.

In addition, there was no overresponse of factor VIII coagulant activity to transfusion and the disease was X-chromosomally transmitted. Because the bleeding was mainly from the skin and mucous membranes and the patients had prolonged bleeding times and a decrease of platelet adhesiveness, they were considered to have von Willebrand's disease rather than hemophilia.

Hensen and colleagues[109] reported patients with an autosomally transmitted bleeding disease that they diagnosed as having hemophilia A because there was no overresponse to transfusion and the bleeding times were normal. Subsequently, Veltkamp and van Tilburg[110] considered these patients to have a variant of von Willebrand's disease rather than hemophilia. Similar patients have been reported by Bloom and colleagues.[111]

Bouma and colleagues[30] reported four patients in three families who had normal factor VIII-related antigen and low factor VIII coagulant activity as in classic hemophilia. Unlike hemophilia, however, there was no abnormality in platelet retention. When cryoprecipitate was made from the plasma of these patients, it corrected the abnormal platelet retention test of other patients with von Willebrand's disease. The authors were not able to exclude the possibility that these patients actually had hemophilia with abnormal platelet function. Similar patients were found in two families who had low factor VIII levels, long Ivy bleeding times, low platelet retention, and evidence of an abnormality in platelet release.[112,113] By immunologic assay there was more than 200% factor VIII-related antigen. It was suggested that these patients had mild hemophilia or were carriers of hemophilia with an additional abnormality in the release of the platelets.

The advent of ristocetin led to descriptions of patients who had normal levels of factor VIII coagulant activity and factor VIII-related antigen but decreased or absent ristocetin-Willebrand factor.[114,115] Kernoff and colleagues[116] reported such a patient who had an overresponse of factor VIII to transfusion. The factor VIII coagulant activity varied between 60 and 80%. She had a long Ivy bleeding time, and although the factor VIII-related antigen showed a line of identity on immunodiffusion with plasma from normals and patients with hemophilia, it exhibited a faster anodal migration on crossed immunoelectrophoresis. It was suggested by these authors that the patient had a variant of the factor VIII-related antigen. Similar patients have subsequently been reported.[117-119]

Table 2
VARIANTS OF VON WILLEBRAND'S DISEASE[a]

	Coagulant VIII	VIII antigen	Ristocetin: Aggreg PRP	Ristocetin: Plasma factor	Bleeding time	Platelet retention	Response to transfusion	Inheritance	Comments	Ref.
Classic patterns: H A	D	N	N	N	N	N	N	Sex-linked		
Classic patterns: vW d	D	D	D	D	Long	D	Overresponse	Autosomal		
Holmberg and Nilsson	D	N	—	—	Long	V	N	Sex-linked	Platelet function normal	106-108
Hensen et al.	D	—	—	—	N	—	N	Autosomal dominant	"Autosomal" hemophilia	109
Veltkamp and van Tilburg	D	D	—	—	N and long	N and D	Over-response	Autosomal	von Willebrand's disease (same family as Hensen et al.[109])	110
Bloom et al.	D	D	Modified D	—	N	—	—	Autosomal	Resembles autosomal hemophilia of Hensen et al.[109]	111
Bouma et al.	D	N	—	—	—	D	—			30
Pechet et al.	D	High	—	—	Long	D	N	Probably sex-linked	Platelet release abnormality	112
Chesney et al.	D	High	—	—	Long	D	N	Probably sex-linked		113
Firkin et al.	N	N	D	Absent	Long	Absent	—	Uncertain		114, 115
Kernoff et al.	D	N	—	—	Long	—	Over-response	Uncertain	VIII antigen abnormal on electrophoresis	116
Stableforth et al.	D	N	D	—	Long	D	N	Probably autosomal	VIII antigen abnormal on electrophoresis	117, 118
	D	N	D	—	Long	D	Over-response	Probably autosomal	Platelet abnormality	
Peake et al.	N or B	N or B	D	—	Long	—	Over-response	Autosomal	VIII antigen abnormal on electrophoresis	119
Meyer et al.	N or B	N and D	D	D	Long	D	—	Autosomal	Different variants including "usual" type in same family	120

Thomson et al.	D to N	D to N	D	D	Long	—	—	Autosomal	Plasma from patients with high antigen did not correct ristocetin aggregation	121
Koutts et al.	D	N	N	N	Long	D	—	Autosomal		122
	D	Incr	D	—	Long	Absent	—	Uncertain		
	N	N	D	—	Long	Absent	—	Uncertain		
	D	N	D	—	Long	Absent	—	Uncertain		
Ruggeri et al.	a. I	I	D	Absent	Long	—	—	Autosomal	After transfusion of vasopressin analog, Willebrand factor rose less in group a than in group b	123
	b. I	I	Incr	I	Long	—	—	Autosomal		
Holmberg et al.	N	D	N	D	Long	—	Over-response	Autosomal	Patient presumably homozygous (parents were first cousins)	124
Bowie et al.	N and D	N and D	N and D	N and long	N and D	—	—	Autosomal	VIII coagulant levels variable in some patients	105

[a] PRP = platelet-rich plasma; H A = hemophilia A; vW d = von Willebrand's disease; D = decreased; N = normal; V = variable; B = borderline; I = intermediate; — = not done.

There are now several patients in the literature in whom the factor VIII coagulant activity is normal, the factor VIII-related antigen is also normal,[117-119] and ristocetin-induced platelet aggregation is abnormal.[114]

Ten members of a family were studied by Meyer et al.[120] Three were normal, four had a severe form of von Willebrand's disease, one had higher antigen than Willebrand factor, and two showed normal levels of factor VIII coagulant activity and factor VIII-related antigen but decreased Willebrand factor. Thus these authors show different patterns of the disease in a single family in contrast to the report of Koutts et al.,[122] who found that the pattern of the disease remained constant in a given family. Ruggeri et al.[123] reported a group of patients with von Willebrand's disease who showed increased aggregation with ristocetin in their platelet-rich plasma. They further differentiated the patients from the usual patterns of von Willebrand's disease by vasopressin infusion, finding that the patients in the group with increased ristocetin aggregation had greater overresponses of factor VIII activities after the infusion. Five patients with variants of von Willebrand's disease have been reported by Stableforth and colleagues.[117,118] Nine patients from five families with variants of von Willebrand's disease were reported by Bowie and colleagues.[105] The most usual variant of von Willebrand's disease in our experience is the one with borderline levels of coagulant factor VIII (which may fluctuate from time to time), commensurate levels of factor VIII-related antigen, and low levels of ristocetin-Willebrand factor.

It is apparent from the foregoing discussion that von Willebrand's disease may be difficult to diagnose. At the present time it would seem that the single most helpful test is an assay for the ristocetin-Willebrand factor and that in most cases of von Willebrand's disease this activity is low. The ristocetin-Willebrand factor may be normal in certain instances, but these are extremely uncommon.

Acquired von Willebrand's Disease

Several patients have now been described as having acquired von Willebrand's disease. As far as could be determined from their clinical histories, especially their response to major operations, the hemostatic mechanism was previously normal, and they subsequently acquired a disease with all the characteristics of von Willebrand's disease.[66,125-131] Unlike inherited von Willebrand's disease, there was a limited or absent response of factor VIII to transfusion of plasma. Three patients had monoclonal gammopathy,[66,126,128] and three other patients had a diffuse increase of immunoglobulins.[126] Two patients with acquired von Willebrand's disease had systemic lupus erythematosus.[126,130] In the cases reported by other workers, no inhibitor to von Willebrand factor could be demonstrated. More recently, a patient has been described with acquired von Willebrand's disease on the basis of an inhibitor (presumably an antibody) directed against von Willebrand factor.[125]

The Nature of von Willebrand's Disease

It has been shown that in normal plasma there is a protein related to factor VIII that has a corrective effect on the abnormal platelet function in von Willebrand's disease. The activity of this protein can be measured by its ability to produce platelet aggregation in the presence of appropriate amounts of ristocetin. This protein, but not coagulant factor VIII, is created in endothelial cells.[28,29,132] Is this protein the same as factor VIII? Is the ristocetin cofactor (Willebrand factor) the same as factor VIII antigen? There is currently no definite answer to these questions because it is quite clear that factor VIII is a complex molecule. Some investigators have suggested that it is a single molecule that has both factor VIII coagulant activity and ristocetin cofactor activity.[133,134]

The one-molecule hypothesis is supported by some samples of the purified factor

VIII molecule which are homogeneous on SDS polyacrylamide gel electrophoresis and have coagulant activity, antigenic effect, and von Willebrand factor activity.[52,65,67,72,97,133] Other workers, however, have compelling evidence that these two activities are represented by two separate molecules that are associated in vitro. In support of the two-molecule theory, factor VIII coagulant activity can be separated from the antigenic effect and von Willebrand factor activity by agarose gel chromatography and sucrose density-gradient ultracentrifugation in high salt concentrations.[40,66,135,136] The activities have also been separated by DEAE ion-exchange chromatography.[137] The activities furthermore are dissociated after transfusion.[70,93,107] Immunologic experiments have also resulted in separation of these entities by double-antibody immunoprecipitation[138] and immunoabsorption assays.[139] Brockway and Fass[140] have separated the two activities by ultracentrifugation on sucrose density gradients using high salt concentrations, by lowering the pH, and by anti-Willebrand factor antibodies. These workers have also separated the activities immunologically by adding an antibody to purified von Willebrand factor.

One could suggest that in von Willebrand's disease, the Willebrand molecule is not made, and in hemophilia, the factor VIII coagulant molecule is not made. The description of variant forms of the disease, however, renders the situation more complex. Although it is possible that in some patients with von Willebrand's disease, the molecule is actually not made, it seems likely in some of these variant forms of the disease that the molecule is made but is abnormal in function.[141] In some of the variant forms of von Willebrand's disease, the molecule migrates with a very rapid electrophoretic mobility on crossed immunoelectrophoresis.[119] Gralnick et al.[142] have found that the von Willebrand factor protein in some of these variants may be present in normal amounts. They have further shown that such molecules are deficient in von Willebrand factor activity and have a reduced content of carbohydrate. Zimmerman et al.[143] have shown that by crossed immunoelectrophoresis, the von Willebrand factor exists in normal human plasma in multiple molecular forms. In patients with von Willebrand's disease, the distribution of these forms, if present, may be abnormal, and the relative proportion of these molecules may vary from time to time in the same patient.

Fass and colleagues[144,145] have studied the von Willebrand factor in the pig model of human von Willebrand's disease. Using 2% agarose gel, they have shown that von Willebrand factor exists as a regular series of polymers with molecular weights varying from 1.1 to 21 million daltons.

Von Willebrand Disease in Animals

A bleeding disease of swine was described by Hogan et al.[146] in 1941. These animals have all the features of human von Willebrand's disease,[147] including variant forms.[148] The disease is inherited as an autosomal recessive trait.[149] The severely affected animals have no detectable von Willebrand factor[150] and the carriers have approximately 40 to 50% of the factor.[150,151]

The pigs show the same overresponse to transfusion as humans do,[84,147] but after transfusion, factor VIII is abnormally thermolabile.[150] The observation that these pigs seem resistant to the development of atherosclerosis[152-154] has opened up a new approach to the study of this important disease. The pig is a particularly suitable model for studying human atherosclerosis because it develops lesions that are almost identical to the human lesion.

A family of German Shepherd dogs with von Willebrand's disease was described by Dodds[155-157] in 1970, and it has now been studied for three generations.[158] The disease in these animals has all the characteristics of the human disease, and since the original description, the disease has also been found in golden retrievers, miniature Schnauzers, Doberman pinschers, and Scottish terriers. The fact that there are also dogs with hemophilia makes the dog a particularly interesting animal model. Studies of the factor VIII-related antigen show increased levels in hemophilic dogs and low levels in von Willebrand dogs.[158,159]

Animal models of a human disease allow investigations that would otherwise be impossible, including controlled genetic studies, organ transplantation and other types of surgery, and studies involving multiple transfusions. The study of these animals has provided information of importance to the understanding of human von Willebrand's disease.

Conclusions

In the last few years, impressive progress has been made in the elucidation of the enigma of von Willebrand's disease. It should be clear from this account that a number of problems remain to be solved. Two of the most important areas for research are the interaction of the platelet and von Willebrand factor in the arterial wall and the nature of the factor VIII coagulant molecule in relationship to von Willebrand factor.

REFERENCES

1. **von Willebrand, E. A.,** Hereditär pseudohemofili, *Finsk. Laekaresaellsk. Handl.,* 68, 87, 1926.
2. **von Willebrand, E. A.,** Über hereditare pseudohamophilie, *Acta Med. Scand.,* 76, 521, 1931.
3. **Alexander, B. and Goldstein, R.,** Dual hemostatic defect in pseudohemophilia, *J. Clin. Invest.,* 32 (Abstr.), 551, 1953.
4. **Larrieu, M.-J. and Soulier, J. P.,** Déficit en facteur antihémophilique a chez une fille, associé a un trouble du saignement, *Rev. Hematol.,* 8, 361, 1953.
5. **Quick, A. J. and Hussey, C. V.,** Hemophilic condition in the female, *J. Lab. Clin. Med.,* 42(Abstr.), 929, 1953.
6. **Geiger, A. J. and Evans, A. G.,** Atypical hereditary hemorrhagic syndromes, *Int. Clin.,* 2, 135, 1938.
7. **Schulman, I., Smith, C. H., Erlandson, M., and Fort, E.,** Vascular hemophilia: a familial hemorrhagic disease in males and females characterized by combined antihemophilic globulin deficiency and vascular abnormality, *Am. J. Dis. Child.,* 90(Abstr.), 526, 1955.
8. **Blombäck, M., Jorpes, J. E., and Nilsson, I. M.,** von Willebrand's disease, *Am. J. Med.,* 34, 236, 1963.
9. **Nilsson, I. M. and Blombäck, M.,** von Willebrand's disease in Sweden—occurrence, pathogenesis and treatment, *Thromb. Diath. Haemorrh.,* 9(Suppl. II), 103, 1963.
10. **Nilsson, I. M., Blombäck, B., Blombäck, M., and Svennerud, S.,** Kvinnlig hämofili och dess behandling med humant antihamofiliglobulin, *Nord. Med.,* 56, 1654, 1956.
11. **Blombäck, M.,** Studies on antihemophilic globulin, *Acta Paediatr. (Stockholm),* 47, 709, 1958.
12. **Blombäck, M., Blombäck, B., and Nilsson, I. M.,** Response to fractions in von Willebrand's disease, in *The Hemophilias,* Brinkhous, K. M., Ed., University of North Carolina Press, Chapel Hill, 1964, 286.
13. **Nilsson, I. M. and Blombäck, M.,** Symposium on hemophilia: the pathogenesis and treatment of v. Willebrand's disease, in *Hemophilia and Other Hemorrhagic States,* Brinkhous, K. M., Ed., University of North Carolina Press, Chapel Hill, 1959, 93.
14. **Nilsson, I. M., Blombäck, M., and Blombäck, B.,** The use of human anti-haemophilic globulin (fraction I-O) in haemophilia A and in von Willebrand's disease, *Acta Haematol. (Basel),* 24, 116, 1960.
15. **Nilsson, I. M., Blombäck, M., Jorpes, E., Blombäck, B., and Johansson, S.-A.,** v. Willebrand's disease and its correction with human plasma fraction I-O, *Acta Med. Scand.,* 159,179, 1957.
16. **Nilsson, I. M., Blombäck, M., and von Francken, I.,** On an inherited autosomal haemorrhagic diathesis with antihaemophilic globulin deficiency and prolonged bleeding time, in *Trans. Sixth Congr. Eur. Soc. Haematol.,* Part 2, Videbaek, A., Ed., S. Karger, Basel, 1958, 629.
17. **Noller, K. L., Bowie, E. J. W., Kempers, R. D., and Owen, C. A., Jr.,** von Willebrand's disease in pregnancy, *Obstet. Gynecol.,* 41, 865, 1973.

18. Magnusson, S., Discussion, *Thromb. Diath. Haemorrh.*, 9(Suppl. 11), 126, 1963.
19. Perkins, H. A., Correction of the hemostatic defects in von Willebrand's disease, *Blood*, 30, 375, 1967.
20. Sutor, A. H., Bowie, E. J. W., and Owen, C. A., Jr., A new method of demonstrating the effect of therapy in von Willebrand's disease, *Mayo Clin. Proc.*, 46, 345, 1971.
21. Bowie, E. J. W. and Owen, C. A., Jr., Platelet abnormalities in von Willebrand's disease, *Ann. N.Y. Acad. Sci.*, 201, 400, 1972.
22. Sutor, A. H., Bowie, E. J. W., and Owen, C. A., Jr., Effect of aspirin, sodium salicylate, and acetaminophen on bleeding, *Mayo Clin. Proc.*, 46, 178, 1971.
23. Quick, A. J., Salicylates and bleeding: the aspirin tolerance test, *Am. J. Med. Sci.*, 252, 265, 1966.
24. Kaneshiro, M. M., Mielke, C. H., Jr., Kasper, C. K., and Rapaport, S. I., Bleeding time after aspirin in disorders of intrinsic clotting, *N. Engl. J. Med.*, 281, 1039, 1969.
25. Leslie, J. and Mason, D. Y., Sensitivity of platelets to aspirin in von Willebrand's disease, *J. Clin. Pathol.*, 23, 526, 1970.
26. Sahud, M. A. and Cohen, R. J., Aspirin-induced prolongation of the Ivy bleeding time: its diagnostic usefulness, *Calif. Med.*, 115(4), 10, 1971.
27. Tschopp, T. B., Weiss, H. J., and Baumgartner, H. R., Decreased adhesion of platelets to subendothelium in von Willebrand's disease, *J. Lab. Clin. Med.*, 83, 296, 1974.
28. Jaffe, E. A., Hoyer, L. W., and Nachman, R. L., Synthesis of antihemophilic factor antigen by cultured human endothelial cells, *J. Clin. Invest.*, 52, 2757, 1973.
29. Jaffe, E. A., Hoyer, L. W., and Nachman, R. L., Synthesis of von Willebrand factor by cultured human endothelial cells, *Proc. Natl. Acad. Sci. U.S.A.*, 71, 1906, 1974.
30. Bouma, B. N., Sixma, J. J., de Graaf, S., Wiegerinck, Y., van Mourik, J. A., and Mochtar, I. A., Factor-VIII antigen and platelet retention in a glass bead column, *Br. J. Haematol.*, 25, 645, 1973.
31. Morawitz, P. and Jürgens, R., Gibt es eine Thrombasthenie? *Munch. Med. Wochenschr.*, 77, 2001, 1930.
32. Jürgens, R., Die erblichen Thrombopathien, *Ergeb. Inn. Med. Kinderheilkd.*, 53, 795, 1937.
33. v. Willebrand, E. A. and Jürgens, R., Über ein neues vererbbares Blutungsübel: Die konstitutionelle Thrombopathie, *Dtsch. Arch. Klin. Med.*, 175, 453, 1933.
34. Borchgrevink, C. F., A method for measuring platelet adhesiveness in vivo, *Acta Med. Scand.*, 168, 157, 1960.
35. Caen, J. and Cousin, C., Le trouble d'adhésivité "in vivo" des plaquettes dans la maladie de Willebrand et les thrombasthénies de Glanzmann: essai d'interpretation, *Nouv. Rev. Fr. Hematol.*, 2, 685, 1962.
36. Cornu, P., Larrieu, M. J., Caen, J., and Bernard, J., Maladie de Willebrand: Étude clinique, génétique et biologique (a propos de 22 observations), *Nouv. Rev. Fr. Hematol.*, 1, 231, 1961.
37. Cornu, P. and Bernard, J., L'allongement du temps de saignement dans la maladie de Willebrand, *Nouv. Rev. Fr. Hematol.*, 3, 321, 1963.
38. Dodds, W. J., Storage, release, and synthesis of coagulation factors in isolated perfused organs, *Am. J. Physiol.*, 217, 879, 1969.
39. Quick, A. J., Hereditary thrombopathic thrombocytopenia and Minot-von Willebrand syndrome: probable co-existence in a family, *Am. J. Med. Sci.*, 250, 1, 1965.
40. Owen, W. G. and Wagner, R. H., Antihemophilic factor: separation of an active fragment following dissociation by salts or detergents, *Thromb. Diath. Haemorrh.*, 27, 502, 1972.
41. Weiss, H. J., The use of plasma and plasma fractions in the treatment of a patient with von Willebrand's disease, *Vox Sang.*, 7,267, 1962.
42. Bowie, E. J. W., Didisheim, P., Thompson, J. H., Jr., and Owen, C. A., Jr., The spectrum of von Willebrand's disease, *Thromb. Diath. Haemorrh.*, 18, 40, 1967.
43. Hellem, A. J., The adhesiveness of human blood platelets in vitro, *Scand. J. Clin. Lab. Invest.*, 12 (Suppl. 51), 1, 1960.
44. Zucker, M. B., In vitro abnormality of the blood in von Willebrand's disease correctable by normal plasma (Letter to the Editor), *Nature (London)*, 197, 601, 1963.
45. Salzman, E. W., Measurement of platelet adhesiveness: a simple in vitro technique demonstrating an abnormality in von Willebrand's disease, *J. Lab. Clin. Med.*, 62, 724, 1963.
46. Meyer, D., Larrieu, M.-J., Maroteaux, P., and Caen, J. P., Biological findings in von Willebrand's pedigrees: implications for inheritance, *J. Clin. Pathol.*, 20, 190, 1967.
47. Murphy, E. A., von Willebrand's disease: statistical evaluation of the glass bead test in diagnosis; preliminary report, *Thromb. Diath. Haemorrh. Suppl.*, 35, 211, 1969.
48. O'Brien, J. R. and Heywood, J. B., Some interactions between human platelets and glass: von Willebrand's disease compared with normal, *J. Clin. Pathol.*, 20, 56, 1967.
49. Bowie, E. J. W., Owen, C. A., Jr., Thompson, J. H., Jr., and Didisheim, P., Platelet adhesiveness in von Willebrand's disease, *Am. J. Clin. Pathol.*, 52, 69, 1969.

50. **Meyer, D. and Larrieu, M.-J.**, von Willebrand factor and platelet adhesiveness, *J. Clin. Pathol.*, 23, 228, 1970.
51. **Weiss, H. J. and Rogers, J.**, Correction of the platelet abnormality in von Willebrand's disease by cryoprecipitate, *Am. J. Med.*, 53, 734, 1972.
52. **Bouma, B. N., Wiegerinck, Y., Sixma, J. J., van Mourik, J. A., and Mochtar, I. A.**, Immunological characterization of purified anti-haemophilic factor A (factor VIII) which corrects abnormal platelet retention in von Willebrand's disease (Letter to the Editor), *Nature London New Biol.*, 236,104,1972.
53. **Mazurier, C., Parquet-Gernez, A., and Goudemand, M.**, Action des anticorps anti-facteur VIII sur la rétention des plaquettes aux billes de verre, *Pathol. Biol. (Paris)*, 21 (Suppl.), 72, 1973.
54. **Meyer, D., Dreyfus, M. D., and Larrieu, M. J.**, Willebrand factor: immunological and biological study, *Pathol. Biol. (Paris)*, 21(Suppl.), 66, 1973.
55. **McPherson, J. and Zucker, M. B.**, Platelet retention in glass bead columns: adhesion to glass and subsequent platelet-platelet interactions, *Blood*, 47, 55, 1976.
56. **Bowie, E. J. W. and Owen, C. A., Jr.**, The value of measuring platelet "adhesiveness" in the diagnosis of bleeding diseases, *Am. J. Clin. Pathol.*, 60, 302, 1973.
57. **Niessner, H.**, Messung der Plättchenadhäsivität mit einer modifizierten Form der Hellem II-methodik unter besonderer Berücksichtigung des von Willebrand-Jürgens-Syndroms, *Thromb. Diath. Haemorrh.*, 27, 434, 1972.
58. **Weiss, H. J.**, Platelet function tests and their interpretation (Editorial), *J. Lab. Clin. Med.*, 87, 909, 1976.
59. **Gangarosa, E. J., Johnson, T. R., and Ramos, H. S.**, Ristocetin-induced thrombocytopenia: site and mechanism of action, *Arch. Intern. Med.*, 105, 83, 1960.
60. **Howard, M. A. and Firkin, B. G.**, Ristocetin — a new tool in the investigation of platelet aggregation, *Thromb. Diath. Haemorrh.*, 26, 362, 1971.
61. **Howard, M. A., Sawers, R. J., and Firkin, B. G.**, Ristocetin: a means of differentiating von Willebrand's disease into two groups, *Blood*, 41, 687, 1973.
62. **Firkin, B. and Howard, M. A.**, Ristocetin — a new approach to the investigation of von Willebrand's disease, *Aust. N.Z. J. Med.*, 1(Abstr.), 279, 1971.
63. **Olson, J. D., Brockway, W. J., Fass, D. N., Magnuson, M. A., and Bowie, E. J. W.**, Evaluation of ristocetin — Willebrand factor assay and ristocetin-induced platelet aggregation, *Am. J. Clin. Pathol.*, 63, 210, 1975.
64. **Barbui, T., Battista, R., and Dini, E.**, Relationship between ristocetin-induced platelet aggregation and factor VIII (activity and antigen) in v. Willebrand's disease, *Blut*, 29, 260, 1974.
65. **Meyer, D., Jenkins, C. S. P., Dreyfus, M., and Larrieu, M.-J.**, Experimental model for von Willebrand's disease (Letter to the Editor), *Nature (London)*, 243, 293, 1973.
66. **Meyer, D. Jenkins, C. S. P., Dreyfus, M. D., Fressinaud, E., and Larrieu, M.-J.**, Willebrand factor and ristocetin. II. Relationship between Willebrand factor, Willebrand antigen and factor-VIII activity, *Br. J. Haematol.*, 28, 579, 1974.
67. **Weiss, H. J., Rogers, J., and Brand, H.**, Defective ristocetin-induced platelet aggregation in von Willebrand's disease and its correction by factor VIII, *J. Clin. Invest.*, 52, 2697, 1973.
68. **Allain, J. P., Cooper, H. A., Wagner, R. H., and Brinkhous, K. M.**, Platelets fixed with paraformaldehyde: a new reagent for assay of von Willebrand factor and platelet aggregating factor, *J. Lab. Clin. Med.*, 85, 318, 1975.
69. **Brinkhous, K. M., Graham, J. E., Cooper, H. H., Allain, J. P., and Wagner, R. H.**, Assay of von Willebrand factor in von Willebrand's disease and hemophilia: use of a macroscopic platelet aggregation test, *Thromb. Res.*, 6, 267, 1975.
70. **Thomson, C., Forbes, C. D., and Prentice, C. R. M.**, Relationship of factor VIII to ristocetin-induced platelet aggregation: effect of heterologous and acquired factor VIII antibodies, *Thromb. Res.*, 3, 363, 1973.
71. **Olson, J. D., Fass, D. N., Bowie, E. J. W., and Mann, K. G.**, Ristocetin-induced aggregation of gel filtered platelets: a study of von Willebrand's disease and the effect of aspirin, *Thromb. Res.*, 3, 501, 1973.
72. **Jenkins, C. S. P., Meyer, D., Dreyfus, M. D., and Larrieu, M.-J.**, Willebrand factor and ristocetin. I. Mechanism of ristocetin-induced platelet aggregation, *Br. J. Haematol.*, 28, 561, 1974.
73. **Weiss, H. J., Hoyer, L. W., Rickles, F. R., Varma, A., and Rogers, J.**, Quantitative assay of a plasma factor deficient in von Willebrand's disease that is necessary for platelet aggregation: relationship to factor VIII procoagulant activity and antigen content, *J. Clin. Invest.*, 52, 2708, 1973.
74. **Van Royen, E. A., Flier, O. T. N., and ten Cate, J. W.**, von Willebrand-factor activity in pregnancy, *Lancet*, 2, 657, 1974.
75. **Sarji, K. E., Stratton, R. D., Wagner, R. H., and Brinkhous, K. M.**, Nature of von Willebrand factor: a new assay and a specific inhibitor, *Proc. Natl. Acad. Sci. U.S.A.*, 71, 2937, 1974.
76. **Howard, M. A., Hutton, R. A., and Hardisty, R. M.**, Hereditary giant platelet syndrome: a disorder of a new aspect of platelet function, *Br. Med. J.*, 2, 586, 1973.

77. Caen, J., Levy-Toledano, S., Sultan, Y., and Bernard, J., La dystrophie thrombocytaire hémorragipare (interaction des plaquettes et du facteur Willebrand), *Nouv. Rev. Fr. Hematol.*, 13, 595, 1973.
78. Jürgens, R., Lehmann, W., Wegelius, O., Ericksson, A. W., and Hiepler, E., Mitteilung über den Mangel an Antihämophilem Globulin (factor VIII) bei der Aaländischen Thrombopathie (v. Willebrand- Jürgens), *Thromb. Diath. Haemorrh.*, 1, 257, 1957.
79. Nilsson, I. M., Blombäck, M., and Blombäck, B., V. Willebrand's disease in Sweden: its pathogenesis and treatment, *Acta Med. Scand.*, 164, 263, 1959.
80. Biggs, R. and Matthews, J. M., The treatment of haemorrhage in von Willebrand's disease and the blood level of factor VIII (AHG), *Br. J. Haematol.*, 9, 203, 1963.
81. Borchgrevink, C. F., Egeberg, O., Godal, H. C., and Hjort, P. F., The effect of plasma and Cohn's fraction I on the Duke and Ivy bleeding times in von Willebrand's disease, *Acta Med. Scand.*, 173, 235, 1963.
82. Cornu, P., Larrieu, M. J., Caen, J., and Bernard, J., Transfusion studies in von Willebrand's disease: effect on bleeding time and factor VIII, *Br. J. Haematol.*, 9, 189, 1963.
83. Fantl, P. and Sawers, R. J., Stimulation of factor VIII (antihaemophilic) activity by transfused serum, *Nature (London)*, 200, 1214, 1963.
84. Chan, J. Y. S., Owen, C. A., Jr., Bowie, E. J. W., Didisheim, P., Thompson, J. H., Jr., Muhrer, M. E., and Zollman, P. E., von Willebrand disease "stimulating factor" in porcine plasma, *Am. J. Physiol.*, 214, 1219, 1968.
85. Zimmerman, T. S., Ratnoff, O. D., and Powell, A. E., Immunologic differentiation of classic hemophilia (factor VIII deficiency) and von Willebrand's disease: with observations on combined deficiencies of antihemophilic factor and proaccelerin (factor V) and on an acquired circulating anticoagulant against antihemophilic factor, *J. Clin. Invest.*, 50, 244, 1971.
86. Bennett, E. and Huehns, E. R., Immunological differentiation of three types of haemophilia and identification of some female carriers, *Lancet*, 2, 956, 1970.
87. Gralnick, H. R., Coller, B. S., and Marchesi, S. L., Immunological studies of factor VIII in haemophilia and von Willebrand's disease (Letter to the Editor), *Nature London New Biol.*, 244, 281, 1973.
88. Gruson, R. and Kernoff, P. B. A., Diagnostik des von-Willebrand-Jürgens-Syndroms mit Hilfe der quantitativen immunologischen Bestimmung des Faktor-VIII assoziierten Antigens, *Dtsch. Med. Wochenschr.*, 99, 1593, 1974.
89. Hoyer, L. W., Immunologic studies of antihemophilic factor (AHF, factor VIII). IV. Radioimmunoassay of AHF antigen, *J. Lab. Clin. Med.*, 80, 822, 1972.
90. Hoyer, L. W., Immunologic properties of antihemophilic factor, *Prog. Hematol.*, 8, 191, 1973.
91. Meyer, D., Lavergne, J.-M., Larrieu, M.-J., and Josso, F., Cross-reacting material in congenital factor VIII deficiencies (haemophilia A and von Willebrand's disease), *Thromb. Res.*, 1, 183, 1972.
92. Stites, D. P., Hershgold, E. J., Perlman, J. D., and Fudenberg, H. H., Factor VIII detection by hemagglutination inhibition: hemophilia A and von Willebrand's disease, *Science*, 171, 196, 1971.
93. Bennett, B., Ratnoff, O. D., and Levin, J., Immunologic studies in von Willebrand's disease: evidence that the antihemophilic factor (AHF) produced after transfusions lacks an antigen associated with normal AHF and the inactive material produced by patients with classic hemophilia, *J. Clin. Invest.*, 51, 2597, 1972.
94. Bloom, A. L., Peake, I. R., and Giddings, J. C., The presence and reactions of high and lower-molecular-weight procoagulant factor VIII in the plasma of patients with von Willebrand's disease after treatment: significance for a structural hypothesis for factor VIII, *Thromb. Res.*, 3, 389, 1973.
95. Bowie, E. J. W., Fass, D. N., Olson, J. D., and Owen, C. A., Jr., Transfusion and autotransfusion of plasma in von Willebrand's disease, *Thromb. Res.*, 5, 479, 1974.
96. Muntz, R. H., Ekert, H., and Helliger, H., Properties of post-infusion factor VIII in von Willebrand's disease, *Thromb. Res.*, 5, 111, 1974.
97. Weiss, H. J. and Sussman, I. I., Synthesis of high-molecular-weight antihaemophilic factor in von Willebrand's disease (Letter to the Editor), *Lancet*, 2, 402, 1974.
98. Bennett, B., Oxnard, S. C., Douglas, A. S., and Ratnoff, O. D., Studies on antihemophilic factor (AHF, factor VIII) during labor in normal women, in patients with premature separation of the placenta, and in a patient with von Willebrand's disease, *J. Lab. Clin. Med.*, 84, 851, 1974.
99. Evans, P. C., Obstetric and gynecologic patients with von Willebrand's disease, *Obstet. Gynecol.*, 38, 37, 1971.
100. Strauss, H. S. and Diamond, L. K., Elevation of factor VIII (antihemophilic factor) during pregnancy in normal persons and in a patient with von Willebrand's disease, *N. Engl. J. Med.*, 269, 1251, 1963.
101. Egeberg, O. and Owren, P. A., Oral contraception and blood coagulability, *Br. Med. J.*, 1, 220, 1963.
102. Glueck, H. I. and Flessa, H. C., Control of hemorrhage in von Willebrand's disease and a hemophiliac carrier with norethynodrel-mestranol, *Thromb. Res.*, 1, 253, 1972.

103. Prentice, C. R. M., Forbes, C. D., and Smith, S. M., Rise of factor VIII after exercise and adrenaline infusion, measured by immunological and biological techniques, *Thromb. Res.,* 1, 493, 1972.
104. Mannucci, P. M., Ruggeri, Z. M., Pareti, F. I., and Capitanio, A., 1-Deamino-8-D-arginine vasopressin: a new pharmacological approach to the management of haemophilia and von Willebrand's disease, *Lancet,* 1, 869, 1977.
105. Bowie, E. J. W., Fass, D. N., Olson, J. D., and Owen, C. A., Jr., The spectrum of von Willebrand's disease revisited, *Mayo Clin. Proc.,* 51, 35, 1976.
106. Holmberg, L. and Nilsson, I. M., Genetic variants of von Willebrand's disease, *Br. Med. J.,* 3, 317, 1972.
107. Holmberg, L. and Nilsson, I. M., Two genetic variants of von Willebrand's disease, *N. Engl. J. Med.,* 288, 595, 1973.
108. Holmberg, L. and Nilsson, I. M., Letter to the Editor, *N. Engl. J. Med.,* 288, 1130, 1973.
109. Hensen, A., Mattern, M. J., and Loeliger, E. A., Haemophilia A with apparently autosomal dominant inheritance: evidence for a second autosomal locus involved in factor VIII production, *Thromb. Diath. Haemorrh.,* 14, 341, 1965.
110. Veltkamp, J. J. and van Tilburg, N. H., 'Autosomal haemophilia': a variant of von Willebrand's disease, *Br. J. Haematol.,* 26, 141, 1974.
111. Bloom, A. L., Peake, I. R., and Giddings, J. C., Factor-VIII-related antigen or von Willebrand factor? (Letter to the Editor), *Lancet,* 1, 576, 1974.
112. Pechet, L., Chesney, C., and Colman, R. W., Variants of von Willebrand's disease (Letter to the Editor), *N. Engl. J. Med.,* 288, 1129, 1973.
113. Chesney, C., Colman, R. W., and Pechet, L., A syndrome of platelet-release abnormality and mild hemophilia, *Blood,* 43, 821, 1974.
114. Firkin, B., Firkin, F., and Stott, L., Von Willebrand's disease type B: a newly defined bleeding diathesis, *Aust. N.Z. J. Med.,* 3, 225, 1973.
115. Firkin, B. and Koutts, J., VIII-Related antigen and von Willebrand factor (Letter to the Editor), *Lancet,* 1, 803, 1974.
116. Kernoff, P. B. A., Gruson, R., and Rizza, C. R., A variant of factor VIII related antigen, *Br. J. Haematol.,* 26, 435, 1974.
117. Stableforth, P., Barrowcliffe, R. W., and Dormandy, K., Von Willebrand factor and factor-VIII-related antigen (Letter to the Editor), *Lancet,* 1, 685, 1974.
118. Stableforth, P., Hughes, J., Wilson, E., and Dormandy, K. M., The von Willebrand syndrome, *Br. J. Haematol.,* 29, 605, 1975.
119. Peake, I. R., Bloom, A. L., and Giddings, J. C., Inherited variants of factor-VIII-related protein in von Willebrand's disease, *N. Engl. J. Med.,* 291, 113, 1974.
120. Meyer, D., Jenkins, C. S. P., Dreyfus, M., and Larrieu, M.-J., Willebrand-factor activity and antigen in von Willebrand's disease (Letter to the Editor), *Lancet,* 1, 512, 1974.
121. Thomson, C., Forbes, C. D., and Prentice, C. R. M., Evidence for a qualitative defect in factor-VIII- related antigen in von Willebrand's disease, *Lancet,* 1, 594, 1974.
122. Koutts, J. Stott, L., Sawers, R. J., and Firkin, B. G., Variant patterns in von Willebrand's disease, *Thromb. Res.,* 5, 557, 1974.
123. Ruggeri, Z. M., Pareti, F. I., Bintadish, P., and Mannucci, P. M., Clotting factors in von Willebrand's disease (Letter to the Editor), *Lancet,* 2, 105, 1974.
124. Holmberg, L., Rašović, N., and Nilsson, I. M., von Willebrand's disease with normal factor VIII activity in a homozygote, *Haemostasis,* 3, 237, 1974.
125. Handin, R. I. and Moloney, W. C., Antibody-induced von Willebrand's disease, *Blood,* 44 (Abstr.), 933, 1974.
126. Ingram, G. I. C., Kingston, P. J., Leslie, J., and Bowie, E. J. W., Four cases of acquired von Willebrand's syndrome, *Br. J. Haematol.,* 21, 189, 1971.
127. Ingram, G. I. C., Prentice, C. R. M., Forbes, C. D., and Leslie, J., Low factor-VIII-like antigen in acquired von Willebrand's syndrome and response to treatment, *Br. J. Haematol.,* 25, 137, 1973.
128. Mant, M. J., Hirsh, J., Gauldie, J., Bienenstock, J., Pineo, G. F., and Luke, K. H., von Willebrand's syndrome presenting as an acquired bleeding disorder in association with a monoclonal gammopathy, *Blood,* 42, 429, 1973.
129. Poole-Wilson, P. A., Acquired von Willebrand's syndrome and systemic lupus erythematosus, *Proc. R. Soc. Med.,* 65, 561, 1972.
130. Simone, J. V., Cornet, J. A., and Abildgaard, C. F., Acquired von Willebrand's syndrome in systemic lupus erythematosus, *Blood,* 31, 806, 1968.
131. Veltkamp, J. J., Stevens, P., Plas, M. v. d., and Loeliger, E. A., Production site of bleeding factor (acquired morbus von Willebrand), *Thromb. Diath. Haemorrh.,* 23, 412, 1970.
132. Booyse, F. M., Quarfoot, A. J., Bell, S., Fass, D. N., Lewis, J. C., Mann, K. G. and Bowie, E. J. W., Cultured aortic endothelial cells from pigs with von Willebrand disease: *in vitro* model for studying the molecular defect(s) of the disease, *Proc. Natl. Acad. Sci. U.S.A.,* 74, 5702, 1977.

133. McKee, P. A., Anderson, J. C., and Switzer, M. E., Molecular structural studies of human factor VIII, *Ann. N.Y. Acad. Sci.*, 240, 8, 1975.
134. Gralnick, H. R. and Coller, B. S., Studies of the human factor VIII/von Willebrand's factor protein. II. Identification and characterization of the von Willebrand protein, *Blood*, 46, 417, 1975.
135. Rick, M. E. and Hoyer, L. W., Immunologic studies of antihemophilic factor (AHF, factor VIII). V. Immunologic properties of AHF subunits produced by salt dissociation, *Blood*, 42, 737, 1973.
136. Weiss, H. J. and Hoyer, L. W., von Willebrand factor: dissociation from antihemophilic factor procoagulant activity, *Science*, 182, 1149, 1973.
137. Austen, D. E. G., Carey, M., and Howard, M. A., Dissociation of factor VIII-related antigen into subunits (Letter to the Editor), *Nature (London)*, 253, 55, 1975.
138. Hougie, C., Sargeant, R. B., Brown, J. E., and Bough, R. F., Evidence that factor VIII and the ristocetin aggregating factor (VIII_{Rist}) are separate molecular entities, *Proc. Soc. Exp. Biol. Med.*, 147, 58, 1974.
139. Zimmerman, T. S. and Edgington, T. S., Factor VIII coagulant activity and factor VIII-like antigen: independent molecular entities, *J. Exp. Med.*, 138, 1015, 1973.
140. Brockway, W. J. and Fass, D. N., The nature of the interaction between ristocetin-Willebrand factor and the factor VIII coagulant activity molecule, *J. Lab. Clin. Med.*, 89, 1295, 1977.
141. Gralnick, H. R., Sultan, Y., and Coller, B. S., von Willebrand's disease: combined qualitative and quantitative abnormalities, *N. Engl. J. Med.*, 296, 1024, 1977.
142. Gralnick, H. R., Coller, B. S., and Sultan, Y., Carbohydrate deficiency of the factor VIII/von Willebrand factor protein in von Willebrand's disease variants, *Science*, 192, 56, 1976.
143. Zimmerman, T. S., Roberts, J., and Edgington, T. S., Factor-VIII-related antigen: multiple molecular forms in human plasma, *Proc. Natl. Acad. Sci. U.S.A.*, 72, 5121, 1975.
144. Fass, D. N., Knutson, G., and Bowie, E. J. W., Agarose Sodium Dodecylsulfate (SDS) Analysis of Porcine Willebrand Factor, Abstr. 19th Annu. Meet. Proc. Am. Soc. Hematol., Boston, 1976, 171.
145. Fass, D. N. and Bowie, E. J. W., Reduced Polymerization of Willebrand Factor in a Family of Pigs with a Variant of von Willebrand's Disease, Abstr. Int. Cong. Thromb. Haemostasis, Philadelphia, 1977, 86.
146. Hogan, A. G., Muhrer, M. E., and Bogart, R., A hemophilia-like disease in swine, *Proc. Soc. Exp. Biol. Med.*, 48, 217, 1941.
147. Bowie, E. J. W., Owen, C. A., Jr., Zollman, P. E., Thompson, J. H., Jr., and Fass, D. N., Tests of hemostasis in swine: normal values and values in pigs affected with von Willebrand's disease, *Am. J. Vet. Res.*, 34, 1405, 1973.
148. Bowie, E. J. W., Fass, D. N., and Owen, C. A., Jr., Variants of von Willebrand's Disease in Pigs, Abstr. Free Commun. 16th Int. Cong. Hematol., Kyoto, Japan, 1976, 331.
149. Owen, C. A. Jr., Bowie, E. J. W., Zollman, P. E., Fass, D. N., and Gordon, H., Carrier of porcine von Willebrand's disease, *Am. J. Vet. Res.*, 35, 245, 1974.
150. Fass. D. N., Bowie, E. J. W., Owen, C. A., Jr., and Mann, K. G., Stability of porcine factor VIII, *Thromb. Res.*, 6, 109, 1975.
151. Griggs, T. R., Webster, W. P., Cooper, H. A., Wagner, R. W., and Brinkhous, K. M., von Willebrand factor: gene dosage relationships and transfusion response in bleeder swine a new bioassay, *Proc. Natl. Acad. Sci. U.S.A.*, 71, 2087, 1974.
152. Bowie, E. J. W., Fuster, V., Owen, C. A., Jr., and Brown, A. L., Resistance to the development of spontaneous atherosclerosis in pigs with von Willebrand's disease, *Thromb. Diath. Haemorrh.*, 34 (Abstr.), 599, 1975.
153. Fuster, V., Lewis, J. C., Bowie, E. J. W., and Brown, A. L., Quantitation and Structural Characterization of Spontaneous and Dietary induced Atherosclerosis in Normal and von Willebrand Pigs, in Proceeding of the Workshop on Platelets, Philadelphia, 1976, U.S. Government Printing Office, Washington, D.C. (in press).
154. Fuster, V., Bowie, E. J. W., and Brown, A. L., Spontaneous arterial lesions in normal pigs and pigs with von Willebrand's disease, *Adv. Exp. Med. Biol.*, 82, 315, 1977.
155. Dodds, W. J., Hereditary and acquired hemorrhagic disorders in animals, *Prog. Hemostasis Thromb.*, 2, 215, 1974.
156. Dodds, W. J., Canine von Willebrand's disease, *J. Lab. Clin. Med.*, 76, 713, 1970.
157. Dodds, W. J., Congenital thrombopathies and related coagulation disorders in dogs, in *Proc. les Mutants Pathologiques chez l'animal, leur Intérêt dans la Recherche Bio-médicale*, Sabourdy, M., Ed., CNRS Press, Paris, 1970, 317.
158. Dodds, W. J., Further studies of canine von Willebrand's disease, *Blood*, 45, 221, 1975.
159. Dodds, W. J., Benson, R. E., and Bouma, B. N., Antihemophilic factor-related antigen in canine hemophilia A and von Willebrand's disease (Abstr.), *Circulation*, 50 (Suppl. 3), 280, 1974.

QUANTITATIVE DISORDERS OF PLATELETS THROMBOCYTOPENIA

Douglas A. Triplett

Thrombocytopenia (less than 100,000 platelets per cubic millimeter) is the most common cause of serious clinical bleeding. There are many causes of thrombocytopenia, but they can be broadly divided into two major groups: those with decreased platelet production and those with increased platelet destruction or utilization. In the majority of cases, one or the other of these mechanisms will be responsible; however, in some instances both may be operative. A precise etiologic diagnosis is of paramount importance for optimal treatment and prognosis.

The clinical importance of thrombocytopenia is related to the bleeding hazard, but this is variable and often is not easily correlated with the platelet count. Patients with counts as low as 20,000 per cubic millimeter and sometimes lower may have little or no clinical bleeding or purpura in contrast to patients with widespread purpura and frank bleeding with platelet counts slightly less than 100,000 per cubic millimeter. This apparent paradox can be explained on the basis of platelet function with respect to platelet age. Young platelets typically are much more hemostatically effective than senescent platelets.[1] Consequently, platelets found in clinical situations associated with increased platelet destruction are hemostatically more effective than the platelets seen in disorders characterized by decreased platelet production.

In Table 1,* the thrombocytopenias are classified according to the major underlying pathophysiologic mechanism. The amegakaryocytic thrombocytopenias are characterized by decreased platelet production due to a loss of megakaryocytes in the bone marrow. The megakaryocytic thrombocytopenias occur as a result of an increased consumption of platelets or ineffective platelet production.

Accelerated platelet destruction may result from either intrinsic abnormalities in the platelet or extracorpuscular abnormalities. Intrinsic abnormalities are relatively rare, but have been demonstrated in certain forms of hereditary thrombocytopenia, such as the Wiskott-Aldrich Syndrome. In most cases, accelerated platelet destruction is due to extrinsic problems including immunologic phenomena, destruction associated with consumptive coagulopathies, or microangiopathic processes (Figure 1).

In the clinical evaluation of any patient with thrombocytopenia, a careful drug history must be taken. Drugs are capable of inducing thrombocytopenia by either directly suppressing megakaryocytic production in the bone marrow or by an immunologic mechanism with accelerated peripheral platelet destruction. Immunologic drug-induced thrombocytopenia appears to be of the "innocent bystander type" similar to the Stibophen-type of drug-induced immune hemolytic anemia (Table 2, Figure 2).

Thrombocytosis and Thrombocythemia

A platelet count greater than normal may be encountered in a variety of clinical circumstances (Table 6). Thrombocytosis refers to a moderate, often short-lived and symptomless elevation of the platelet count that occurs in association with a number of well-defined clinical states. Thrombocythemia refers to a marked and persistent elevation in the platelet count occurring as a manifestation of an underlying myeloproliferative disorder. By definition, thrombocythemia implies an unregulated proliferation of megakaryocytes with an associated increase in platelet production in contrast to the reactive megakaryocytic proliferation and platelet production of thrombocytosis. Clinically, a clear-cut distinction between thrombocytosis and thrombocythemia

* All figures and tables for this chapter follow text.

may prove difficult. However, because of the diagnostic, prognostic, and therapeutic implications, an attempt at differentiating these states is important (Table 7).

Thrombocytosis is frequently a chance finding. The underlying cause is often readily detectable. Platelet function in thrombocytosis has not been well studied, although in the past, an increased platelet retention in glass bead columns has been demonstrated in postoperative states (Table 8).

To establish the diagnosis of thrombocythemia, one should rule out the clinical states associated with thrombocytosis. It should also be possible to define features of a myeloproliferative disorder. The typical bone marrow findings in myeloproliferative thrombocythemias include the presence of an increased number of megakaryocytes with increased cytoplasmic size and nuclear lobe count. There should also be evidence of abnormalities of the other cell series, i.e., myeloid and erythroid.

Patients with thrombocythemia may have either thrombotic or hemorrhagic problems, although hemorrhagic symptoms are more common. The abnormal bleeding has been attributed to a variety of qualitative platelet defects. The finding of platelet functional abnormalities, particularly with respect to aggregation, is helpful in separating thrombocythemias from thrombocytoses. Abnormalities of epinephrine-induced platelet aggregation have been the most frequently described (Table 8).

Table 1
CLASSIFICATION OF THROMBOCYTOPENIA

Amegakaryocytic thrombocytopenia

- Congenital hypoplasia
  - Fanconi's syndrome (constitutional anemia)[2,3]
  - Thrombocytopenia with absent radii (TAR baby syndrome)[4]
  - Deficiency of thrombopoietin[5]
  - Rubella and other viral illnesses[6]
  - Neonatal thrombocytopenia resulting from maternal ingestion of thiazid diuretics[7]
  - Hereditary thrombocytopenias
    - May-Hegglin anomaly
    - Bernard-Soulier syndrome
- Infiltrative diseases
  - Metastatic carcinoma
  - Leukemias
  - Lymphomas
  - Myelofibrosis
  - Osteopetrosis
  - Miliary tuberculosis
  - Histiocytosis
- Acquired hypoplasia
  - Radiation and myelosuppressive drugs
  - Drugs (thiazides,[8] estrogens,[9] alcohol[10,11])
  - Tidal platelet dysgenesis[12]
  - Aplastic anemia

Megakaryocytic thrombocytopenia

- Ineffective thrombopoiesis
  - Vitamin B_{12} deficiency
  - Folate deficiency
  - Preleukemia
  - Acute myelomonocytic leukemia
  - Paroxysmal nocturnal hemoglobinuria
  - Cyclic thrombocytopenia[13]
  - Di Guglielmo's syndrome
  - Iron deficiency anemia

Table 1 (continued)

Altered distribution of platelets
- Splenomegaly (e.g., cirrhosis, Gaucher's disease, etc.)
- Hypothermia[14]

Nonimmunologic destructive thrombocytopenia
- Disseminated intravascular coagulation
- Bacterial,[15] viral,[16] rickettsial, mycotic, and protozoal infection
- Infectious mononucleosis[17,18]
- Thrombotic thrombocytopenic purpura[19,20]
- Hemolytic uremic syndrome[21]
- Kasabach-Merrit syndrome
- Acute hemolytic reactions (e.g., erythroblastosis fetalis)
- Waring® blender syndrome
- Ristocetin induced

Immunologic thrombocytopenia
- Isoimmune thrombocytopenia[22]
  - Newborns[23]
  - Following multiple transfusions[24]
- Drug-induced thrombocytopenia[25,26]
- Post-transfusion purpura[27,28]
- Idiopathic thrombocytopenic purpura[29-32]
- Acute
- Recurrent
- Chronic

Loss of platelets

Multiple blood transfusions
Extracorporeal circulation

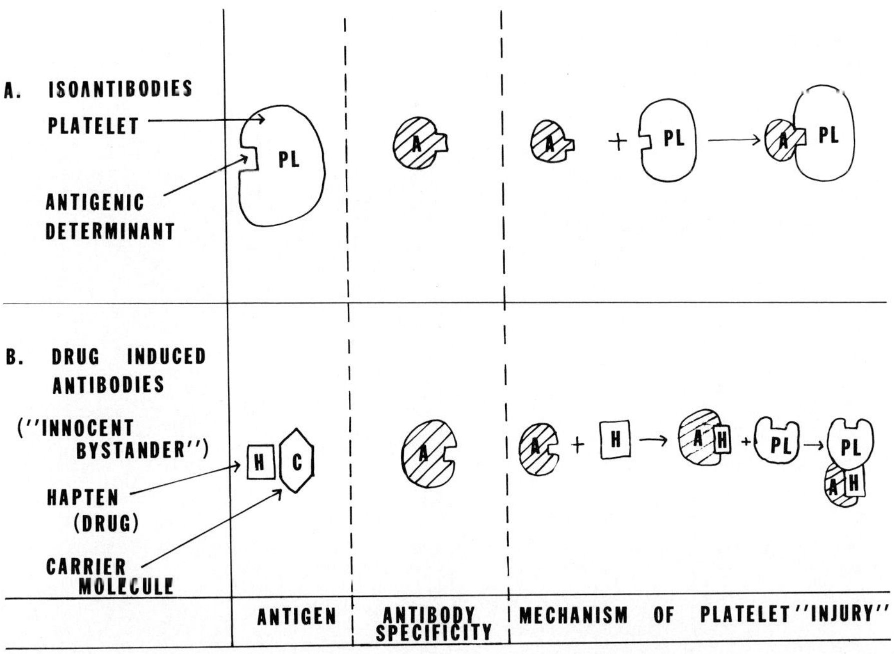

FIGURE 1. Reactions involved in immunologic platelet injury.[75]

Table 2
DRUGS ASSOCIATED WITH IMMUNOLOGIC THROMBOCYTOPENIA

	Ref.
Analgesics	
Salicylates[a]	33
Acetaminophen	34
Phenylbutazone[a]	35
Antipyrine	36
Antibiotics	
Cephalothin	37
Penicillin	38
Streptomycin	39
Para-amino salicylic acid (PAS)	40
Rifampin	41
Novobiocin	42
Various sulfa drugs[a]	43—45
Cinchona alkaloids	
Quinidine[a]	46—48
Quinine[a]	49—51
Hypnotics	
Phenobarbital	52
Meprobamate[a]	53
Sedormid[a]	54, 55
Dilantin®	56
Chlorpromazine	57
Oral hypoglycemics	
Chlorpropamide[a]	58
Tolbutamid	59
Heavy metals	
Gold	60, 61
Mercury	62
Bismuth	63
Organic arsenicals[a]	64
Diuretics	
Acetazolamide	—
Chlorothiazide[a]	53, 65—67
Mercurial diuretics	62
Others	
Digitoxin[a]	68
Ergot	69
Methyldopa	70
Propylthiouracil	71
Disulfiram (Antabuse)	72
Chloroquine[a]	33
Stibophen (Fuadin)	73
Heparin	74

[a] Drugs most frequently associated with immunologic thrombocytopenia.

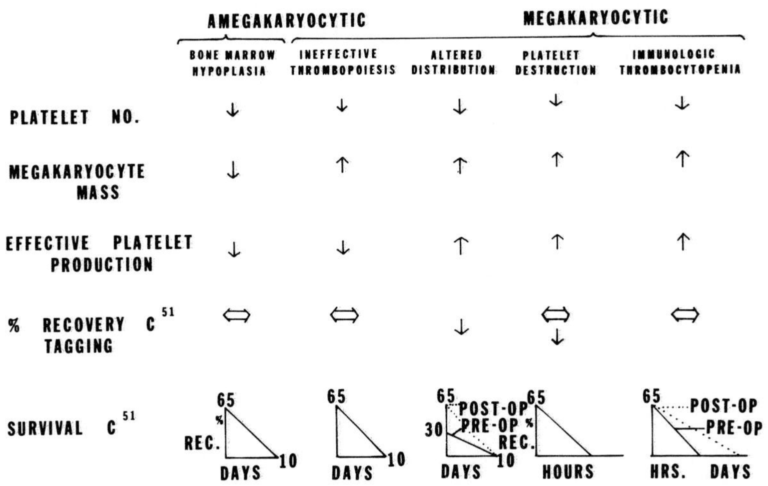

FIGURE 2. Platelet kinetics in thrombocytopenic states.

Table 3
CLINICAL PICTURE OF ACUTE AND CHRONIC IDIOPATHIC THROMBOCYTOPENIA

	Acute	Chronic
Age	Less than 8 years old	20 to 40 years old
Sex predilection	None	Female over male 3:1
Prior infection	Common	Unusual
Onset of bleeding	Abrupt	Insidious
Platelet count	<20,000/mℓ mm^3	30,000 to 80,000/mℓ mm^3
Splenomegaly	Absent	Absent
Duration	2 to 6 weeks	Months to years
Spontaneous remissions	Occur in 90% of patients	Uncommon, fluctuating clinical course
Therapy		
Steroids	70% Response	30% Response
Splenectomy	70% Response	90% Response under age 45 40% Response over age 45

Table 4
LABORATORY TESTS FOR PLATELET ANTIBODIES

	Ref.
Platelet precipitation	76
Passive hemagglutination	77
Platelet lysis	78
Platelet complement fixation	79
Platelet agglutination	80
Antihuman globulin (AHG) techniques	81
Direct	
Indirect	
AHG agglutination	81
Mixed antiglobulin reaction	82
Antiglobulin consumption test	81
Fluorescent antibody techniques	83

Table 4 (continued)

Platelet electrophoresis	84
Platelet factor 3 availability test	85, 86
Immunofluorescence microphotometry (IFMP)	87
^{14}C Serotonin release	88
^{51}CR Release from PNH platelets	89
^{131}I-FAB-anti F $(ab)_2$ test for quantitation of platelet bound immunoglobulin	90
Inhibition of anti-IgG-dependent lysis of sheep erythrocytes	91
Platelet indirect radioactive Coombs test	92
Platelet migration inhibition	93
Inhibition of platelet aggregation	94, 95

Table 5
THE HEREDITARY THROMBOCYTOPENIAS[75]

Sex-linked recessive inheritance

Wiskott-Aldrich syndrome
  Variants without eczema, etc.
"Isolated" thrombocytopenia[96,97]
Thrombocytopenia with increased IgA immunoglobulins and renal disease[98]

Autosomal dominant inheritance

May-Hegglin anomaly[99,100]
Hemoglobin Köln[101]
"Isolated" Thrombocytopenia[102,103]
"Thrombopathic" thrombocytopenia

Autosomal recessive inheritance

Bernard-Soulier syndrome
Chediak-Steinbrink-Higashi Anomaly
Fanconi syndrome
Cystathioninuria[104]
Hyperglycinemia[105]
Methylamalonic acidemia[105]
Isovaleric acidemia[105]
Sidbury syndrome[106]
Schwachmann syndrome[107]

Unclassified forms

In association with qualitative abnormalities of platelet function[108-112]
In association with other heritable hemostatic defects
  Von Willebrand's syndrome[113]
  Factor IX deficiency[114]

Table 6
CAUSES OF AN ELEVATED PLATELET COUNT[115]

Thrombocytosis

Secondary or reactive — transient
  Acute blood loss[116]
  Postpartum
  Infection

Table 6 (continued)

- Post-traumatic
- Post-splenectomy[117]
- Exercise
- Post-operative state
- Drugs — epinephrine
- Following thrombocytopenia
  - Pernicious anemia (after treatment)
  - Acute thrombocytopenic purpura
  - Alcohol-induced thrombocytopenia
  - Drug-induced thrombocytopenia
- Ovulation
- Sarcoidosis
- Adrenal hyperplasia
- Osteoporosis
- Vinblastine therapy
- Oral contraceptives
- 7-Beta-17-Alpha-Dimethyl testosterone
- Citrovorum factor therapy

Chronic

- Inflammatory bowel disease
  - Ulcerative colitis
  - Granulomatous colitis
- Rheumatoid arthritis
- Neoplasms[118]
  - Hodgkin's disease
  - Carcinoma
  - Osteogenic sarcoma
  - Retinoblastoma
  - Mesothelioma
- Iron deficiency (late in iron deficiency may see thrombocytopenia)[119]
- Chronic hemolytic anemia with splenectomy
- Splenic atrophy

Thrombocythemia

As a predominant feature — essential thrombocythemia[120-122]

As an accompanying feature of myeloproliferative disorder

- Polycythemia rubra vera[123]
- Myeloid metaplasia[124]
- Chronic myelocytic leukemia[125]
- Myelomonocytic leukemia

Table 7
DIFFERENTIATION OF REACTIVE THROMBOCYTOSIS AND THROMBOCYTHEMIA[75]

	Reactive thrombocytosis	Thrombocythemia
Platelet kinetics		
Total megakaryocyte mass	Slightly increased	Greatly increased
Megakaryocyte number	Increased	Increased
Megakaryocyte volume	Decreased	Increased
Platelet turnover or production rate	Increased	Increased
Total platelet mass	Increased	Increased
Platelet survival	Normal	Normal to slightly decreased
Clinical and laboratory features		
Thromboembolism and hemorrhage	Uncommon	Common
Duration	Often transitory	Persistent
Spenomegaly	Absent	80% of Cases
Platelet count	Usually $<1000 \times 10^9/\ell$	Usually $>1000 \times 10^9/\ell$
Bleeding time	Normal	Prolonged
Aggregation studies	Normal	Abnormal
Platelet morphology	Normal	Abnormal
Leukocyte count	Usually normal	Increased in 90% of cases

Table 8
PLATELET FUNCTION IN THROMBOCYTOSIS AND THROMBOCYTHEMIA

Number of patients tested	Aggregation: ADP[a]	Aggregation: Epinephrine	Aggregation: Collagen	Aggregation: Thrombin	Platelet retention	Platelet factor 3	Serotonin uptake	Clot retraction	Bleeding time	Tourniquet test
Polycythemia rubra vera[b]										
8 PRV[126]	0/5	6/6	0/6	—	1/4	0/6	—	—	0/4	—
47 PRV[127]	29/62[c]	32/62	23/62[c]	20/54[c]	—	—	—	—	10/49[c]	—
7 PRV[128]	5/7	6/7	—	—	—	3/10[d]	—	—	3/11	—
8 PRV[129]	7/8	Abnormal aggregation patterns	Abnormal aggregation patterns	Abnormal aggregation patterns	7/8	4/8	—	—	2/8	—
6 PRV[130]	14/33	20/33	11/33	15/26	—	4/6	—	—	3/33	—
10 PRV[131]	—	—	—	—	↓[e]	—	↓	—	5/14[d]	—
4 PRV[132]	—	—	—	—	—	—	—	—	—	—
22 PRV[125]	14/22	↓	Abnormal aggregation patterns	Abnormal aggregation patterns	Abnormal aggregation patterns	—	—	—	—	—
1 PRV[133]	—	—	—	—	—	—	—	1/1	0/1	—
7 PRV[134]	4/7	Spontaneous aggregation	Spontaneous aggregation	—	—	—	—	—	—	—
Chronic myelocytic leukemia[f]										
3 CML[126]	0/3	1/3	1/3	—	—	0/1	—	—	—	—
9 CML[129]	7/9	Abnormal aggregation patterns	Abnormal aggregation patterns	Abnormal aggregation patterns	4/8	4/9	—	—	1/9	—
19 CML[130]	14/33	20/33	11/33	15/26	—	14/19	—	—	3/33	—
5 CML[128]	0/5	1/5	1/5	—	—	3/10	—	—	3/11	—
12 CML[132]	S1↓	Severely impaired	↓	—	—	—	—	—	—	—
2 CML[133]	—	—	—	—	—	—	—	0/2	0/2	0/2
10 CML[134]	6/10	Spontaneous aggregation	Spontaneous aggregation	—	—	—	—	—	—	—

Table 8 (continued)

					Essential thrombocythemia[g]					
3ET[126]	0/1	1/1	0/1	—	1/1	0/2	—	—	0/2	—
3 ET[135]	3/3	3/3	0/3	—	1/3↓, 2/3↓	0/3	2/2	0/3	0/3	—
7 ET[128]	7/7	7/7	4/7	—	—	3/10	—	—	3/11	—
5 ET[131]	—	—	—	—	↓[e]	—	↓	—	5/14	—
4 ET[132]	Disaggregation ↓	↓	↓	—	—	—	—	—	—	—
1 ET[134]	1/1	Spontaneous aggregation	Spontaneous aggregation	—	—	—	—	—	—	—
					Agnogenic myeloid metaplasia[h]					
4 AMM[126]	0/3	3/3	0/3	—	0/1	1/2	—	—	—	—
1 AMM[129]	1/1	Spontaneous aggregation	Spontaneous aggregation	—	1/1	1/1	—	—	1/1	—
4 AMM[130]	14/33	20/33	11/33	15/26	—	0/4	—	—	3/33	—
1 AMM[131]	—	—	—	—	↓[e]	—	↓	—	5/14	—
10 AMM[136]	—	—	—	—	3/10[e]	3/10	—	2/10	9/10	3/10
5 AMM[134]	2/5	Spontaneous aggregation	Spontaneous aggregation	—	—	—	—	—	—	—
					Miscellaneous myeloproliferative disorders					
5 MPD[137i] (with hemorrhage or thrombosis)	2/5[j]	5/5	Reaction time prolonged	—	2/5	2/5	—	—	3/5	—
7 MPD[137i] (without hemorrhage or thrombosis)	0/7	1/7	—	—	1/7	2/7	—	—	0/7	—
1 EL[130k]	14/33	20/33	11/33	15/26	—	1/1	—	—	3/33	—
3 UMD[130l]	14/33	20/33	11/33	15/26	—	2/3	—	—	3/33	—
					Secondary thrombocytosis[m]					
4 11° T[126]	0/3	0/3	0/3	—	—	0/1	—	—	—	—
1 11° T[138]	1/1	1/1	0/1	—	—	1/1	—	—	0/1	—
16 11° T[128]	1/13	2/15	1/15	—	—	1/8	—	—	0/9(Mielke)	—

Table 8 (continued)

5 11° T[137]	0/5	0/5	Reaction time shortened	—	0/5	0/5	—	—	0/4	—
16 11° T[131]	—	—	—	—	0/16	—	—	—	2/9	—
4 11° T[133]	—	—	—	—	—	—	—	0/4	0/4	0/4

Note: Results of platelet function tests are expressed as the number of abnormal results/total number tested. Methods used for testing varied from study to study.

[a] Concentration of aggregating agents may vary.
[b] PRV = polycythemia rubra vera.
[c] Abnormalities especially associated with elevated hemocrits.
[d] Results enclosed in boxes represent group studies in which the results obtained were not differentiated for each specific disorder in the myeloproliferative syndrome.
[e] Both in vivo and in vitro.
[f] CML = chronic myelocytic leukemia.
[g] ET = essential thrombocythemia.
[h] AMM = agnogenic myeloid metaplasia.
[i] MPD = myeloproliferative disorder (not identified as to type).
[j] Decreased magnitude.
[k] EL = erythroleukemia.
[l] UMD = undifferentiated myeloproliferative disorder.
[m] 11° T = secondary thrombocytosis.

REFERENCES

1. Shulman, N. R., Watkins, S. P., Jr., Itscoitz, S. B., and Students, A. B., Evidence that the spleen retains the youngest and hemostatically most effective platelets, *Trans. Assoc. Am. Physicians,* 81, 302, 1968.
2. Dacie, J. B. and Gilpin, A., Refractory anaemia (Fanconi type), *Arch. Dis. Child.,* 19, 155, 1944.
3. O'Neill, E. M. and Varadi, S., Neonatal aplastic anemia in Fanconi's anemia, *Arch. Dis. Child.,* 38, 92, 1963.
4. Eisenstein, E. M., Congenital amegakaryocytic thrombocytopenic purpura, *Clin. Pediatr.,* 5, 143, 1966.
5. Schulman, I., Pierce, M., Lukens, A., and Currimbhoy, Z., Studies on thrombopoiesis. I. A factor in normal human plasma required for platelet production, chronic thrombocytopenia due to its deficiency, *Blood,* 16, 943, 1960.
6. Vossaugh, P., Leikin, C. S., Avery, G., Monif, G., and Sever, J., Neonatal thrombocytopenia in association with rubella, *Acta Haematol. (Basel),* 35, 158, 1966.
7. Rodriquez, S. U., Leikin, S., and Hiller, N. P., Neonatal thrombocytopenia associated with antepartum administration of thiazide drugs, *N. Engl. J. Med.,* 270, 881, 1964.
8. Kutti, J. and Linefield, A., The frequency of thrombocytopenia in patients with heart disease treated with oral diuretics, *Acta Med. Scand.,* 183, 245, 1968.
9. Cooper, B. A. and Bigelow, F. S., Thrombocytopenia associated with the administration of diethylstilbestrol in man, *Ann. Intern. Med.,* 52, 907, 1960.
10. Lindebaun, J. and Hargrove, R. L., Thrombocytopenia in alcoholics, *Ann. Intern. Med.,* 68, 526, 1968.
11. Lindebaun, J. and Lieber, P. S., Hematologic effects of alcohol in man in the absence of nutritional deficiency, *N. Engl. J. Med.,* 281, 333, 1969.
12. Engström, K., Lindquist, A., and Söderström, N., Periodic thrombocytopenia or platelet dysgenesis occurring in man, *Scand. J. Haematol.,* 3, 290, 1966.
13. Wilkinson, T. and Firkin, B., Idiopathic cyclical acute thrombocytopenic purpura, *Med. J. Aust.,* 1, 217, 1966.
14. Villalobos, T. J., Adelson, E., Riley, P. A., Crosley, W. H., and technical assistance of Glaucke, H., A cause of the thrombocytopenia and leukopenia that occurs in dogs during deep hypothermia, *J. Clin. Invest.,* 37, 1, 1958.
15. Wilhelm, D. J. and Cherubin, C., Hypofibrinogenemia and thrombocytopenia with meningococcemia, *Am. J. Dis. Child.,* 113, 494, 1967.
16. McKay, D. G. and Margaretten, W., Disseminated intravascular coagulation in virus diseases, *Arch. Intern. Med.,* 120, 129, 1967.
17. Carter, R. L., Platelet levels in infectious mononucleosis, *Blood,* 25, 817, 1965.
18. Radel, E. B. and Schorr, J. B., Thrombocytopenic purpura with infectious mononucleosis, *J. Pediatr.,* 63, 486, 1963.
19. Moschcowitz, E., An acute febrile pleiochromic anemia with hyaline thrombosis of terminal arterioles and capillaries: an undescribed disease, *Arch. Intern. Med.,* 36, 89, 1925.
20. Amorosi, E. L. and Ultmann, J. E., Thrombotic thrombocytopenic purpura: report of 16 cases and review of the literature, *Medicine (Baltimore),* 45, 139, 1966.
21. Brain, M. C., The hemolytic uraemic syndrome, *Semin. Hematol.,* 6, 162, 1969.
22. Pearson, H. A., Shulman, N. R., Marder, V. J., and Cone, T. E., Jr., Isoimmune neonatal thrombocytopenia purpura: clinical and therapeutic considerations, *Blood,* 23, 154, 1964.
23. Poley, J. R. and Stickler, G. B., Petechiae in the newborn infant, *Am. J. Dis. Child.,* 102, 365, 1961.
24. Shulman, N. R., Marder, J., and Hiller, M. C., Platelet and leukocyte isoantigens and antibodies: serologic, physiologic, and clinical studies, *Prog. Hematol.,* 4, 222, 1964.
25. Vipan, W. H., Quinine as a cause of purpura, *Lancet,* 2, 37, 1865.
26. Shulman, N. R., A mechanism of cell destruction in individuals sensitized to foreign antigens and implications in autoimmunity, *Ann. Intern. Med.,* 50, 506, 1964.
27. Morrison, F. S. and Mollison, P. L., Post-transfusion purpura, *N. Engl. J. Med.,* 275, 243, 1966.
28. Howard, J. E., Glassberg, A. B., and Perkins, H. A., Post-transfusion thrombocytopenic purpura: a case report, *Am. J. Hematol.,* 1, 339, 1976.
29. Rabinowitz, U. and Dameshek, W., Systemic lupus erythematosus after "idiopathic" thrombocytopenic purpura, *Ann. Intern. Med.,* 52, 1, 1960.
30. Marshall, J. S., Weisberger, A. S., Levy, R. P., and Breckenridge, R. T., Co-existent idiopathic thrombocytopenic purpura and hyperthyroidism, *Ann. Intern. Med.,* 67, 411, 1967.
31. Baldini, M., Idiopathic thrombocytopenic purpura, *N. Engl. J. Med.,* 274, 1245, 1969.
32. Mueller-Eckhardt, C., Idiopathic thrombocytopenic purpura (ITP): clinical and immunologic considerations, *Semin. Thromb. Hemostasis,* 3, 125, 1977.

33. Niewig, H. O., Bouma, H. G., DeVries, K., and Jansz, A., Haematological side effects of some anti-rheumatic drugs, *Ann. Rheum. Dis.*, 22, 440, 1963.
34. Heading, R. C., Purpura and paracetamol, *Br. Med. J.*, 3, 743, 1968.
35. Feldman, L., Cohnen, F., and Hirsch, H., Fatal thrombocytopenic purpura following phenylbutazone therapy, *Ill. Med. J.*, 105, 83, 1954.
36. Malinvaud, G., Dausset, J., and Layani, F. Purpura thrombopénique aigue aux dérivés de l'antipyrine, *Sang*, 26, 130, 1955.
37. Gralnick, H. R., McGinniss, M., and Halterman, R., Thrombocytopenia with sodium cephalothin therapy, *Ann. Intern. Med.*, 77, 401, 1972.
38. Hsi, Y. J., Kuo, H. Y., and Ouyang, A., Thrombocytopenia following administration of penicillin, *Chin. Med. J.*, 85, 249, 1966.
39. Oppenhelm, M. and de Meyer, G., Granulound Thrombocytopenie infolge streptomycin Behandlung, *Schweiz. Med. Wochenschr.*, 79, 1187, 1949.
40. Wurzel, H. A. and Mayock, R. L., Thrombocytopenia induced by sodium paraaminosalicyclic acid: report of case, *J.A.M.A.*, 153, 1094, 1953.
41. Blajchman, M. A., Lowry, R. C., Pettit, J. E., and Stradling, P., Rifampicin-induced immune thrombocytopenia, *Br. Med. J.*, 3, 24, 1970.
42. Day, H. J., Conrad, F. G., and Moore, J. E., Immunothrombocytopenia induced by novobiocin, *Am. J. Med. Sci.*, 236, 475, 1958.
43. Ackroyd, J. F., Allergic purpura, including purpura due to food, drugs and infections, *Am. J. Med.*, 14, 605, 1953.
44. Hurd, R. W. and Jacox, R. F., Thrombopenic purpura developing as a complication of sulfathiazole and sulfadiazine therapy, *J.A.M.A.*, 122, 296, 1943.
45. MaCaulay, D., Thrombocytopenia following sulphadimidine, *Br. Med. J.*, 2, 1269, 1954.
46. Bishop, R. C., Spencer, H. H., and Bethell, F. H., Quinidine purpura, *Ann. Intern. Med.*, 50, 1227, 1959.
47. Bolton, F. G. and Damashek, W., Thrombocytopenic purpura due to quinidine, *Blood*, 11, 527, 1956; *Blood*, 11, 547, 1956.
48. Schen, R. J. and Rabinovitz, M., Thrombocytopenic purpura due to quinidine, *Br. Med. J.*, 2, 1502, 1958.
49. Belkin, G. A., Cocktail purpura: an unusual case of quinine sensitivity, *Ann. Intern. Med.*, 66, 583, 1967.
50. Bolton, F. G. and Young, R. V., Observations on cases of thrombocytopenic purpura due to quinine, sulphamezathine, and quinidine, *J. Clin. Pathol.*, 6, 320, 1953.
51. Helmly, R. B., Bergin, J. J., and Shulman, N. P., Quinine-induced purpura, *Arch. Intern. Med.*, 120, 59, 1967.
52. Boas, E. P. and Erf, L. A., Thrombocytopenic purpura following medication with Sedormid and with phenobarbital, *N.Y. State J. Med.*, 36, 491, 1936.
53. Karpatkin, S., Strick, N., Karpatkin, M., and Siskind, G. W., Cumulative experience in the detection of anti-platelet antibody in 234 patients with idiopathic thrombocytopenic purpura, systemic lupus erythematous and other clinical disorders, *Am. J. Med.*, 52, 776, 1972.
54. Ackroyd, J. F., The pathogenesis of thrombocytopenic purpura due to hypersensitivity to Sedormid, *Clin. Sci.*, 7, 249, 1949.
55. Borrie, P., A purpuric drug eruption caused by carbromal, *Br. Med. J.*, 1, 645, 1955.
56. Weintraub, R. M., Pechet, L., and Alexander, B., Rapid diagnosis of drug-induced thrombocytopenic purpura, *J.A.M.A.*, 180, 528, 1962.
57. Horowitz, H. I. and Nachman, R. L., Drug purpura, *Semin. Hematol.*, 2, 287, 1967.
58. Grace, W. J., Thrombocytopenia in a patient taking chlorpropamide, *N. Engl. J. Med.*, 260, 711, 1959.
59. Schiff, D., Aranda, J. V. and Stern, L., Neonatal thrombocytopenia and congenital malformations associated with administration of tolbutamide to mother, *J. Pediatr.*, 77, 457, 1970.
60. Hazlett, B. E. and Yendt, E. R., Thrombocytopenia following gold therapy with successful treatment, *Can. Med. Assoc. J.*, 79, 31, 1958.
61. Thompson, M., Sinclair, R. J. G., and Duthie, J. J. R., Thrombocytopenic purpura after administration of gold, *Br. Med. J.*, 1, 899, 1954.
62. Butt, E. M. and Simonsen, D. G., Mercury and lead storage in human tissues with special reference to thrombocytopenic purpura, *Am. J. Clin. Pathol.*, 20, 716, 1950.
63. Bianchi, A. E., Comments on a case of purpura, *Rev. Assoc. Med. Argent.*, 46, 1566, 1932.
64. Falconer, E. H. and Epstein, N. N., Purpura haemorrhagica following neoarsphenamine and bismarsen therapy, *Arch. Intern. Med.*, 65, 1158, 1940; *Arch. Intern. Med.*, 66, 319, 1940.
65. Bettman, J. W., Drug hypersensitivity purpura, *Arch. Intern. Med.*, 112, 840, 1963.
66. Eisner, E. V. and Crowell, E. R., Hydrochlorothiazide dependent thrombocytopenia due to IgM antibody, *J.A.M.A.*, 215, 480, 1971.

67. Gesink, M. H. and Bradford, H. A., Thrombocytopenic purpura associated with hydrochlorothiazide therapy, *J.A.M.A.*, 172, 556, 1960.
68. Young, R. C., Nachman, R. L., and Horowitz, H. I., Thrombocytopenia due to digitoxin, *Am. J. Med.*, 41, 605, 1966.
69. Peshkin, M. M. and Miller, J. A., Quinine and ergot allergy and thrombocytopenic purpura, *J.A.M.A.*, 102, 1737, 1934.
70. Benraad, A. H. and Schoenaker, A. H., Thrombopenia after use of methyldopa, *Lancet*, 2, 292, 1965.
71. Fewell, R. A., Engel, E. F., and Zimmerman, S. L., Acute thrombocytopenic purpura associated with propylthiouracil, *J.A.M.A.*, 143, 891, 1950.
72. Leibetseder, F., Akute thrombopenische Purpura nach Antabus-Behandlung, *Klin. Wochenschr.*, 64, 431, 1952.
73. Kahn, H. R. and Brod, R. C., Thrombocytopenia due to stibophen, *Arch. Intern. Med.*, 108, 496, 1961.
74. Natelson, E., Lynch, E. C., Alfrey, C. P., and Gross, J. B., Heparin induced thrombocytopenia, *Ann. Intern. Med.*, 71, 112, 1969.
75. Wintrobe, M. M., Clinical Hematology, 7th ed., Lea & Febiger, Philadelphia, 1974, 1093, 1100, 1104.
76. Dausset, J., Colin, M., and Colombani, J., Immune platelet iso-antibodies, *Vox Sang.*, 5, 4, 1960.
77. Dausset, J. and Colombani, J., Reactions immunologiques au cours du purpura thrombopenique idiopathique, *Sem. Hop. (Paris)*, 40, 387, 1964.
78. Miescher, P. A., Autoantibodies against thrombocytes and leukocytes, in *Textbook of Immunopathology*, Vol. 2, Miescher, P. A. and Muller-Eberhard, M. J., Eds., Grune & Stratton, New York, 1969, 500.
79. Dausset, J., Colombani, J., and Colombani, M., Studies of leukopenias and thrombocytopenias by the direct antiglobulin consumption test on leukocytes and/or platelets, *Blood*, 18, 672, 1961.
80. Corn, M. and Upshaw, J. D., Evaluation of platelet antibodies in idiopathic thrombocytopenic purpura, *Arch. Intern. Med.*, 109, 157, 1962.
81. Kissmeyer-Nielsen, F. and Jensen, K. G., Immunology of platelets, *Prog. Clin. Pathol.*, 2, 141, 1969.
82. Coombs, R. R. A., Marks, J., and Bedford, D., Specific mixed agglutination: mixed erythrocyte platelet antiglobulin reaction for the detection of platelet antibodies, *Br. J. Haematol.*, 2, 84, 1956.
83. van Boxtel, C. J., Oosterhof, F., and Engelfriet, C. P., Immunofluorescence microphotometry for the detection of platelet antibodies. III. Demonstration of autoantibodies against platelets, *Scand. J. Immunol.*, 4, 657, 1975.
84. Seidl, S. and Holtz, G., Der Einfluss des Serums von Patienten mit Thrombocytopenie auf die elektrophoretische Beweglichkeit normaler menschlicher Thrombozyten, *Klin. Wochenschr.*, 45, 588, 1967.
85. Spaeth, T. H. and Cintron, J., Studies on platelet factor 3 availability, *Br. J. Haematol.*, 11, 269, 1965.
86. Horowitz, H. I., Rappaport, H. I., Young, R. C., and Fujimoto, M. M., Change in platelet factor 3 as a means of demonstrating immume reactions involving platelets: its use as a test for quinidine-induced thrombocytopenia, *Transfusion*, 5, 336, 1965.
87. Denk, H., Fischer, M., Pilgerstorfer, H. W., and Schnack, H., Immunofluoreszenzmikrophotometrie zur quantitativen Erfassung antithrombozytärer Autoantikörper, *Thromb. Diath. Haemorrh.*, 21, 387, 1969.
88. Bridges, J. M., Baldini, M., Fischera, C., and Dameshek, W., Effect of anti-platelet antibodies on the in vitro uptake of 5-hydroxytryptamine by blood platelets, *Nature (London)*, 197, 364, 1963.
89. Aster, R. H., A platelet membrane defect in paroxysmal nocturnal hemoglobinuria (PNH): usefulness in detecting platelet antibodies in thrombocytopenic purpuras, *J. Clin. Invest.*, 47, 2 (Abstr.), 1968.
90. McMillan, R., Smith, R. S., Longmire, R. L., Yelenosky, R., Reid, R. T., and Craddock, C. G., Immunoglobulins associated with human platelets, *Blood*, 37, 316, 1971.
91. Dixon, R., Rosse, W., and Ebert, L., Quantitative determination of antibody in idiopathic thrombocytopenic purpura: correlation of serum and platelet-bound antibody in clinical response, *N. Engl. J. Med.*, 292, 230, 1975.
92. Soulier, J. P., Patereau, C., and Drouet, J., Platelet indirect radioactive Coombs test. Its utilization of PLA_1 grouping, *Vox Sang.*, 29, 253, 1975.
93. Duquesnoy, R. J., Lorentzen, D. F., and Aster, R. H., Platelet migration inhibition: a new method for detection of platelet antibodies, *Blood*, 45, 741, 1975.
94. Heinrich, D., Stephinger, U., and Mueller-Eckhardt, C., Specific interaction of HLA antibodies (eluates) with washed platelets, *Br. J. Haematol.*, in press.
95. Mueller-Eckhardt, C. and Mönch, H., The effect of platelet-specific allo-antibodies on the aggregation of human thrombocytes induced by ADP and collagen, *Thromb. Diath. Haemorrh.*, 25, 379, 1971.

96. **Chiaro, J. J., Dharmkreng-at, A., Bloom, G. E.,** X-linked thrombocytopenic purpura, *Am. J. Dis. Child.,* 123, 565, 1972.
97. **Schaar, F. E.,** Familial idiopathic thrombocytopenic purpura, *J. Pediatr.,* 62, 546, 1963.
98. **Gunterberger, J., Trygstad, C. W., Stiehm, E. R., Opitz, J. M., Thatcher, L. G., Bloodworth, J. M. B., and Setzkorn, J.,** Familial thrombocytopenia, elevated serum IgA levels and renal disease, *Am. J. Med.,* 49, 729, 1970.
99. **Beck. E. A. and Baumgartner, H. R.,** Zur Frage der Thrombopathie bei May-Hegglin-Anomalie, *Schweiz. Med. Wochenschr.,* 7, 330, 1970.
100. **Davis, J. W. and Wilson, S. J.,** Platelet survival in the May-Hegglin anomaly, *Br. J. Haematol.,* 12, 61, 1966.
101. **Hutchison, H. E., Pinkerton, P. H., Waters, P., Douglas, A. S., Lehmann, H., and Beale, D.,** Hereditary Heinz-body anemia, thrombocytopenia, and hemoglobinopathy (Hb Koln) in a Glasgow family, *Br. Med. J.,* 2, 1099, 1964.
102. **Bithell, T. C., Didisheim, P., Cartwright, G. E., and Wintrobe, M. M.,** Thrombocytopenia inherited as an autosomal dominant trait, *Blood,* 25, 231, 1965.
103. **Schaison, G., Najean, Y., Saugier, J., Ardaillov, N., and Bernard, J.,** Thrombopenie familiale chronique, *Nouv. Rev. Fr. Hematol.,* 8, 397, 1968.
104. **Mongeau, J., Hilgartner, M., Worthen, H. G., and Frimpter, G. W.,** Cystathioninuria: study of an infant with normal mentality, thrombocytopenia, and renal calculi, *J. Pediatr.,* 69, 1113, 1966.
105. **Morrow, G., III, Barnes, L. A., Auerbach, V. H., DiGeorge, A. M., Ando, T., and Nyhan, W. L.,** Observations on the coexistence of methylmalonic acidemia and glycinemia, *J. Pediatr.,* 74, 680, 1968.
106. **Sidbury, J. B., Smith, E. K., and Harlan, W.,** An inborn error of short-chain fatty acid metabolism, *J. Pediatr.,* 70, 8, 1967.
107. **Shwachman, H., Diamond, L. K., Oski, F. A., and Khaw, K.,** The syndrome of pancreatic insufficiency and bone marrow dysfunction, *J. Pediatr.,* 65, 645, 1964.
108. **Raccuglia, G.,** Gray platelet syndrome. A variety of qualitative platelet disorder, *Am. J. Med.,* 51, 818, 1971.
109. **Rozenszain, L. and Medin, T.,** Thrombocytopathy and transitory forms between thrombocytopathy and thrombocytopenia, *Acta Haematol.,* 22, 255, 1959.
110. **Seip, M. and Kjaerheim, A.,** A familial platelet disease — hereditary thrombasthenic — thrombopathic thrombocytopenia, *Scand. J. Clin. Lab. Invest.,* 17, 159, 1965.
111. **Sheth, N. K. and Prankerd, T. A. J.,** Inherited thrombocytopenia with thrombasthenia, *J. Clin. Pathol.,* 21, 154, 1968.
112. **Stavem, P., Jeremic, M., Hjort, P. F., Wisloff, F., Vogt, E., Oyen, R., Abrahamsen, A. F., and Sovde, A.,** Hereditary thrombocytopenia with excessively prolonged bleeding time, *Scand. J. Haematol.,* 6, 250, 1969.
113. **Nielsen, E. G. and Svejgaard, A.,** von Willebrand's disease associated with intermittent thrombocytopenia, *Lancet,* 2, 966, 1967.
114. **Harms, D. and Sachs, V.,** Familial chronic thrombocytopenia with platelet autoantibodies, *Acta Haematol. (Basel),* 34, 30, 1965.
115. **Triplett, D. A.,** Quantitative platelet disorders, in *Platelet Function: Laboratory Evaluation and Clinical Application,* Triplett, D. A., Ed., American Society of Clinical Pathology Press, Chicago, 1978.
116. **Desforges, J. F., Bigelow, F. S., and Chalmers, T. C.,** The effects of massive gastrointestinal hemorrhage on hemostasis, *J. Lab. Clin. Med.,* 43, 501, 1954.
117. **Hirsh, J. and Dacie, J. V.,** Persistent post-splenectomy thrombocytosis and thromboembolism: a consequence of continuing anemia, *Br. J. Haematol.,* 12, 44, 1966.
118. **Levin, J. and Conley, D. L.,** Thrombocytosis associated with malignant disease, *Arch. Intern. Med.,* 114, 497, 1964.
119. **Schloesser, L. L., Kipp, M. A., and Wenzel, F. J.,** Thrombocytosis in iron deficiency anemia, *J. Lab. Clin. Med.,* 66, 107, 1965.
120. **Davis, W. M. and Ross, A. O. M.,** Thrombocytosis and thrombocythemia, *Am. J. Clin. Pathol.,* 59, 243, 1973.
121. **Gunz, F. W.,** Hemorrhagic thrombocythemia: a critical review, *Blood,* 15, 706, 1960.
122. **Ozer, F. L., Truax, W. E., Miesck, D. C., and Levin, W. C.,** Primary hemorrhagic thrombocythemia, *Am. J. Med.,* 28, 807, 1960.
123. **Wasserman, L. R.,** Polycythemia vera — its course and treatment: relation to myeloid metaplasia and leukemia, *Bull. N.Y. Acad. Med.,* 3, 343, 1954.
124. **Bouroncle, B. A. and Doan, C. A.,** Myelofibrosis: clinical, hematologic and pathologic study of 110 patients, *Am. J. Med. Sci.,* 243, 697, 1962.
125. **Gilbert, H. S.,** A reappraisal of the "myeloproliferative disease" concept, *M. Sinai J. Med. N.Y.,* 37, 426, 1970.

126. Neemah, J. A., Bowie, E. J. W., Thompson, J., Didisheim, P., and Owen, C., Quantitation of platelet aggregation in myeloproliferative disorders, *Am. J. Clin. Pathol.*, 57, 336, 1972.
127. Berger, S., Aledort, L. M., Gilbert, H. S., Hanson, J. P., and Wasserman, L. R., Abnormalities of platelet function in patients with polycythemia, *Cancer Res.*, 33, 2683, 1973.
128. Ginsburg, A. D., Platelet function in patients with high platelet counts, *Ann. Intern. Med.*, 82, 506, 1975.
129. Cardamone, J., Edson, J. R., McArthur, J. R., and Jacob, H. S., Abnormalities of platelet function in the myeloproliferative disorders, *J.A.M.A.*, 221, 270, 1972.
130. Tangun, Y., Platelet aggregation and platelet factor 3 in myeloproliferative disorders, *Thromb. Diath. Haemorr.*, 25, 241, 1971.
131. McClure, P. D., Ingram, G. I. C., Stacey, R. S., Glass, U. H., and Matchett, M. O., Platelet function tests in thrombocythaemia and thrombocytosis, *Br. J. Haematol.*, 12, 478, 1966.
132. Caen, J. P., Sultan, Y., and Delobel, J., Les thrombopathies acquires, *Nouv. Rev. Fr. Hematol.*, 9, 553, 1969.
133. Niewiarowski, S., Zywicka, H., and Latallo, Z., Coagulation disorders in thrombocythemia, a study of seven cases, *Thromb. Diath. Haemorrh.*, 7, 114, 1962.
134. Barbui, T., Battista, R., and Dini, E., Spontaneous platelet aggregation in myeloproliferative disorders, *Acta Haematol.*, 50, 25, 1973.
135. Spaet, T., Lejnieks, I., Gaynor, E., and Goldstein, M., Defective platelets in essential thrombocythemia, *Arch. Intern. Med.*, 124, 135, 1969.
136. Didisheim, P. and Bunting, D., Abnormal platelet function in myelofibrosis, *Am. J. Clin. Pathol.*, 45, 566, 1966.
137. Zucker, S. and Mielke, C. H., Classification of thrombocytosis based on platelet function tests: correlation with hemorrhagic and thrombotic complications, *J. Lab. Clin. Med.*, 80, 385, 1972.
138. Dube, B., Bajpai, H. S., Chawla, S. C., and Gupta, Y. N., Platelet defects in post-splenectomy thrombocythaemia, *Acta Haematol.*, 46, 221, 1971.

Index

INDEX

A

Abnormalities and disorders, effects of, see also Normal values; Variation and variants; specific disorders by name
amino acid residues
general positions and, 161—163
heme groups in contact with, 154—156
subunit contacts and, 157—160
bleeding time procedures, 374—378
coagulation measurements, 11
erythrocyte measurements, 6—7
anemia and, 237—239
globin synthesis, genetic mechanisms accounting for, 57—63
hematopoietic-related factor measurement, 13—14
hemoglobins, see Chains; Chains and chain variants; Hemoglobinopathies; Variations and variants, hemoglobins; specific variants by name
iron metabolism
deficiencies, see also Anemia; Iron, deficiency, 237—239
storage in body, 231—233
leukocyte measurements, 7—8
maturation, iron and, 237—239
nuclear, anemia and, 238—239
platelets
acquired, see also Qualitative abnormalities, platelets, 463—469
aggregation testing, 334—335, 339—344, 381—394
bleeding time, 331—332, 374—378
function, 329—347, 355—357
glass bead column retention test, see Glass bead column retention test, biologic and physiologic variations and
hereditary, see also Qualitative abnormalities, platelets, 447—459
kinetics and, 263—270
measurement of, 9
production, 255—259
qualitative, see Qualitative abnormalities, platelets
quantitative, see Quantitative disorders, platelets
release (secretion) reaction, 343—344, 394, 439—442
retention, see Platelets, Retention, abnormalities
sizing techniques, 425—432
thrombocytopenia, see Thrombocytopenia
von Willebrand's disease, see von Willebrand's disease
proliferation, anemia and, 237—238
variable blood volume, 35—38
Absorbance monitor, use in hemoglobin chromatography, 78
Absorption
hemoglobincyanide system, 212, 214—215
iron, see Iron, absorption of
ACD, platelet kinetics and, 264—265, 440
Acetylsalicylic acid, see Aspirin
Acid hydrolase secretion, in platelets, 290
Acid mucopolysaccharides, in platelet coat, 313
Acquired platelet abnormalities, see Qualitative abnormalities, platelets, acquired; specific disorders by name
Actin, platelet structure and function, role in, 274—278, 280—281, 288, 290, 314, 324
α-Actinin, in platelets, 281
Actomyosin, platelet structure and function, role in, 274—278, 280—281, 288—294, 296
Acyl-CoA activity, in platelets, 279—280
Adenine nucleotides, platelet functions and, see also specifice adenine nucleotides by name, 273—277, 280—281, 287—291, 315, 435, 454—457, 463
Adenine uptake, in platelets, 275, 289
Adenosine diphosphate, platelet functions and abnormalities, 450—452, 463, 465, 468—469, 494—496
aggregation, 381—394
biochemistry, 273, 276—277, 279—280, 286—287, 289—291, 295
bleeding time procedures, 369
coagulation activities, 353—354, 403—405
kinetics, labeled platelets, 264
secretory proteins, assay of, 435—437, 440
sizing, 415—417
tests, laboratory, 329, 334, 337—341, 343—346
Adenosine monophosphate, platelet response to, 273
cyclic, 275, 294—297, 440
Adenosine triphosphate, platelet functions and, 273, 275—281, 285—287, 294—296, 314, 324, 344, 454
Adenosine uptake, in platelets, 275
Adenyl cyclase, in platelets, 295
Adhesion, platelet, see Platelets, adhesion; Platelets, aggregation; Platelets, retention
ADP, see Adenosine diphosphate
Affinity, oxygen, hemoglobins, see Bohr effect; Oxygen, affinity
Aging, platelet, effects of, see Platelets, senescence
Agglutination, platelet, see Platelets, agglutination
Aggregation, platelet, see Platelets, adhesion; Platelets, aggregation; Platelets, retention
Aggregometer, use in platelet aggregation studies, 342, 346, 381—394, 463
Allopurinol, role in iron metabolism, 229
Allosteric binding, hemoglobin structure and, 109
Alpha chains, see α-Chains and α-chain variants
Alpha cistron, globin, activity at, 55—58
Alpha contacts, see Contacts, α β

Alpha classes, globins and hemoglobins, see α-Chains; α-Globins
Alpha dimers, see Dimers, α β
Alpha subunits, see α-Subunits
Amberlite® polystyrene resin, in hemoglobin chromatography, 68
Amega karocytic thrombocytopenia, characteristics of, 487—489, 491
Amino acids
chains, distance from heme, hemoglobin structure and, 137—139
contacts within quaternary structures, hemoglobinopathies, see Contacts, α β hemoglobin structure and
iron metabolism, role in, 221, 226
metabolism, in platelets, 273
residues, hemoglobin structure and
chain variants, 90—94, 178—194
deleted, see Deleted amino acid residues
general positions, 161—163
helical segments of globin fold, presence in, 105—106, 112—125
heme groups, contact with, 154—156
hydrogen bonds, presence in, 105—106, 126—127
hydrophilic and hydrophobic, 128—131
interatomic contacts of heme groups and, 136
numbering system, 105
subunit contacts and, 145—146, 157—160
three-dimensional hemoglobin structure and, 105—171
variability, species difference causing, 106, 131
sequences
globins, 51—52, 58—63, 105
hemoglobin chains, 45—48, 105, 112—117, 129—131
myoglobin chains, 105, 112—117
three-dimensional hemoglobin structure related to, 110, 164—171
transferrin molecule, 226
substitutions, hemoglobin chains and chain variants, 90—94, 178—187, 189—194
AMP, see Adenosine monophosphate
cAMP, see Adenosine monophosphate, cyclic
Anemia, see also Iron, deficiency
iron metabolism and, 221, 224—225, 227, 231—232, 237—243
categories, determination of, 237—239
platelet functions and, 255, 426, 467—469, 487
Anion exchangers, hemoglobin chromatography, 67—70, 73
Antibodies, platelet, tests for, 491—492
Anticaogulants, see also specific anticoagulants by name
coagulation tests, use in, 10—11
evacuated collection tubes, use with, 28
platelet studies
aggregation, 339—340, 388—389
glass bead column retention, 334
release studies, 441—442
sizing techniques, 409—410, 412—414, 416, 418—419, 426
survival, 264
Antigen, factor VIII, see Coagulation factors I-XIII, factors VIII antigen
Antihemophilic factor, see Coagulation factors, factor VIII
Antiheparin factor, platelet, see Platelet factor 4
Antiheparin proteins, platelet secretion of, 437—440
Antihistamines, platelet functions and, 375—376, 464
Anti-Lepore β δ fusion gene, characteristics of, 56
Antithrombin II, coagulation and, 355
Antithrombin III
coagulation and, 11, 355
plasma, sensitivity to heparin and, 439
α_1-Antitrypsin, platelet function of, 355, 436—437
Aplastic anemia, iron metabolism and, see also Anemia, 240, 243
Apoferritin, role in iron metabolism, 229
Arachidonate, platelet function and, 337, 339, 342
liberation, 290
lipoxygenase activity, 293
oxygenation of, 287—294
Arachidonic acid, platelets and, 287—294
Arrowhead complexes, platelet, see Platelets, arrowhead complexes
Ascorbic acid, role in iron metabolism, 221, 229, 231—232
Aspirin and aspirin-like effects on platelet function, 268—270, 287, 332, 334, 336, 339, 341—344, 346, 375—378, 392, 448, 453, 463—464
von Willebrand's disease and, 471
Aspirin tolerance test, von Willebrand's disease measured by, 464, 471
Assays, see Tests
Atherosclerosis, platelet function and, 329, 336, 346
Atomic absorption spectroscopy, estimation of serum transferrin by, 229
Atomic coordinates, rigid-body fitting and, hemoglobin structure, 141
Atoms, number involved in hemaglobin contacts, 136
ATP, see Adenosine triphosphate
Autoimmune thrombocytopenic purpura, platelet activities and, 425—432, 447, 453—457, 468, 489, 493
Automated and semiautomated platelet counters, 361, 365
Autoradiography, transferrin studies using, 226

B

Backwashing, hemoglobin chromatographic systems, 78

Bactericidal factor, platelet secretion of, 437
Bacto Agar®, use in electrophoretic mobility studies of mutant hemoglobins, 89
Bart's hemoglobin, see Hemoglobin Bart's
Baumgartner's platelet adhesion and aggregation tests, qualitative abnormalities measured by, 450—452
Benzidine reagent, starch gel electrophoresis of hemoglobins, 100
Bernard-Soulier syndrome, platelet functions and, 332, 336, 340, 344, 357, 378, 394, 448, 450, 457, 488, 492
  von Willebrand's disease and, 473
Beta chains, see β-Chains and β-chain variants
Beta contacts, see Contacts, α β
Beta dimers, see Dimers, α β
Beta subunits, see β-Subunits
Beta-thromboglobulin, see β-Thromboglobulin
Bilirubin, platelet functions and, 467
Binding
  allosteric, hemoglobin structure and, 109
  diphosphoglycerate, hemoglobins, see Diphosphoglycerate, binding of
  iron, see Iron, binding capacity
  isotopic labeling of platelets, 267
  oxygen, hemoglobins, see Oxygen, binding of
  transferrin, see Transferrin, iron-binding activity of
Biochemistry
  globins, 51, 57—63
  platelets, 279—312
BIO/DATA® aggrogometer, characteristics of, 385—387
Biologic and physiologic variation, see Abnormalities and disorders; Normal values; Variation and variants; specific diseases and disorders by name
Biosynthesis, see Production
Bleeding
  easy, blood defects noted by, 447, 463
  iron absorption augmented by, 224
  thrombocyopenia and, see also Thrombocytopenia, 487—497
Bleeding time procedures, platelet studies utilizing, 329—332, 345—347, 369—380, 397
  Duke method, 331—332, 369—370, 471
  Ivy method, 331—332, 369—370, 471, 475
  platelet abnormalities and, 450—453, 463—469, 494—496
  standardized template method, 331—332, 370—378
  von Willebrand's disease and, 471—472, 474—478
Blood
  ferrokinetic profiles of, 243
  flow rate
    blood sampling and, 28
    Bowie's platelet retention test, importance in column, 401
    glass bead column platelet retention test, effect on, 335
    hemoglobin chromatography, effect in column, 68, 74—75, 77—79
  properties of, in measuring total concentration of hemoglobin, 24
  volume, measurement of, 33—39
    expression of, 36
    formulas for predicting, 37
    variable, clinical effects of, 35
Body hematocrit, measurement of, 33
Body surface area, see Surface area, body
Bohr effect, hemoglobin
  defined and described, 44, 51—54, 108—109
  three-dimensional structure and, 105, 108—109, 151, 164—171
Bone marrow, role in iron metabolism, 221, 224—225, 231—232, 236—240, 242—243
Borchgrevink test
  bleeding time, 331
  platelet retention, 330, 397
  von Willebrand's disease, 472
Bottom screen replacement, hemoglobin chromatographic systems, 80
Bowie test, platelet retention, see Glass bead column platelet retention test, Bowie method
Bridges
  platelet, see Platelets, bridges
  salt, see Salt bridges
Brilliant cresyl blue, staining with, platelet counting, 361
Bruising, easy, blood defects and, 447
Brush borders, iron-binding capacity of, 222—224
BT, see Bleeding time
Buffers
  chromatography of hemoglobins, 69—70, 76
  starch gel electrophoresis of hemoglobins, 97—98
Buried residues, see Internal residues

C

Calcium, platelet structure and function, role in, 294—297, 329, 333—334, 337, 339, 344, 352, 355, 403—406, 454—457
Calcium^{2+}, platelet biochemistry and, 294—297
Calibration graph, use in hemoglobincyanide system, 212
Canalicular system, platelets, see Platelets, canalicular system
Capillary blood sampling, equipment and procedures, 23—24, 27—28
Capillary platelet counts, method, 366
Capillary tubes, information about, 27
Carbamate groups, activity of, in hemoglobin structure, 109
α-Carbon backbones, globins, stereo-pair drawings, 118
Carbon determinations, hemoglobins, 213
Carbon dioxide
  carbamino compounds formed from, 109

platelet function and
aggregation, 340
production in, 275, 289
Carbonmonoxyhemoglobin, defined, 43
Carboxyhemoglobin, defined, 43
Carboxymethyl ion exchangers, titration curves, hemoglobin chromatography, 72—73
Catabolism
hemoglobin, in reticuloendohelial cells, 222
transferrin, 227
Cationic exchangers, hemoglobin chromatography, 67—70, 73
Cationic proteins, in platelets, 283—284
CATP III, see Connective tissue-activating peptide II
Cell counting, platelets, see Platelet counts
Celloscope® 401, platelet counting with, 364
Cells see Red blood cells; White blood cells
Cellulose acetate, use in electrophoretic mobility studies of mutant hemoglobins, 87—94
Cellulose ion exchangers, hemoglobin chromatography, 68—70, 72,77—80, 80—83
Centrifugation
differential techniques, platelet sizing studies, 418—425
platelet-rich plasma, effect on, 388
Cerebrospinal fluid, transferrin in, 227
Ceruloplasmin, cellular iron release and, 229
Chains
amino acid, distance from heme, hemoglobin structure and, 137—139
globin
imbalance of production, 57—58
Lepore, origin of, 56—57
hemoglobin, see also Chain variants; Hemoglobinopathies; Variation and variants, hemoglobin; specific variants by name
abnormalities of, 178—194
amino acid residues, sequences, and substitutions, 105, 112—117, 129—130, 177—194
chromatographic analysis of, 83
difference from myoglobin chains, 105, 121
distances from heme to surrounding amino acid side-chains, 137—139
electrophoretic mobilities of, 90—94
extended, see Extended chain variants
Gower, 45
Portland, 45
postsynthetic changes, 48
relative electrophoretic mobilities of, 90—94
relative electrophoretic positions on starch gel electrophoresis, 101—103
separation by starch gel electrophoresis, 101—103
stereochemistry, 133
structure of, 43, 45—48, 105—110, 112—118, 121, 126—127, 129—130, 133, 140, 142, 148, 153—163
unstable, characteristics of, 190, 192—193
methemoglobin, structure of, 106, 127—128
myoglobin
amino acid sequences of, 105, 112—117, 129—130
difference from α- and β-chains of hemoglobins, 105, 121
transferrin, structure of, 226
α-Chains and α-chain variants, hemoglobins, see also α-Subunits
abnormalities, 178—181, 194
amino acids and
sequences and positions of, 112—117
substitutions, 90—91, 178—181
contacts, 178—181, 190, 194
formation of, mRNA triplet codon deletion and, 177—181, 190, 194
oxygen affinity of, 190
relative electrophoretic mobilities, 90—91
relative electrophoretic positions on starch gel electrophoresis, 101—103
structure of, 43, 45—46
three-dimensional, studies of, 105—110, 112—118, 121, 126, 129—130, 133, 140, 142, 148, 153—157, 161
unstable, characteristics of, 190
$\alpha_2\varepsilon_2$ Chain variants, hemoglobin, in fetus, 45
α-Chains and β-chain variants, hemoglobins, see also β-Subunits
abnormalities, 182—186, 194
amino acids and
sequences and positions, 112—117
substitutions, 91—93, 182—186, 191—194
contacts, 182—186, 191—194
formation of, mRNA triplet codon deletion and, 177, 182—186, 191—194
oxygen affinity of, 191—192
relative eletrophoretic mobilities of, 91—93
relative electrophoretic positions on starch gel electrophoresis, 103
structure of, 43, 46
three-dimensional, studies of, 105—110, 112—118, 121, 127, 129—130, 133, 140, 142, 148, 153—155, 158—163
unstable, characteristics of, 192—193
γ-Chains and γ-chain variants, hemoglobins
amino acids and
sequences and positions of, 112—117
substitutions, 94, 187
contacts, 187
formation of, mRNA triplet codon deletion and, 177, 187
relative electrophoretic mobilities of, 94
relative electrophoretic positions on starch gel electrophoresis, 103
structure of, 43, 47, 108
δ-Chains and δ-chain variants, hemoglobins
amino acids and
sequences and positions of, 112—117
substitutions, 94, 186
contacts, 186
formation of, mRNA triplet codon deletion and, 177, 186
relative electrophoretic mobilities of, 94
relative electrophoretic positions on starch gel electrophoresis, 102

structure of, 43, 47—48
Chandler loop technique, bleeding time test, 330, 337
Characterization, platelet secretory proteins, 435—446
Chart recorders, use on aggrogometers, 385
Chediak-Higashi syndrome, platelet function and, 294, 344, 448, 451, 454
Chelating agents, use in estimating body iron stores, 232—233
Chemical determination, of hepatic iron, 233—236
Chemotactic factor, platelet secretion of, 437
Chesapeake oxyhemoglobin, see Oxyhemoglobin Chesapeake
Cholesterol, in platelets, 274
Choline, in platelets, 280
Cholinephosphotransferase activity, in platelets, 279
Chromatography, hemoglobin, see Ion exchange chromatography, hemoglobin
^{51}Chromium, use in labeling platelets, 263—269, 424, 441
Chronic thrombocytopenic purpura, platelet functions and, 425—432, 447, 453—457
Chrono-log aggrogometer, characteristics of, 386—387
Cirrhosis, iron metabolism and, 232
Cistrons, globin, see Alpha cistron; Nonalpha cistron
Citrate, anticoagulant in platelet studies, see also Sodium citrate, 339—340, 388—389, 440
Citrate agar, use in electrophoretic mobility studies of mutant hemoglobins, 87—94
Clinical effects, see Abnormalities and disorders
Clinical measurements, see Tests
Clotting, see Coagulation
Clotting factors, see Coagulation factors
Coagulation
  anticoagulants, see Anticoagulants
  bleeding time, see Bleeding time
  platelets and
    bleeding time procedures, 369—380
    clot retraction, 288—294, 329—330, 345, 450—452, 465, 469, 494—496
    clotting process, 314, 322, 403—404
    intrinsic, contributions to, 351—357, 403—406
    laboratory evaluation of activities, 403—407
    plasma deficiencies and, 403—406, 447, 449, 453
    structure and, 313—315, 322, 345
  tests, 9—11
  thrombocytopenia and, see also Thrombocytopenia, 487—497
Coagulation factors I-XIII
  abnormalities and deficiencies of, 11, 449, 452
  activation of, platelet, 329
  factor VII deficiency, platelet abnormalities and, 464
  factor VIII activity
    anti-factor VIII antibody activity, platelet abnormalities and, 466
    von Willebrand's disease and, 471—479
  factor VIII antigen, platelet function and, 336, 352, 397, 463, 467
    von Willebrand's disease and, 471—478
  factor-X activator, 352—353
  factor Xa inactivation by heparin, 439
  intrinsic coagulation, platelets and, 351—357, 403—406
  stability of, 10—11
  tests utilizing, 10—11
Coat, platelet, see Platelets, coat
Cocktails, anticoagulant, in platelet secretory protein studies, 441—442
Coefficient of variation, platelets, 9
Cohn fraction I, von Willebrand's disease and, 471
Cohort label, platelet volume studies, 420—424
Colchicine, platelet response and, 294, 314, 464—465
Collagen, platelet functions and
  abnormalities, 448, 450—452, 463—464, 494—496
  aggregation, 381—396
  biochemistry, 284, 287, 289—291
  coagulation activities, 353—355, 357, 403—406
  secretory proteins, assay of, 436—437, 440
  sizing, 415—417
  tests, laboratory, 329, 337—338, 340—345
  ultrastructure, 313
Collection and preparation procedures, blood specimens
  drawing techniques, 21—26
  equipment, 27—29
  general discussion, 3
  platelet studies
    aggregation, 385—392
    glass bead column retention, 335
    kinetic, 269
    release, 442
  tests, types used, described, 5—20
Color coding, evacuated blood collection tubes, 28
Column size and preparation, hemoglobin chromatography, 70—76
Compartmentalization, of adenine nucleotides, in platelets, 273—277
Compartments, iron turnover, 241
Concentration, total, of hemoglobin in blood, measurement of
  errors in systems, 212, 215—217
  hemoglobincyanide, 211—217
  other systems, 211
Conformational changes, during oxygenation, heme-heme interactions, 109—110, 152—153
Conformational parameters, globin-fold helices, 121
Connective tissue, platelet function and, see Collagen
Connective tissue-activating peptide II, platelet secretion and, 438
Conservation, of residues in globin fold, 131
Constant Spring hemoglobin, see Hemoglobin Constant Spring

Contact product forming activity, platelet coagulent activities and, 353—355, 403—405
Contacts, α β, hemoglobin structure and, 107—108, 110, 126, 136, 144—150, 153—160, 177-194
Containers, specifications for, in sampling procedures, 24, 27
Contractile proteins, platelet, see Platelets, contractile proteins
Coulter Counter®, platelet counting with, 364—366, 410, 412—413, 416, 429
Counters, platelet, 361—366, 410, 412—413, 416, 429
Counterstaining procedure, electrophoretic mobility studies of mutant hemoglobins, 89
Counting methods, see specific counts by name
Crossing over, genetic material, during meiosis, see also Fusion hemoglobins, 177
Cryoprecipitate, von Willebrand's disease and, 471, 473
Crystallography, see X-ray crystallography
CTP activity, in platelets, 279
CV, see Coefficient of variation
Cyanide solutions, see Hemoglobincyanide system, measuring total hemoglobin concentration in blood
Cyclic AMP, see Adenosine monophosphate, cyclic
Cyclic GMP system, platelet response and, 294—297
Cyclic nucleotide phosphodiesterase, in platelets, 295
Cyclooxegenase, platelets functions and, 293, 332, 448, 451, 456
Cytidine diphosphate diglyceride activity, in platelets, 279
Cytochrome oxidase, iron absorption and, 224
Cytoplasm, platelet, disorders of, 454—457

D

DEAE ion exchanger, hemoglobin chromatography, 68—70, 73, 80—83
Deficiency, iron, see Iron, deficiency, effects of
Deleted amino acid residues, in hemoglobin structure
  abnormalities, 189
  formation of, 153, 177, 189
  globin and hemoglobin synthesis and, 62
  relative electrophoretic mobilities of, 93
Deletion, in formation of hemoglobin variants, see Deleted amino acid residues
Delta chains, see δ-Chains and δ-chain variants
Dense granules, see Platelets, granules, dense
Dense tubular system,see Platelets, tubular system
Deoxyhemoglobin
  defined, 43
  three-dimensional structure, studies of, 106—110, 135, 137—141, 143, 146, 148—149, 151
  contact regions, 108, 149
Deoxyhemoglobin Kansas, functional properties of 110, 166
Desferrioxamine, use in estimating body iron stores, 232—233
Destruction, platelet, see Platelets, destruction of
Detergent, nonionic, reagent in hemoglobincyanide system 212—214
Dextran ion exchangers, hemoglobin chromatography, 68
DF, see Desferrioxamine
DFP- see ^{32}P-Diisopropylfluorophosphate
DG, see Platelets, granules, dense
Diabetes mellitus, platelet function and, 346, 425, 427
Diacyl glycerophosphate-cytidyl transferase, in platelets, 279
Dialysis, use in sample preparation, hemoglobin chromatography, 73
DIC, see Disseminated intravascular coagulation
Didisheim and Bunting test, platelet retention, 397—398
Diethylaminoethyl ion exchangers, titration curves, hemoglobin chromatography, 72
Diethylene-triamine pentaacetic acid, use in estimating body iron stores, 232—233
Differential centrifugation techniques, platelet studies using, 418—425
Diglyceride O-acyltransferase, in platelets, 279
Diglyceride kinase activity in platelets, 279
^{32}P-Diisopropylfluorophosphate, use in labeling platelets, 263, 267, 425—426
Dimers, α β, methemoglobin, structure and, 107—108, 143, 147, 149
Diphosphoglycerate, binding of, hemoglobins, 108, 151—152
2, 3-Diphosphoglyceric acid, concentration of, hemoglobin function parameter, 44—45
Diribonucleic acid, see DNA
Disease, effect of, see Abnormalities and disorders; specific diseases by name
Disorders, see Abnormalities and disorders; specific disorders by name
Disseminated intravascular coagulation, platelet size and, 425—427
Distances, heme to surrounding side chains, 137—139
Distribution transferrin, in body, 227
DNA
  globin activity of 55—56, 58, 63
  platelets and, 273, 437
Dog, studies of, von Willebrand's disease, 479—480
Donnan equilibrium, hemoglobin chromatography, 73
DPG, see Diphosphoglycerate
2,3-DPG, see 2,3-Diphosphoglyceric acid
Drabkin's solution, reagent in hemoglobincyanide system, 214
Drawing techniques, blood, see also Collection procedures, 21—29
^{59}Fe DRBC, see Erthrocytes, ^{59}Fe-labeled
Drugs, effects on platelet functions, see also

specific drugs by name, 341—342, 375—378, 392, 448, 464—465, 487—491, 493
DTPA, see Diethylene-triamine pentaacetic acid
Duke method, bleeding time test, see Bleeding time procedures, Duke method
Duplication, genes, globins 53—55, 57
Dysfunctional states, platelets, see Abnormalities and disorders, platelets
Dysproteinemias, platelet abnormalities and, 466—467

E

Edema fluid, transferrin in, 227
EDTA, see Ethylenediamine tetracetic acid
Ehlers-Danlos syndrome, bleeding time and, 331, 448, 451
EIT, see Erythrocyte iron turnover
Electronic particle counting, platelets, see Platelet counts, electronic particle methods
Electrophoresis, hemoglobin, 67
  starch gel technique, see Starch gel electrophoresis of hemoglobins
Electrophoretic mobilities, mutant hemoglobins, 71, 87—95, 101—103
Electrophoretic positions, relative, of chain variants on starch gel electrophoresis, 101—103
Embryonic globins, structure of, 55
Endotoxin, platelet functions and, 355, 440
Energy metabolism, platelets, see Platelets, energy metabolism of
Epinephrine
  factor VIII activity and, 474
  platelet functions and
    abnormalities, 450—452, 463, 488, 493—496
    aggregation, 390—392
    biochemistry, 287, 289—291, 295
    laboratory tests, 337—345
    secretory proteins, assay of, 437
    sizing, 415—417
Epithelial cell, role in iron metabolism, 222—224
Equipment, see also specific types of equipment by name
  bleeding time procedure, 331—332, 369—378
  blood drawing, 21—29
  electrophoretic mobility studies, mutant hemoglobins, 88—89
  hemoglobin chromatographic systems, 74—75, 80—82
  hemoglobincyanide system, measuring total concentration of hemoglobin in blood, 211—217
  leukocyte counting, automated, 8
  platelet studies
    aggregation, 342, 381—394
    bleeding time, 331—332, 369—378
    counting, 361—366
    glass bead column retention, 333—335
    labeling, 264—265
    platelet-rich plasma studies, 341
    retention procedures, 397—401
    secretory protein studies, 437—442
    sizing, 409—412
    von Willebrand's disease, 472
  starch gel electrophoresis of hemoglobins, 97
  transferrin, quantitative measurement of circulating, standard method 227—229
Erythrocyte counts, see also Erythrocytes, measurement of, 6
Erythrocyte iron turnover, iron metabolism and, see also Iron, turnover; Plasma iron, turnover 237—239
Erythrocytes
  indices, 6
  iron metabolism, role in, 221—222, 230, 236—240, 242—243
    ^{59}Fe-labeled, 240, 242
  mature, disorders of, 237—239
  measurement of, 5—7
  platelets and
    secretory proteins and, 439
    separation from, techniques, 361—366
Erythrocyte Sedimentation Rate, normal values, 7
Erythropoiesis, iron metabolism and, 221—222, 230—231, 235, 239—241, 243
Erythropoietin, iron metabolism and, 225, 237—238
ESR, see Erythrocyte Sedimentation Rate
Ethanolamine activity, in platelets, 279—280
Ethanolamine-phosphotransferase activity, in platelets, 279
Ethylenediamine tetracetic acid, platelet functions and, 264, 340, 363—364, 366, 399, 440, 464, 468
  direct smear technique, platelet sizing studies, 409—410, 413
  sizing, 409—410, 412—414, 416, 418—419, 426
Evacuated tubes, specifications and procedures for using, 27—28
Evolution, globins and hemoglobins, 51—54
Exhangers, ion, in hemoglobin chromatography, 67—69
Expression, blood volume, 36
Extended chain variants
  formation of, 177, 188
  relative electrophoretic mobilities of, 94
Extinction coefficient, hemoglobincyanide system, 211—213

F

Factors
  clotting, see Coagulation factors
  coagulation, see coagulation factors I-XIII
  hematopoietic-related, see Hematopoietic-related factors
  platelet, see Platelet factor 3; Platelet factor 4; Platelet factor 5
Fatty acids, platelets and, 274, 276, 296

Ferrireductase, iron metabolism and, 229, 231
Ferritin
 iron metabolism, role in, 221—224, 229—231, 233—236
  serum ferritin measurements, 233—236
  synthesis, iron storage and, 229
 peripheral blood concentrations of, 13
 platelet responses and, 313, 318
Ferrokinetic techniques, see Iron, kinetic studies of
Fetal hemoglobin, properties and activity of, 43—48, 55, 58
 γ-chain, 108
Fibrin, platelet functions and, 329, 344, 369, 466—467
Fibrinogen, platelet functions and, 329, 331, 333—334, 344, 351, 435—436, 439, 466—467
Filaments, platelet, see Platelets, filaments
Filamin, in platelets, 280
Films, blood, preparation of, 25, 464
Flow rate, blood, see Blood, flow rate; Plasma, flow rate
Folate, concentrations in peripheral blood, 13
Fold, globin, see Globins, fold
Food, iron absorption from, 225
Formulas
 blood volume, normal, prediction of, 37
 hemoglobin subunit structure, 43
Fraction collectors, use in hemoglobin chromatography, 78
Fragments, red blood cell and platelet, detection of, 429—432
Free fatty acids, in platelets, 274
Freeze-fractured platelets, see Platelets, freeze-fractured
Fructose, role in iron metabolism, 221
Function
 hemoglobin, see Hemoglobin, functional properties
 platelet, see Platelets, functions
Fusion hemoglobins
 formation of, 177, 187
 relative electrophoretic mobilities of, 93

G

Gamma chains, see γ-Chains and γ-chain variants
Gamma-globulin, platelet functions and, 333, 439
Gastric juice, iron-binding capacity of, 224
Gel electrophoresis, starch, of hemoglobin, see Starch gel electrophoresis of hemoglobins
Gel filtration, hemoglobins, 67
Gene duplication, globins, 53—55, 57
General position, effect on hemoglobin structure, 112—117
 changes in, 110, 161—163
Genes, globin, organization of, 55—57
Genetic mechanisms, abnormal globin synthesis, 57—63
Genetics, hemoglobin, 51—66
Giant platelets, see Megathrombocytes
Glanzmann's disease, platelet functions and, 447—448, 450
Glass bead column platelet retention test, description and uses of, 329—330, 333—336, 346, 415, 463, 472—473, 494—496
 Bowie method, 333—334, 398—401
  flow rate, blood, importance of, 401
  von Willebrand's disease, 472
 Hellem method, 333—335
  von Willebrand's disease, 472
 Salzman method, 333, 398
  von Willebrand's disease, 472
 Variabless affecting, 334—336
Globins, see also specific globins by name
 chain elecrophoresis, in mutant hemoglobin studies, 87
 fold, characteristics of, 105—106, 111—128, 131
  helices, see Helices, globin-fold
 genetics of, 51—63
  genes, organization of, 55—57
 monomeric, structure of, 105, 111
 sequences, 105
α-Globins, occurrence of, 54—57
Glucose uptake, in platelets, 275, 289
Glutathion metabolism, in platelets, 275
sn-Glycero-3-phosphate O-acyl-transferase, in platelets, 279
Glycine-NaCl buffers, use in hemoglobin chromatography, 70
Glycogen, platelet structure and, 275, 315, 448
Glycogenolysis, in platelets, 275, 289
Glycolysis, platelet responses and, 276, 289, 313, 319
Glycopeptides, platelet size and, 424
Glycoproteins
 iron metabolism and, 226
 platelet biochemistry and, 278—283, 313
Glycosphingolipid, platelets and, 273
Gower chains, hemoglobin, in fetus, 45
Gradients, hemoglobin chromatography, 70—73
Grady hemoglobin, see Hemoglobin Grady
Granules, platelet, see Platelets, granules
Gray platelet syndrome, platelet functions, and 344, 449, 452, 455
Guanidosuccinic acid, uremic and, 465

H

Hageman trait, platelet functions and, 355—357
Haptoglobin, concentrations in peripheral blood, 13
Hb, see Hemoglobin for all subjects with this prefix
Hct, see Hematocrit
Heavy meromyosin, platelet response to, 314, 324
Heavy platelets, characteristics and activity of, 419—425

Helices, globin fold, 105, 107—109, 118—125, 143, 147
  conformational parameters, 121
3_{10}-Helix, in globin fold, 105, 120
α-Helix, in globin fold, 105, 119, 122
π-Helix, in globin fold, 105, 120, 122
Helix C, globin fold, structure of, 105—106, 150
Helix E, globin fold, structure of, 105—106, 123—124
Helix F, globin fold, structure of, 105—106, 122, 125
Hellem method, glass bead column platelet retention test, see Glass bead column platelet retention test, Hellem method
Hemagglutination inhibition method, measurement of platelet production, 255—256
Hematocrit
  body, 33
  measurement of, 6, 33
  venous, 33
Hematology procedures, see Collection procedures; Tests
Hematoma prevention in blood sampling, 23
Hematopoietic-related factors, concentrations in peripheral blood, 11—14
Heme groups, structure and environment of, hemoglobins, 106—107, 132—141, 154—156
  center, distances involving, 137—140
  interatomic contacts of and residues, 136
  stereochemistry, 133
Heme-heme interactions, three-dimensional structure of hemoglobin and, 107, 109—110, 152—153
Heme iron, iron metabolism and, see also Nonheme iron, 223, 225
Hemochromatosis, iron metabolism and, 231—232, 235, 238—239, 242
Hemocytometer platelet counts, method, 361—362
Hemoglobin
  abnormal, see Chains; Chains and chain variants, Hemoglobinopathics; Mutations, hemoglobin; Variations and variants, hemoglobins; specific variants by name
  chains, see Chains, hemoglobins; Chains and chain variants, hemoglobin
  chromatography of, see Ion exchange chromatography, hemoglobin
  concentration, total, in blood, measurement of
    errors in systems, 212, 215—217
    hemoglobincyanide system, 211—217
    other systems, 211
  deleted, see Deleted amino acid residues
  derivatives and their spins, 132
  electrophoretic mobilities of mutant, 71, 87—95
  evolution of, 51—54
  extinction coefficient, 211—213
  fetal, see Fetal hemoglobin
  functional properties, 43—45, 51—54, 177
    altered, abnormal hemoglobins, 110, 164—171
  fusion, see Fusion hemoglobins
  gene duplication, 53—55, 57
  general discussion, 43—49
  genetics of, 51—66
  hemoglobinometry, 211—219
  hemoglobinopathies, see Hemoglobinopathies
  instability of, 110, 153, 190, 192—193
  iron metabolism and, 221—251
  mean cell, see Mean cell hemoglobin
  mean corpuscular concentration, see Mean corpuscular hemoglobin concentration
  measurement of, 6, 211—219
  molecular weight, 43
  mutant, see Variation and variants, hemoglobin
  nomenclature, 43
  normal values, 6
  oxygenation of, changes during, 140, 150, 152—153
  production of, 51—66
  properties and activity of, 43—48
    quaternary structure and, see Quaternary structure, hemoglobins
  species difference in, residue variabilities caused by, 106, 131
  starch gel electrophoresis of, see Starch gel electrophoresis of hemoglobins
  stereochemistry, 133
  structure, see Structure, hemoglobins
  subunit, see Subunit
  synthesis, impaired, iron metabolism and, 238—239
  time course in individual, 45
  variants, see Chains; Chains and chain variants Hemoglobinopathies; Variation and variants, hemoglobin; specific variants by name
Hemoglobin A
  electrophoretic mobility of, 87
  properties and activity of, 43—48, 57
Hemoglobin A_2, properties and activity of, 43, 57
Hemoglobin A-like variants, chromatography of, 68, 82
Hemoglobin Bart's, starch gel electrophoresis of, 98
Hemoglobin C
  chromatography of, 68
  electrophoretic mobility of, 87
Hemoglobin C-like variants, chromatography of, 68, 80
Hemoglobin Constant Spring, synthesis of, 63
Hemoglobincyanide system, measuring total hemoglobin concentration in blood, 211—217
  error possibilities, 215—217
  reagent, 212— 214
  reference solutions, 214—215
    optical density of, 215—216
    stability of, 215—216
  turbidity, prevention of, 213—214
Hemoblogin D variants, chromatography of, 68
Hemoglobin E variants, chromatography of, 68
Hemoglobin F, electrophoretic mobility of, 87
Hemoglobin G variants, chromatography of, 68
Hemoglobin — Gower — 1 chains, in fetus, 45

Hemoglobin — Gower — 2 chains, in fetus, 45
Hemoglobin Grady, synthesis of, 63
Hemoglobin H variants, chromatography of, 68
chromatography of, 68
starch gel electrophoresis of, 98
Hemoglobin I-like variants, chromatography of, 68, 82
Hemoglobin J-like variants, chromatography of, 68, 82
Hemoglobin Kenya, characteristics of, 57
Hemoglobin Lepore, characteristics of, 56—57, 63
Hemoglobin O-like variants, chromatography of, 68
Hemoglobinometry, 211—219
Hemoglobinopathies, see also Chains; Chains and chain variants; Variation and variants, hemoglobin; specific variants by name, 177—194
Hemoglobin — Portland — 1 chains, in fetus, 45
Hemoglobin Porto Alegro, gel filtration studies, 67
Hemoglobin S
harmfulness of, 110
subunit status of, 43
variants, chromatography of, 68, 81
Hemoglobin Wien, instability of, 110, 162
Hemolysates, starch gel electrophoresis of, 99
Hemolysis
causes of, 7
coagulation tests and, 10
Hemolytic anemia, iron metabolism and, see also Anemia, 224—225, 227, 238—243
Hemophilia, platelet functions and, 357, 378, 447, 464, 467
antihemophelia factor, see Coagulation factors, factor VIII
von Willebrand's disease and, 471—480
Hemosiderin, role in iron metabolism, 222, 231
Hemostasis, platelet function and, 283, 329—347, 355—357, 397, 435, 447
bleeding time prodedures, see Bleeding time procedures,
Hemostatic deficiency states, platelet functions and, 335—336, 355—357
Heparin, platelet function and 335, 339—340, 355, 375—376, 399—400, 437—440
Hepatosplenomegaly, platelet size and, 427—429
Hereditary platelet abnormalities, see Qualitative abnormalities, platelets, hereditary; specific disorders by name
Hermansky-Pudlak syndrome, platelet function and, 344, 448, 450, 459
Hexose monophosphate shunt, in platelets, 275
HiCN, see Hemoglobincyanide system
High spin, see Spin states
Hill equation, n of, hemoglobin function parameter, 49
Histidine, effect on hemoglobin structure, 108—109
HMM, see Heavy meromyosin
Homocystinuria, platelet function and, 329, 346
Horse methemoglobin, three-dimensional structure, studies utilizing, 105—108, 118, 122—128, 134, 137—139, 143—145, 147
hydrogen bonding network of molecule, 105—106, 126—127
Human deoxyhemoglobin, three-dimensional structure, studies utilizing, 106—110, 135, 137—141, 143, 146, 148—149, 151
Human globin, for discussion of topics concerning, see Globins
Human hemoglobin, for discussion of topics concerning, see Hemoglobin
Humoral factors
intestinal iron absorption and, 225
platelet production and, see Thrombopoietin
Hydrogen bonds, hemoglobin structure, 105—108, 123—128, 144, 147—148
network of horse methemoglobin model, 105—106, 126—127
Hydrolases, platelet function and, 436—437
Hydrophobic and hydrophilic residues, hemoglobin structure and, 106, 128, 147
Hydrophobic interactions, hemoglobin structure and, 106—107, 128—131, 147
Hydroxyphenolic acids, uremia and, 465
Hyperaggregable platelets, see Platelets, aggregation, hyperaggregable forms
Hyperfibrinogenemia, platelet abnormalities and, 466—467
Hypersplenism, platelet production and, 259, 427—429
Hypertransfusion, of platelets, effect of, 258
Hypothyroidism, platelet abnormalities and, 463—464, 467

I

ICSH, see International Committee for Standardization in Hematology
Idiopathic thrombocytopenic purpura, see Autoimmune thrombocytopenic purpura
Imbalance, of chain production, globin synthesis, 57—58
Immunoassay, lysosomal elastase, 439
Immunodiffusion, estimation of serum transferrin by, 226, 229
Immunoelectrophoresis
platelet studies, 440, 467, 479
transferrin studies, 226
Immunoradiometric assay, hepatic iron determination by, 233—235
Indices, erythrocyte, 6
^{111}Indium, use in labeling platelets, 263, 266—268
Infection, iron metablism and, 227, 231, 237—238
Inflammation, caused by infection, iron metabolism and, 235—238, 242
Inherited platelet disorders, see Qualitative abnormalities, platelets, hereditary; specific disorders by name
Instability, hemoglobin, 110, 153, 190, 192—193

Interatomic contacts, heme groups and residues, 136
Internal residues, hemoglobin structure and, 106, 129, 131
International Committee for Standardization in Hematology
blood sampling standards, 21
blood volume measurement standards, 33
hemoglobin, total concentration in blood, standards of measurement, 212, 214—215
iron metabolism testing standards, 227—229
platelets, labeling procedure for, 265—267
International hemoglobincyanide reference solution, 214—215
optical density of, 215—216
stability of, 215—216
Intestinal iron absorption, mechanism and regulation of, 221—225
Intracellular regulation, platelet responses, see Platelets, intercellular regulation of responses
Intrinsic coagulation, platelets and, see Coagulation, platelets and, intrinsic
Iodine^{125}, platelet labeling with, 424
Ion exchange chromatography, hemoglobin, 67—83
buffer, choice of, 69—70, 76
column size and preparation, 70—76
diagrams of systems, 74—75, 80—82
flow rate and pumping, 68, 74—75, 77—79
gradients, 70—73, 76
ion exchanger, choice of, 67—69
monitoring and fraction collection, 78
sample preparation, 73
systems, 74—75, 80—83
trouble shooting, 79—80
Inophores, platelet secretion and, 440
Iron
absorption of, intestinal, 221—225
atom, distance from porphyrin ring, effect of, hemoglobin structure, 106—107
average daily intake, 225
binding capacity
binding protein, location of, 223
brush borders, 222—224
compounds, iron-binding, 221—222
epithelial cell, 222—224
gastric juice, iron absorption and, 224
plasma, related to iron release, se also Plasma iron turnover, 225
serum-unsaturated, see Serum-unsaturated iron-binding capacity
transferrin, binding sites, figure, 230
transferrin, serum-unsaturated, 228—229
concentrations in peripheral blood, 13
deficiency, see also Anemia
iron metabolism, effects on, 221—225, 231—232, 235—242
platelet abnormalities and, 468
determinations, hemoglobins, 213
enzymes containing, 221—222, 231
exchange in body, studies of, 240—243
heme, see Heme iron; Nonheme iron
kinetic studies of, 236—243
labeling of, 236—243
metabolism of
intestinal absorption process, 221—225
iron turnover, isotopes used to study, 236—243
storage iron, 229—236
transferrin metabolism, 225—229
mobilizable, total, estimations of, 233, 235
overload, effects of, on iron metabolism, 222, 224—225, 232, 235—236, 241
oxidation of ferrous, 229
plasma, see Plasma iron
receptors, on mucosal cells, 222
spin states, see Spin states
standard solution, 228
storage in body, iron metabolism and, 221, 223—224, 229—236
clinical evaluation of, 231—233
hepatic iron, chemical determination of, 233—236
regulation of, 229—231
total body, locations of, 221—222
transport, mechanism of, 221—222
turnover, studies using isotopes, see also Erythrocyte iron turnover; Plasma iron, turnover, 236—243
compartments, 241
^{59}Fe iron, studies utilizing, 231, 236—243
Iron-binding capacity, normal values of, 13
Isoelectric point, transferrin, 226
Isolation, platelet, 265—266
Isotopes
blood volume measurement techniques utilizing, 33—38
radioactive
blood measurement techniques utilizing, 33—34
forms used in platelet labeling, 263—264
iron turnover studies utilizing, 236—243
nonradioisotope technique, platelet kinetics, 266—270
platelet production and kinetics, 257, 259, 263—270
platelet volume-platelet senescence studies using, 419—425
Isotopically labeled platelets, see Platelets, isotopically labeled
Ivy method, bleeding time test, see Bleeding time procedures, Ivy method

J

Jejunum, role in iron metabolism, 221—224

K

Kansas deoxyhemoglobin, see Deoxyhemoglobin Kansas
Kaolin, platelet activity and, 344, 403—405

Kenya hemoglobin, see Hemoglobin Kenya
Kidney, site of platelet production, 255
Kininogen, platelet functions and, 357
Koshland-Nemethy-Filmer model heme-heme interaction, 109

L

^{59}Fe-Labeled iron, see ^{59}Fe-Iron
Labeling
  iron, see Isotopes, radioactive, iron turnover studies
  platelets, see Platelets, labeling
Lancets, optimal design of, 27
LA-PF_4, see Low-activity platelet factor 4
Large platelets, see Megathrombocytes
Latex, platelet responses and, 313, 319
Lepore hemoglobin, see Hemoglobin Lepore
Leukemia, platelet abnormalities and, 464—465
  von Willebrand's disease and, 473
Leukocyte counts, see also Leukocytes, measurement of, 7—8
Leukocytes
  measurement of, 7—8
  platelets and
    coagulation activities, 355
    secretory proteins and, 439
    separation from techniques, 361—364
Leukocytosis, causes of, 8
Life span, platelets, 263—270
Ligands, effect of
  hemoglobin structure, 43, 106, 132, 153
  iron metabolism, 223
Light microscopy, platelet counting by, 362
Light platelets, characteristics and activity of, 419—425
Light scattering, measurement of platelet structure and function, 337—339, 364—366
Light transmission studies, platelet aggregation, 337—339, 342, 381
Linkage between alpha and nonalpha cistrons, globin, 55—57
Lipids, platelets and
  coagulation and, 351—352, 355
  metabolism, 273—274, 278—280
  peroxidation, platelet kinetics measured by, 268—270
Liver
  iron metabolism in, 221, 223, 226—227, 231—236, 242—243
  platelet functions in
    abnormalities in diseased states, 468—469
    sequestration and, 264
Low-activity platelet factor 4, 435—442
  antigen, 440—442
Low spin, see Spin states
Lupus erythematosis, see Systemic lupus erythematosis
Lymph, transferrin in, 227
Lymphocytes, transferrin synthesis in, 227
Lysosomal enzymes, in platelets, 329
Lysosomes, platelet structure and, 315, 326, 435—437, 439

M

Macroglobulinemia, platelet abnormalities and, 466—467
Marrow, see Bone marrow
Mass, red blood, see Red blood cells, mass
Maturation, disorders of, anemia and, 237—239
Maximum parsimony method, hemoglobin evaluation, 51—52
May-Hegglin anomaly, platelet function and, 344, 448, 451, 455, 488, 492
MCH, see Mean cell hemoglobin
MCHC, see Mean corpuscular hemoglobin concentration
MCV, see Mean cell volume
Mean cell hemoglobin, normal values of, 6
Mean cell volume, erythrocytes, hemoglobin, and hematocrit, normal values of, 6
Mean corpuscular hemoglobin concentration, normal values of, 6
Mean platelet volume, measurement of, 411—413, 415
Mean values, red cell mass and plasma volume related to body surface area, 37—38
Measurements, see Tests; specific testing and measuring devices and systems by name
Mechanisms, genetic, abnormal globin synthesis, 57—63
Median hepatic storage iron concentrations, 234
Megakarocytes
  labels, platelet kinetics, 263
  megathrombocytes and, 425—426
  thrombocytopenia and, 487—488
    amegakarocytic forms, 487—488, 491
Megakaryocytopoiesis, platelet production and, 255—256
Megathrombocytes, characteristics and activity of, 314, 320, 409—432
  index, platelet count and, 412—413, 415—417
  megakarocytes and, 425—426
Membrane, platelet, see Platelets, membrane
Messenger RNA, see mRNA
Metabolism
  adenine nucleotide, see Adenine nucleotides, metabolism
  amino acids, in platelets, 273
  energy, see Platelets, energy metabolism and
  hemoglobin, see topics listed under Hemoglobin
  iron, see Iron, metabolism of
  lipids, 273—274, 278—280
  red blood cell, iron release and, 230
  transferrin, 225—229
Metastatic carcinoma, platelet function and, 346
Methemoglobin
  chains, see Chains, methemoglobin
  defined, 43

dimers, $\alpha\beta$, structure and, 107—108, 143, 147, 149
starch gel electrophoresis of, 98
three-dimensional structure, studies of, 105—108, 118, 122—128, 134, 137—140, 143—145, 147
hydrogen bonding network of molecule, 105—106, 126—127
Micro-blood-collection equipment, standards for, 27
Microtubules, platelet, see Platelets, microtubules
Mitochondria, platelet, see Platelets, mitochondria
Mitochondrial iron, characteristics of, 224
MK-45 counter, platelet counting with 364-365
Mobilities, electrophoretic, of mutant hemoglobins, see Electrophoretic mobilities of mutant hemoglobins
Mobilizable iron estimations, total, 233, 235
Molecular pathology, human hemoglobin, 110
Molecular weight
hemoglobin, 43
membrane glycoproteins, 282
platelet proteins, 280—281
transferrin, 226
Monitors, use in hemoglobin chromatography, 78
Monoclonal gammopathy, von Willebrand's disease and, 478
Monod-Wyman-Changeux model, heme-heme interactions, 109
Monomeric globins, structure of, 105, 111
Morphologic abnormalities, platelets, see also Abnormalities and disorders, platelets, 467—468
MPV, see Mean platelet volume
Mucoprotein of gastric juice, role in iron metabolism, 221
Mucosal block theory, iron metabolism and, 223
Mucosal cells, role in iron metabolism, 222—225, 230
Multichamber gradient, hemoglobin chromatography, 72—73
Multiple convex gradient, hemoglobin chromatography, 72—73
Multiple myeloma, platelet function and, 335, 466-467
Mutant hemoglobins, see Mutations, hemoglobins; Variation and variants, hemoglobins; specific mutants by name
Mutations, see Variation and variants
Myelofibrosis, iron metabolism and, 238—239
Myeloid metaplasia, platelet abnormalities and, 465—466
Myeloproliferative syndrome, platelet functions and, 259, 335, 378, 442, 463—466, 468, 488
Mylar®, use in electrophoretic mobility studies of mutant hemoglobins, 89
Myocardial infarction, platelet secretion and, 439, 442
Myoglobin
chains, see Chains, myoglobin
iron metabolism and, 221—222, 225, 231
species difference in, residue variabilities caused by, 106, 131
structure of, 105, 111, 118, 128, 133, 136
Myoinositol, in platelets, 279
Myosin, platelet structure and function, role in, 274—278, 280—281, 290, 294, 296, 314, 324
Myosin light chain kinase, in platelets, 281

N

n, of Hill equation, hemoglobin function parameter, 44, 164—171
National Committee for Clinical Laboratory Standards, recommended standards for blood collection procedures and equipment, 21, 27
NCCLS, see National Committee for Clinical Laboratory Standards
Needles, specifications for, in sampling procedures, 28
Nephrosis, iron metabolism and, 227
Network, hydrogen bonding, of horse methemoglobin model, 105—106, 126—127
Neutral lipids, platelets and 274
Nitrogen
atom, covalent bond between and iron atom, hemoglobin structure, 106
determinations, hemoglobin, 213
Nomenclature, hemoglobin, 43
Nonalpha cistron, globins, activity at, 53—57
Nonalpha classes, globins and hemoglobins, 43, 46—48, 54—57
Nonheme iron, iron metabolism and, see also Heme iron, 224—225, 232
Nonionic detergent, reagent in hemoglobincyanide system, 212—214
Nonpolar residues, hemoglobin structure and, 106, 130—131
Nonradioisotope technique, platelet kinetics, 266—270
Nonstorage pool deficiency, platelet release and, see also Storage pool deficiency, 343—344
Normal values, see also Abnormalities and disorders; Variation and variants
bleeding time procedures, 332, 374—377
blood volume, 33, 36—38
coagulation, 9—11
erythrocyte count, 6
Erythrocyte Sedimentation Rate, 7
hematocrit, 6
hematopoietic-related factors, 11—14
hemoglobin, 6
platelet studies
aggregation, 342, 394
bleeding time, 332, 374—377
counts, 8—9, 365
kinetics, 266, 269—270
sizing techniques, 413, 427
red blood cells, 6

reticulocyte counts, 6—7
white blood cells, 7—8
Nuclear abnormality, anemia and, 238—239

O

Old platelets, see Platelets, senescence
Optical density, hemoglobincyanide reference solutions, 215—216
Optical light scattering, see Light scattering
Oral contraceptives, factor VIII activity and, 474
Organelles, platelet, disorders of, 454—457
Organization, globin genes, 55—57
Osmotic fragility, red blood cells, 7
Overload, iron, see Iron, overload, effects of
Oxidation, of ferrous iron, 229
Oxidative phosphorylation, in platelets, 276
Oxygen
affinity, hemoglobins, 67, 105, 108—109, 164—171, 177, 190—192
binding of, hemoglobins, related to oxygen affinity, 105, 109
consumption, in platelets, 276
dissociat ion of, see Oxygen, equilibrium data
equilibrium data, hemoglobins, 43—44, 51—54, 109
O_2 uptake, 289
Oxygenation
arachidonate, see Arachidonate oxygenation
hemoglobin, changes during, 140, 150, 152—153
Oxyhemoglobin
defined, 43
structure of, 106—107, 109—110, 151—152
Oxyhemoglobin Chesapeake, functional properties of, 110, 164

P

p_{50}, hemoglobin function parameter, 44—45
Packed cell volume technique, use in platelet sizing studies, 411—412
Packed platelet volume, 412—415
Packing, column, hemoglobin chromatography, 76
Pancreatic secretion, iron metabolism and, 224
Paper chromatography, hemoglobins, 67
Parenchymal cells, role in iron metabolism, 221—222, 229—232, 235, 240, 242—243
Payton aggregometer, characteristics of, 386—387
PCV, see Venous hematocrit
Peripheral blood
erythrocyte measurements in, 5—7
films of, preparation, 25
hematopoetic-related factor concentrations in, 11—14
leukocyte measurements in, 7—8
lymphocytes, transferrin synthesis in, 227
platelet measurements in, 8—9, 425—432
Peripheral platelets, see Young platelets
Peristaltic pump, use in hemoglobin chromatography, 77
Pernicious anemia, iron metabolism and, see also Anemia, 232, 238
Peroxidase, platelet responses and, 293, 313, 318, 325
Peroxidation, lipid, see Lipid peroxidation
Perutz theory, stereochemistry of heme-heme interactions, 109—110, 152—153
PF, see Platelet factors 3, 4, and 5
PGD, see Prostaglandins
PGF, see Platelet growth factor
pH, effect of
hemoglobin
chromatography, 69—73, 75—76, 79
function parameter, 44
gradients, in chromatography, 71—73
platelet aggregation studies, effect of, 340, 390—391
Phase microscopy, platelet counting by, 361—362
Phenols, uremia and, 465
Phlebotomy, measuring body iron stores with, 233, 235
Phosphates, role in iron metabolism, 221
Phosphate system, starch gel electrophoresis of hemoglobins, 97—98
Phosphatidate phosphatase activity, in platelets, 279
Phosphatidyl—transferase, in platelets, 279
Phosphoinositide kinase activity, in platelets, 279
Phosphoinositide synthesis, in platelets, 290
Phospholipase A_2 activity, in platelets, 280, 293, 448
Phospholipid acyltransferase, in platelets, 280
Phospholipids, platelet structure and, 313, 330
factor 3, see Platelet factor 3
intrinsic coagulation activities, 351—357
metabolism of, 273—274, 278—280
Physiologic variation, see Abnormalities and disorders; Normal values; Variation and variants
Phytates, role in iron metabolism, 221
Pig, studies of, von Willebrand's disease, 479
Piston pump,use in hemoglobin chromatography
PIT, see Plasma iron, turnover
pK_a, in hemoglobin chromatography, 67
Plasma
flow rate, in blood sampling, 28
heparin, sensitivity to, 439
iron-binding capacity of, related to iron release, see also Plasma iron, 225
platelets and
coagulant activities, 403—406, 447, 449, 453
function studies, 329—347
membrane, structure and, 273—274, 283, 285, 295, 313—314
plasmatic factor, in von Willebrand's disease, 472—473, 476—477
platelet-poor plasma, see Platelet-poor plasma
platelet-rich, see Platelet-rich plasma

production in, 255—259
storage in, 264—265
protein
glass bead column platelet retention test, importance in, 333—334
platelet protein, similarity to, 283—284, 435—436, 439, 447
precipitation of, in hemoglobincyanide system, 213—214
thrombosis and, 336
radioiron disappearance from, 236—243
transferrin in, 227
transport of iron in, see also Plasma iron, turnover, 225—229
volume, measurement of, 33—38
mean values, related to body surface area, 37—38
variation in, 36
Plasma iron
concentration, measurement of, 236—237
turnover, characteristics of, see also Erythrocyte iron turnover, Iron, turnover, 221—222, 227, 230, 236—243
total, defined, 240
Plasminogen, coagulation and, 11
Plastic tubing, use in glass bead column retention test 334
Platelet counts, see also Platelets, measurement of
abnormalities in, 366, 450—452, 463, 492—493
adjustment, in aggregation studies, 388—389
automated methods, 361, 365
capillary methods, 366
counters, types, 361—366
Didisheim and Buntingg platelet retention test, 397—398
electronic particle methods, 361—364, 366, 410—414, 429—432
elevated, causes of, 492—493
error, sources of, 366
hemocytometer method, 361—362
megathrombocyte index and, 412—413, 415—417
methods, 361—366
optical light scattering method, 364—366
packed cell volume technique, 411—412
peripheral blood platelet content, 8—9
platelet production, 255—256, 259
platelet-rich plasma platelet aggregation tests, 341
platelet sizing, use in, 409—432
thrombocytopenia, 487, 492—493
visual methods, 361—362, 366
Platelet factor 3, activity of, 313, 329—330, 344—345, 403—405
abnormalities in, 447—448, 450—452, 465, 468—469
defined, 352
intrinisic coagulation and, 351—357
tests for, 463
Platelet factor 4, structure and activity of, 284, 329, 346, 355, 435—442
antigens, 440—442
low-activity type, 435—442
primary structure of human, 437—438
tests for, 463
Platelet factor 5, activity of, 436
Platelet growth factor, release of, 437
Platelet phospholipid, see Platelet factor 3
Platelet-poor plasma, use in platelet studies, 265, 381—383, 388—389, 403—404, 435—442
preparation of, assay of secretory proteins, 441—442
Platelet-rich plasma, use in platelet studies, 265, 294, 330, 336—344, 346, 381—394, 403—405, 410—412, 415—419, 440—441, 474—478
storage, effect of, 340—341, 390—391
Platelets
abnormalities, see Abnormalities and disorders, platelets; Qualitative abnormalities, platelets. Quantitative disorders, platelets; Thrombocytopathies; Thrombocytopenia
adenine nucleotides and, see Adenine nucleotides, platelets and
adhesion, characteristics of, see also Platelets, aggregation; Platelets, retention, 313, 334
abnormalities of, 447—448, 450—452
tests, see also listings under Platelets, retention, test, 329—330, 333—336, 397—401
von Willebrand's disease and, see also von Willebrand's disease, 471—472
agglutination, effect of, 287, 336—344
von Willebrand's disease and, see also von Willebrand's disease, 473
aggregation, effect of, see also Platelets, adhesion; Platelets, retention
abnormalities of, 9, 346, 447—448, 450—452, 458, 463—469, 488, 494—496
ADP, collagen, and ristocetin affecting, 381—396
aggregometers, use of, 342, 346, 381—397, 463
biochemistry of, 283—296
bleeding time test, see Bleeding time
drugs, effect of, 341—342, 464—465
glass bead column retention, see Glass bead column platelet retention test
hyperaggregable forms, detection of, 346
intraindividual variation in, 9
mechanism of, 337
secretion and, 435—442
tests, see also listings under Platelets, retention, test, 329—330, 336—344, 397—401, 463
theoretical model, 381, 384
ultrastructure and, 313—314, 317, 323, 325—326
velocity of, megathrombocyte index and, 416
von Willebrand's disease and, see also von Willebrand's disease, 472—479
antibodies, tests for, 491—492
arrowhead complexes, characteristics of, 314, 324
biochemistry, of, 273—312

bleeding time procedures for, see Bleeding time
bridges, characteristics of, 313, 317
canalicular system, characteristics of, 313—314, 318—320, 325
clumping, causes of, 287
coagulation and, see Coagulation, platelets and
coat, characteristics of, 313, 316
collagen and, see Collagen
contact-forming product activity of, 353—354, 403—405
contractile proteins, characteristics and function of, 274—278, 296, 314
cytoplasm, abnormalities of, 454—457
dense bodies, abnormalities of, 454—457
dense granules, see Platelets, granules, dense
density, volume related to, 415—416, 421
destruction of, 259, 487—489
disorders, see Abnormalities and disorders, platelets; Biologic and physiologic variation, platelets; Qualitative abnormalities, platelets; Quantitative disorders, platelets
drugs, effect on, see Drugs
EDTA and, see Ethylenediamine tetracetic acid, use in platelet studies
energy metabolism of, 273—274, 287—291
erythrocytes, separation from, techniques, 361—366
factors, see Platelet factor 3; Platelet factor 4; Platelet factor 5
filaments, characteristics and types of, 288—294, 313—314, 317—325
fragments, detection of, 429—432
freeze-fractured, characteristics of, 315, 327
functions
  abnormalities, see Abnormalities and disorders, platelets; Qualitative abnormalities, platelets; Quantitative disorders, platelets
  aggregation, agglutination, adhesion, release, and retention, see Platelets, adhesion; Platelets, agglutination; Platelets, aggregation; Platelets, release; Platelets, retention
biochemisty of, 287—291
bleeding time procedures and, see Bleeding time procedures
disorders of, see Abnormalities and disorders, platelets; Qualitative abnormalities, platelets; Quantitative disorders, platelets
drugs, effect of, see Drugs
interrelationships among, measured by sizing, 415—425
qualitative abnormalities of, see Qualitative abnormalities, platelets
quantitative abnormalities of, see Quantitative disorders, platelets
tests, 329—349, 450—457, 463—469, 494—496
thrombocytopenia and, see Thrombocytopenia
thrombocytosis and thrombocythemia, see Thrombocythemia; Thrombocytosis
volume and, 415—417
giant, see Megathrombocytes
glass bead column retention test, see Glass bead column platelet retention test
granules, characteristics and activity of, 273, 278, 283—286, 290, 294, 314—315, 326, 337, 435—437
  abnormalities of, 454—457, 468
  coagulation factors in, 351—352
  dense granules, 273, 283, 285—286, 290, 294, 315, 326
  α-granules, 273, 284, 290, 435, 437
heavy, characteristics and activity of, 419—425
hemostasis and, see Hemostasis, platelets and
inhibition of, 285—288, 292—296
intracellular regulation of responses, 294—297
intrinsic coagulation activities, see also Coagulation, platelets and, 351—357
isolation of, 265—266
isotopically labeled, kinetics of, see also Platelets, labeling of, 263—270
kinetics of labeled, 263—270
  nonradioactive system, 266—270
labeling of, 257, 259, 263—270, 278—284
  cohort label, volume studies, 420—424
  nonradioactive system, 266—270
large, see Megathrombocytes
leukocytes and, see Leukocytes, platelets and
life spans of, 263—270
light, characteristics and activity of, 419—425
lipids and, see Lipids, platelets and
loss of, see Platelets, destruction of
lysosomes and, see Lysosomes, platelets and
measurement of
  cell counting, see also Platelet counts, 361—368
  in peripheral blood, 8—9
  production, 255—259
megathrombocytes, characteristics and activity of, 314, 320, 409—432, 448
  index, platelet counts and, 412—413, 415—417
  megakarocytes and, 425—426
membranes, characteristics of, 278—284, 297, 345, 352, 435
  abnormalities of, 448, 450—452, 454—457
  plasma membrane and, 273—274, 283, 285, 295, 313—314, 352
metabolism, 273—297
microtubules, characteristics of, 274—278, 280—281, 288—294, 296, 314, 321—323
  proteins, 274—278, 280—281, 288—294
mitochondria, characteristics of, 273, 290, 315
  abnormalities of, 454—457
morphologic abnormalities of, 467—468
number of, see Platelet counts
old, see Platelets, senescence
organelles, abnormalities of, 454—457
peripheral, see Platelets, young
phospholipids and, see Phospholipids
plasma and, see Plasma, platelets and
production, 255—261

protective function, 355, 357
proteins, 274—278, 280—281, 283—284, 288—294, 435—442
pseudopods, characteristics of, 273, 288, 314, 322—323, 338
  abnormalities of, 466, 468
qualitative abnormalities of, see Qualitative abnormalities, platelets
quantitative disorders of, see Quantitative disorders, platelets
regulatory proteins, 274—278, 280—281
release, characteristics of, see also Platelets, retention, 283—294, 296, 313, 315, 329—330, 338—339, 343—344, 435—442
  abnormalities of, 343—344, 394, 439—442, 447—448, 450—452, 456
  defect, see Storage pool deficiency
resting, biochemistry of, 273—287
retention, see also Platelets, adhesion; Platelets, aggregation; Platelets, release
  abnormalities of, 343—344, 394, 447, 450—452, 494—496
  defined, 334, 398—399
  procedures, 397—401
  test, 397—401
  test: Bowie, see Glass bead column platelet retention test, Bowie method
  test: Berchgrevink, see Borchgrevink test, platelet retention
  test: Didisheim and Bunting, see Didisheim and Bunting test
  test: glass bead column, see Glass bead column platelet retention test
  test: Salzman, see Glass bead column platelet retention test, Salzman method
  von Willebrand's disease and, see also von Willebrand's disease, 472—478
ristocetin and, see Ristocetin
secretion, see Platelets, release
secretory proteins
  assay of, 439—442
  characterization of, 283—284, 435—439
senescence, effects of, 419—425, 487
serotonin and, see Serotonin
shape of, 273, 283, 285, 287—288, 291, 295, 313, 315—316, 337—339, 343, 409—410
size
  abnormalities of, 425—432, 448, 450—452
  clinical significance of measurements, 425—432
  interrelationships among platelet functions and structure measured by, 412—425
  sizing techniques, 409—412
small, characteristics and activity of, 419—425
splenic sequestration of, 259, 415—418, 426—429, 468
stimulated, biochemistry of, 287—297, 436—437, 441
storage, 285—286, 388—390
structure, 313—328
survival studies, 264—270, 346—347, 420, 425—426
temperature, effect of, 383, 389—390
tabular system, characteristics of, 314
  abnormalities of, 454—457
ultrastructure, 313—328
  abnormalities of, 454—457
uptake, 285—286
volume, platelet size related to, 409—432
  density and, 415—416, 421
  function and, 415—417
  mean volume, 411—413, 415
  packed platelet volume, 412—415
  recovery from whole blood and, 418—419
  senescence and, 418—425
  splenic sequestration and, 415—418
von Willebrand's disease and, see von Willebrand's disease
whole blood, recovery from, 418—419
young, characteristics and activity of, 419—425, 448, 487
Polarity, linked globin genes in alpha and nonalpha cistrons, 56—57
Polar residues, hemoglobin structure and, 106, 131
Polycythemia
  iron metabolism and, 238—239
  platelet abnormalities and, 465—466
Polyethylene bottles, use in hemoglobincyanide system, 217
Polypeptide chain
  hemoglobin, more than one point mutation in, 177, 189
  transferrin, 226
Polystyrene ion exchangers, use in hemoglobin chromatography, 68, 73, 77
Porphyrin ring
  hemoglobin structure and, 106—107, 137—139
  iron metabolism and, 223
Portland chain, hemoglobin, see Hemoglobin — Portland chains
Porto Alegro hemoglobin, see Hemoglobin Porto Alegro
Position, hemoglobins, see General position
Postsynthetic changes, hemoglobin chains, 48
PPP, see Platelet-poor plasma
PPV, see Packed platelet volume
Predicting normal blood volume, formulas for, 37
Pregnancy
  factor VIII activity and, 474
  iron loss in, 225
Prekallikrein, platelet function and, 354
Pressure, column, effect of, hemoglobin chromatography, 74, 77
Production
  abnormal globin synthesis, 57—63
  hemoglobin, 51—66
  chain, globin, imbalance of, 57—58
  iron, 221—243
  phospholipids, in platelets, 273—274, 278—280
  platelets, 255—261
  transferrin, 226—227
Profiles, ferrokinetic, blood and tissues, 243
Profilin, in platelets, 281
Proliferative disorders

anemias, 237—238
myeloproliferative, see Myeloproliferative disorders
platelet production and, 259
Prostacyclin, in platelets, 288, 292—293
Prostaglandins, platelet functions and, 440, 450—452, 464
biochemistry, 274, 287—288, 290, 292—294, 296
tests, laboratory, 329, 332, 337—338, 344, 346
Protective function, platelet, 355, 357
Protein kinases, in platelets, 297
Proteins
contractile, platelet, see Platelets, contractile proteins
elution of, hemoglobin chromatography, 70—71
evolutionary rates, 53
iron-binding, location of, 223
iron metabolism, role in, 221, 223—225, 227
mutant, see Variation and variants, proteins
plasma, see Plasma, protein
platelet, see Platelets, proteins
secretory, see Platelets, secretory proteins
Prothrombinase, platelet function and, 344
Prothrombin, platelet coagulant activities and, 351, 403—404
consumption test, 403—404, 463
PRP, see Platelet-rich plasma
Pseudopods, platelet, see Platelets, pseudopods
Pumping, use in hemoglobin chromatography, 77—78
Puncture procedures, see Capillary blood sampling; Venipuncture
Purpural disorders, platelet function and, 425—432, 447, 453—457, 468, 473, 487, 489, 493
PV, see Plasma, volume

Q

Qualitative abnormalities, platelets, see also Thrombocytopathies; Thrombocytopenia; specific disorders by name, 331, 447—459, 463—469
acquired, 463—469
hereditary states and, 448
von Willebrand's disease, 478
diagnosis of, flow diagram for, 459
hereditary, 447—459
acquired states and, 448
classification of, 447—459
screening tests, 447, 458—459
von Willebrand's disease, see von Willebrand's disease
Quality control, see Standards
Quantitation, platelet aggregation studies, 392—394
Quantitative disorders, platelets, see also Thrombocytopathies; Thrombocytopenia; specific disorders by name, 331, 378, 487—496
Quantitative estimation, transferrin, 227—229
Quaternary structure, hemoglobins
amino acid contacts in, see Contacts, $\alpha\beta$, hemoglobin structure and
three-dimensional structure, effect on, 107—110, 142—150, 152

R

Radialimmunodiffusion techniques, platelet secretory studies, 440
Radioactive isotopes, see Isotopes, radioactive
Radioimmunoassay, antiheparin factors in platelet secretion, 440—441
Radioiron, studies of, 236—243
Radioisotopes, see Isotopes, radioactive
RBC, see Red blood cell
RBCU, see Red blood cell utilization
RCM, see Red blood cells, mass
RE, see Reticuloendothelial cells
Reagents
electrophoretic mobility studies of mutant hemoglobins, 88—89
hemoglobincyanide system, 212—214
platelet tests
aggregation, 337—339, 391—392
factor 3 availability, 344—345
retention, 399
starch gel electrophoresis of hemoglobins, 100
transferrin measurements
serum iron, 227—228
serum-unsaturated iron-binding capacity, 228
Recycling, hemoglobin chromatographic systems, 80
Red blood cells, see also Erythrocytes; Reticulocytes
fragments, detection of, 429—432
iron metabolism, role in, 221, 230, 236—237, 239, 241—243
mass, measurement of, 33—38
mean values, related to body surface area, 37—38
variation in, 35
normal values, 6
platelet function and, 334, 345—346
Red blood cell utilization, iron metabolism and, 237
Red cell folate, concentration in peripheral blood, 13
"Reduced" hemoglobin, defined, 43
Reference solution, hemoglobincyanide system, 214—215
optical density, 215—216
stability of, 215—216
Reflux, iron into plasma, 239—242
Refractory anemias, iron metabolism and, see also Anemia, 238—239
Relative electrophoretic mobilities of mutant hemoglobins, 90—94
Relative electrophoretic positions of chain variants on starch gel electrophoresis, 101—103

Renal failure, iron metabolism and, 235
Replacements, among internal sites, hemoglobins, 129—130
Residues, amino acid, see Amino acids, residues; Deleted amino acid residues
Resin, use in hemoglobin chromatography, 67—68, 73, 76, 80
Resting platelet, biochemistry of, 273—287
Retention, platelet, see Platelets, adhesion; Platelets, aggregation; Platelets, retention
Reticulocyte counts, normal values of, 6—7
Reticuloendothelial cells, role in iron metabolism, 221—222, 229—233, 235, 240, 242—243
Retinitis, platelet size and, 425, 427
Rheumatic heart disease, platelet size and, 425, 427
Ribonucleic acid, see RNA
Rigid-body fitting, model atomic coordinates and, hemoglobin structure, 141
Ristocetin, platelet functions and
  abnormalities, 450—452, 463, 467, 489
  aggregation studies, methodology, 381—394
  biochemistry, 278, 287
  tests, laboratory, 337—338, 342—344
  von Willebrand factor and, 474—479
  von Willebrand's disease and, 473—478
RNA, platelets and, 273
mRNA
  ferritin subunits derived from, 229
  globin genetics, role in, 55—56, 58, 63
  triplet codons, changes in, hemoglobin variants from, 177—187
Russell's viper venum, platelet studies utilizing, 344, 352, 403—405
Russell's viper venum

S

SA, see Surface area
Salt bridges, hemoglobin structure, 107—109, 148, 151—152
Salzman test, see Glassbead column platelet retention test, Salzman method
Sample capacity, hemoglobin chromatography, 74
Sampling techniques, see Capillary blood sampling; venipuncture
Saturated serum iron, see Serum iron, saturated
Schroeder developers, properties and composition of, 83
Screening tests, plateletqualitative disorders, 447, 458—459
Scurvy, platelet abnormalities and,476
Secretory proteins, platelet, see Platelets, secretory proteins
Sedimentation constant, transferrin, 226
  tests, laboratory, 329, 337, 342,344
Selenium^{75}-selenomethionine, platelet studies using, 255—259, 263,420—423
Senescence, platelet, effects of, see Platelets, senescence
Separation, chain, by starch gel electrophoresis, 101—103
Sephacel® buffer,use in hemoglobin chromatography, 68—69
Sephadex chromatography, hemoglobins, 67—69, 77, 80—83
Sequences, see Amino acids, sequences
Serine transferan, in platelets, 280
Serotonin, platelet functions and, 263, 267, 315, 435
  abnormalities, 454—457, 463, 494—496
  biochemistry, 277, 283—287, 289—291
  tests, laboratory, 329, 337, 342, 344
^{14}C-Serotonin, platelet studies and, 263, 267, 334
Serum ferritin measurements, 233—236
Serum folate, concentrations in peripheral blood, 13
Serum iron
  isotopic studies of, 236—243
  saturated, in transferrin, measurement of, 227—228
Serum protein electrophoresis, platelet abnormalities measured by, 467
Serum-unsaturated iron-binding capacity, transferrin, measurement of, 228—229
SI, see Serum iron, saturated
Sialic acid, platelet weight and, 425
Side chains, see Chains
Sideroblastic anemia, iron metabolism and, see also Anemia, 224—225
Sienco® aggregometer, characteristics of, 386—387
Sizing, platelet, see Platelets, size
Skin puncture sampling, see Capillary blood sampling
Slurry, choice of, hemoglobin chromatography, 76
Small platelets, characteristics and activity of, 419—425
Smears, blood see Films, blood
^{51}Cr-Sodium chromate, use in labeling platelets, 263—269
Sodium citrate, anticoagulant in platelet studies, see also Citrate, 264, 388—389
Sodium heparin, reagent in Bowie platelet retention test, 399—400
Sodium^{+} — potassium^{+} transport, in platelets, 277
^{35}S-Sodium sulfate, use in labeling platelets, 255—256, 263
Species difference, myoglobins and hemoglobins, residue variability caused by, 106, 131
Specimens, blood, collection procedures, see Collection procedures
Spectrofluorometry, estimation of serum transferrin by, 229
Spectrophotometers, use in hemoglobincyanide system, 211—217
Spin states, effect on hemoglobin structure, 106, 109—110, 132, 153
Spleen
  iron metabolism, role in, 221, 231, 243
  platelet sequestration by, 259, 415—418, 426—429

Stability, hemoglobincyanide reference solutions, 215—216
Stainable marrow iron, studies of, 231—232
Staining, see also specific staining agents by name
hemoglobin starch gel electrophoresis, 100—101
platelet studies
coat, 313, 316
counting, 361
Standardized template bleeding time test, description of, see Bleeding time procedures, standardized template method
Standards
blood collection procedures and equpment, 21, 27, 33
hemoglobin, total concentration in blood, measurement of, 211—215
iron metabolism testing, 227—229
platelet studies
aggregation, 381, 385—388, 394
counting, 364—360
labeling, 265—267
Starch gel electrophoresis of hemoglobins, 97—104
chain separation, 101—103
electrophoretic conditions, 100
electrophoretic mobilities of hemoglobin variants, 101—103
equipment, 97
gel preparation, 98—100
gel slicing, 100
preservation of gels, 101
sample insertion, 100
source of starch, 97
staining, 100—101
Stereochemical theory, of heme-heme interactions, 109—110, 152—153
Sterox®, use in reagent in hemoglobincyanide system, 212—214
Stimulated platelet, biochemistry of, 287—297
Stir bars, used in platelet aggregation studies, 385
Stirring conditions, effect on platelet-rich plasma platelet aggregation studies, 341
Stirring speed, platelet aggregation and, 383—385
Storage
blood specimens, see Collection procedures
iron, see Iron, storage
platelet-rich plasma, see Platelet-rich plasma, storage
platelets, see Platelets, storage
Storage pool deficiency, platelet functions and, see also Nonstorage pool deficiency, 271, 283, 294, 336, 343—344, 378, 448, 450—451, 454—456, 463, 473
Stripping, hemoglobin chromatographic systems, 80
Structure
chains, see Chains, hemoglobin, structure of
globin, altered, 58—63
hemoglobins
altered, 58—63, 164—171
changes in general position, effect of, 110, 161—163
quaternary, see Quaternary structure, hemoglobins
subunit structural formula, 43
three-dimensional, see Three-dimensional structure, hemoglobin
platelet ultrastructure, 313—328
transferrin, 225—226
Stypven, see Russell's viper venom
Submembranous filaments, platelets, see Platelets, filaments
Substitution, in formation of hemoglobin variants, 90—94, 177—194
Subunit
ferritin, 229
hemoglobin
α- and β-, see α-subunit, hemoglobin; β-subunit, hemoglobin
contacts, see Contacts
status, 43
structure and activity of, 105—110, 122—125, 127—128, 134—139, 141, 143, 147, 149—150, 152, 157—160
α-Subunit, hemoglobin three-dimensional stucture of, see also α-Chains and α-chain variants, 105—110, 123, 125, 127, 134—138, 141, 149—150, 152, 157—160
β-Subunit,hemoglobin, three-dimensional structure of, see also β-Chains and β-chain variants, 105—110, 122, 124, 128, 134—136, 138—139, 141, 149—150, 152, 157—160
Succinic dehydrogenase, iron absorption and, 224
Sulfhemoglobin, measurement of, 211
Surface area
body, mean values for red cell mass and plasma volume related to, 37—38
subunit contacts, buried in, hemoglobin structure and, 107, 143
Surface residues, hemoglobin structure and, 106-108, 130-131, 145-146
Survival studies, platelet, see Platelets, survival studies
Swine, see Pig
"Swiss-cheese" platelet disorder, platelet functions, 344, 449
Synthesis, see Production
Syringe system, venipuncture procedure, 23
Systemic lupus erythematosis, platelet functions and, 425—427, 468
von Willebrand's disease and , 478

T

TBT, see Template bleeding time
Technicon® AutoCounter system, platelet counting with, 364—366
Temperature, effect on platelet kinetics, 264
Template bleeding time, platelets and, 370—378
Template system, bleeding time, see Bleeding time procedure, standardized template method

Tertiary structure, hemoglobin, see Three-dimensional structure, hemoglobin
Tests, see also specific testing and measuring devices and systems by name
  blood collection, 5—20, 27, 33
  blood volume, 33—38
  coagulation, 9—11, 403—406
  erythrocyte measurement, 5—7
  hematopoietic-related factors, 11—14
  hemoglobin, total concentration in blood, standards for, 211—215
    iron
    hepatic, determination of, 233—236
    metabolism, standards for, 227—229
    storage, 231—233
    turnover, isotopes used in, 236—243
  leukocyte measurement, 7—8
  platelets
    abnormalities and disorders, see also Abnormalities and disorders, platelets, 447—459, 463—469
    aggregation, see Platelets, aggregation, tests
    antibodies, 491—492
    coagulant activities, 403— 406
    counting, see Platelet counts
    differential centrifugation techniques, 418—425
    electronic particle size counts, see Platelet counts, electronic particle methods
    functions, see Platelets, function, tests
    glass bead column retention, see Glass bead column platelet retention test
    kinetics, isitopic labeling and, 263—270
    packed cell volume technique, 411—412
    peripheral blood, measurement in, 8—9
    production, 255—259
    retention procedures, see Platelets, retention, test
    secretory proteins, 439—442
    sizing, 409—432
    thrombocytopenia, 487—497
  serum ferritin measurements, 233—236
  transferrin metabolism, 226
  von Willebrand's disease, 471—480
Tetrametric hemoglobins, structure of, 111
βTG, see β-Thromboglobulin
Thalassemia
  globin chain production and, 58
  iron metabolism and, 224—225, 235, 238—239
Three-dimensional structure, hemoglobin, 105—176
  Bohr effect and, 105, 108—109, 151, 164—171
  diphosphoglycerate, binding of 108, 151—152
  globin fold, characteristics of, 105—106, 111—128, 131
  heme groups, structure and environment of, 106—107, 132—141, 154—156
  heme-heme interactions, 107, 109—110,152—153
  hydrophobic interactions, 106—107, 128—131, 147
  mutations, mechanism of, 110, 153—171
  quaternary structure, effect of, 107-110, 142-150, 152
Thrombasthenia, platelet functions and, 343, 345, 357, 378, 392, 457
  von Willebrand's disease and, 473
Thrombin, platelet functions and,284, 287, 289-291, 337-338, 340, 342, 344, 352, 378, 435-437, 439-440, 463, 494-496
Thrombocounter®, platelet counting with, 364-366
Thrombocythemia, platelet functions and, 439, 465-466, 494-496
  thrombocytosis, differentiated from, 487-488, 493
Thrombocytin, platelet secretion and, 440
Thrombocytolytic state, increased megathrombocytes and, 425-428
Thrombocytopathies, platelet function and, see also Qualitative aanormalities, platelets; Thrombocytopenia; specific disorders by name, 331-332, 345, 403
  inaccuracy of term, 447
Thrombocytopenia, platelet functions and, see also Quantitative disorders, platelets; Thrombocytopathies; specific disorders by name, 255-259, 263, 270, 331-332, 337, 344, 378, 425-432, 447-448, 451, 454-457, 463-464, 468-469, 473, 487-496
  acute and chronic idiopathic, clinical picture of, 491
  classification of, 487-489
  drug-induced, 487-491, 493
  hereditary, 488, 492
  megaKarocytes and, 487-489, 491
Thrombocytopoiesis, platelet functions and, 314-315
Thrombocytosis, platelet functions and, 209, 255-256, 335, 468, 494-496
  thrombocythemia, differentiated from, 487-488, 493
β-Thromboglobulin, platelet secretory proteins, studies of, 346, 435—442
  antigen, 440—442
Thromboplastin generation test, platelet coagulant activity measured by, 403—404
Thromboplastin generation test, platelet abnormalities measured by, 469
Thrombopoiesis-stimulating factors, role in platelet production, 255
Thrombopoietin, role in platelet production, 255—259
Thrombosis and thrombotic tendencies, platelet function and, 329, 333, 336, 346—347, 357, 442, 488
Thromboxames, platelet function and, 274, 287—288, 290, 292—294, 337, 339, 448, 451, 456
TIBC, see Total iron-binding capacity
Time course, hemoglobins in individual, 45
Tissue cluture method, measurement of platelet production, 255—256
Tissues, ferrokinetic profiles of, 243
Titration curves, ion exchangers, hemoglobin chromatography, 72—73
Total iron binding capacity, transferrin, 228

Tourniquet, use in venipuncture procedure, 22—23
Tourniquet test, platelet functions measured by, 494—496
Transferrin
  catabolism, 227
  distribution, 227
  iron-binding activity of, 225—229
  iron metabolism, role in, 221—223, 225—230, 233, 236, 240—243
  isoelectric point, 226
  metabolism, 225—229
  molecular weight, 226
  quantitative estimation of circulating, 227—229
  sedimentation constant, 226
  structure of, 225—226
  synthesis, 226—227
  turnover, 227
  ^{59}Fe uptake of, 240—243
Transport
  blood specimens, see Collection procedures
  iron, in plasma, see Iron, transport; Iron, turnover
Triglycerides, in platelets, 274
Triplet codons, mRNA, changes in, hemoglobin variants from, 177—187
Tris-citrate-borate system, starch gel electrophoresis of hemoglobins, 97—98
Tris-EDTA-borate system, starch gel electrophoresis of hemoglobins, 97—98
Tropomyosin, in platelets, 281
Troponin, in platelets, 281
Trouble shooting, hemoglobin chromatographic systems, 78—80
Trypsin, platelet activity and, 287
Tubes, evacuated collection, specifications and procedures for using, 27—28
Tubular system, platelet, see Platelets, tubular system
Tubulin, in platelet structure, 278, 281, 314
Turbidity, prevention of, hemoglobincyanide system, 213—214
Turnover, iron, see Erythrocyte iron turnover; Iron, turnover; Plasma iron, turnover
Turpentine abscesses, iron absorption and
Two-chamber gradient, hemoglobin chromatography, 71—72, 74

U

UIBC, see Serum-unsaturated iron-binding capacity
Ultrastructure, platelet, 313—328
  hereditary abnormalities and, 454—457
Unsaturated iron-binding capacity, see Serum-unsaturated iron-binding capacity,abnormalities, platelets; Quantitative disorders, platelets
Unstable chains, hemoglobins, characteristics of, 190, 192-193
Uremia, platelet abnormalities and, 465

V

Valine E 11, position of, importance in hemoglobin structure, 107
Values, normal, see Normal values
VAriation and variants, see also Abnormalities and disorders; Normal values; specific variants by name
  blood volume, clinical effects, 35
  chain variants, see Chains and chain variants
  coefficient, see Coefficient of variation
  glass bead column platelet retention test, 334-335
  globin genes, 58-63
    altered functional properties of, 110, 164-171
  hemoglobins, see also Chains, Chains and chain variants; hemoglobinopathies; specific variants by name
    altered structure of, 58-63
    Bohr effect and, 109
    chromatography of, 68, 80-83
    current list of, source, 178
    deleted, see Deleted hemoglobins
    electrophoretic mobilities of, see Electrophoretic mobilities of mutant hemoglobins
    extended chain, see Extended chain hemoglobins
    fusion, see Fusion hemoglobins
    more than one in some polypeptide chain, 177, 189
    three-dimensional structure and, 110, 154-171
  iron metabolism, see Abnormalities and disorders, iron metabolism
  plasma volume, 36
  platelets, see Abnormalities and disorders, platelets; Qualitaaive aanormalities, platelets; Quantitative disorders, platelets
  protein, types of, 110, 154—171
  Red cell mass, 35
Vascular permeability factor, in platelets, 329, 437
Vasculitis, platelet size and, 425
Vasopressin
  factor VIII activity and, 474
  platelet functions and, 287, 289
Vein puncture sampling, see Venipuncture
Venipuncture, equipment and procedures for, 10, 22—23, 28, 335, 388, 442
Venous blood sampling, see Venipuncture
Venous hematocrit, measurement of, 33
Vincristine, platelet response and, 314, 465
Visual platelet counts, method, 361—362, 366
Vitamin B12, concentrations in peripheral blood, 13—14
Vitamin C deficiency, platelet abnormalities and, 468
Vitamin E, iron metabolism and, 232
Vitamin K, effect on coagulation, 11, 351—352

Volumes, blood, see Blood volume; Plasma, volume; Red cells, mass
von Willebrand factor, platelet functions and, 331, 334, 336—337, 342, 344, 394, 397, 463, 472, 478
ristocetin and, 474—479
von Willebrand's disease, platelet functions and
in animals, 479—480
in humans, 332, 335—337, 378, 394, 397, 448, 450, 463—464, 471—480, 492
acquired form, 478
discovery of, 471
diagnosis of, 474—478
hemophilia and, 471—480
nature of, 478—479
vWF, see von Willebrand factor

W

WBC, see White blood cell
Wet digestion technique, estimation of serum transferrin by, 229
White blood cells, see also Leukocytes
normal values, 7—8
platelet function and, 334, 345—346
WHO, see World Health Organization
Whole blood, platelet recovery from, 418—419
Wien hemoglobin, see Hemoglobin Wien
Willebrand factor, see von Willebrand factor
Wiskott-Aldrich syndrome, platelet function and, 344, 448, 450, 455, 487, 492
World Health Organization
hemoglobin, total concentration in blood, standards for measuring, 212, 214
international hemoglobincyanide reference solution, 214—215

X

Xanthine oxidase, role in iron metabolism, 229
X-ray crystallography, of hemoglobin structure, 105, 108—111
abnormal hemoglobins, 164—171

Y

Young platelets, characteristics and activity of, 419—425